AF327168

*Atlas of* **GENITOURINARY ONCOLOGY**

# *Atlas of* GENITOURINARY ONCOLOGY

**Benjamin Movsas, MD**

Vice-Chairman, Department of Radiation Oncology
Fox Chase Cancer Center
Philadelphia, Pennsylvania

**Gary Hudes, MD**

Director, Genitourinary Malignancies
Department of Medical Oncology
Fox Chase Cancer Center
Philadelphia, Pennsylvania

**Carl Olsson, MD**

John K. Lattimer Professor and Chairman
Department of Surgery
Division of Urology
College of Physicians and Surgeons of Columbia University
New York, New York

**W.B. SAUNDERS COMPANY**
*A HARCOURT HEALTH SCIENCES COMPANY*

Philadelphia  London  New York  St. Louis  Sydney  Toronto

**W.B. SAUNDERS COMPANY**
*A Harcourt Health Sciences Company*

The Curtis Center
Independence Square West
Philadelphia, Pennsylvania 19106

**Library of Congress Cataloging-in-Publication Data**

Atlas of genitourinary oncology/[edited by] Benjamin Movsas, Gary Hudes, Carl Olsson.

p.; cm.

ISBN 0–7216–8738–5

I. Genitourinary organs—Cancer—Atlases.    I. Movsas, Benjamin.
II. Hudes, Gary.    III. Olsson, Carl

[DNLM: 1. Urogenital Neoplasms—Atlases. WJ 17 A88148 2002]
RC280.G4 A855 2002

616.99′46—dc21                                        2001020606

*Acquisitions Editor:*  Stephanie Donley
*Production Editor:*  Edna Dick
*Production Manager:*  Guy Barber
*Illustration Specialist:*  Robert Quinn

ATLAS OF GENITOURINARY ONCOLOGY                    ISBN 0–7216–8738–5



Printed in the United States of America

Last digit is the print number:    9    8    7    6    5    4    3    2    1

*To my dear wife, Tammy, my wonderful children, Shoshana, Avielle, Shira, and Aviva, and to my friend and mentor, Gerald Hanks.*

**Benjamin Movsas**

---

*To my wife, Debra, and to Ellis, Rachel, and Jennifer, for your patience and support.*

**Gary Hudes**

# Contributors

**Matthew T. Ballo, M.D.**
Assistant Professor of Radiation Oncology, University of Texas MD Anderson Cancer Center, Houston, Texas
*Radiotherapy in the Management of Seminoma*

**Arie Belldegrun, M.D.**
Professor of Urology and Chief, Division of Urologic Oncology; Director, Urologic Research, University of California, Los Angeles School of Medicine, Los Angeles, California
*Renal and Adrenal Carcinoma: Genetics, Staging, and Surgical Management*

**Mitchell C. Benson, M.D.**
George F. Cahill Professor of Urology, College of Physicians and Surgeons of Columbia University; Director of Urologic Oncology, Columbia-New York Presbyterian Hospital, New York, New York
*Nonseminomatous Germ Cell Tumors: Surgical Management*

**Ronald Bukowski, M.D.**
Director, Experimental Therapeutics Program, Cleveland Clinic Taussig Cancer Center, Cleveland, Ohio
*Systemic Therapy of Renal Cell Carcinoma*

**Diane Carter, M.D.**
Department of Pathology, University of California Los Angeles School of Medicine, Los Angeles, California
*Renal and Adrenal Carcinoma: Genetics, Staging, and Surgical Management*

**C. J. Davis, Jr., M.D.**
Staff Pathologist, Department of Genitourinary Pathology, Armed Forces Institute of Pathology, Washington, D.C.
*Pathology and Staging of Genitourinary Cancer*

**Elliot Fagelman, M.D.**
Chief Resident, Department of Urology, Columbia-New York Presbyterian Hospital, New York, New York
*Nonseminomatous Germ Cell Tumors: Surgical Management*

**Gary M. Freedman, M.D.**
Associate Member, Fox Chase Cancer Center, Philadelphia, Pennsylvania
*Radiotherapy for Prostate Cancer*

**Erik T. Goluboff, M.D.**
Assistant Professor of Urology, College of Physicians and Surgeons of Columbia University; Director of Urology, Columbia-Presbyterian Medical Center, New York, New York
*Radical Prostatectomy for the Treatment of Prostate Cancer*

**Sarel Halachmi, M.D.**
Department of Urology, Bnai Zion Medical Center, Haifa, Israel
*Bladder and Other Urothelial Malignancies—Surgical Management*

**Gerald E. Hanks, M.D.**
Chairman, Department of Radiation Oncology, Fox Chase Cancer Center, Philadelphia, Pennsylvania
*Radiotherapy for Prostate Cancer*

**Gary Hudes, M.D.**
Director, Genitourinary Malignancies, Department of
   Medical Oncology, Fox Chase Cancer Center,
   Philadelphia, Pennsylvania
*Bladder Cancer: Radiotherapy and Chemotherapy;
   Nonseminomatous Germ Cell Tumors: Systemic Issues*

**Philip W. Kantoff, M.D.**
Director, Lank Center for Genitourinary Oncology,
   Dana-Farber Cancer Institute, Department of
   Urinary Oncology, Boston, Massachusetts
*Biology of Prostate Cancer*

**Aaron E. Katz, M.D.**
Assistant Professor of Urology, Columbia-Presbyterian
   Medical Center, New York, New York
*Radical Prostatectomy for the Treatment of Prostate Cancer*

**John S. Lam, M.D.**
Resident, Department of Urology, Columbia-
   Presbyterian Medical Center, New York, New York
*Radical Prostatectomy for the Treatment of Prostate Cancer*

**Jürgen F. Linn, M.D.**
c/o Horst Linn, Muhlenstr. 52, D-53859, Germany
*Bladder and Other Urothelial Malignancies—Surgical
   Management*

**F. K. Mostofi, M.D.**
Chairperson, Department of Genitourinary Pathology,
   Armed Forces Institute of Pathology, Washington,
   D.C.
*Pathology and Staging of Genitourinary Cancer*

**Benjamin Movsas, M.D.**
Vice Chairman, Department of Radiation Oncology,
   Fox Chase Cancer Center, Philadelphia,
   Pennsylvania
*Radiotherapy for Prostate Cancer*

**John Naitoh, M.D.**
Clinical Instructor, Department of Surgery, University
   of California, San Diego School of Medicine; Vice
   Chairman, Section of Urology, Scripps Memorial
   Hospital, La Jolla, California
*Renal and Adrenal Carcinoma: Genetics, Staging, and
   Surgical Management*

**Carl Olsson, M.D.**
John K. Lattimer Professor and Chairman,
   Department of Surgery, Division of Urology,
   College of Physicians and Surgeons of Columbia
   University, New York, New York
*Radical Prostatectomy for the Treatment of Prostate Cancer*

**Alan Pollack, M.D., Ph.D.**
Professor of Radiation Oncology, University of Texas
   MD Anderson Cancer Center, Houston, Texas
*Radiotherapy in the Management of Seminoma*

**Marvin Rotman, M.D.**
Professor and Chairman, Department of Radiation
   Oncology, State University of New York Health
   Science Center, SUNY HSCB, Brooklyn, New York
*Bladder Cancer: Radiotherapy and Chemotherapy*

**Ihor S. Sawczuk, M.D.**
Professor of Urology, College of Physicians and
   Surgeons, Columbia University; Attending
   Urologist, Columbia-New York Presbyterian
   Hospital, New York, New York
*Nonseminomatous Germ Cell Tumors: Surgical
   Management*

**Scott Saxman, M.D., F.A.C.P.**
Senior Investigator, Cancer Therapy Evaluation
   Program, National Cancer Institute, Bethesda,
   Maryland
*Nonseminomatous Germ Cell Tumors: Systemic Issues*

**Mark P. Schoenberg, M.D.**
Associate Professor of Urology and Oncology, Johns
   Hopkins University School of Medicine; Director of
   Urologic Oncology, Johns Hopkins Medical
   Institutions, Baltimore, Maryland
*Bladder and Other Urothelial Malignancies—Surgical
   Management*

**Alan R. Schulsinger, M.D.**
Assistant Professor of Radiation Oncology, State
   University of New York Health Science Center,
   SUNY-HSCB; Senior Attending, Long Island
   College Hospital, Brooklyn, New York
*Bladder Cancer: Radiotherapy and Chemotherapy*

**I. A. Sesterhenn, M.D.**
Senior Pathologist, Department of Genitourinary
   Pathology, Armed Forces Institute of Pathology,
   Washington, D.C.
*Pathology and Staging of Genitourinary Cancer*

**Kathleen M. Shadle, M.D.**
Private Practice, Memorial Hermann Health Care
   System, Houston, Texas
*Radiotherapy in the Management of Seminoma*

**Matthew R. Smith, M.D., Ph.D.**
Assistant Professor, Division of Hematology-
   Oncology, Harvard Medical School; Assistant
   Physician, Massachusetts General Hospital, Boston,
   Massachusetts
*Biology of Prostate Cancer*

**Ramesh Vedula, M.D.**
Clinical Instructor, Department of Radiation Oncology,
   State University of New York Health Science
   Center, SUNY-HSCB; Brooklyn, New York
*Bladder Cancer: Radiotherapy and Chemotherapy*

# Foreword

This thoroughly illustrated Atlas of Genitourinary Oncology clearly demonstrates the power of visual images and text to teach complex concepts. Herein, Drs. Movsas, Hudes, and Olsson have cleverly combined vivid caricatures and illustrations with concise and precise textual statements to explain the biology and treatment of urologic malignancies. The images and illustrations are, by themselves, quite vivid and transmit the required information with accuracy and clarity. The written text is well-referenced and reinforces the message of the illustrations in a meticulous manner. As the text is supported by the illustrations, the content is not burdened by tedious and confusing descriptions. The end result is a clear, concise, and accurate presentation of the problems that exist in the diagnosis and therapy of genitourinary malignancies.

DAVID F. PAULSON, M.D.

## NOTICE

Oncology is an ever-changing field. Standard safety precautions must be followed, but as new research and clinical experience broaden our knowledge, changes in treatment and drug therapy may become necessary or appropriate. Readers are advised to check the most current product information provided by the manufacturer of each drug to be administered to verify the recommended dose, the method and duration of administration, and contraindications. It is the responsibility of the treating physician, relying on experience and knowledge of the patient, to determine dosages and the best treatment for each individual patient. Neither the Publisher nor the editor assume any liability for any injury and/or damage to persons or property arising from this publication.

THE PUBLISHER

# Preface

"We will draw the curtain and show you the picture."
*Twelfth Night,* William Shakespeare.

Genitourinary (GU) oncology is a vast discipline, encompassing multiple primary sites including the prostate, bladder, kidney, and testicle. With the advent of newer diagnostic imaging techniques to the exponential growth of molecular oncology and to ever-changing treatment strategies, investigators in this field have developed a wealth of information. Simply open any of the classic textbooks in GU oncology and you will find a collection of minutiae often spanning more than a thousand pages. At times this detail can create a virtual "curtain of confusion." How does one integrate and synthesize this information overload?

The purpose of this Atlas is to present the key concepts of GU oncology in a visual format. Rather than detailing an exhaustive work-up, the book contains classic diagnostic images. The concepts underlying molecular biology have been crystallized into simple diagrams. Treatment strategies are presented as algorithms, with results and complications systemically tabulated. This Atlas presents the fundamental concepts, clinical pearls, and key images of this field in order to create an everlasting picture in the reader's mind.

The underlying strength of this Atlas is that it provides access to the personal slide collections of internationally recognized experts in the field. Each slide is accompanied by a focused text that explains the underlying theme. It is as though the authors are conversing directly with the reader at Grand Rounds, using their prized collection of slides.

This Atlas is organized according to the major primary sites of GU oncology, arranged in order of their prevalence: prostate, bladder, kidney, and testis. Because prostate cancer is the leading cause of cancer in men in this country, a separate chapter has been devoted to the biology of prostate cancer, which has exploded in its scope over the last decade. Separate chapters devoted to both the surgical and the radiotherapeutic management of prostate cancer follow this. After this, the next set of chapters is devoted to the surgical and chemoradiotherapeutic management of bladder cancer. For easy accessibility, a chapter highlighting the pathology and staging of GU oncology has been placed in the very center of this Atlas. In this way, one can flip to this section while in the middle of any other chapter to refer to the key pathologic features. The pathology chapter itself has been organized in the same order as the overall Atlas. Following the pathology chapter, the next two chapters are dedicated to the surgical versus systemic management of renal cell carcinoma. Finally, the last three chapters review the management of nonseminomatous versus seminomatous germ cell tumors.

The Atlas is targeted for urologists, medical oncologists, and radiation oncologists who are involved in the management of patients with GU cancers. We hope that these specialists will find this visual format refreshing and use it as an educational tool as they teach others about this fascinating field. Residents and fellows in these fields can literally use this Atlas as a "visual aid" in their training. As this Atlas builds on the fundamental building blocks of GU oncology, it is also an appropriate guide for medical students and nurses.

The editors would like to take this opportunity to thank the many contributing authors, who spent a great deal of time finding, choosing, and creating the images presented. We also would like to thank our editor, Stephanie Donley, without whom this project would not have been possible. A special thanks to Louise Marcewicz for her tireless efforts in meticulously preparing the manuscript. We would also like to thank our families, who supported us wholeheartedly in this worthwhile project. Finally, thanks to all our patients, whose courage and determination continue to inspire us.

So, sit back, relax, and let us "draw the curtain and show you the picture."

BENJAMIN MOVSAS, M.D.
GARY HUDES, M.D.
CARL OLSSON, M.D.

# Contents

1 **Biology of Prostate Cancer** *Matthew R. Smith/Philip W. Kantoff* — 1

2 **Radical Prostatectomy for the Treatment of Prostate Cancer** *Erik T. Goluboff/John S. Lam/Aaron E. Katz/Carl Olsson* — 17

3 **Radiotherapy for Prostate Cancer** *Gary M. Freedman/Benjamin Movsas/Gerald E. Hanks* — 45

4 **Bladder and Other Urothelial Malignancies—Surgical Management** *Jürgen F. Linn/Sarel Halachmi/Mark P. Schoenberg* — 75

5 **Bladder Cancer: Radiotherapy and Chemotherapy** *Alan R. Schulsinger/Ramesh Vedula/Marvin Rotman/Gary Hudes* — 95

6 **Pathology and Staging of Genitourinary Cancer** *F. K. Mostofi/C. J. Davis, Jr./I. A. Sesterhenn* — 117

7 **Renal and Adrenal Carcinoma: Genetics, Staging, and Surgical Management** *John Naitoh/Diane Carter/Arie Belldegrun* — 143

8 **Systemic Therapy of Renal Cell Carcinoma** *Ronald Bukowski* — 167

9 **Nonseminomatous Germ Cell Tumors: Surgical Management** *Elliot Fagelman/Ihor S. Sawczuk/Mitchell C. Benson* — 189

10 **Nonseminomatous Germ Cell Tumors: Systemic Issues** *Gary Hudes/Scott Saxman* — 199

**11 Radiotherapy in the Management of Seminoma** *Matthew T. Ballo/Kathleen M. Shadle/Alan Pollack* 205

**Index** 217

# 1

# Biology of Prostate Cancer

*Matthew R. Smith*

*Philip W. Kantoff*

## INTRODUCTION

Prostate cancer is the most common noncutaneous malignancy and the fourth leading cause of cancer death among men worldwide. In 2001, there were approximately 198,100 new cases of prostate cancer and 31,500 prostate cancer deaths.

Prostate-specific antigen (PSA) screening has dramatically increased the detection of early stage prostate cancers. Many aspects of the management of early stage prostate cancer remain controversial. Because prostate cancer is prevalent in older men and often clinically indolent, a significant proportion of men diagnosed with localized prostate cancer will die from other causes. The ability to identify the men most likely to benefit from potentially curative therapy is imprecise and central to the management controversy.

Androgen ablation is the mainstay of treatment for men with metastatic disease. Androgen ablation by either orchiectomy or androgen blockade results in disease regression in the vast majority of patients, but the median response duration is less than 2 years. There are currently no life-prolonging treatments for men with androgen-refractory disease.

Future advances in the field of prostate cancer will be based on an improved understanding of the molecular basis for prostate cancer growth and progression. This chapter presents the fundamentals of prostate cancer biology. It is not meant to be a comprehensive review but rather focuses on subjects with relevant clinical correlations and emphasizes topics that are likely to produce future innovations in prostate cancer prevention, diagnosis, and treatment.

**Figure 1–1:** Glandular anatomy of the prostate. The functional unit of the prostate is the glandular acinus, composed of epithelial and stromal compartments. The

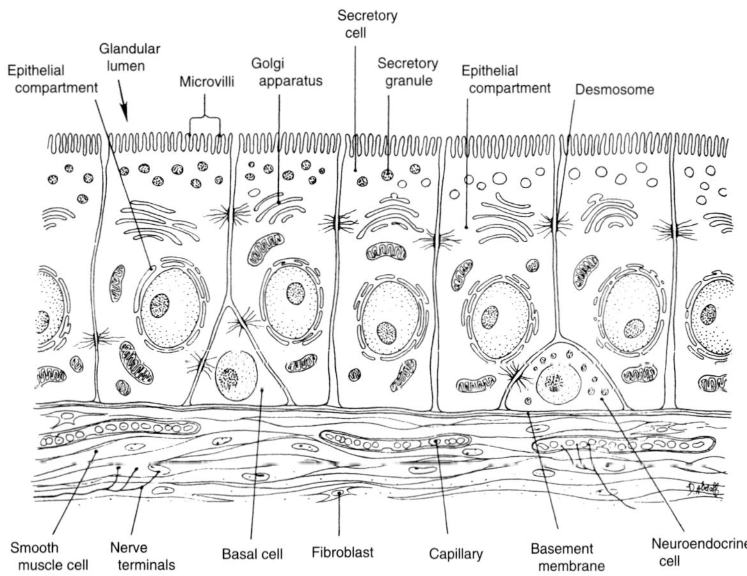


**Figure 1–1**

epithelial compartment consists of secretory epithelial cells, basal epithelial cells, and neuroendocrine cells. The secretory epithelial cells constitute the predominant cell type of the epithelial compartment. These exocrine cells synthesize and secrete prostate-specific antigen (PSA) and prostate-specific acid phosphatase (PAP) into the glandular lumen, producing the prostatic fluid of the ejaculate. The secretory epithelial cells express androgen receptors and depend upon androgenic stimulation for their secretory ability and growth. The epithelial compartment is separated from the stromal compartment by the basement membrane.

## PATHOLOGY OF PROSTATE CANCER

**Figure 1–2:** Malignant neoplasms of the prostate. Adenocarcinomas account for more than 95% of all primary malignancies of the prostate. Uncommon primary malignancies of the prostate include adenoid cystic carcinomas, adenosquamous carcinomas, squamous carcinomas, small cell neuroendocrine carcinomas, transitional cell carcinomas, sarcomas, carcinosarcomas, and lymphomas. Involvement of the prostate by metastases from distant primary sites is rare, although bladder and rectal malignancies may involve the prostate by direct extension.

**Figure 1–3:** Model of prostate carcinogenesis. There appears to be a morphologic continuum from normal prostate epithelium to invasive adenocarcinoma of the prostate. The diagnosis of invasive prostate cancer is based on abnormal glandular histologic changes. Cytologic atypia in the absence of these diagnostic histologic changes has been termed *prostatic intraepithelial neoplasia* (PIN). PIN is characterized by nuclear pleomorphism and nucleolar prominence similar to that seen in prostate cancer. High-grade PIN is distinguished from low-grade PIN on the basis of the severity of cytologic changes and disruption of the basal cell layer. PIN is thought to be a premalignant condition because of its morphologic similarities to invasive pros-

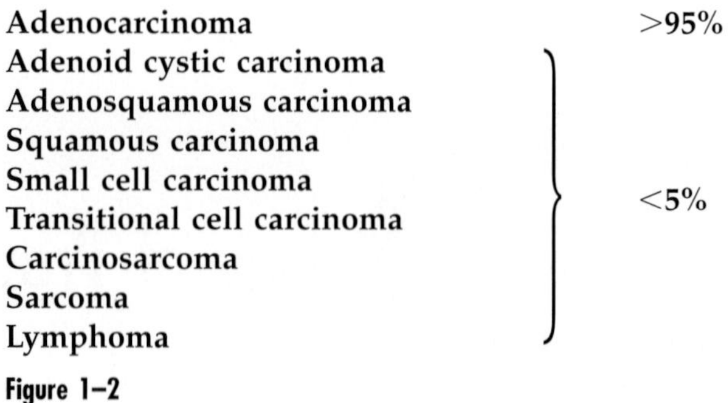

| Adenocarcinoma | >95% |
| Adenoid cystic carcinoma | |
| Adenosquamous carcinoma | |
| Squamous carcinoma | |
| Small cell carcinoma | |
| Transitional cell carcinoma | <5% |
| Carcinosarcoma | |
| Sarcoma | |
| Lymphoma | |

**Figure 1–2**

tate cancer and the greater incidence, extent, and severity of PIN associated with concomitant invasive prostate cancers. (Adapted from Bostwick DG, Brawer MK: Prostatic intraepithelial neoplasia and early invasion in prostate cancer. Cancer 59:788–794, 1987.)

**Figure 1–4:** The Gleason grading system is the most widely used histologic method for classifying adenocarcinoma of the prostate and is based on glandular architecture. The primary pattern of adenocarcinoma is assigned a score of 1 to 5, with 1 describing the most differentiated with discrete glandular formation and 5 representing the most undifferentiated and nearly complete loss of glandular architecture. The second most common pattern is also assigned a score of 1 to 5/5. The combination of these two scores, termed the *Gleason sum,* is correlated with probability of extracapsular extension, pelvic lymph node involvement, and distant metastases. (Adapted from Gleason DF: The Veterans Administration Cooperative Research Group: Histological grading and clinical staging of prostatic carcinoma. In Tannenbaum M [ed]: Urologic Oncology: The Prostate. Philadelphia, Lea & Febiger, 1977, pp 171–174.)

## EPIDEMIOLOGY OF PROSTATE CANCER

**Figure 1–5:** Worldwide variation in prostate cancer mortality rate (age-adjusted death rates per 100,000

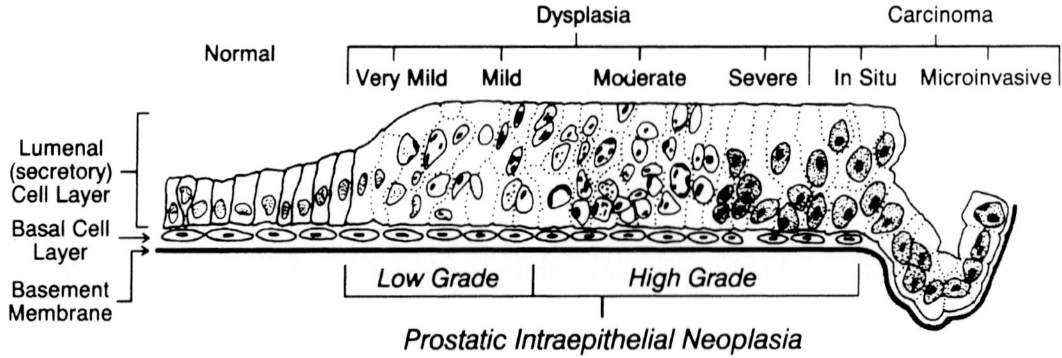


**Figure 1–3**

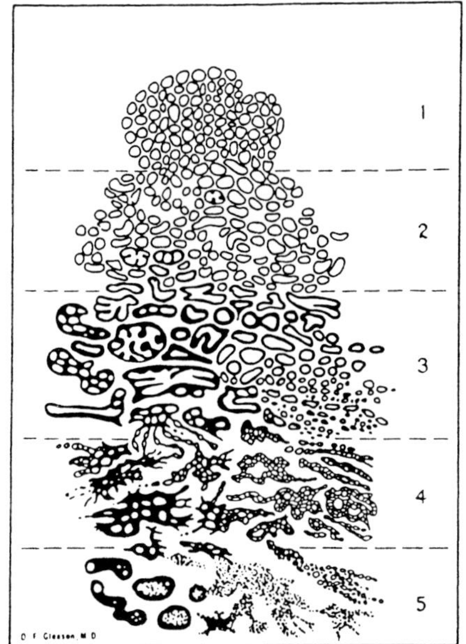

**Pattern 1**: closely packed, single, separate, round, uniform glands

**Pattern 2**: single, separate, round, less uniform glands, separated by stroma up to one gland diameter

**Pattern 3**: single, separate, irregular glands of variable size; masses with cribriform or papillary pattern

**Pattern 4**: fused glands, cords, or small glands of papillary, cribriform, or solid patterns

**Pattern 5**: few or no glands; masses with comedo pattern; cords or sheets of tumor cells

**Figure 1–4**

population per year). The mortality rate from prostate cancer is highly variable worldwide. Norwegian men have the highest reported age-adjusted mortality rates from prostate cancer, with 23.8 deaths per 100,000 population per year. American men also have high rates of death from prostate cancer, with 17.3 deaths per 100,000 population per year. The Japanese have among the lowest prostate cancer mortality rates, with 4.2 deaths per 100,000 population per year. Worldwide variation in prostate cancer incidence closely parallels the geographic differences in prostate cancer mortality rates. (Data from Landis SH, Murray T, Bolden S, Wingo PA: Cancer Statistics, 1998. CA A Cancer Journal for Clinicians 48:6–48, 1998.)

**Figure 1–6:** Age and race are risk factors for prostate cancer. Prostate cancer incidence rates in American men from the surveillance, epidemiology, and end result database are stratified by age and race. Black

American men have significantly higher incidence of prostate cancer than their white American counterparts. Black American men also have higher prostate cancer mortality rates. The racial variation in prostate cancer incidence and mortality rates is likely explained by a combination of environmental and genetic differences. The incidence of clinical prostate cancer dramatically increases with age. The rate of this age-dependent increase in prostate cancer incidence is greater than that of any other malignancy. The basis for the distinctive age-dependent incidence of prostate cancer is unknown. (Data from Pienta KJ, Esper PS: Risk factors for prostate cancer. Ann Intern Med 118:793, 1993.)

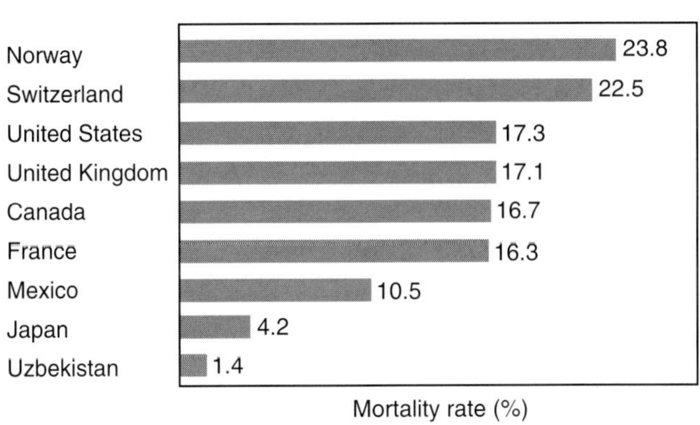


**Figure 1–5**

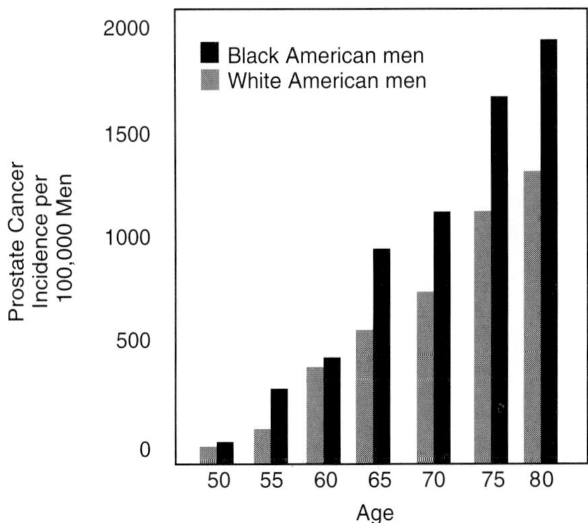


**Figure 1–6**

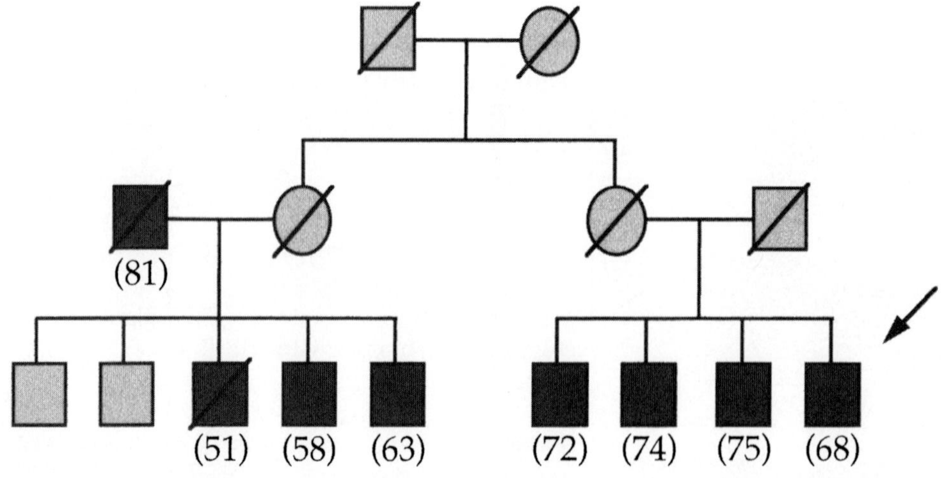

Figure 1–7

## Determinants of Prostate Cancer Risk

Epidemiologic studies have identified several potential determinants of prostate cancer risk. After age, family history of prostate cancer appears to be the most important risk factor for prostate cancer. Family history may increase the risk of prostate cancer through inheritance of rare, highly penetrant cancer susceptibility genes. In addition, germline polymorphisms in the androgen receptor gene, vitamin D receptor gene, and 5α-reductase gene may contribute to familial clustering of prostate cancer. Several dietary factors also appear to influence prostate cancer risk. High dietary intake of fat is associated with an increased prostate cancer risk. In contrast, diets rich in selenium or lycopene, a carotenoid derived from tomatoes, are associated with decreased prostate cancer risk.

**Figure 1–7:** Familial prostate cancer. The eight cases of prostate cancer identified in this typical prostate cancer family are represented in the dark shaded boxes, with the ages at diagnosis noted in parentheses below them. Familial prostate cancer is characterized by an autosomal dominant pattern of inheritance and early onset of disease. Segregation analyses suggest that at least one dominant susceptibility locus is responsible for familial prostate cancer. Mutations in these loci may account for approximately 9% of all prostate cancers and 43% of early onset prostate cancers. On the basis of these estimates, we can deduce that prostate cancer has a genetic component similar to that of breast and colon cancer.

**Figure 1–8:** Hereditary prostate cancer 1 locus. Genetic analyses performed on members of 91 high-risk prostate cancer families from the United States and Sweden have provided evidence for linkage to the long arm of chromosome 1 (1q24-25). This locus, called hereditary prostate cancer 1 (HPC1), spans approxi-

mately 10 million base pairs of DNA. The *hpc1* gene has not yet been identified, and its function remains unknown. However, prostate cancer cells sometimes contain extra copies of the region of chromosome 1 that contains the HPC1 locus, suggesting that the *hpc1* gene may be a tumor-promoting oncogene rather than a tumor-suppressor gene. The identification of the *hpc1* gene and other prostate cancer susceptibility genes may provide important insights into the prevention, diagnosis, and treatment of prostate cancer.

## ENDOCRINOLOGY OF PROSTATE CANCER

**Figure 1–9:** The hypothalamic-pituitary-gonadal axis. The testosterone synthesized by the Leydig cells of the testis is the primary source of androgens in men. Ley-

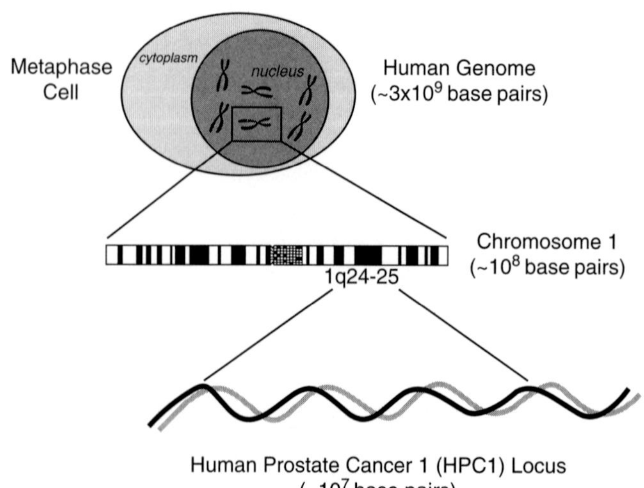


Figure 1–8

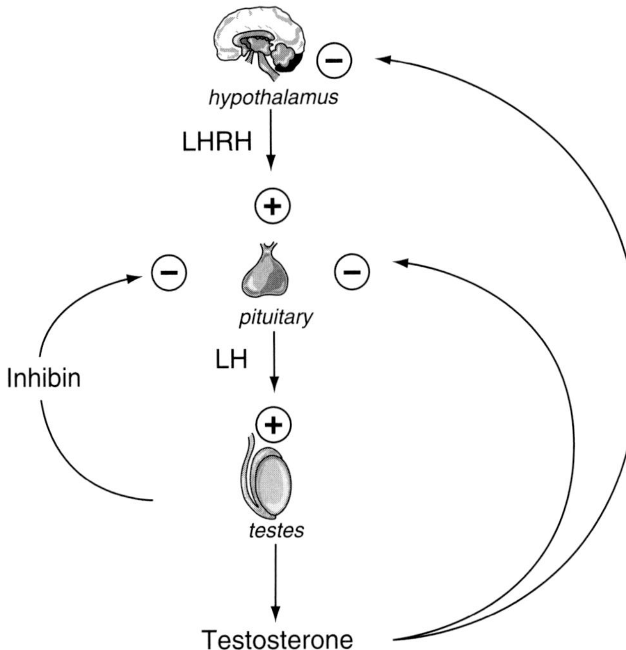



**Figure 1–9**

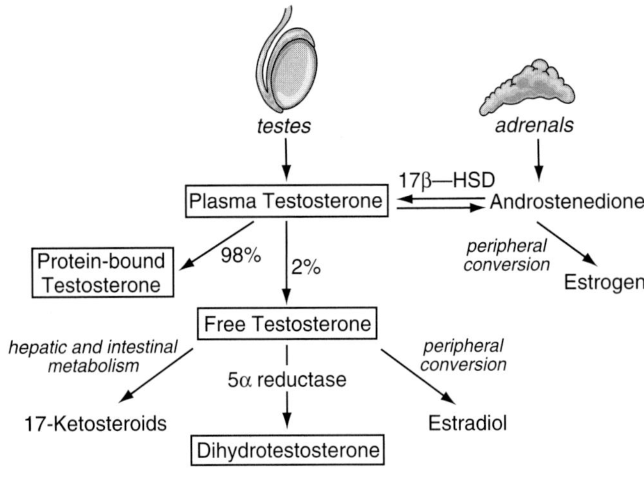



**Figure 1–11**

dig cell synthesis of testosterone is regulated by luteinizing hormone (LH) of pituitary origin. The release of luteinizing hormone is regulated by luteinizing hormone–releasing hormone (LHRH) from the hypothalamus. Levels of circulating testosterone are maintained within normal limits by negative feedback at the level of the hypothalamus and pituitary.

**Figure 1–10:** Adrenal androgen production. Under the influence of pituitary adrenocorticotropic hormone (ACTH), the adrenal glands produce androstenedione, dehydroepiandrosterone (DHEA), and dehydroepiandrosterone sulfate (DHEA-S). These compounds, collectively known as the adrenal androgens, have relatively weak androgenic activity. However, androstenedione can be converted to testosterone in peripheral tissues and in the prostate. In normal men, the adrenal cortex is a minor source of androgen production. However, residual adrenal androgens may be important in pro-

moting disease progression in men with advanced prostate cancer following medical or surgical castration.

**Figure 1–11:** Metabolic fate of testosterone. Approximately 98% of plasma testosterone is present in a biologically inactive protein-bound form. Free testosterone enters cells by diffusion across the cell membrane. In some tissues, including the brain, pituitary, and kidney, unmodified testosterone is bound by the androgen receptor. In other tissues, including the prostate, seminal vesicles, epididymis, adrenal glands, liver, and skin, testosterone is efficiently converted to dihydrotestosterone (DHT) by membrane-bound 5α-reductase type II. DHT binds the androgen receptor with approximately threefold greater affinity than testosterone. In adipose tissue, testosterone is converted to estradiol by cytochrome P450-dependent aromatization. In the liver and intestines, testosterone and other steroids are converted to inactive 17-ketosteroids. These compounds are then conjugated and excreted in the urine.

**Figure 1–12:** Model of androgen-dependent transcriptional activation. The action of androgens is mediated by nuclear androgen receptors. After diffusing across the cell membrane, testosterone (T) is efficiently converted to dihydrotestosterone (DHT) by membrane-bound 5α-reductase type II. DHT diffuses into the nucleus and associates with unbound androgen receptor. Binding of DHT to the androgen receptor induces conformational changes that result in dissociation from heat shock proteins (hsp), unmasking of the DNA binding domain, and dimerization. The androgen receptor dimer binds to the palindromic androgen response elements (ARE) present within the promoters of target genes, resulting in transcriptional activation of various androgen-regulated genes. The activity of the androgen receptor is modulated by a variety of transcriptional cofactors. Transcriptional activation results in increased expression of several proteins, including epidermal

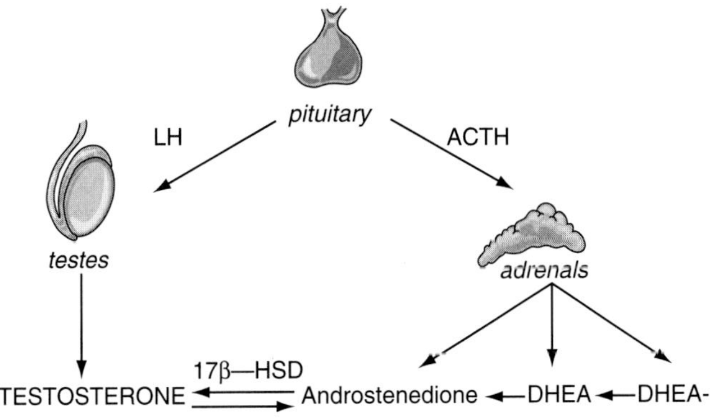



**Figure 1–10**

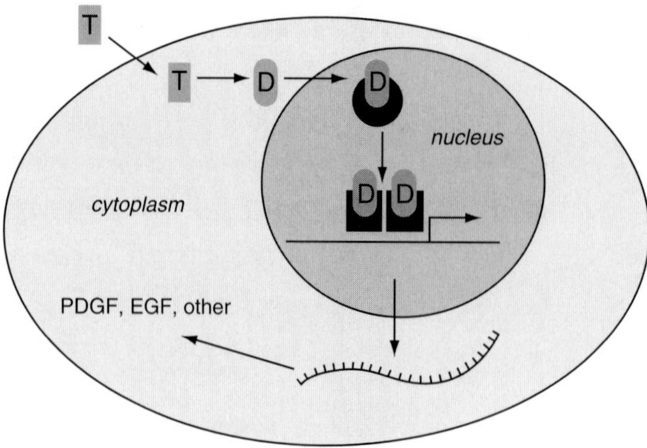



**Figure 1–12**

growth factor (EGF) and platelet-derived growth factor (PDGF).

**Figure 1–13:** Mechanisms of androgen deprivation. The mainstay of treatment for metastatic prostate cancer is androgen ablation. This procedure has an 80% response rate but ultimately fails to prevent disease progression. Permanent androgen deprivation can be accomplished by bilateral orchiectomy. Reversible methods of androgen ablation include the administration of a luteinizing hormone–releasing hormone (LHRH) agonist or diethylstilbestrol (DES). Administration of LHRH agonists causes an initial stimulation of pituitary luteinizing hormone (LH) production and a rise in serum testosterone levels. Chronic administration of LHRH agonists causes the pituitary to become resistant to endogenous LHRH, resulting in suppression of testicular androgen production similar to that observed after surgical castration. Similarly, DES suppresses pituitary LH production, resulting in castration levels of testosterone. Cardiovascular toxicity associated with DES has resulted in the preferential use of LHRH agonists for reversible androgen ablation. Adrenal androgen production is unaffected by administration of either DES or LHRH agonists.

**Figure 1–14:** Mechanism of antiandrogen action. Nonsteroidal antiandrogens including bicalutamide, flutamide, and nilutamide competitively inhibit the binding of testosterone and dihydrotestosterone to the androgen receptor. These nonsteroidal antiandrogens bind to the androgen receptor with less than 2% of the affinity of dihydrotestosterone. Monotherapy with nonsteroidal antiandrogens is inferior to androgen ablation for metastatic prostate cancer, probably because of their relatively low binding affinity. Combination therapy with an LHRH agonist and a nonsteroidal antiandrogen, termed *combined androgen blockade*, has the theoretical advantage of inhibiting testicular androgen production and blocking the action of residual adrenal androgens. Results of randomized trials have called into question the clinical utility of combined androgen blockade.

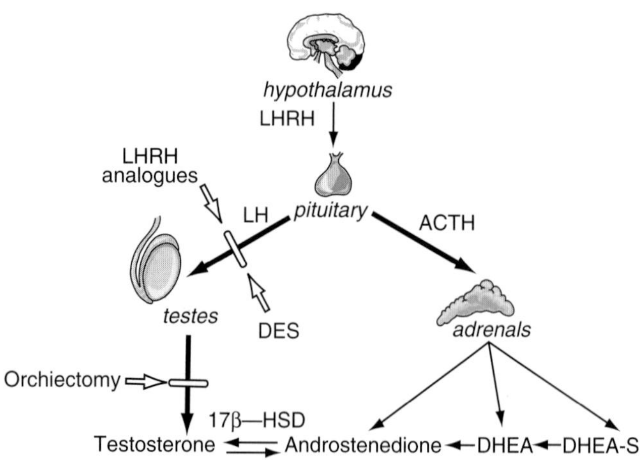



**Figure 1–13**

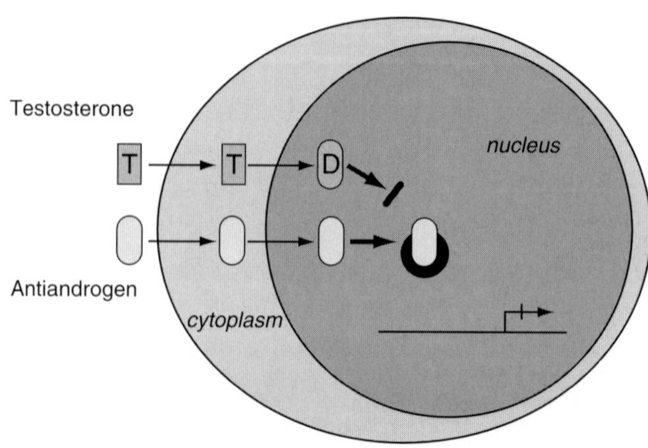



**Figure 1–14**

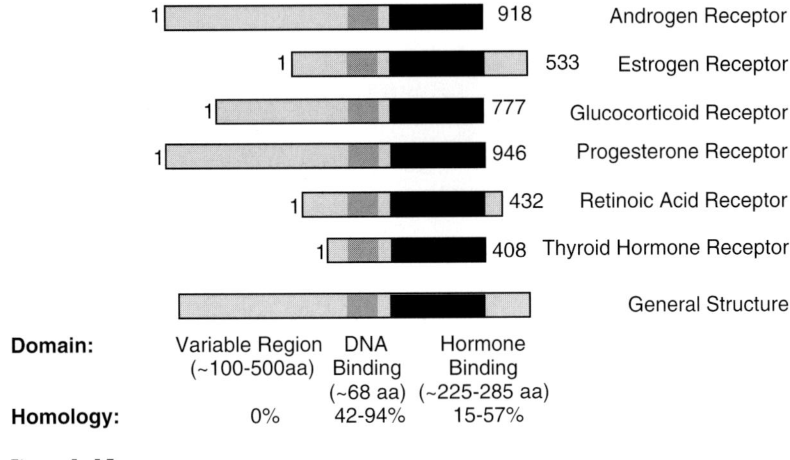



**Figure 1–15**

## BIOLOGY OF EARLY PROSTATE CANCER

**Figure 1–15:** Steroid receptor superfamily of nuclear transcription factors. This gene superfamily includes specific receptors for androgen, estrogen, glucocorticoids, mineralocorticoids, progesterone, retinoic acid, thyroid hormone, and vitamin D. The steroid receptor proteins contain three common domains. The amino-terminal domain varies in length and contains regions involved in transcriptional activation. The highly conserved central domain is responsible for DNA binding. The carboxy terminal domain mediates hormone binding.

**Figure 1–16:** The human androgen receptor gene is located on the X chromosome. This single copy gene contains a total of eight exons. The large first exon encodes an amino-terminal domain that is responsible for modulating the transcriptional activity of the androgen receptor. The second and third exons encode the two zinc finger motifs that form the DNA binding domain. Exons 5 through 8 encode the steroid-binding domain.

**Figure 1–17:** Trinucleotide (CAG) repeats in the androgen receptor gene. The first exon of the androgen receptor gene contains a stretch of repeated CAG codons that are translated into a region of consecutive glutamine (Gln) residues within the amino-terminal modulatory domain of the androgen receptor protein. The length of the CAG repeat sequence is polymorphic and varies between 8 and 39 codons in normal men.

The number of CAG repeats is inversely correlated with strength of transcriptional activation by the androgen receptor. A small number of CAG repeats appears to be associated with increased risk of prostate cancer and death from prostate cancer due to increased activation of androgen-dependent genes. Conversely, an abnormally large number of CAG repeats (40 to 60 repeats) results in Kennedy syndrome, an X-linked neurologic syndrome of spinal and bulbar muscular dystrophy characterized by relative androgen insensitivity.

## CAG Trinucleotide Repeats in Human Disease

Several neurologic diseases are characterized by the abnormal expansion of polymorphic CAG repeat regions in the mutant causal gene. This class of molecular diseases includes Kennedy syndrome, Huntington's disease, type 1 spinocerebellar ataxia, dentato-rubro-pallido-luyasian atrophy, and Machado-Joseph disease. In each of these conditions, the expanded CAG repeat involves a coding region of the affected gene and is expressed as an expanded polyglutamine region in the

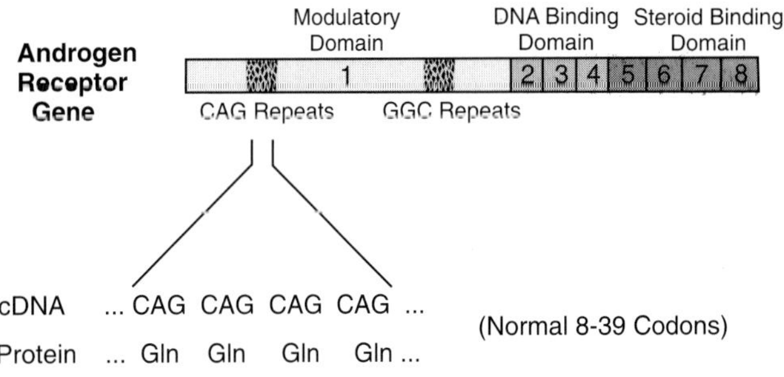



**Figure 1–17**

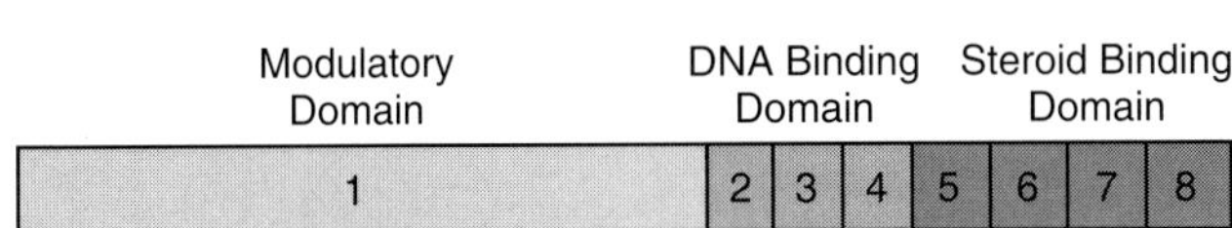



**Figure 1–16**

**TABLE 1–1**

## CAG TRINUCLEOTIDE REPEAT-LENGTH POLYMORPHISMS IN HUMAN DISEASE

| | | | | | REPEAT LENGTH | |
|---|---|---|---|---|---|---|
| **DISEASE** | **REPEAT** | **INHERITANCE** | **LOCUS** | **GENE** | **Normal** | **Disease** |
| Prostate cancer | CAG | X-linked | Xq11-12 | Androgen receptor | 8–39 | Reduced |
| Kennedy syndrome | CAG | X-linked | Xq11-12 | Androgen receptor | 8–39 | 40–62 |
| Huntington's disease | CAG | Autosomal dominant | 4p16.3 | Huntington | 11–30 | 36–121 |
| Spinocerebellar ataxia, type 1 | CAG | Autosomal dominant | 6p22–p23 | Ataxin | 19–36 | 40–81 |
| Dentato-rubro-pallido-luyasian atrophy | CAG | Autosomal dominant | 12p12-ter | — | — | Expanded |
| Machado-Joseph disease | CAG | Autosomal dominant | 14q24.3–q32 | — | 12–37 | 61–84 |

mutant protein. The mechanism of disease progression is not known. In contrast to these neurologic conditions, some forms of prostate cancer may represent a novel CAG repeat disease characterized by a short CAG repeat region in the androgen receptor gene. The excess risk of prostate cancer associated with a short CAG repeat region appears to result from the cumulative and lifelong increase in androgen receptor activation.

**Figure 1–18:** Role of 5α-reductase in prostate cancer. Dihydrotestosterone has an important role in prostate development, growth, and carcinogenesis. The intracellular levels of dihydrotestosterone are controlled by the activity of the membrane-bound 5α-reductase type II. Population studies have demonstrated that Japanese men have significantly lower 5α-reductase activity than black and white American men. The gene encoding the 5α-reductase type II gene is polymorphic, and certain alleles may account for racial differences in 5α-reductase activity and prostate cancer incidence.

## BIOLOGY OF PROSTATE CANCER PROGRESSION

**Figure 1–19:** Several characteristic androgen receptor mutations have been identified in metastatic lesions of some men with androgen-refractory prostate cancer. Many of these mutations (*indicated with arrows*) are located in the ligand-binding domain encoded by exons 5 through 8. Some of these mutations can alter the ligand-binding specificity of the androgen receptor. For example, missense mutations at codon 877 result in a mutant androgen receptor with the novel ability to bind and proliferate in response to flutamide, estrogen, and progesterone. Mutations of this type may provide a selective growth advantage following androgen ablation. In addition, the altered ligand-binding specificity of some mutant androgen receptors may explain why some androgen-refractory prostate cancers are sensitive to secondary hormonal treatments, including antiandrogen withdrawal.

**Figure 1–20:** Inactivation of tumor suppressor genes is associated with a variety of human malignancies, including prostate cancer. Cells that are defective in only the maternal or paternal copy of a tumor suppressor gene usually demonstrate normal patterns of growth control. Progression to the malignant phenotype requires inactivation of both copies of a tumor suppressor gene by one or more mechanisms, including chromosomal loss, regional chromosomal deletion, mutation, and hypermethylation. Primary and metastatic prostate cancers are characterized by the frequent loss of specific chromosomal regions that include 8p, 13q, 5q, and 6q. The identification of these characteristic regional chromosomal deletions suggests that tumor suppressor genes at these locations are involved in prostate carcinogenesis and prostate cancer progression.

**Figure 1–21:** DNA hypermethylation in prostate cancer. Methylation of CpG dinucleotides in the regulatory regions of genes is associated with decreased gene

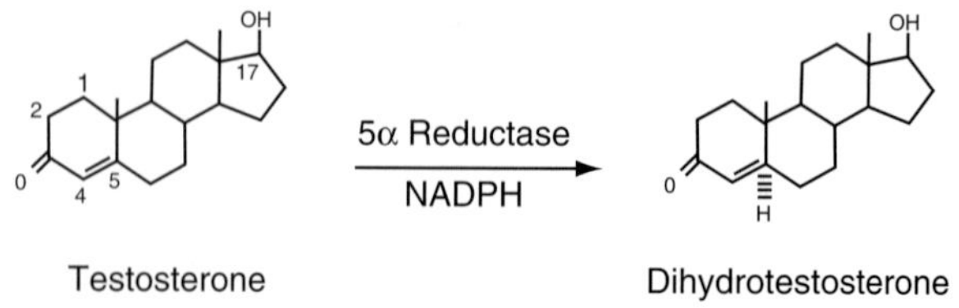

Testosterone

5α Reductase / NADPH

Dihydrotestosterone

**Figure 1–18**

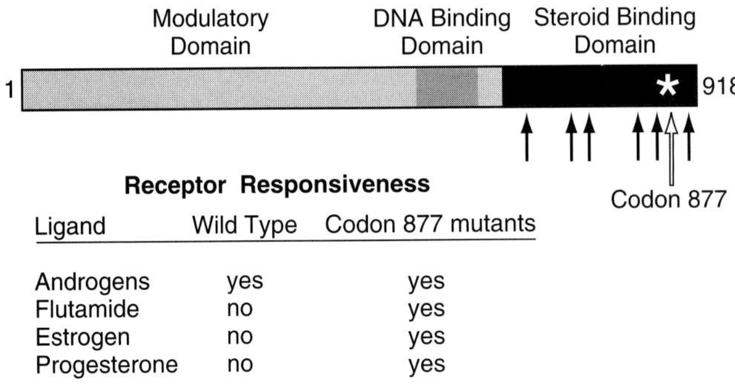



| Ligand | Wild Type | Codon 877 mutants |
|---|---|---|
| Androgens | yes | yes |
| Flutamide | no | yes |
| Estrogen | no | yes |
| Progesterone | no | yes |

**Figure 1–19**

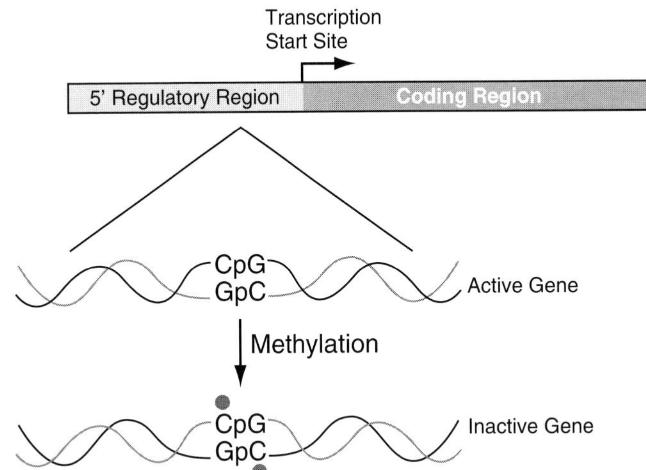



**Figure 1–21**

expression. Approximately 4% of cytosine residues are normally methylated, and only cytosine residues present in the dinucleotide CpG are substrates for methylation. Methylation is involved in the phenomena of X chromosome inactivation and genomic imprinting that result in differential gene expression based on parental origin of alleles. Alterations in patterns of DNA methylation are associated with a variety of human neoplasms, including prostate cancer. The regulatory regions of both the endothelin B receptor gene and the glutathione S-transferase π gene are hypermethylated in most prostate cancers but not in normal or hypertrophic prostate epithelium. Because decreased expression of both of these genes is associated with prostate cancer, DNA hypermethylation may represent an additional mechanism contributing to prostate cancer progression.

**Figure 1–22:** Retinoblastoma and the cell cycle. The retinoblastoma gene (Rb) plays a pivotal role in the cell cycle. In early G1, hypophosphorylated Rb protein tightly binds the E2F family of transcription factors. Following phosphorylation by cyclin-dependent kinases in late G1, the Rb protein releases the E2F proteins, resulting in transcriptional activation of regulatory genes and entry into S phase. Disruption of the normal Rb regulatory pathway is associated with the pathogenesis of many human malignancies. Allelic loss and mutations of Rb have been described in 27% to 60% of prostate cancers. Other components of the Rb

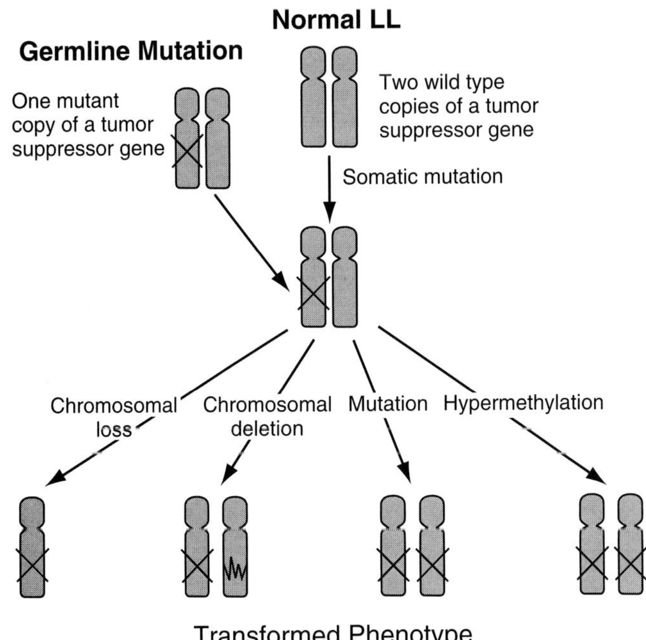



**Figure 1–20**

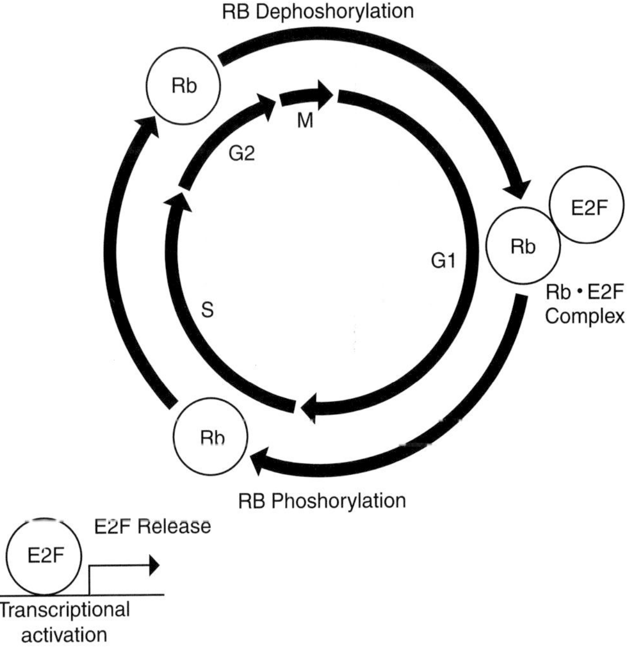



**Figure 1–22**

pathway have also been implicated in prostate cancer. The p21 and p27 gene products are inhibitors of the G1 cyclin-dependent kinases. Abnormal expression of p21 and p27 is common in prostate cancers. Absent or low levels of p27 expression are associated with a poor prognosis. Specific polymorphisms of the p21 gene are overrepresented in prostate cancer and other malignancies.

**Figure 1–23:** PTEN is a tumor suppressor gene. Cowden syndrome (CS) is an autosomal dominant inherited syndrome characterized by hamartoma development in multiple organs and an increased risk of breast, thyroid, and other cancers. This syndrome results from germline mutations in the PTEN tumor suppressor gene. Somatic mutations and deletion in the PTEN gene are common in prostate cancer, endometrial carcinomas, and glioblastoma multiforme. The PTEN gene encodes a dual specificity protein phosphatase that regulates the phosphatidylinositol-3-kinase (PI3K) Akt signaling pathway. PTEN inhibits conversion of PI-4,5-diphosphate to PI-3,4,5-triphosphate. Loss of PTEN function results in accumulation of PI-3,4,5-triphosphate, leading to activation of Akt. Activation of Akt results in cell survival and proliferation. (Contributed by William Sellers, M.D., Dana-Farber Cancer Institute.)

**Figure 1–24:** Apoptosis, or programmed cell death, is a normal cellular mechanism to eliminate damaged or unnecessary cells. This electron photomicrograph shows an apoptotic cell characterized by a disinte-

grating nuclear envelope and dark clumps of condensed chromatin. The p53 tumor suppressor gene product promotes apoptosis in cells that are disorganized or have damaged DNA. Loss of normal p53 function is common in most human malignancies. In contrast, p53 mutations are infrequent in primary prostate cancers. Mutations of the p53 gene are more common in metastatic and androgen-independent cancers, suggesting that inactivation of the p53 gene product is a late event in prostate cancer progression. Abnormal p53 expression correlates with high histologic grade, high stage, clinical disease progression, and a decreased survival rate following local treatment. (From Alberts B: Molecular Biology of the Cell. New York, Garland, 1994, p 1174.)

**Figure 1–25:** The *bcl-2* oncogene is an inhibitor of apoptosis. The t(14;18) chromosomal translocation that is characteristic of follicular B-cell lymphomas moves the *bcl-2* oncogene into the immunoglobulin locus. Recombination of this locus in mature B cells results in a chimeric bcl-2-immunoglobulin gene and overexpression of the *bcl-2* gene product. The bcl-2 protein normally functions as an inhibitor of apoptosis. In damaged or disorganized cells, bcl-2 is downregulated. Inappropriate overexpression of the bcl-2 results in malignant transformation by decreasing the rate of cell death. Bcl-2 is not usually expressed in primary prostate cancers. However, bcl-2 is commonly expressed in androgen-refractory prostate cancers, suggesting that

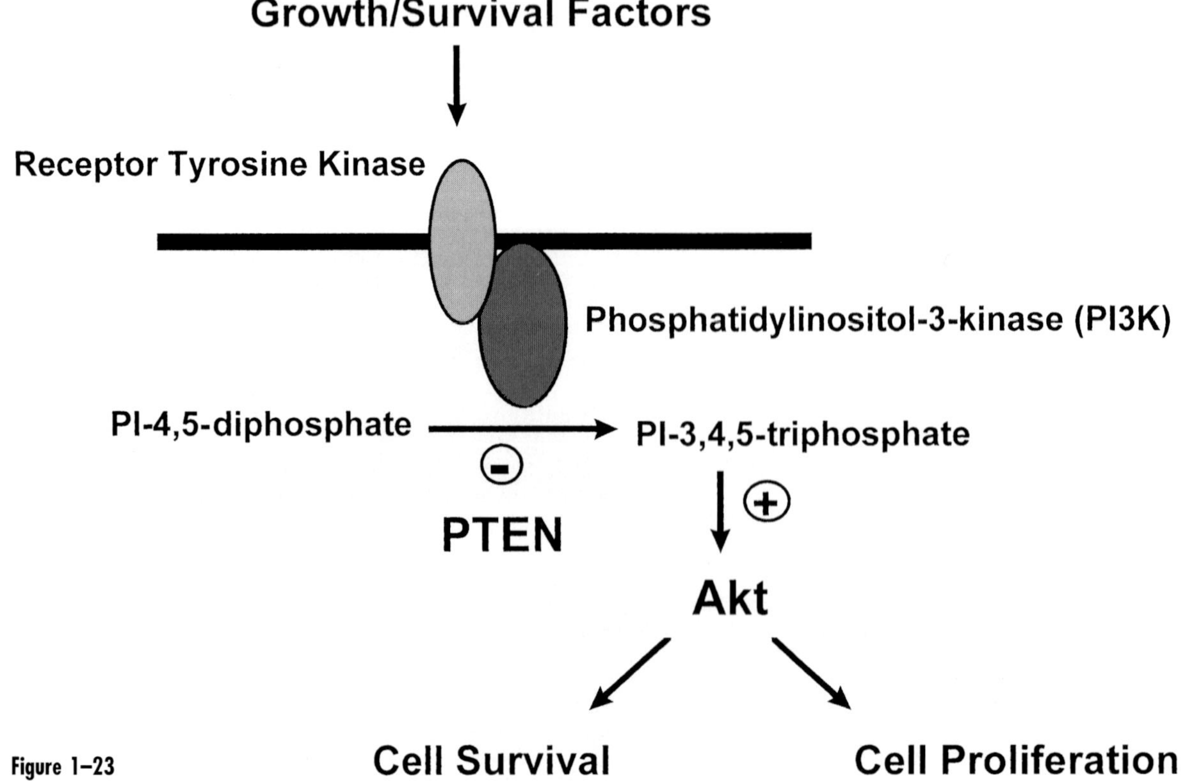


Figure 1–23

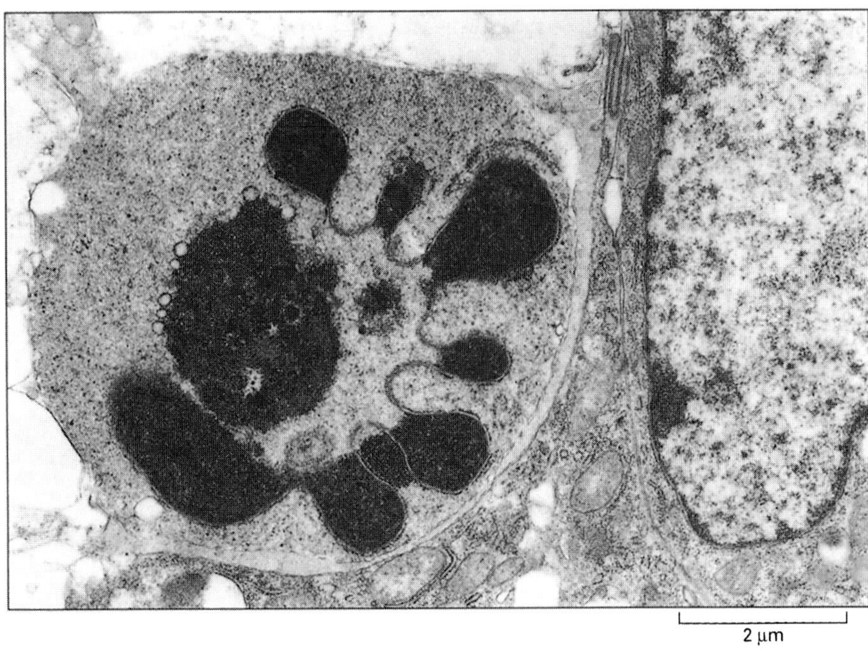



**Figure 1–24**

overexpression of the *bcl-2* gene is associated with the transition to androgen independence. The mechanism of bcl-2 overexpression in prostate cancer appears to be distinct from that of human lymphoid malignancies.

**Figure 1–26:** Growth factors implicated in prostate cancer progression. A variety of polypeptide growth factors appear to influence prostate cancer progression. These factors include members of the families of transforming growth factor β, epidermal growth factor, fibroblast growth factor, and insulin-like growth factor. These growth factors promote prostate cancer growth by both paracrine and autocrine mechanisms. Most of the receptors for these growth factors are transmembrane tyrosine-specific protein kinases. This observation suggests that these polypeptides influence prostate cancer growth through common intracellular signalling pathways. Androgens regulate the expression of some of these growth factors, including amphiregulin and fibroblast growth factor 7 (FGF-7).

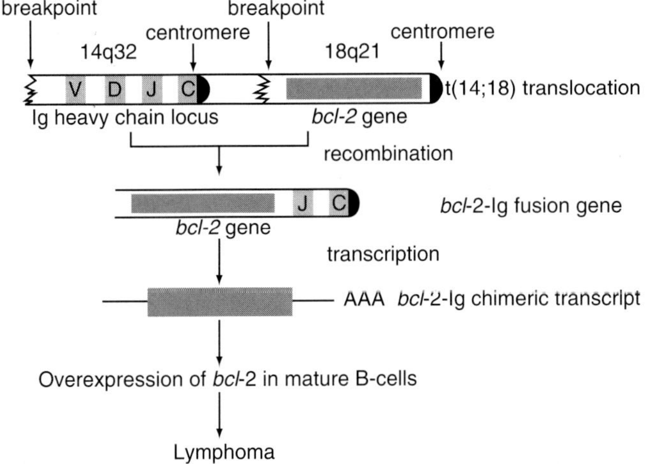



**Figure 1–25**

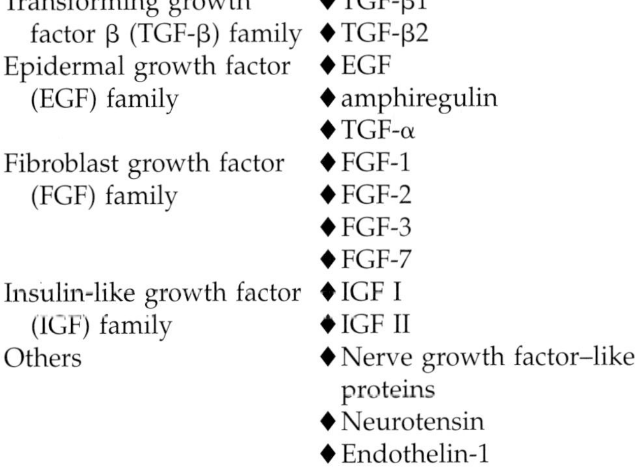

### GROWTH FACTORS WITH POTENTIAL ROLES IN PROSTATE CANCER PROGRESSION

| | |
|---|---|
| Transforming growth factor β (TGF-β) family | ◆ TGF-β1 <br> ◆ TGF-β2 |
| Epidermal growth factor (EGF) family | ◆ EGF <br> ◆ amphiregulin <br> ◆ TGF-α |
| Fibroblast growth factor (FGF) family | ◆ FGF-1 <br> ◆ FGF-2 <br> ◆ FGF-3 <br> ◆ FGF-7 |
| Insulin-like growth factor (IGF) family | ◆ IGF I <br> ◆ IGF II |
| Others | ◆ Nerve growth factor–like proteins <br> ◆ Neurotensin <br> ◆ Endothelin-1 |

**Figure 1–26**

**Figure 1–27:** Ras mutations in prostate cancer. Most growth factor receptors are transmembrane tyrosine-specific protein kinases that stimulate proliferation through a complex signal pathway. Ras is an important intracellular transduction protein involved in relaying signals from receptor tyrosine kinases to the nucleus through the mitogen-activating protein (MAP) kinase cascade. Ras belongs to the GTPase superfamily of switch proteins that cycle between active and inactive states. Mutations in the *ras* gene that result in continuous activation of the Ras protein are common in many human malignancies. In primary and metastatic prostate cancers from Japanese men, activating *ras* gene mutations have been identified in approximately 20% of cases. In contrast, activating *ras* gene mutations are relatively uncommon (<5% of cases) in prostate cancers from American men. These observations suggest that there may be fundamental racial differences in prostate cancer pathogenesis.

**Figure 1–28:** Endothelin-1 and endothelin receptors. Endothelin-1 is a normal ejaculate protein produced by the prostate epithelium. Men with metastatic prostate cancer have increased plasma levels of endothelin-1. Endothelin-1 stimulates increased osteoblast activity and may enhance the osteoblastic response of bone to metastatic prostate cancer. In addition, endothelin-1 induces bone pain associated with metastatic disease. Endothelin-1 has weak direct effects on cell growth but can greatly increase the mitogenic effects of other growth factors. The growth-promoting effects of endothelin-1 are mediated by the isotype-selective $ET_A$ receptor. The $ET_B$ receptor attenuates the activity of endothelin-1 by decreasing endothelin-1 secretion, increasing endothelin-1 clearance, and activating inhibitory pathways. Compared with normal prostate epithelium, primary and metastatic prostate cancers have

decreased expression of the inhibitory $ET_B$ receptor. The regulatory regions of the $ET_B$ receptor gene are hypermethylated in prostate cancer, suggesting that methylation-induced transcriptional silencing of the inhibitory $ET_B$ receptor gene contributes to the increased expression of endothelin-1 in prostate cancer. (Contributed by Joel Nelson, M.D., Johns Hopkins Hospital.)

**Figure 1–29:** Multistep process of metastases. Metastases represent the major cause of illness and death due to prostate cancer. The development of metastases is a multistep process involving an array of host–tumor interactions. In order to successfully metastasize, prostate cancer cells must gain entry to the circulation, travel to a distant vascular bed, adhere, extravasate, and proliferate. The ability to metastasize appears to involve multiple molecular events, including alterations in expression of tumor suppressor genes, motility factors, cell–cell adhesion molecules, proteases, angiogenesis factors, growth factors, and growth factor receptors. Animal models suggest that only a small fraction of circulating tumor cells develop into detectable metastases. However, the ability of tumor cells to enter the circulation appears to be clinically important because the detection of circulating prostate cancer cells by sensitive reverse transcriptase and polymerase chain reaction (RT-PCR) assays predicts a poor prognosis in men with advanced prostate cancer. (From Alberts B: Molecular Biology of the Cell, 2nd ed. New York, Garland, 1989, p 1200.)

**Figure 1–30:** E-cadherin mediates cell–cell recognition and adhesion. The cadherins are a family of integral membrane glycoproteins that play an important role in normal vertebrate development and cellular differentiation by mediating cell–cell recognition and adhesion. The conserved extracellular domain of the

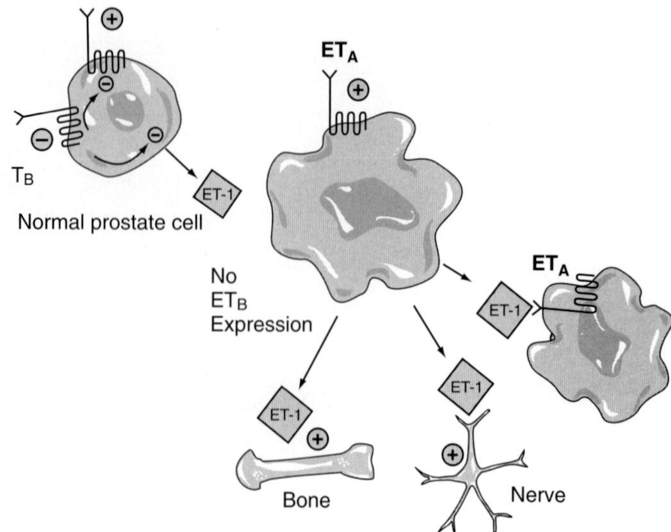


**Figure 1–28**

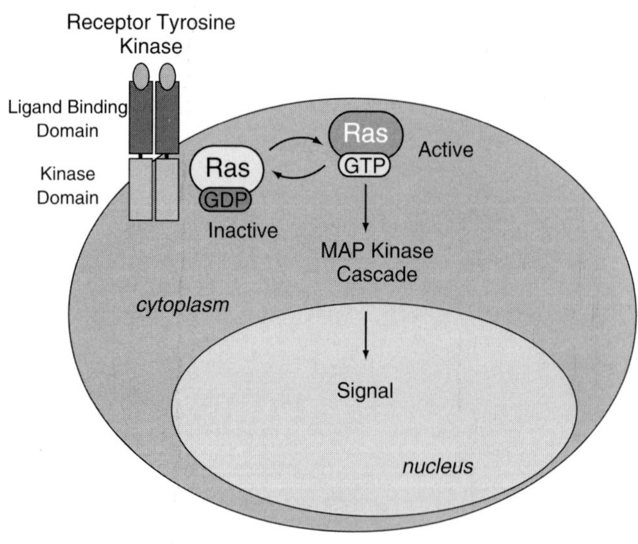


**Figure 1–27**

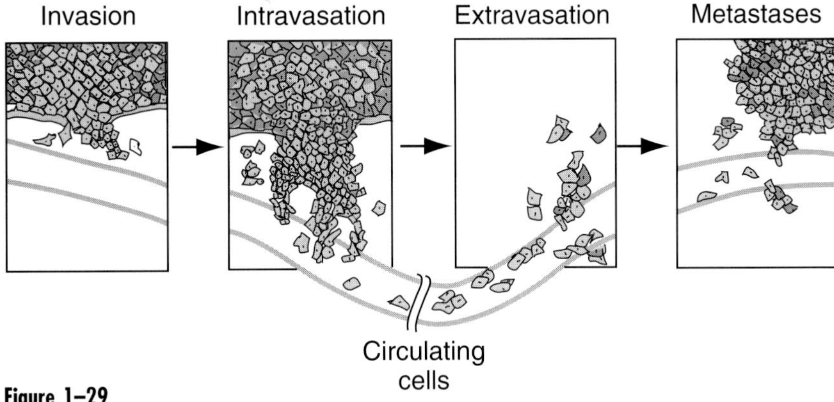


**Figure 1–29**

cadherins is responsible for cell–cell recognition and adhesion processes. The cytoplasmic tail interacts with the actin cytoskeleton by association with intracellular attachment proteins termed catenins. E-cadherin is expressed on many types of epithelial tissues, including the normal prostate. However, E-cadherin expression is aberrant or absent in many prostate cancers. Loss of normal E-cadherin expression is correlated with high Gleason grade and poor clinical outcome. In addition, the expression of the α-catenin is reduced or absent in some prostate cancer cell lines. These observations suggest that loss of normal cadherin-mediated cell–cell recognition may result in prostate cancer progression. (From Alberts B: Molecular Biology of the Cell. New York, Garland, 1994, p 966.)

**Figure 1–31:** Tumor-associated angiogenesis. The growth of a solid tumor is limited by its blood supply. To grow beyond a certain size, a tumor must induce the formation of a capillary network that invades the expanding tumor mass. Angiogenesis, the process of new blood vessel formation, is regulated by a complex combination of signals, including angiogenic factors elaborated by tumor cells. Tumor-associated angiogenesis has been studied in prostate cancer by measurement of microvessel density in pathologic specimens. Microvessel density is greater in prostate cancers with higher Gleason scores. In addition, microvessel density in primary prostate cancers of men with metastatic disease is significantly higher than in the primary tumors of men without metastasis. These findings suggest that the ability of prostate cancer cells to induce angiogenesis may contribute to prostate cancer progression and metastasis.

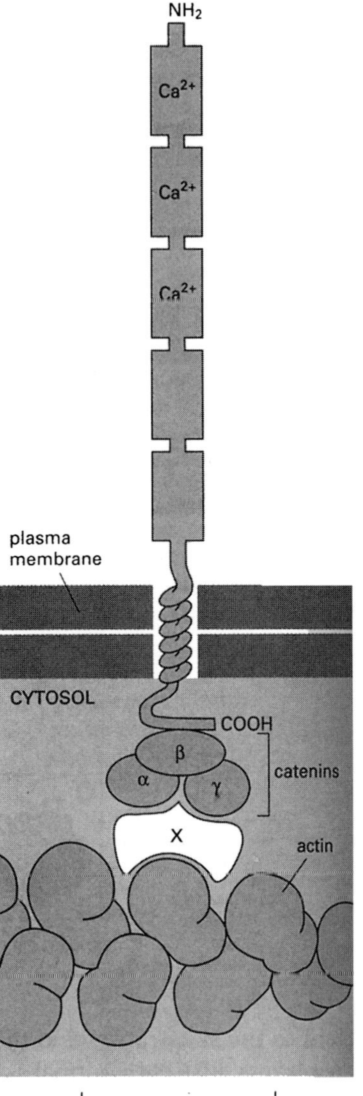


**Figure 1–30**

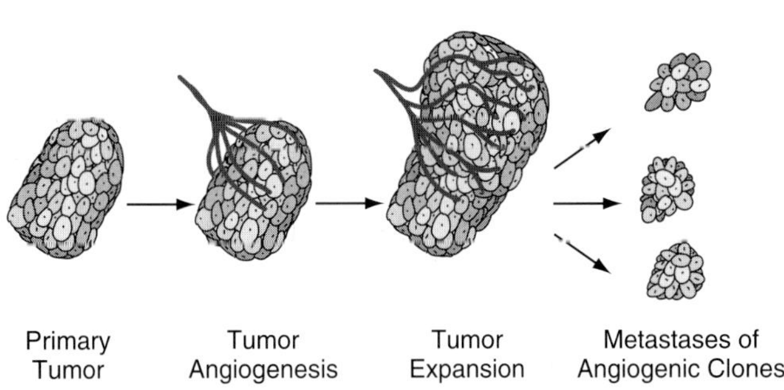


**Figure 1–31**

25
20
15
10
5
0
(%)
0 5 10 15 20 25 30 35 40 45 50 55 60 65 70 75 80 85 90 95
A
Tissue oxygen pressure (mmHg)
25
20
15
10
5
0
(%)
0 5 10 15 20 25 30 35 40 45 50 55 60 65 70 75 80 85 90 95
B
Tissue oxygen pressure (mmHg)
40
30
20
10
0
Average median pO$_2$ (mm Hg)
982
951
212
403
186
418
372
161
190
All T1C T2A T2B
C
Stage
Tissue
Pathologically involved prostate
Normal muscle
Pathologically normal prostate

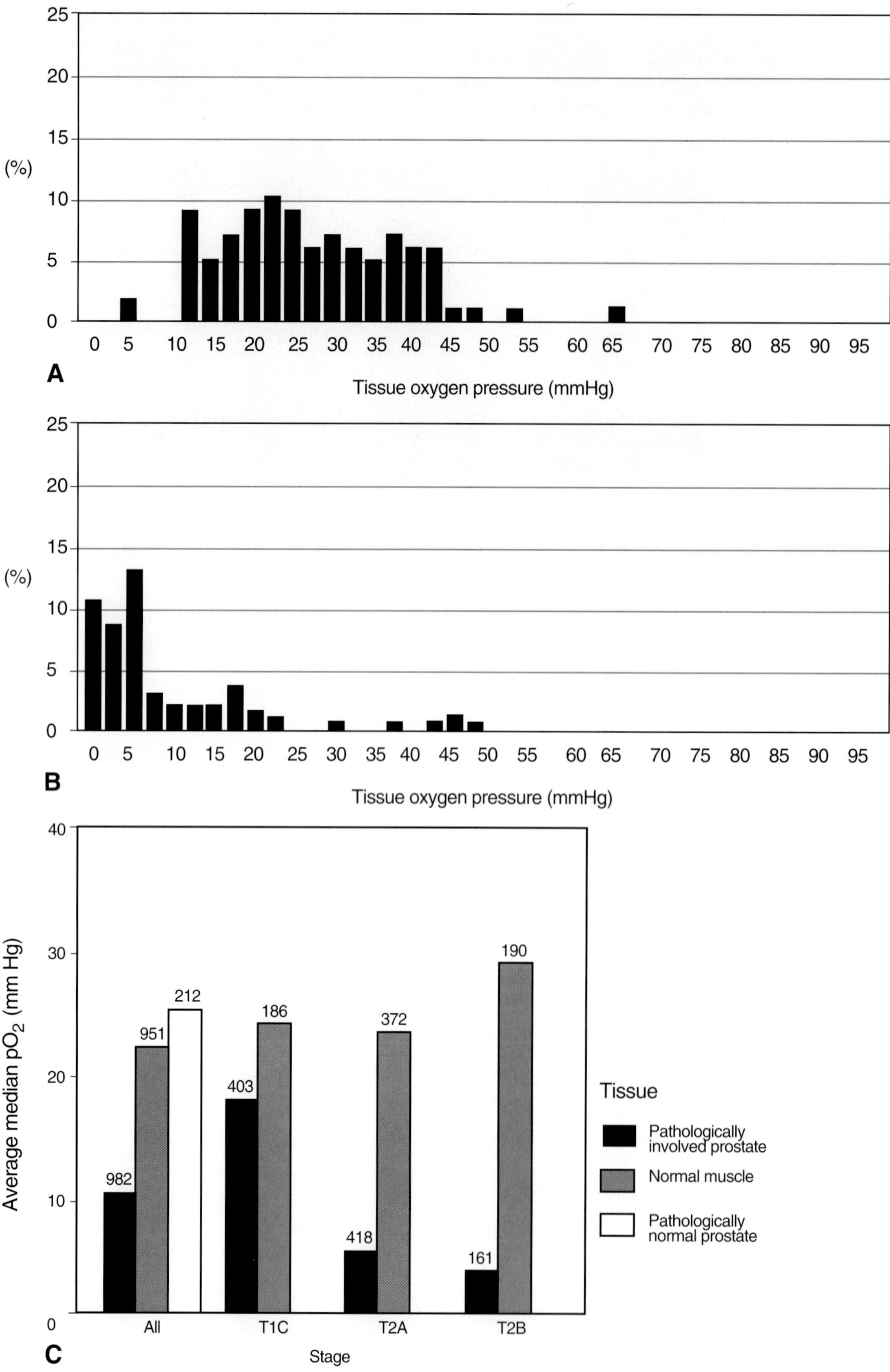

**Figure 1–32**

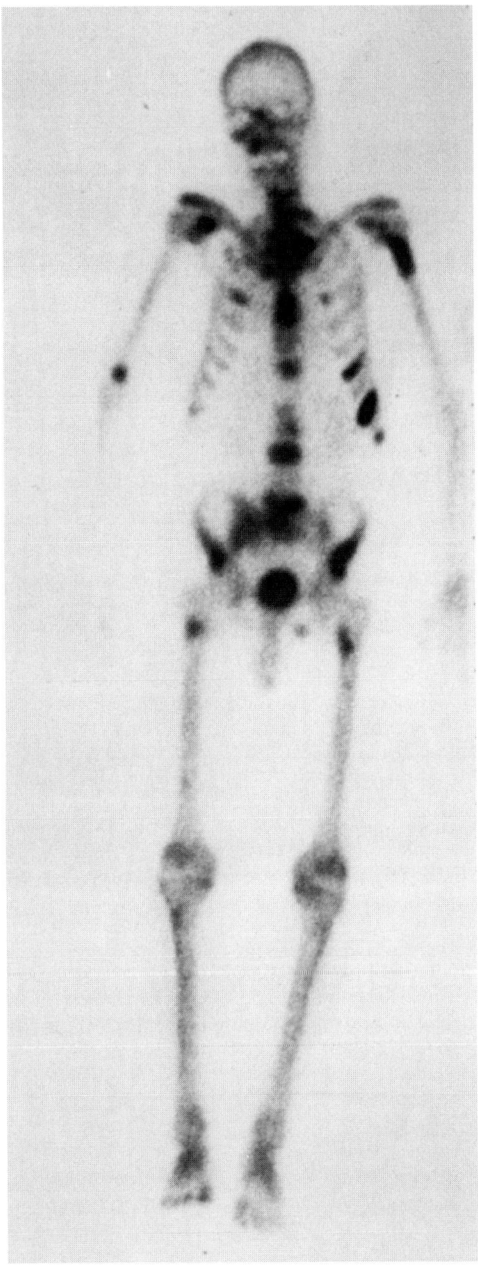

**Figure 1–33**

Increasing levels of hypoxia were observed with increasing clinical stage (C)—the numbers above the bars indicate the number of separate $pO_2$ measurements taken in that group of patients.

This study, suggesting that hypoxic regions exist in human prostate carcinoma, may have important prognostic implications. Prior studies have shown a significant relation between the extent of hypoxia and treatment outcome of tumors after radiotherapy. The biologic findings of increased levels of hypoxia with increasing clinical stage (C) suggests that hypoxia may be a factor underlying the high β rate of treatment failure in patients with locally advanced disease. Studies suggest that hypoxia may be a significant force that drives cells toward a more aggressive phenotype. Indeed, there may be a link between tumor hypoxia and angiogenesis. Hypoxia-induced factor 1 (HIF-1), a transcription factor involved in the cellular response to hypoxia, leads to increased transcription of vascular endothelial growth factor (VEGF), a key angiogenesis factor. (From Semenza G: Hypoxia-inducible factor 1: master regulator of $O_2$ homeostasis. Curr Opin Genet Dev 8:588–594, 1998.)

**Figure 1–33:** Bone metastases in prostate cancer. This bone scan demonstrates multiple areas of increased tracer uptake at the sites of osteoblastic bone metastasis in a man with advanced hormone-refractory prostate cancer. Prostate cancer preferentially metastasizes to the axial and appendicular skeleton and tends to form osteoblastic rather than osteolytic metastases.

**Figure 1–34:** Biology of bone metastases. Bone is a dense, specialized connective tissue. The increase in size and mass of the skeleton during childhood and adolescence involves bone growth and bone modeling. The maintenance of bone strength in adulthood involves bone remodeling, a regulated process of bone resorption followed by new bone formation. During bone remodeling, the bone matrix is resorbed by osteoclasts, and new bone matrix is secreted by osteoblasts.

**Figure 1–32:** Hypoxia in human prostate carcinoma. A recent study suggests that hypoxia exists in human prostate carcinoma. Using the Eppendorf $pO_2$ microelectrode (which measures the partial pressure of oxygen in tissue), Movsas and colleagues (1999) found that oxygen measurements from the pathologically involved portion of the prostate were significantly lower than those for normal muscle. Illustrative histograms of the $pO_2$ measurements for normal muscle versus a prostatic nodule are shown in $A$ and $B$, respectively. The median $pO_2$ from the psoas muscle was 26.5 mm Hg (with only 2% of the measurements <10 mm Hg) versus a median $pO_2$ of 6.1 mm Hg in the prostatic nodule (with 70% of the measurements <10 mm Hg).

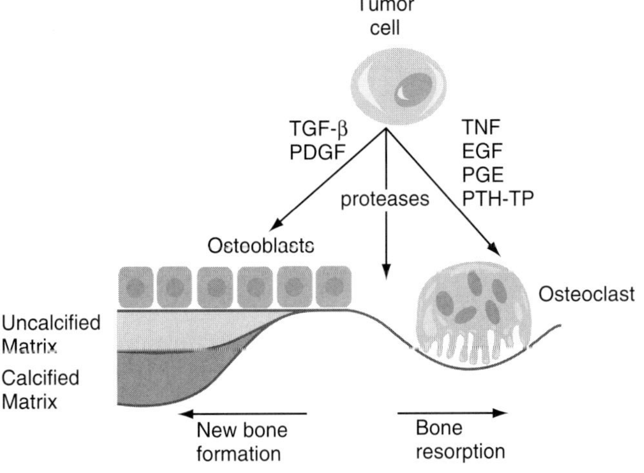


**Figure 1–34**

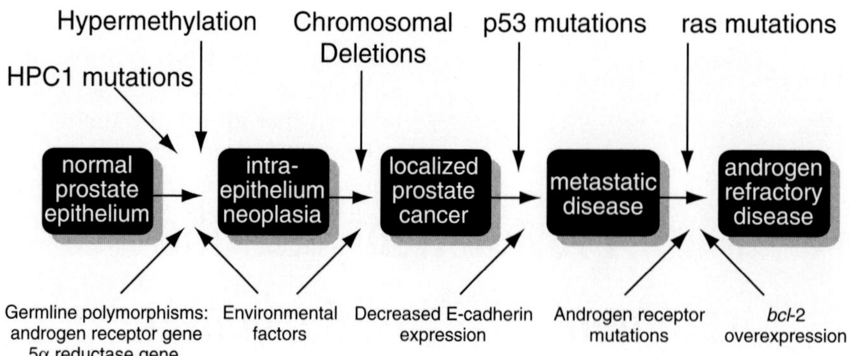


**Figure 1–35**

Malignant cells produce a variety of factors that influence bone remodeling, including hormones, growth factors, and proteases. The tendency of prostate cancer to form osteoblastic rather than osteolytic metastases may result from secretion of specific osteoblast growth factors by prostate cancer cells. These factors include transforming growth factor β (TGF-β), platelet-derived growth factor (PDGF), and endothelin-1.

**Figure 1–35:** Multistep model of prostate carcinogenesis. Multiple processes influence the development of clinical prostate cancer and the subsequent progression to metastatic androgen-refractory disease. Germline polymorphisms and mutations in prostate cancer susceptibility genes increase the lifetime risk of prostate cancer. Environmental factors and additional genetic events appear to be required for transformation to the neoplastic phenotype. A distinct set of molecular events appears to promote the progression of some clinically localized prostate cancers to metastatic and androgen-refractory disease. This figure summarizes the current understanding of these complex events.

## BIBLIOGRAPHY


Bostwick DG, Brawer MK: Prostatic intraepithelial neoplasia and early invasion in prostate cancer. Cancer 59:788–794, 1987.

Giovannucci E, Stampfer MJ, Krithivas K, et al: Proc Natl Acad Sci 1997.

Gleason DF: The Veterans Administration Cooperative Research Group: Histological grading and clinical staging of prostatic carcinoma. In Tannenbaum M (ed): Urologic Oncology: The Prostate. Philadelphia, Lea & Febiger, 1977, pp 171–174.

Greenlee RT, Hill-Harmon M, Murray T, Thun M: Cancer Statistics. CA Can J Clinicians 51:15–36, 2001.

Movsas B, Chapman JD, Horwitz EM, et al: Hypoxic regions exist in human prostate carcinoma. Urology 53(1):11–18, 1999.

Pienta KJ, Esper PS: Risk factors for prostate cancer. Ann Intern Med 118:793, 1993.

Smith JR, Freije D, Carpten JD, et al: Major susceptibility locus for prostate cancer on chromosome 1 suggested by a genome-wide search. Science 274:1371–1374, 1996.

Taplin ME, Bubley GJ, Shuster TD, et al: Mutation of the androgen receptor gene in metastatic androgen-independent prostate cancer. N Engl J Med 332:1393–1398, 1995.

Vogelzang NJ, Scardino PT, Shipley WU, Coffey DS (eds): Comprehensive Textbook of Genitourinary Oncology. Baltimore, Williams & Wilkins, 1996.

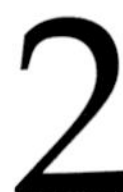
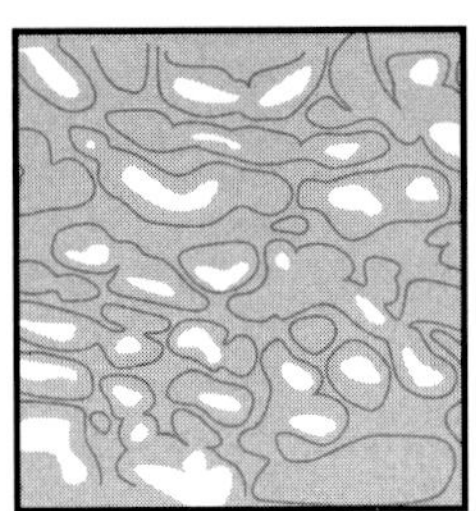

# Radical Prostatectomy for the Treatment of Prostate Cancer


*Erik T. Goluboff*

*John S. Lam*

*Aaron E. Katz*

*Carl Olsson*


The history of prostate cancer surgery dates back to the late 1800s, but it was not until 1904 that Hugh Hampton Young performed the first radical operation with the intent to remove the prostate, cuff of urinary bladder, and seminal vesicles en bloc for the cure of prostate cancer.[1] Young had developed the technique of simple perineal prostatectomy for the treatment of benign prostatic hyperplasia (BPH) in 1902.[2] In 1904, William H. Halsted referred a patient with presumed BPH to Young. Upon examination, Young found the patient's prostate to be firm, consistent with carcinoma, and to have an induration that appeared to be confined to the gland. Young theorized that, through a perineal approach, the entire prostate with its fascial coverings and both seminal vesicles could be removed with anastomosis of the bladder neck to the urethral stump. Young, with Halsted assisting him, performed his radical perineal prostatectomy technique without complications. The patient lived for another 6½ years and eventually died of other causes. An autopsy performed on this patient revealed no evidence of residual prostate cancer.

Although the radical perineal prostatectomy has undergone minor modifications, it is essentially the same operation performed today as when it was first performed by Young over 90 years ago. The radical perineal prostatectomy remains the oldest treatment for prostate cancer in existence. In 1945, Millin pioneered the retropubic approach to radical prostatectomy, which is the most popular approach in the United States today.[3] Since the introduction of this technique,

it has been adopted and modified by others.[4-6] Despite the efficacy of radical prostatectomy in curing prostate cancer, it never gained widespread popularity prior to the early 1980s because of the complications associated with this operation, most notably bleeding, incontinence, and impotence.

The rebirth of radical prostatectomy to treat prostate cancer has primarily occurred due to important modifications in surgical technique. Over the past 20 years, a series of anatomic discoveries have improved the urologic surgeon's ability to remove all tumor and reduced the perioperative morbidity associated with this operation. In 1979, Reiner and Walsh described the anatomy of the dorsal vein complex, which has resulted in a substantial reduction of operative blood loss.[7] The minimization of blood loss has permitted a more precise apical dissection and coaptation of the mucosal surfaces when the vesicourethral anastomosis is created. This reduces the chance of postoperative incontinence.

In 1982, Walsh and Donker elucidated the course of the cavernous nerves in the pelvis to travel dorsolaterally to the prostate along the anterior rectal wall.[8] The realization that impotence following radical prostatectomy resulted from inadvertent injury to these nerve bundles has led to modifications in surgical technique to preserve potency.[8, 9] Defining the relationship of the cavernous nerves to the capsular vessels of the prostate and prostatic fascia has also made it possible to obtain wider margins of resection when it is necessary to remove all the tumor. These recent advances have resulted in a much wider acceptance and application of radical prostatectomy.[10]

The number of radical prostatectomies to treat men with newly diagnosed prostate cancer has quadrupled over the last decade.[11] Several reasons have accounted for the rise in the number of radical prostatectomies performed to treat men with prostate cancer. The increase in the detection of localized disease has primarily been attributed to the use of serum prostate-specific antigen (PSA) testing in conjunction with digital rectal examination (DRE).[12] This approach has resulted in a higher proportion of newly detected and clinically organ-confined tumors that are potentially amenable to radical prostatectomy.[13] The use of early detection strategies for younger men in their forties and fifties (as recommended by the American Cancer Society and the American Urological Association) has also increased the proportion of men who are suitable surgical candidates.[14] The increased and earlier detection of prostate cancer has coincided with a substantial increase in the understanding of the male pelvic anatomy. This has led to the development of surgical techniques that allow for the removal of the prostate with a low risk of comorbidities, especially impotence and urinary incontinence.[8, 15] Thus, radical prostatectomy to treat localized prostate cancer has become much more acceptable to both the patient and the urologist.[16, 17]

Radical prostatectomy is most effective when the disease is organ- or specimen-confined at the time of surgery. Currently, approximately 60% of men with newly diagnosed prostate cancer are believed to be organ-confined based on current staging modalities.[18] Unfortunately, at the time of surgery, up to 50% of these men are ultimately found to have non–organ-confined disease on final pathologic examination.[19, 20] Patients undergoing radical prostatectomy for clinically localized prostate cancer and organ-confined disease demonstrate markedly improved biochemical disease-free survival when compared with men who have extraprostatic disease.[19] Serum PSA, clinical stage, and Gleason score have been used in the preoperative prediction of final pathologic stage for patients with clinically localized prostate cancer in order to assist urologists in clinical decision making.[20] Serum PSA is also used in the follow-up evaluation of men who have been treated for prostate cancer. The gold standard for tumor-free status in men following radical prostatectomy is an undetectable serum PSA level.[21]

Men diagnosed with clinically localized prostate cancer should be considered for definitive treatment if they are in good health and have a life expectancy of 10 years or longer.[22] The experience with radical prostatectomy reported in the past 5 years demonstrates that this operation effectively eradicates the cancer in a large proportion of patients. Long-term follow-up of patients treated with radical prostatectomy for clinically localized prostate cancer have 50 to 80% disease-free recurrence rates, depending on the grade and stage of tumor found pathologically.[19, 20, 23–26] The use of preoperative autologous blood donation and improved surgical techniques has decreased the incidence of homologous blood transfusion to less than 10%, with the majority of patients losing less than 750 cc of blood.[26–31] Urinary continence, defined as not using incontinence pads, has been preserved in over 90% of patients at most major medical centers.[26, 30, 32–40] Maintenance of erectile function has been described in up to 60% of selected patients.[30, 39–42] Hospital stays have decreased from over 7 days to a median of 3 days. Radical prostatectomy is a difficult operation. It remains a challenge to the skills of modern surgeons to perform this operation without blood transfusions, with the complete removal of cancer and negative surgical margins, and with the preservation of continence and erectile function in those patients who were continent and potent prior to the operation.

**Figure 2–1:** This timeline shows the historical milestones in prostate cancer surgery over the past century.

**Figure 2–2:** Incidence of prostate cancer in the United States. Prostate cancer is the most common cancer diagnosed in American men, followed by cancers of the

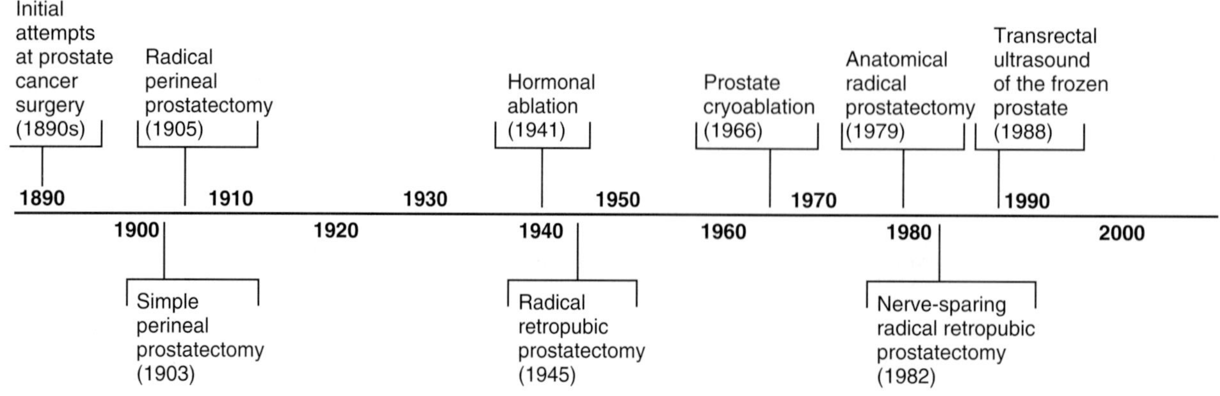


**Figure 2–1**

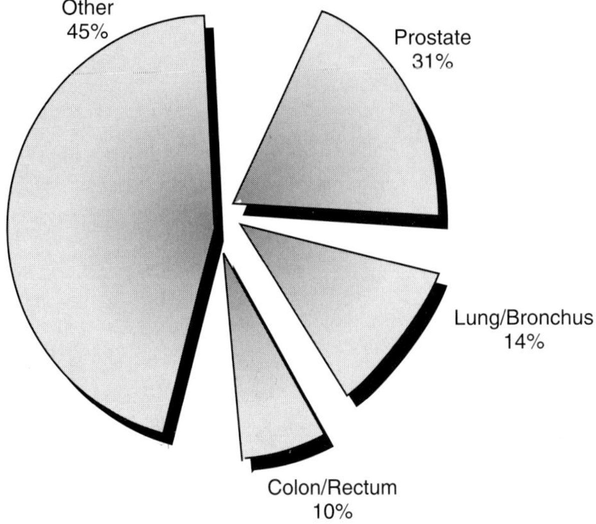


**Figure 2–2**

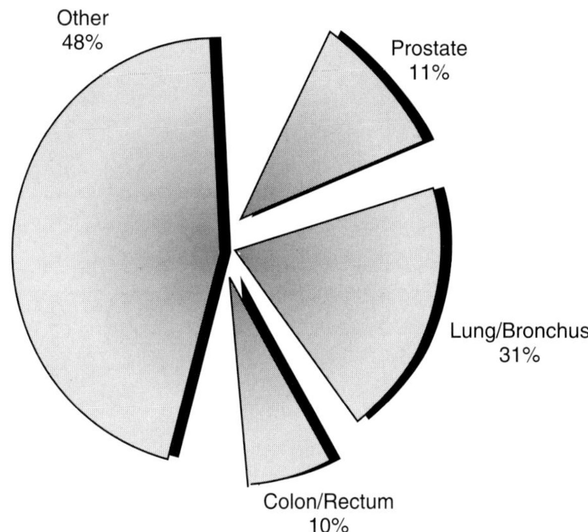


**Figure 2–3**

lung and bronchus and colon and rectum. In 2001, approximately 198,100 new cases of prostate cancer will be diagnosed in the United States,[18] accounting for 31% of the new cancer cases diagnosed in American men.

**Figure 2–3:** Mortality rate of prostate cancer in the United States. Prostate cancer is second only to lung cancer as a cause of cancer deaths in American men. In 2001, approximately 31,500 cancer deaths are estimated to be attributed to prostate cancer in the United States,[18] accounting for 11% of the cancer deaths in American men that year.

## BACKGROUND AND EPIDEMIOLOGY

In the United States, the lifetime chance of a man developing invasive prostate cancer is 1 in 6,[18] higher than for any other invasive cancer in American men **(Table 2–1)**. In addition, the probability of developing prostate cancer increases with age.

Prostate cancer incidence and mortality rates by race and ethnicity in the United States are charted in **Table** 2–2. African-American men have the highest incidence (225 per 100,000 population) and mortality (54.1 per 100,000 population) rates for prostate cancer.[18]

Risk factors for the development of prostate cancer are listed in **Table 2–3**. Age is the most important risk factor. It has been estimated that 70% of men over 80 years old have some histologic evidence of cancer in their prostates.[43] After the age of 50, prostate cancer incidence and mortality rates increase exponentially.[18] Family history is also a risk factor. Several studies have suggested that the incidence of prostate cancer is increased in the male relatives of prostate cancer patients.[44–46] In addition, genetic predisposition to developing prostate cancer is believed to account for 9% of the cancers diagnosed in the United States.[46] Race and ethnicity also play a role in the development of prostate cancer. The incidence of prostate cancer has been reported to be low in Asian men and higher in Scandinavian men.[47] African-American men have a higher incidence of prostate cancer than white men of similar education and socioeconomic classes; this has been demonstrated in age-matched studies.[48] Another reported risk factor is a diet high in saturated fats.[49]

## TABLE 2–1

### PROBABILITY OF DEVELOPING INVASIVE CANCERS AT CERTAIN AGES IN THE UNITED STATES

| SITE | BIRTH TO 39 YEARS | 40 TO 59 YEARS | 60 TO 79 YEARS | LIFETIME |
|---|---|---|---|---|
| Prostate | <1/10,000 | 1/49 | 1/7 | 1/6 |
| Lung and bronchus | 1/2499 | 1/80 | 1/16 | 1/12 |
| Colon and rectum | 1/1531 | 1/115 | 1/25 | 1/17 |

**TABLE 2–2**

**PROSTATE CANCER INCIDENCE AND MORTALITY RATES BY RACE AND ETHNICITY IN THE UNITED STATES**

| | WHITE | AFRICAN-AMERICAN | ASIAN/PACIFIC ISLANDER | AMERICAN INDIAN | HISPANIC |
|---|---|---|---|---|---|
| Incidence* | 145.8 | 225 | 80.4 | 45.8 | 101.6 |
| Mortality rate (%) | 23.3 | 54.1 | 10.4 | 14.2 | 16.2 |

*Per 100,000 population.

**Figure 2–4:** Percentage of indolent (clinically unimportant) prostate cancers detected in patients undergoing radical prostatectomy for clinically localized prostate cancer. In men who have undergone radical prostatectomy, the percentage of indolent prostate cancers detected has been reported to range from 3% to 27%.[50–53] Tumors defined as indolent were impalpable, had a tumor volume less than 0.5 cm³, were organ-confined, and had no Gleason grade ≥ 6. Indolent tumors make up only a small percentage of prostate cancers detected; the majority of prostate cancers detected are clinically important and potentially curable with surgery.

**Figure 2–5:** Long-term risk of death from clinically localized prostate cancer treated conservatively. The natural history of prostate cancer recently has been documented by two large series. *A*, Chodak and colleagues performed a pooled analysis of 828 patients with clinically localized prostate cancer from six medical centers.[54] The 10-year disease specific mortality rate was 13% for well-differentiated cancers, 33% for moderately differentiated cancers, and 66% for poorly differentiated cancers. The corresponding 10-year metastases development rate was 19% for well-differentiated cancers, 42% for moderately differentiated cancers, and 74% for poorly differentiated cancers. It must be stressed that at 10 years following diagnosis, 42% of patients with moderately differentiated tumors had metastatic disease. This finding might indicate a decreased survival rate after a longer period of observation. *B*, Albertsen and colleagues reported the results of a population-based study of 451 men, between the ages of 65 and 75, with clinically localized prostate

cancer treated conservatively.[55] The cancer-specific mortality rate at 10 years was 9%, 24%, and 46% for men with well-differentiated, moderately differentiated, and poorly differentiated cancers, respectively. Men with localized prostate cancer lost an estimated 3.8 to 5.2 years of life when compared with age-matched control subjects. Prostate cancer is a progressive disease when managed conservatively and poses a threat to health and life expectancy except in elderly men or those with serious comorbid conditions.

## Evaluation of a Patient Prior to Surgery

Several elements of the patient history and physical examination are particularly relevant to the urologic surgeon. The age and general health of the patient are important because of the protracted course of prostate cancer. Death from untreated localized prostate cancer is not likely to occur for 8 to 10 years; however, the risk of death from cancer continues to increase for at least 15 to 20 years or more.[54–56] A thorough assessment of the life expectancy of a patient with prostate cancer is necessary to determine whether the patient is a good surgical candidate. Potency status is also an important factor; patients who are impotent or who have significant erectile dysfunction may not benefit from nerve-sparing surgery.

Prostate cancer may cause obstructive voiding symptoms, irritative voiding symptoms, hematospermia, impotence, bone pain, anemia, or lower extremity edema. However, prostate cancer rarely causes symptoms because the majority of adenocarcinomas arise in the periphery of the gland distant from the urethra. The presence of symptoms as a result of prostate cancer suggests locally advanced or metastatic disease.

Physical findings are usually limited to the rectal examination. *Digital rectal examination* (DRE) provides prognostic information on size, location, and volume of tumor. This information is based on the induration and firmness of the abnormal area, as well as the presence of extracapsular extension, such as extension laterally to the pelvic sidewall, superiorly to the semi-

**TABLE 2–3**

**RISK FACTORS FOR PROSTATE CANCER**

Age
Family history
Race and ethnicity
Dietary fat

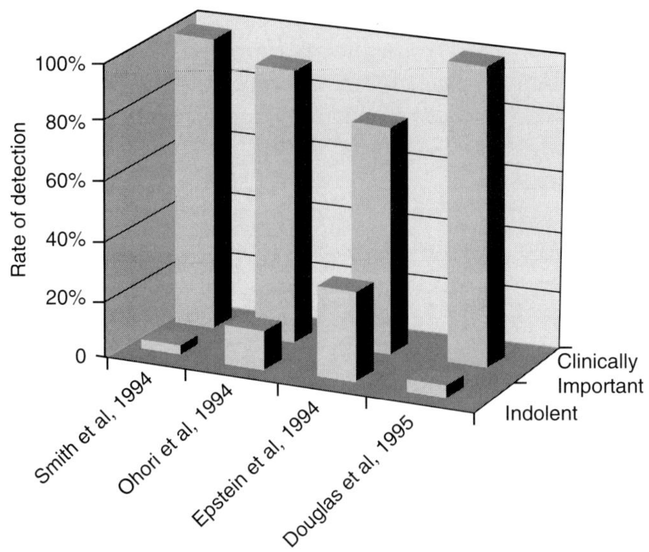

**Figure 2–4**

nal vesicles, or inferiorly at the apex to the pelvic floor diaphragm. For all men who have DRE abnormalities, a prostate biopsy is recommended regardless of the PSA level because 25% of men with prostate cancer have PSA levels below 4.0 ng/ml.[57–59]

*Serum PSA* level remains the most useful test available to detect prostate cancer while it is still organ-confined and potentially curable. The most effective method for early detection of prostate cancer is the combined use of DRE and PSA to assess prostate cancer risk.[57–59] Although 4.0 ng/ml traditionally has been used as the upper limit of normal for PSA testing,[12] a recent study reports that 22% of men with a benign DRE and a PSA level of 2.6 to 4.0 ng/ml have cancer detected on prostate biopsy.[60] Of these biopsy-detected cancers, 81% were pathologically organ-confined and thus potentially curable.[60] This finding suggests that a PSA cutoff point of 2.5 ng/ml may be more appropriate, especially among younger men.

Since the introduction of serum PSA, research efforts have focused on optimizing the measurement of serum

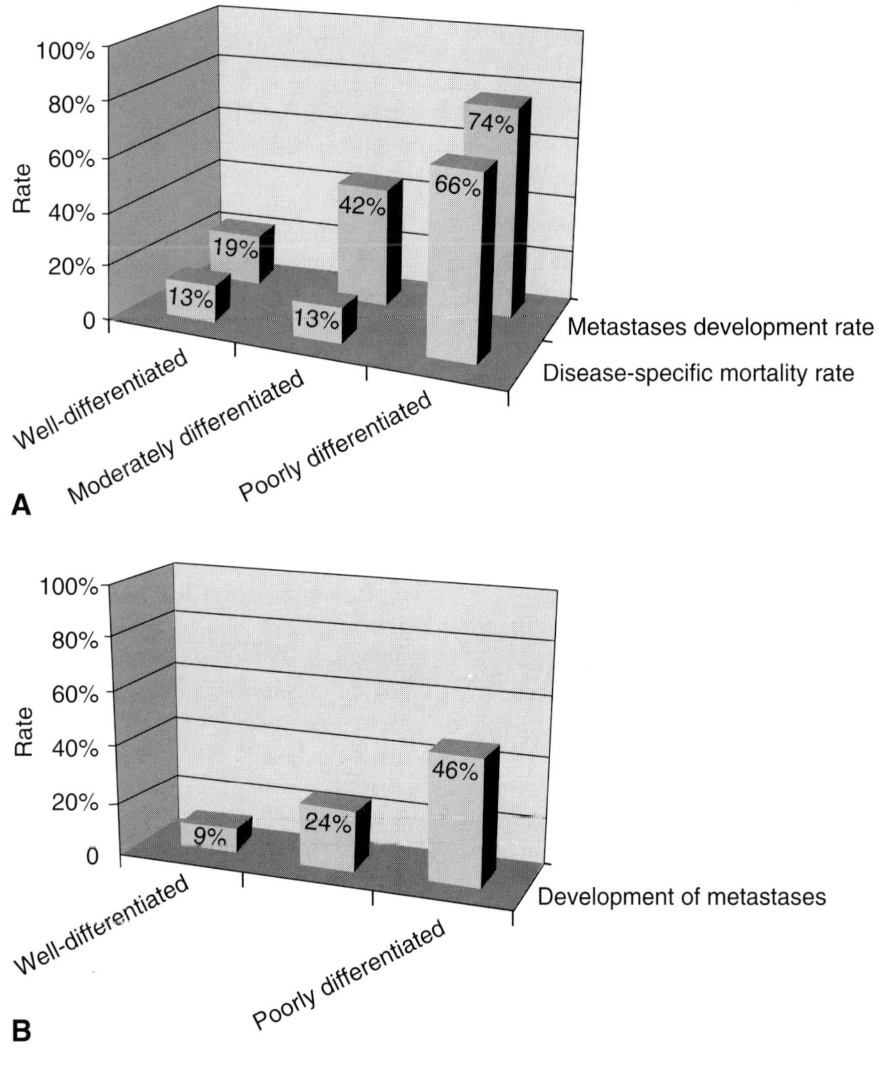

**Figure 2–5**

PSA for the early detection of prostate cancer. These methods have included the use of PSA density, PSA velocity, age-specific PSA reference ranges, and the molecular forms of PSA. PSA density is defined as the total serum PSA level (ng/ml) divided by the transrectal ultrasound-determined prostate volume (ml). PSA density is intended to provide improved differentiation between men with benign prostatic hyperplasia (BPH) and those harboring prostate cancer.[61] PSA velocity measures the rate of change of PSA over time, allowing longitudinal measurements of PSA. Substantial changes or variability in serum PSA can occur between measurements in the presence or absence of prostate cancer.[62] The age-specific PSA reference range is used to improve the sensitivity of prostate cancer detection in younger men while improving the specificity of prostate cancer detection in older men.[63] The age-related effect on the volume of the prostate and changes in PSA levels were not taken into account when the standard PSA reference range (0.0 to 4.0 ng/ml) was initially determined. Various molecular forms of PSA exist within the circulation. PSA is primarily bound in the sera by $\alpha_1$-antichymotrypsin (PSA-ACT). A smaller fraction of PSA is unbound, or "free," or bound to another endogenous protease inhibitor $\alpha_2$-macroglobulin (PSA-A$_2$M). Several studies have demonstrated that the percentage of free PSA decreases as the probability of having prostate cancer increases.[64–66]

*Bone scintigraphy* (radionuclide bone scan) is a very sensitive method to assess prostate cancer tumor spread to bone.[67] However, a positive bone scan is not specific for prostate cancer and should be confirmed by other studies, such as a bone survey or magnetic resonance imaging (MRI).

In general, nonhistologic studies have limited ability to detect capsular penetration and to predict the involvement of the neurovascular bundles by tumor. The staging accuracy of *transrectal ultrasound* (TRUS), MRI, or computed tomography (CT) is low.[68–69] Pelvic imaging for lymph node assessment may be warranted in men at higher risk of metastases when suspected by locally advanced disease on DRE, marked PSA elevations (>20 ng/ml), or the presence of poorly differentiated cancer on needle biopsy. MRI provides better imaging of capsular margins and pelvic lymph nodes; it has largely replaced CT in the local staging of prostate cancer.

TRUS is now the most common imaging modality for evaluating the prostate. TRUS allows an estimation of gland volume, definition of anatomy and the margins of the prostate, and evaluation of the seminal vesicles and the base of the bladder, and it facilitates placement of the needle biopsy.[70] *TRUS-guided biopsy* is generally indicated when there is an abnormality on DRE or an elevation in the serum PSA level. It is recommended that six biopsy cores be taken from the apex, middle, and base of both lobes.[70] Additional cores should also be taken from any abnormal foci found on TRUS, and if clinically indicated, a separate biopsy of the transition zone should be taken.[70] Others have reported that taking 12 or 20 core biopsies improved overall cancer detection by 30% to 35% compared to standard sextant biopsies.[71, 72] Studies have also shown that transition zone biopsies are useful in cancer detection only among men who have previously undergone a negative sextant biopsy and have a persistently elevated PSA.[73, 74]

The pathologic features should be carefully reviewed for Gleason scoring and the presence of perineural invasion. Preoperative biopsy tumor grade correlates with pathologic stage, and the presence of organ-confined disease decreases with higher grade.[75] However, if high-grade cancers are detected early and remain confined to the prostate, the prognosis is excellent.

*Pelvic lymphadenectomy* is the most accurate technique for detecting lymph node involvement in prostate cancer. The objective is to sample the areas of primary and secondary lymphatic drainage of the prostate to determine the presence of lymph node metastases. In the past, lymph node staging has been performed by an open operation, either as a staging procedure prior to radiotherapy or radical perineal prostatectomy, or as part of radical retropubic prostatectomy. Pelvic lymphadenectomy can now be performed laparoscopically. However, only a small proportion of patients undergoing radical prostatectomy are now found to have positive lymph nodes.[84–86] This reduction has been attributed primarily to the use of PSA screening. Pelvic lymph node dissection should be considered in individuals with either higher Gleason score (>6) prostate cancer on biopsy or a PSA greater than 20 ng/ml who have no other evidence of metastatic disease and are candidates for curative therapy by virtue of tumor stage and their life expectancy.

**Figure 2–6:** A multi-institutional model combining serum PSA level, clinical stage, and Gleason score has been developed to predict pathologic stage for men with clinically localized prostate cancer.[75] This study combines the clinical and pathologic data of 4133 men in order to predict organ-confined disease, isolated capsular involvement, seminal vesicle involvement, and pelvic lymph node involvement. *A,* The likelihood of organ-confined disease decreases with increasing serum PSA levels. Ranges of serum PSA levels were 0 to 4.0 ng/mL (64%), 4.1 to 10.0 ng/mL (50%), and above 10 ng/mL (29%). *B,* Clinical stage also influences the pathologic stage after radical prostatectomy. In this study, 80% of men with clinical stage T1a were found to have organ-confined disease. Conversely, only 13% of men with palpably non-organ-confined disease (clinical stage T3a) were subsequently found to have organ-confined disease. Overall, 61% of men with stage T1c (PSA-detected nonpalpable tumors) were found to have organ-confined disease on final pathologic analysis. *C,* Preoperative biopsy tumor grade also correlates with pathologic stage. The presence of organ-confined disease decreases with higher grades. This study reported a pathologically organ-confined rate of 74% for Gleason scores 2 to 4, 48% for Gleason scores 5 to 7, and 17% for Gleason scores 8 to 10. *D*, Risk of positive lymph nodes for men with clinically localized prostate cancer based on the serum PSA level and Gleason score. (*D* from Thompson IM, Rozanski TA: Regionally advanced adenocarcinoma of the prostate (T3a − TNx + M0): Management and prognosis. In Oesterling JE, Richie JP (eds): Urologic Oncology. Philadelphia, WB Saunders, 1997, p 386.)

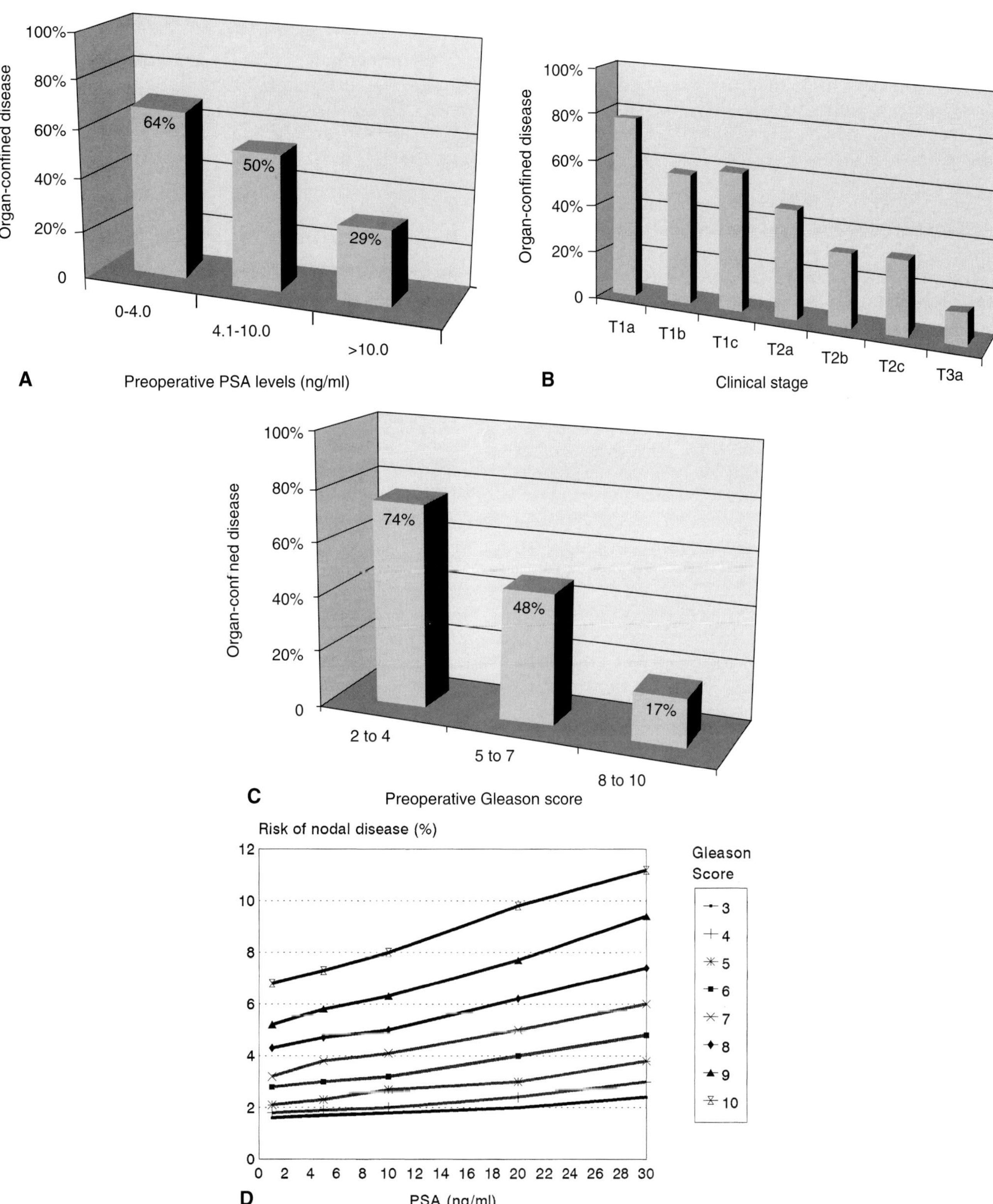


**Figure 2–6**

## Candidates for Surgical Therapy

The goal of treatment for localized disease is cure. Cure by radical prostatectomy requires that all tumor has been excised prior to the advent of micro- or macrometastases. Candidates for radical prostatectomy include all patients with stage T1 or T2 prostate cancer,[22] especially young and healthy men (life expectancy greater than 10 years) with impalpable, clinically organ-confined low- or moderate-grade disease.[14] Some investigators have also attempted to extend indications for surgery to patients with clinical stage T3 or even D1 disease; however, treatment results have been variable for these patients.[76]

## LOCATION AND PATTERNS OF SPREAD

**Figure 2–7:** Location of prostate cancer. The peripheral zone is the palpable portion of the gland on digital rectal examination. It surrounds the central zone, consists of 70% of the glandular tissue, and 70% of cancers occur in this location.[77] The transition zone surrounds the prostatic urethra and occupies 5% of the glandular tissue; however, 20% of cancers develop in this region.[77] The central zone occupies 15% to 20% of the gland, but only 5% to 10% of prostate cancers occur in this zone.[77] Prostate cancer is multifocal in more than 85% of cases.[77]

## Patterns of Prostate Cancer Spread

Prostate cancer may spread by local extension, via the lymphatics, or hematogenously. Local extension tends to be into and through the prostatic capsule, the bladder base, and seminal vesicles, whereas extension into the urethra and rectum is uncommon.[79] Prostate cancer spreads along the tissue planes of least resistance. Tumor often escapes through potential spaces around nerves, arteries, at the apex, around ejaculatory ducts, and through the muscle bundles of Denonvilliers' fascia.[79]

The most frequent sites of metastatic prostate cancer are lymph node metastases, followed by bone metastases. Lymphatic metastases occur most often in the obturator and internal iliac nodes followed by the presacral, presciatic, and external iliac nodes.[79] Spread to supradiaphragmatic nodes is uncommon.[80] Bone metastases most commonly involve the spine, followed by the femur, pelvis, rib cage, skull, and humerus. Following in frequency after lymph nodes, bones, and lung, the next most common regions of spread of prostate cancer at autopsy are bladder, liver, and adrenal glands.[79]

## SURGICAL ANATOMY

**Figure 2–8:** Regarding its anatomic relationships, the prostate is referred to as having anterior, posterior, and lateral surfaces, with a narrowed apex inferiorly and a broad base superiorly that is contiguous with the base of the bladder. Microscopic bands of smooth muscle extend from the posterior surface of the capsule to fuse with Denonvilliers' fascia. On the anterior and anterolateral surfaces of the prostate, the capsule blends with the visceral continuation of the endopelvic fascia. Toward the apex, the puboprostatic ligaments extend anteriorly to fix the prostate to the pubic bone. The superficial branch of the dorsal vein lies outside this fascia in the retropubic fat and pierces it to drain into the dorsal vein complex. Laterally, the prostate is cradled by the pubococcygeal portion of the levator ani and is directly related to its overlying endopelvic fascia. During a radical retropubic prostatectomy, the endopelvic fascia should be divided lateral to the arcus

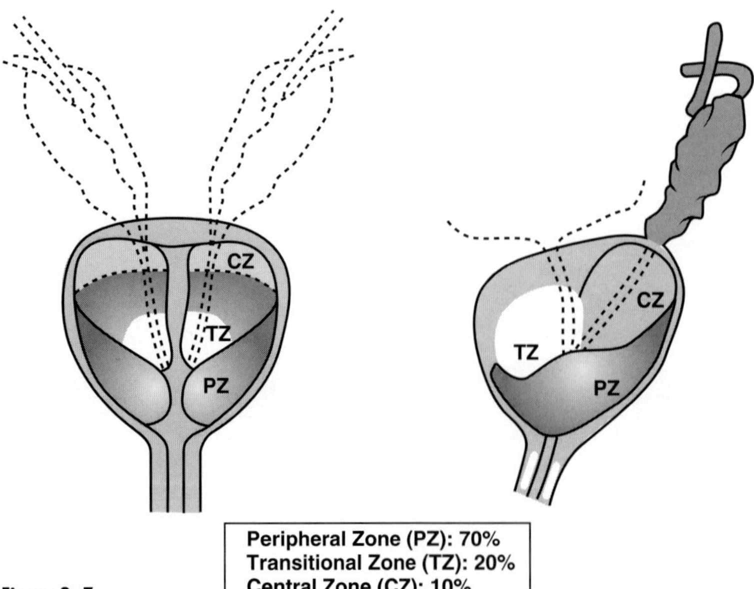


Figure 2–7

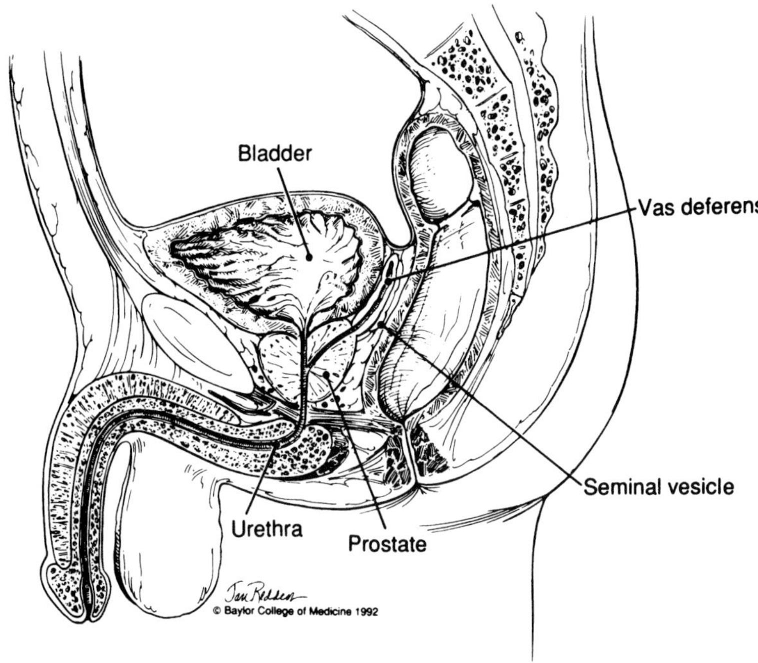


**Figure 2–8**

tendinous fasciae pelvis to avoid injury to the venous complex. The cavernosal nerves run posterolateral to the prostate in the substance of the parietal pelvic fascia. Thus, to preserve these nerves, this fascia must be incised lateral to the prostate and anterior to the neurovascular bundle.[82] The apex of the prostate is continuous with the striated urethral sphincter. At the base of the prostate, outer longitudinal fibers of the detrusor muscle fuse and blend with the fibromuscular tissue of the capsule. (From Oesterling JE, Richie JP (eds): Urologic Oncology. Philadelphia, WB Saunders, 1997, p 370.)

**Figure 2–9:** Vascular supply to the prostate. The primary vascularization of the prostate is from the prostatic artery, derived from the inferior vesical artery. Two main groups of arteries occur—capsular and urethral. Some accessory vessels to the prostate are supplied from the middle hemorrhoidal and internal pudendal arteries. The venous drainage of the prostate is through a prostatic plexus that joins the venous drainage of the penis in Santorini's plexus and then drains into the hypogastric veins. The prostatic lymphatics primarily drain to the obturator and internal iliac nodes. A small portion of drainage may initially pass through the presacral group or, less commonly, the external iliac nodes. (From Walsh PC, Retik AB, Vaughn ED Jr, Wein AJ (eds): Campbell's Urology, 7th ed. Philadelphia, WB Saunders, 1998, p 2567.)

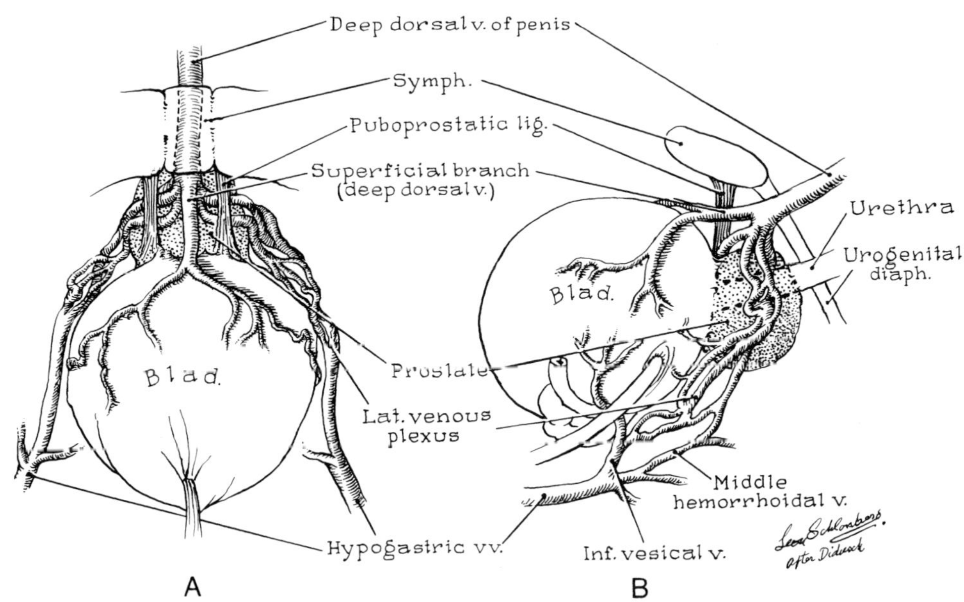


**Figure 2–9**

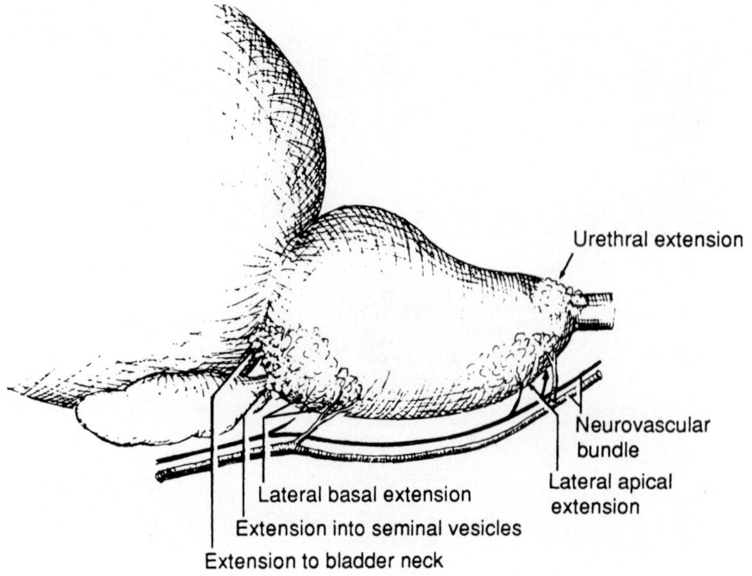



**Figure 2–10**

**Figure 2–10:** Nerve supply to the prostate. The autonomic innervation of the pelvic organs and external genitalia arises from the pelvic plexus, which is formed by parasympathetic visceral efferent preganglionic fibers that arise from the sacral center (S3–S4) and sympathetic fibers from the thoracolumbar center (T11–L2).[8, 9] The most caudal portion of the pelvic plexus gives rise to the innervation of the prostate and the cavernous nerves. The cavernous nerves travel at the posterolateral border of the prostate on the surface of the rectum and are lateral to the prostatic capsular arteries and veins, which serve as the surgical landmark for the course of these nerves (neurovascular bundles). During radical prostatectomy, the nerves are most vulnerable at the apex of the prostate, where they approach the prostatic capsule at the 5- and 7-o'clock positions. (From Lee CT, Oesterling JE: Cancer of the prostate: Diagnosis and staging. In Oesterling JE, Richie JP (eds): Urologic Oncology. Philadelphia, WB Saunders, 1997, p 368.)

**Figure 2–11:** Striated urethral sphincter of the bladder. The striated sphincter is related anteriorly to the dorsal vein complex and laterally to the levator ani. The fibers at the apex of the prostate are horseshoe-shaped and form a tubular striated sphincter surrounding the membranous urethra. In the midline posteriorly, the edges fuse with the perineal body. The striated sphincter contains fatigue-resistant, slow-twitch fibers that are responsible for passive urinary control. Active continence is achieved by voluntary contractions of the levator ani, which surrounds the apex of the prostate and membranous urethra. The pudenal nerve provides the major nerve supply to the striated sphincter and levator ani. (From Walsh PC, Retik AB, Vaughn ED Jr, Wein AJ (eds): Campbell's Urology, 7th ed. Philadelphia, WB Saunders, 1998, p 2569, Fig. 86–5.)

## ANATOMIC RADICAL RETROPUBIC PROSTATECTOMY

### Preoperative Preparation

Surgery is deferred for 6 to 8 weeks after the needle biopsy of the prostate and for 12 weeks after transurethral resection of the prostate. This delay allows the resolution of inflammatory adhesions or hematoma so that the anatomic relationships between the prostate and surrounding structures return to a near normal state before surgery. During this delay, patients are offered the opportunity to donate 2 or 3 units of autologous blood. Ness and colleagues showed no difference in the tumor recurrence rates in patients with prostate

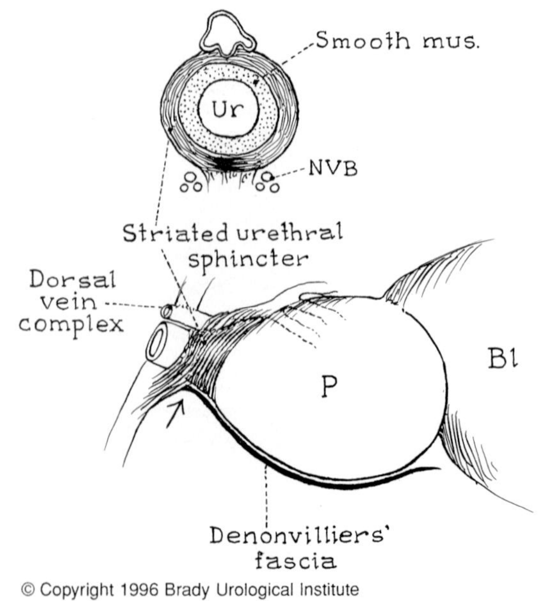





**Figure 2–11**

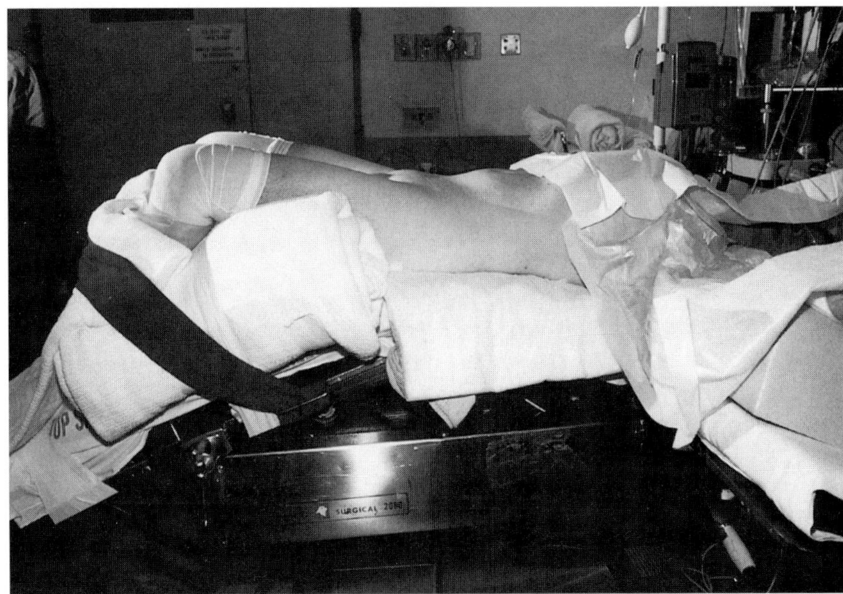

Figure 2–12

cancer who received autologous versus homologous blood.[82] Before surgery, the patient will require medical clearance from his internist. Patients should avoid taking aspirin or nonsteroidal anti-inflammatory agents, which interfere with platelet function. Patients undergo a limited bowel preparation prior to surgery. Most patients are routinely admitted to the hospital on the same day of surgery.

**Figure 2–12:** Positioning of the patient. The patient is initially placed supine with the symphysis pubis just below the break in the table. The table is broken at the umbilicus to extend the distance between the pubis and umbilicus. The table is then tilted in Trendelenburg position. Most surgeons position their patients in this manner; however, variations occur depending on the surgeon's preference.

The skin is prepped in the usual sterile manner. At Columbia, an O'Connor drape is placed in order to allow access to the rectum during the surgery. The remainder of the abdomen is draped in the usual fashion. A Foley catheter is placed sterilely into the bladder and inflated with 30 ml of water.

**Figure 2–13:** Incision for limited pelvic lymphadenectomy. An incision is made from the umbilicus to the symphysis pubis and brought through the fascia in the midline. The rectus bellies are retracted laterally. The peritoneum is swept superiorly on either side of the bladder in the space of Retzius in order to expose the external iliac veins and obturator nerves on each side. The boundaries of dissection for the lymphadenectomy are the external iliac vein, the obturator nerve, the symphysis pubis, the bifurcation of the iliac vessels, and the pelvic side wall. At Columbia, the lymph nodes are sent for frozen section; if they are free of tumor, the prostatectomy continues, but if they are involved with tumor, the prostatectomy is aborted.

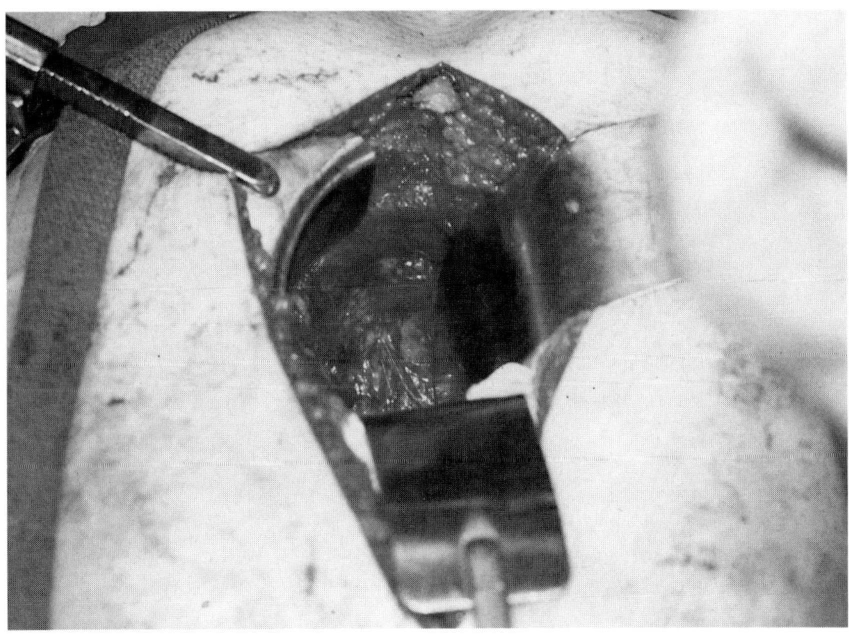

Figure 2–13

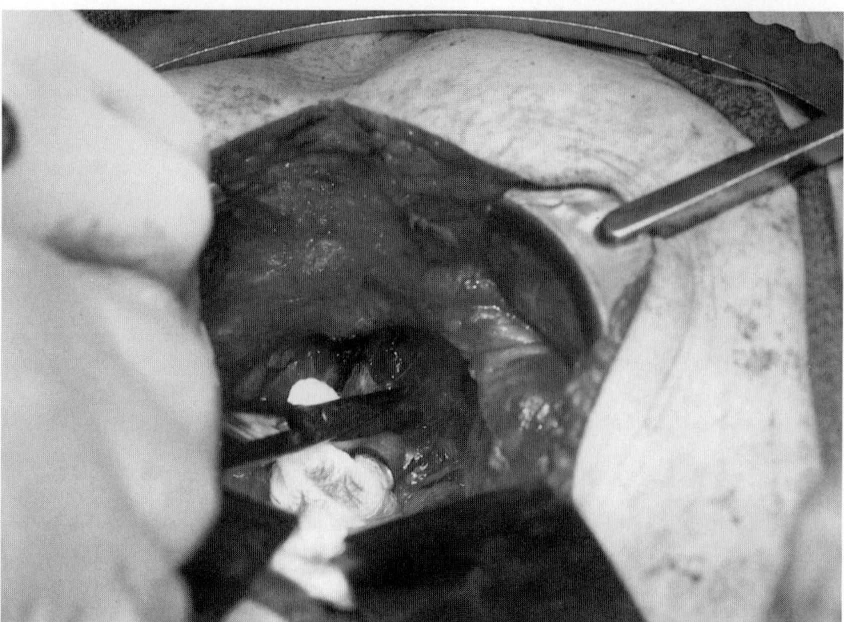

**Figure 2–14**

**Figure 2–14:** Incision in endopelvic fascia. The fibroadipose tissue covering the prostate is carefully dissected away to expose the pelvic fascia, puboprostatic ligaments, and superficial branch of the dorsal vein. The prostate is retracted laterally and the endopelvic fascia is opened on each side exposing the lateral surface of the prostate.

**Figure 2–15:** Division of puboprostatic ligaments. The puboprostatic ligaments attach the prostate to the symphysis pubis. These structures are first cleaned and isolated, and then divided. Some surgeons omit this step in the belief that it will improve continence.

**Figure 2–16:** Division of dorsal vein complex. A right-angle clamp is passed beneath the dorsal vein complex just anterior to the urethra and distal to the apex of the prostate. The dorsal vein is then ligated and divided. Once the dorsal vein complex has been securely ligated and divided, and backbleeding con-

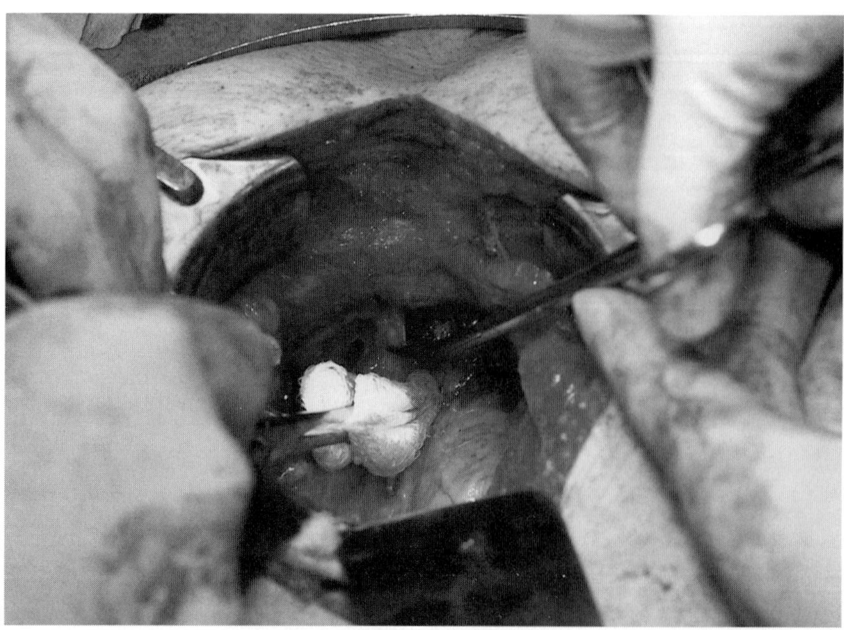

**Figure 2–15**

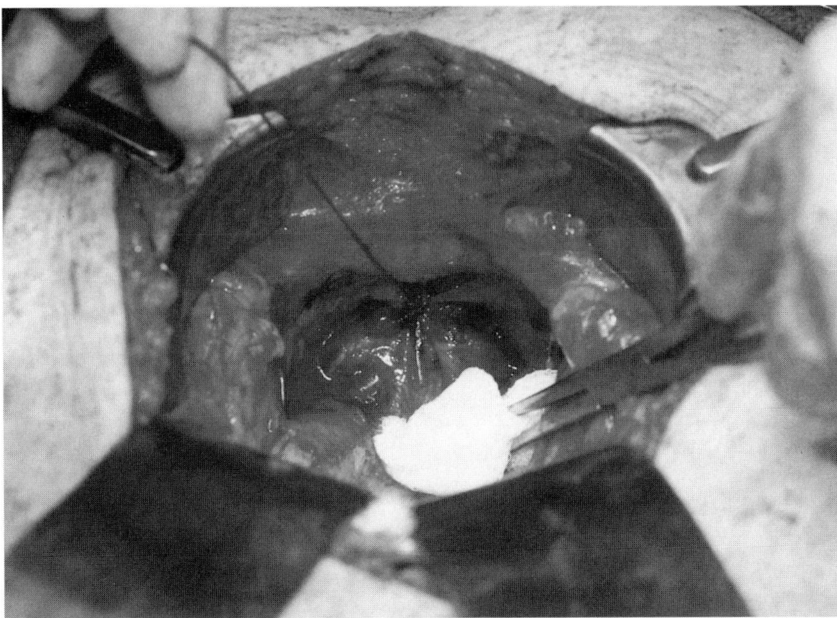

**Figure 2–16**

trolled, the apex of the prostate and adjacent neurovascular bundles can be identified.

**Figure 2–17:** Division of urethra. After division of the dorsal vein complex, the prostate is retracted cephalad and the urethra defined. On either side of the urethra there is a groove, and lateral to each groove are the neurovascular bundles. A large right-angle clamp is placed between the urethra and the neurovascular bundles. The anterior part of the urethra is divided.

Some surgeons place some or all of the anastomotic sutures in the urethra at this time. The Foley catheter is exposed, pulled cephalad into the wound as far as it will permit, clamped, and divided distal to the clamp. The posterior part of the urethra is then divided, exposing the anterior surface of the rectum. Some surgeons use stay sutures to facilitate retracting the urethral stump when the vesicourethral anastomosis is performed.

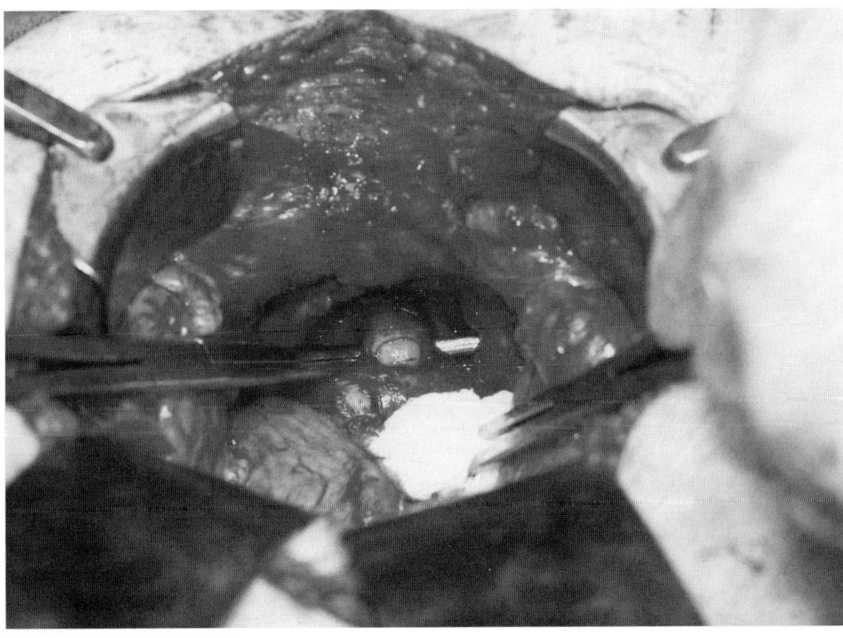

**Figure 2–17**

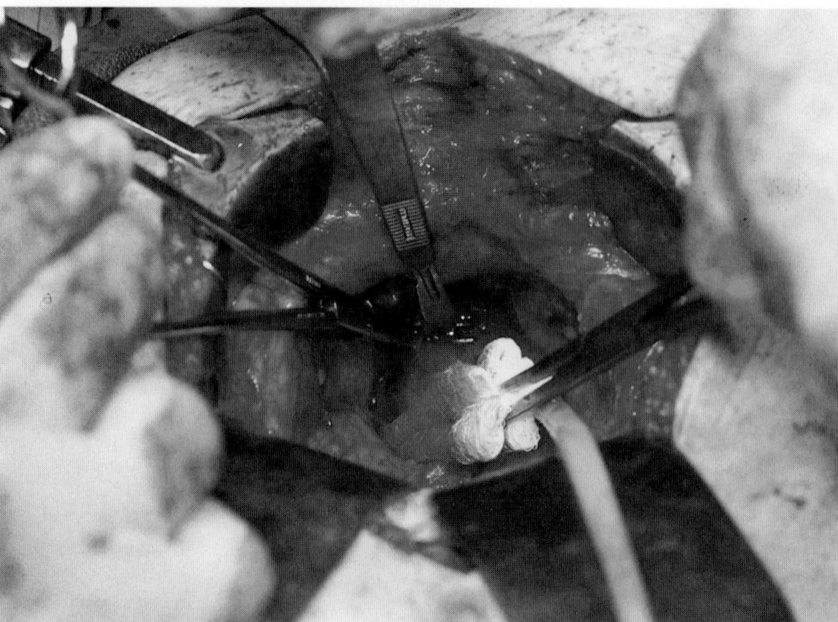

**Figure 2–18**

**Figure 2–18:** Identification and preservation of the neurovascular bundles. Using a fine right-angle clamp, the rectourethralis fibers are divided. A plane posterior to the prostate and anterior to the rectum is developed first sharply and then bluntly to extend the plane to the seminal vesicles. The Foley catheter is occasionally used as a retractor. For patients in whom nerve-sparing prostatectomy is to be performed, these structures are identified and avoided. If nerve-sparing is not planned, the neurovascular bundle is taken at this point so that it can be retracted superiorly with the rest of the prostate.

**Figure 2–19:** Posterior dissection and division of lateral pedicles. The vascular pedicles running posterolaterally from the prostate are ligated and divided. The dissection is carried cephalad until the lateral surface of the seminal vesicle can be seen on either side. For patients with low-grade, low-stage, and nonpalpable tumors, the neurovascular bundle can be preserved by hugging the prostate closely during this dissection. For patients with high-grade, high-stage, high-PSA, or palpable disease, a wide excision sacrificing this bundle can be performed.

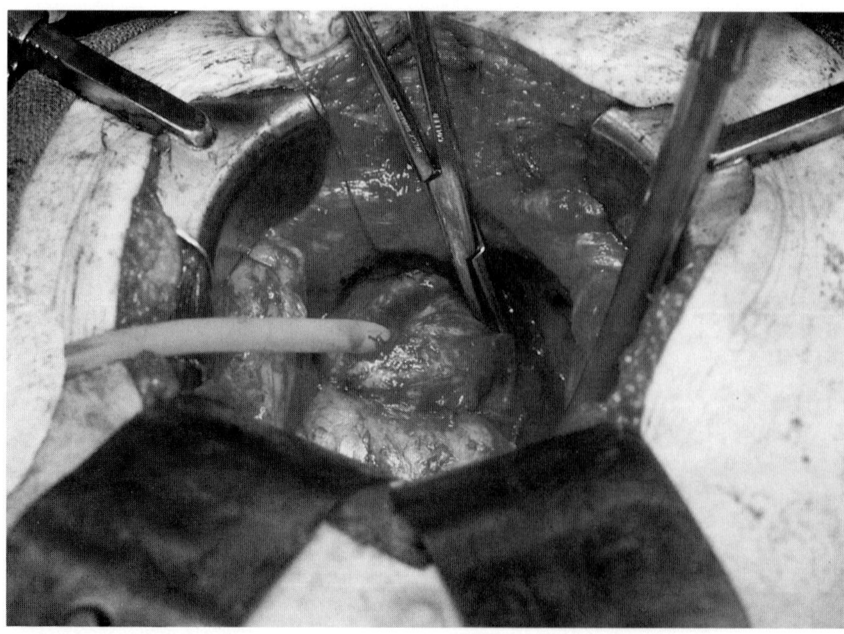

**Figure 2–19**

The decision to excise the lateral pelvic fascia and neurovascular bundles completely on one or both sides should be based on preoperative evaluation and the findings at surgery. The neurovascular bundles should be widely excised in impotent patients if there are any questions; however, these bundles are often preserved because they may play a minor role in the recovery of urinary control.[80] The ipsilateral neurovascular bundle in patients with palpable apical lesions is more commonly excised than in patients with lesions at the base. A wide excision of the ipsilateral neurovascular bundle is performed either if there is induration in the lateral pelvic fascia after the endopelvic fascia has been opened or if the neurovascular bundle is not easily separated from the prostatic capsule.

**Figure 2–20:** Division of bladder neck and excision of seminal vesicles. *A,* The prostate is placed back into its anatomic position, and the anterior bladder neck is opened to expose the Foley balloon. The Foley balloon is brought out of the bladder and clamped to the distal Foley catheter. The ureteral orifices may be catheterized to prevent ureteral damage. A long right-angle clamp is passed just cephalad (posterior) to each of the seminal vesicles and spread widely. This space is between the posterior bladder neck and the seminal vesicles. *B,* The clamp is then passed from one side to the other and the posterior bladder neck is divided. The seminal vesicles can be separated free from other structures, and the vasa can be clipped either before or after opening the bladder. The specimen is then removed.

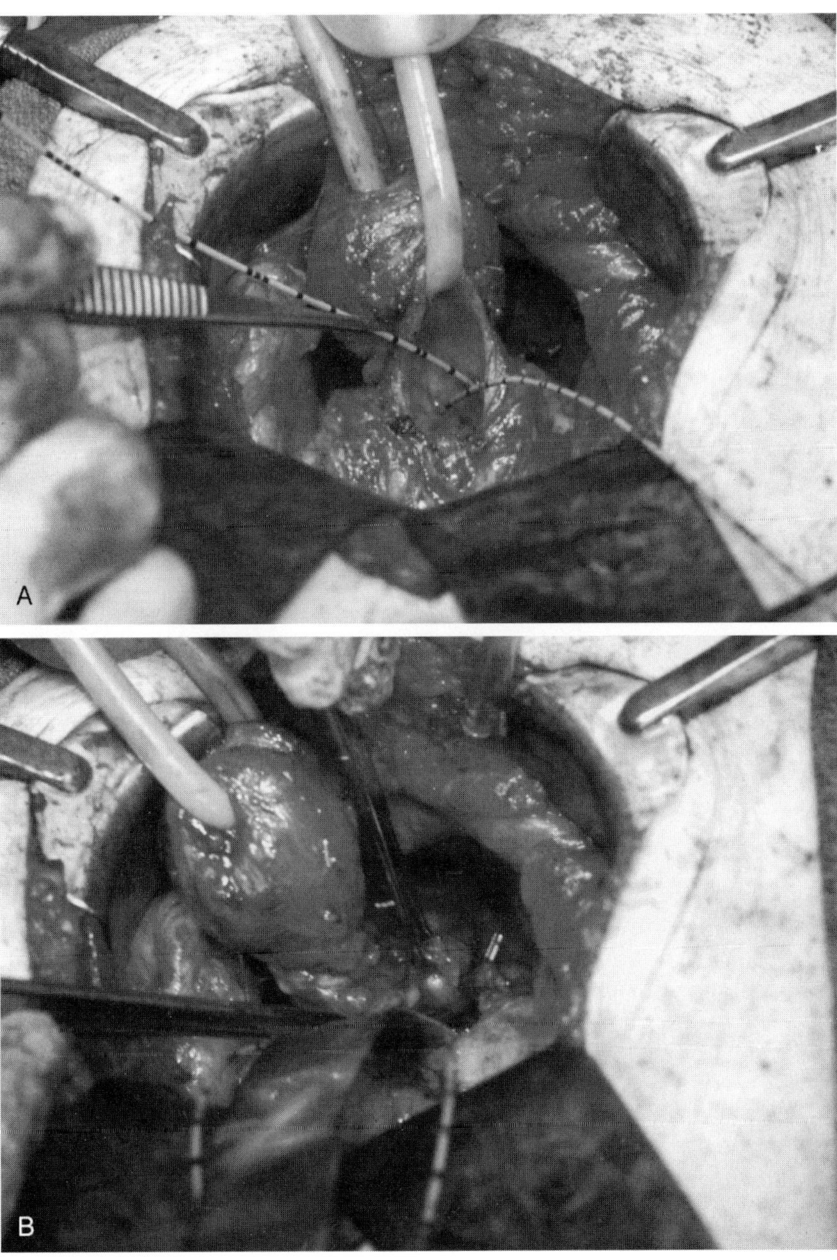

**Figure 2–20**

**Figure 2–21:** Bladder neck reconstruction and anastomosis. *A,* Some surgeons use a bladder neck–sparing procedure, as this has been reported by some to have improved urinary continence. Various methods have been described to expose the urethral stump. These methods include catheter guides, coudé catheters, and placement of the urethral sutures at the time of opening the anterior urethra. A tennis racket–shaped bladder neck closure is used by some surgeons. *B,* The urethral sutures are now placed into the bladder neck. The

retractors are relaxed, and sutures are tied over a catheter. The wound is irrigated. A Jackson-Pratt drain is placed near the anastomosis. The fascia is closed with a running suture. The subcutaneous tissue is closed with interrupted sutures. The skin is closed with staples.

**Figure 2–22:** Postoperative management. The patient remains hospitalized until he is ambulating and tolerating a regular diet. The Foley catheter is left in place for 2 to 3 weeks after the surgery. The drain is left until

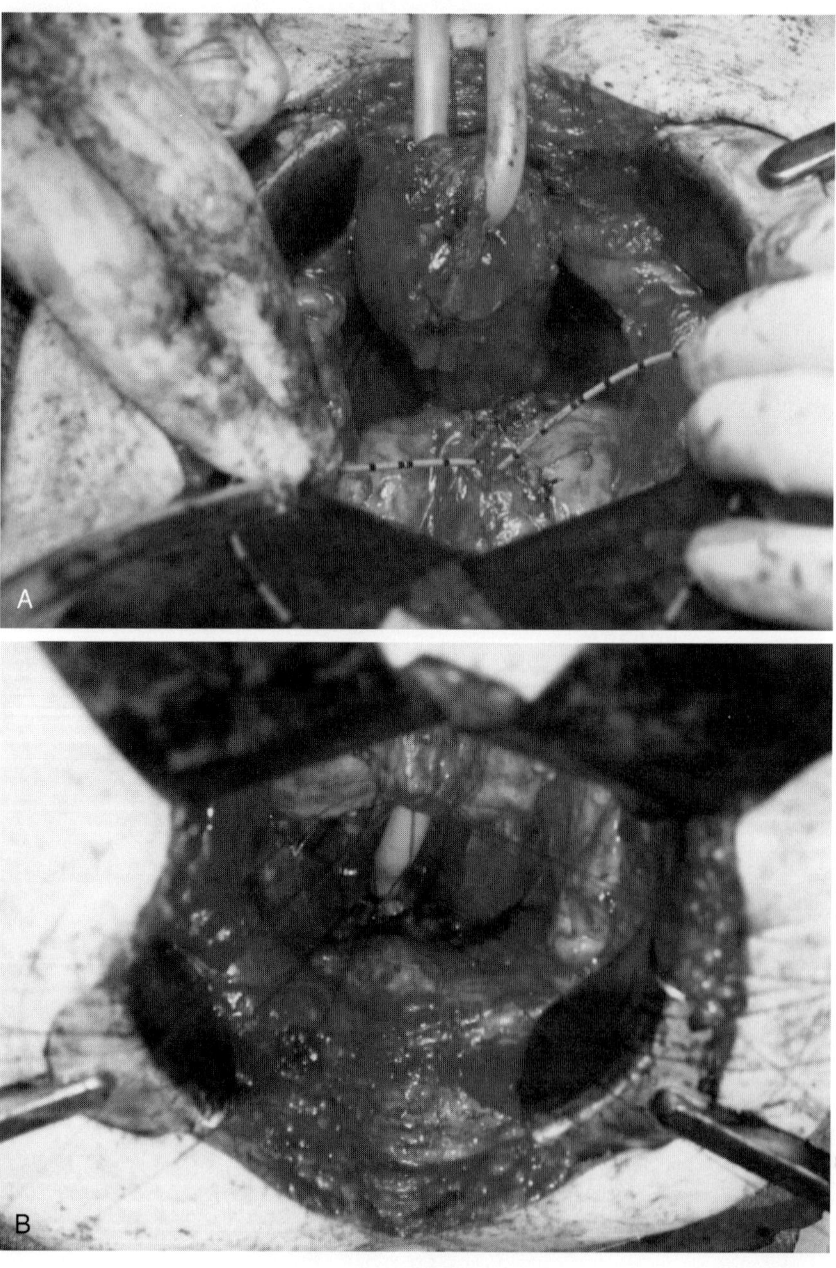

**Figure 2–21**

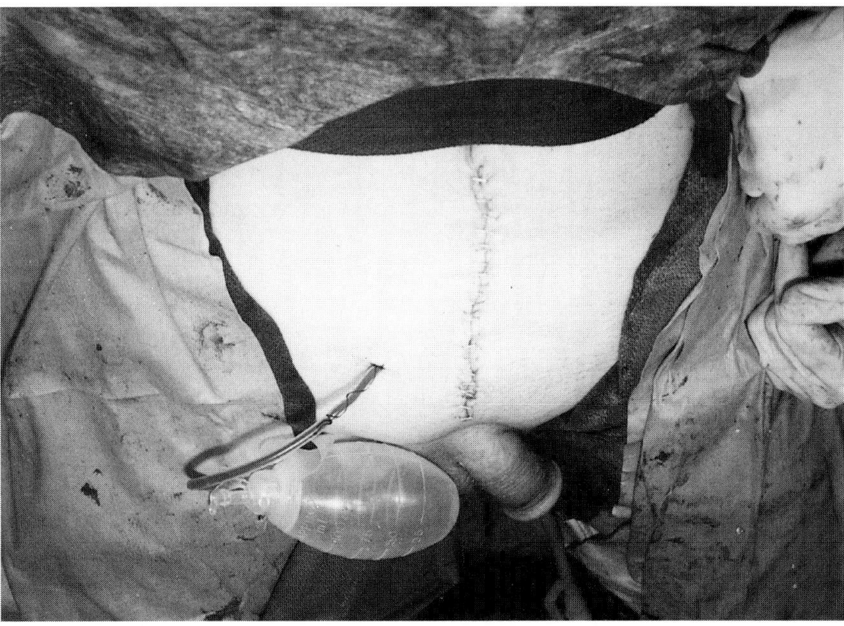

**Figure 2–22**

there is less than 20 ml of drainage per shift. Staples are removed just prior to discharge, usually on postoperative days 3 to 5.

## RADICAL PERINEAL PROSTATECTOMY

### Advantages and Disadvantages

Traditionally, the main advantage of this technique has been less postoperative pain as compared with the radical retropubic prostatectomy. Also, postoperative appetite, bowel function, and resumption of activity return more rapidly. There are several technical advantages of the perineal approach to radical prostatectomy. The operation usually can be accomplished relatively quickly, with low blood loss because the deep dorsal veins are generally avoided.[83] This approach also provides clear exposure and access to the apex of the prostate, allowing the complete removal of this critical margin and a precise transection of the urethra.[83] In addition, the surgeon is able to tie the vesicourethral anastomotic sutures under direct vision in order to perform a watertight closure that is without tension.

The main disadvantage of this technique is the need for a preliminary approach to the pelvic lymph nodes in patients at risk for nodal disease. However, the advent of laparoscopic pelvic lymph node dissection and the low incidence of nodal disease in contemporary patients may obviate this problem.[84–86] The exaggerated lithotomy position may also be a problem for patients with hip ankylosis or marked obesity. Other concerns are the increased risk of rectal injury and that a nerve-sparing prostatectomy may be more difficult to accomplish compared to the retropubic approach.

**Figure 2–23:** *A* and *B*, Technique of radical perineal prostatectomy. The procedure is undertaken with the patient in the exaggerated lithotomy position. (*A*) An inverted U-shaped perineal incision or some variation is made. (*B*) Deepening of this incision is accomplished by careful transection of the central muscles of the perineum, which connect the external anal sphincter to the transverse perineal and bulbospongiosus muscles at the perineal body. The rectourethralis muscle is divided. The membranous urethra is exposed and then divided. The lateral pedicles are then divided close to the gland. The posterior vesical neck musculature can then be divided. The seminal vesicles and ampullary portions of the vasa are dissected free and the vasa divided. The urethra and bladder neck are anastomosed with interrupted sutures over a catheter. The anastomosis is completed with a closure of the bladder neck itself. (From Walsh PC, Retik AB, Vaughn ED Jr, Wein AJ (eds): Campbell's Urology, 7th ed. Philadelphia, WB Saunders, 1998, p 2591, Fig. 87–1 (*A*) and p 2594, Fig. 87–4 (*B*).)

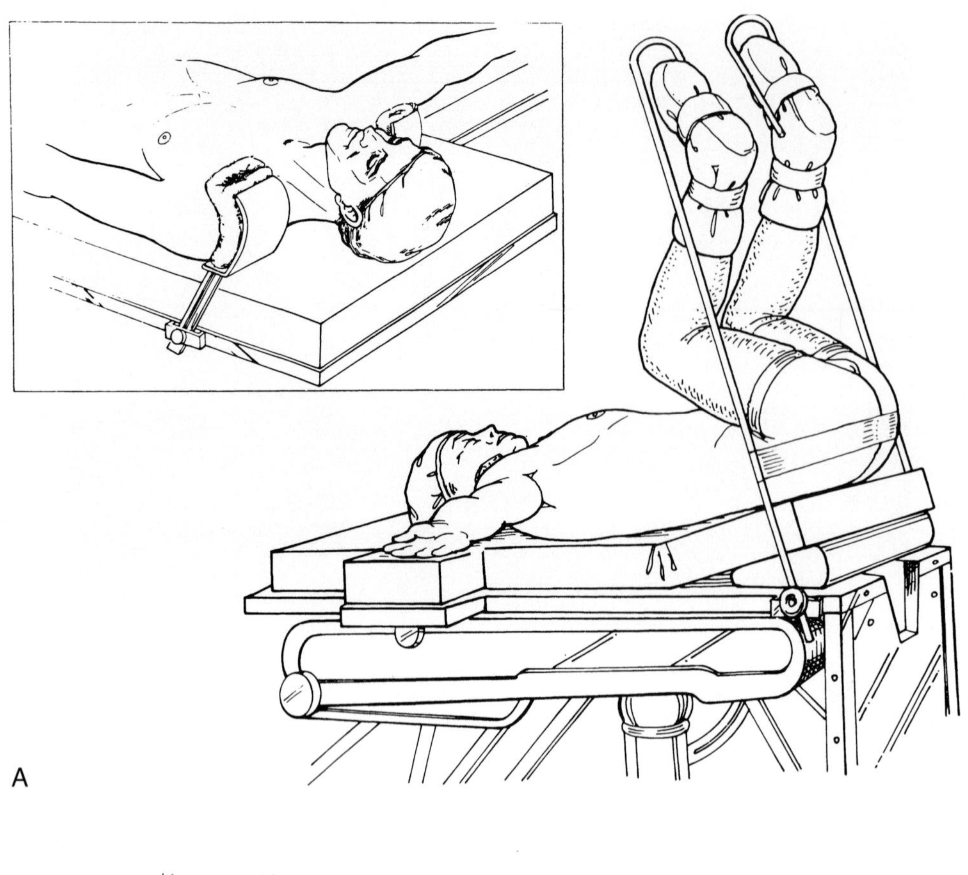

A

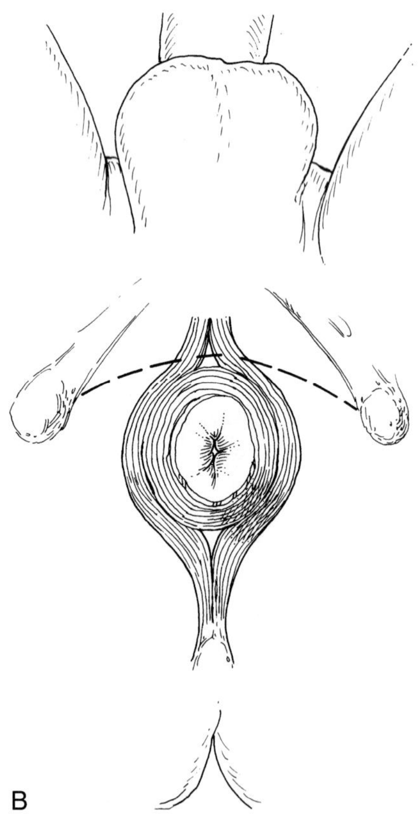

B

Figure 2–23

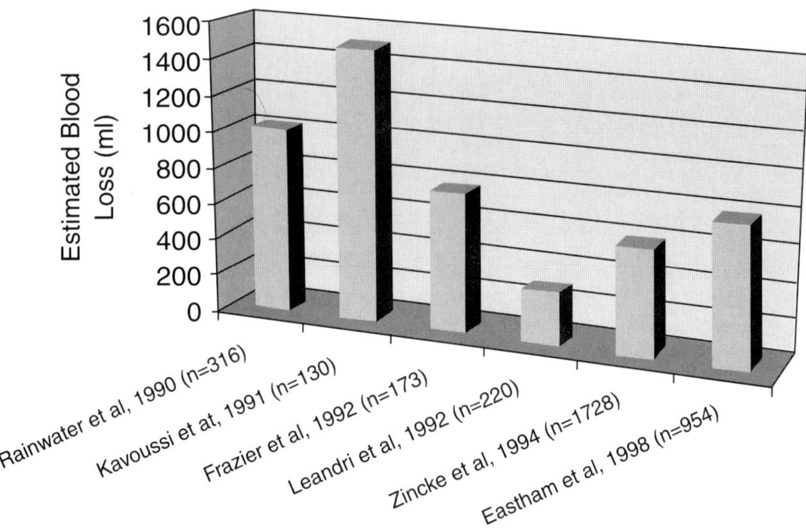


**Figure 2–24**

## COMPLICATIONS FROM RADICAL PROSTATECTOMY

### Early Complications

**Figure 2–24:** Estimated blood loss for patients undergoing radical prostatectomy. Historically, the most common intraoperative complication during radical prostatectomy has been hemorrhage. This has frequently resulted in substantial blood loss and the need for transfusions.[26] The average blood loss during a radical prostatectomy has been minimized with careful surgical technique and a thorough knowledge of the anatomy. The mean estimated blood loss during radical prostatectomy from several large series is shown in this graph.[26–31]

**Figure 2–25:** Perioperative complications and mortality rate of radical retropubic prostatectomy. Several large contemporary series have shown that the perioperative morbidity and mortality rates of radical retropubic prostatectomy have diminished in recent years.[87–90] Intraoperative complications are now less frequent than in previous decades. The operative mortality rate from several large series was 14 of 4262 (0.3%) patients. Rectal injury during radical prostatectomy occurs in less than 1% of patients. Deep venous thrombosis (DVT) and pulmonary embolism occurs in 1.1% to 1.2% of patients undergoing radical prostatectomy.

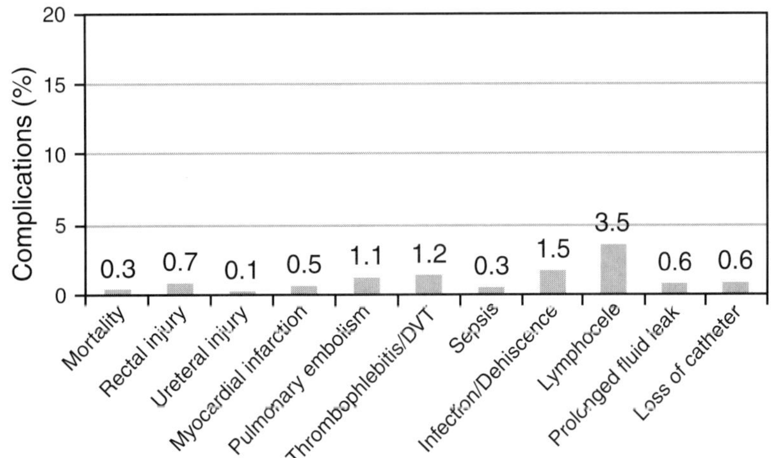


**Figure 2–25**

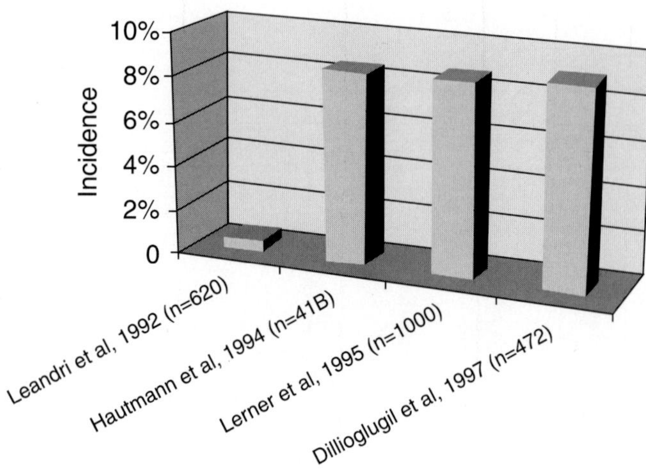


**Figure 2–26**

**Figure 2–26:** Incidence of anastomotic stricture following radical prostatectomy. Anastomotic stricture has been reported in 0.5% to 9% of patients following radical prostatectomy, with one series reporting strictures in 80 of 456 (17.5%) patients.[90] In order to maintain an adequate urine flow, most anastomotic strictures require cold knife incision or periodic dilation.

Urinary incontinence remains one of the most troubling side effects following radical prostatectomy **(Table 2–4)**. Although improved surgical technique has resulted in a decrease in the incidence of incontinence, the reported rates of this complication vary widely. Series from patient surveys report 19% to 32% of patients to be incontinent after radical prostatectomy.[38–40] However, most centers of excellence with broad exper-

tise in radical prostatectomy report 5% to 20% of patients to be incontinent after surgery.[26, 30, 32–40] Despite the relatively high rates of urinary incontinence reported in population surveys, the majority of patients were satisfied with their treatment and would make the same treatment choice again.[40]

Incontinence after radical prostatectomy can be attributed to a variety of mechanisms. These causes include damage to the distal sphincter mechanism, individual variation in the length of the distal urethral segment, bladder neck contracture, denervation, and bladder instability. Patients should be encouraged to perform pelvic floor (Kegel) exercises after catheter removal. Improvement in continence is common up to 1 year and may occur up to 2 years following surgery.[26] Thus, it is best to defer invasive treatments for incontinence for at least 1 year after prostatectomy. However, if incontinence continues to persist following radical prostatectomy, a cause should be sought. Patients with a bladder neck contracture usually have a dribbling urinary stream or symptoms of overflow incontinence. Flexible cystoscopy can be used to evaluate the anastomotic site after ultrasound measurement of residual urine after voiding. If no anastomotic stricture is identified, urodynamic studies are warranted.[91, 92] Based on urodynamic findings, patients with bladder dysfunction should be treated medically, whereas those with sphincteric damage should be treated surgically.

Potency following anatomic radical retropubic prostatectomy. The return of erections after radical prostatectomy has been correlated with patient age, pathologic tumor stage, and extent of preservation of the neurovascular bundles (NVB) **(Table 2–5)**. Before the nerve-sparing radical prostatectomy was developed,

## TABLE 2–4

### INCIDENCE OF INCONTINENCE AFTER RADICAL PROSTATECTOMY

| SERIES | n | INCONTINENCE (%) | DEFINITION OF INCONTINENCE |
|---|---|---|---|
| **From Centers of Excellence** | | | |
| Steiner et al, 1991[32] | 593 | 8 | Leaks with moderate activity |
| Leandri et al, 1992[30] | 398 | 5 | Leaks with moderate activity |
| Catalona et al, 1993[33] | 435 | 6 | Regular use of pads |
| Zincke et al, 1994[26] | 1728 | 5 | Regular use of pads |
| Hautmann et al, 1994[34] | 191 | 19 | Regular use of pads |
| Geary et al, 1995[35] | 458 | 20 | Regular use of pads |
| Eastham et al, 1996[36] | 581 | 9 | Leaks with moderate activity |
| Goluboff et al, 1998[37] | 480 | 8 | Regular use of pads |
| **From Patient Surveys** | | | |
| Fowler et al, 1995[38] | 738 | 31 | Regular use of pads or clamps |
| Murphy et al, 1994[39] | 1796 | 19 | Regular use of pads |
| Litwin et al, 1995[40] | 98 | 25 | "Bother" score |

## TABLE 2–5

### POTENCY FOLLOWING ANATOMIC RADICAL RETROPUBIC PROSTATECTOMY

| SERIES | n | OVERALL POTENCY (%) | NVB STATUS AND POTENCY | |
|---|---|---|---|---|
| **From Centers of Excellence** | | | | |
| Quinlan et al, 1991[41] | 503 | 68 | Bilateral | 76 |
| | | | Unilateral | 63 |
| Leandri et al, 1992[30] | 106 | 71 | N/A | |
| Catalona, 1995[42] | 295 | 59 | Bilateral | 63 |
| | | | Unilateral | 41 |
| **From Patient Surveys** | | | | |
| Murphy et al, 1994[39] | 1059 | 27 | N/A | |
| Litwin et al, 1995[40] | 214 | 29 | N/A | |

NVB = neurovascular bundles.

virtually all patients were impotent after surgery. Quinlan and colleagues reported that for men under the age of 50, 90% were potent if one or both NVB were preserved.[41] For men 50 years or older, potency was better if both NVB were preserved. These workers also reported that 70% of men with pathologically confined prostate cancer were potent if both NVB were preserved compared with only 50% of patients with seminal vesicle involvement.[41] Thus, pathologic stage influences potency.

The recovery of potency after radical prostatectomy in the population surveys is much lower than when compared with the results from centers of excellence.[30, 39–42] However, the median age (65 to 69 years) and pathologic stage (39% C or D) were higher than those reported from the centers of excellence.[39, 40] In addition, preoperative potency status of the men in the population surveys was unknown. Erectile function can be preserved after radical prostatectomy, but the probability of recovery depends on the potency before the operation, the age of the patient, the stage of tumor, and the preservation of the NVB.

## RESULTS FOLLOWING RADICAL PROSTATECTOMY

Serum PSA measurement is the most useful and reliable test to diagnose recurrent prostate cancer after radical prostatectomy **(Table 2–6)**. A detectable serum PSA level after radical prostatectomy is evidence of residual or recurrent prostate cancer, and a rising PSA level usually precedes clinical recurrence by about 3 to 5 years.[94, 95] Prostate cancer recurrence has been documented in patients without a detectable PSA level; however, it is rare.[96, 97] Several series report that following radical prostatectomy, approximately 80% of patients at 5 years and 70% at 10 years have no evidence of cancer as documented by an undetectable PSA level.[18, 19, 61, 80–82]

## TABLE 2–6

### PSA PROGRESSION-FREE RATES FOLLOWING RADICAL PROSTATECTOMY FOR CLINICALLY LOCALIZED PROSTATE CANCER

| SERIES FROM CENTERS OF EXCELLENCE | n | MONTHS OF FOLLOW-UP MEAN (RANGE) | T1 (%) | T2 (%) | 5-YEAR PSA PROGRESSION-FREE RATES (%) | 10-YEAR PSA PROGRESSION-FREE RATES (%) |
|---|---|---|---|---|---|---|
| Johns Hopkins (1993)[20] | 894 | 53 (12–120) | 17 | 83 | 87 | 77 |
| Washington Univ. (1994)[23] | 925 | 28 (0–123) | 21 | 79 | 78 | 65 |
| UCLA (1994)[25] | 601 | 34 (12–237) | 27 | 73 | 69 | 47 |
| Mayo Clinic (1994)[26] | 3170 | 60 (N/A) | 7 | 93 | 70 | 52 |
| Baylor (1995)[96] | 500 | 37 (1–110) | 22 | 78 | 76 | 73 |
| Johns Hopkins (1997)[19] | 1623 | 60.4 (12–156) | 31 | 66 | 80 | 68 |

**Figure 2–27:** Actuarial (PSA-based) 5-year nonprogression rates after radical prostatectomy for clinical stage T1 and T2 disease according to preoperative serum PSA (*A*), clinical stage (*B*), biopsy Gleason score (*C*), and pathologic stage (*D*). Using PSA nonprogression rates, there is an increase in risk of disease recurrence correlated with higher clinical stage, higher Gleason score, higher preoperative PSA levels, and higher pathologic stage.[19, 20] The pathologic stage of the cancer is the single most powerful prognostic factor.[51] When prostate cancer is pathologically confined to the prostate, the 5-year disease-free recurrence measured by serum PSA is over 90%.[50] The prognosis is poor when the cancer involves the seminal vesicles or pelvic lymph nodes. In addition, as with the results for the Gleason score in the preoperative biopsy specimen, the Gleason score for the radical prostatectomy specimen also correlates with disease progression.[51] A recent analysis has demonstrated that perineural invasion on a preoperative prostate needle biopsy is a strong independent predictor of PSA recurrence in patients treated with radical prostatectomy.[52] The issue of radiation after prostatectomy (for various risk factors or a rising PSA) is discussed in Chapter 3 (Radiotherapy for Prostate Cancer).

## SALVAGE RADICAL PROSTATECTOMY

### Candidates for Salvage Radical Prostatectomy

A salvage prostatectomy may be performed on a patient whose cancer is refractory to treatment with radiotherapy. Patients should be selected carefully because of the higher complication rates of salvage surgery after full-dose radiation therapy. Patients should have a life expectancy of greater than 10 years and minimal comorbidity. Accurate restaging following

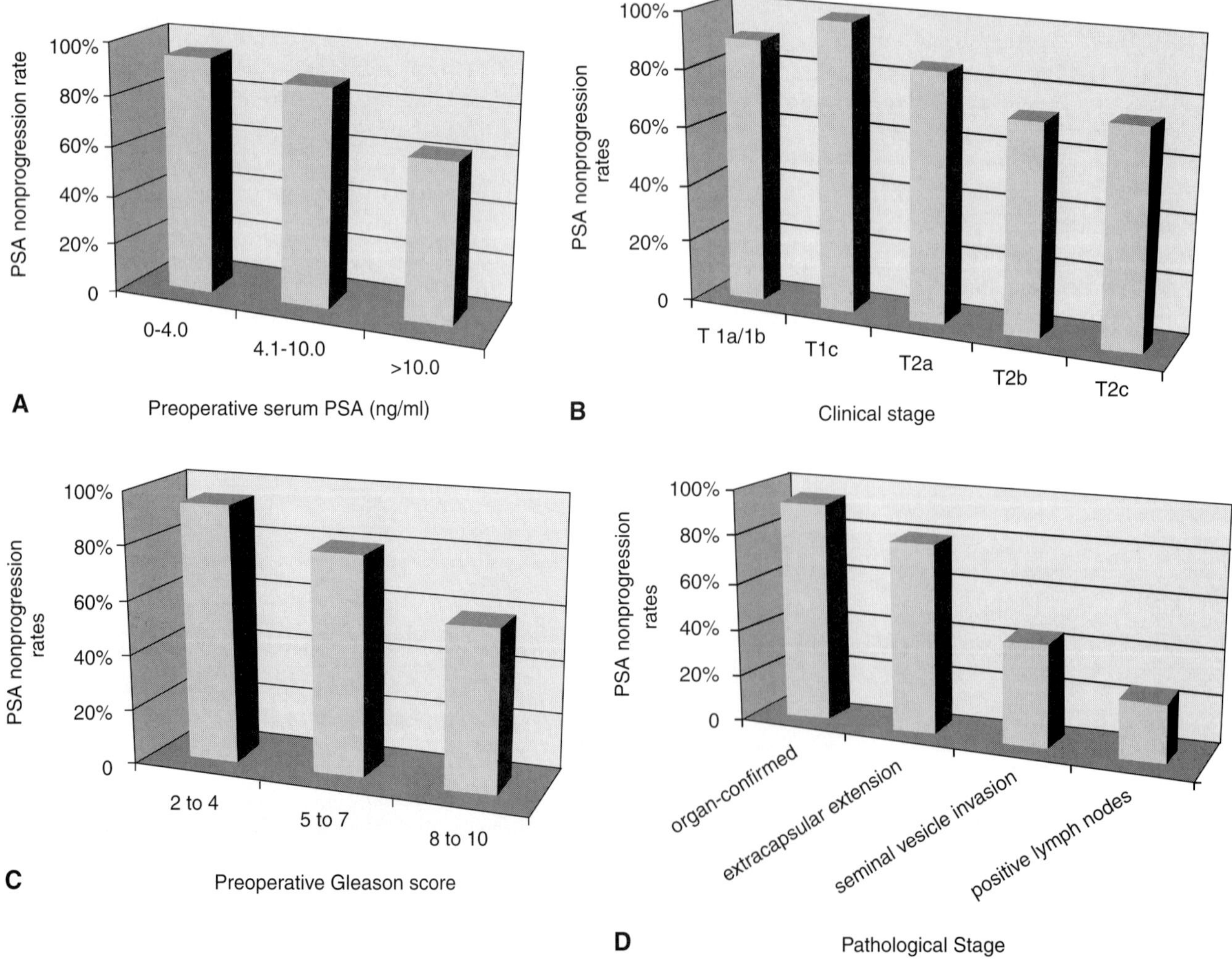


Figure 2–27

TABLE 2–7

## RESULTS FOLLOWING SALVAGE RADICAL PROSTATECTOMY

| SERIES FROM CENTERS OF EXCELLENCE | n | MONTHS OF FOLLOW-UP MEAN (RANGE) | 5-YEAR PSA PROGRESSION-FREE RATES (%) | 5-YEAR CANCER-SPECIFIC SURVIVAL RATES (%) | 10-YEAR CANCER-SPECIFIC SURVIVAL RATES (%) |
|---|---|---|---|---|---|
| USC (1992)[100] | 34 | 109 (43–154) | N/A | N/A | 79 |
| Cleveland Clinic (1993)[99] | 43 | N/A (1–10) | N/A | 80 | N/A |
| Baylor (1995)[97] | 40 | 39 (2–97) | 55 | 95 | N/A |
| Mayo Clinic (1995)[98] | 86 | 70 (12–182) | N/A | 91 | 64 |

the detection of local recurrence should also be performed. Presently, candidates should also have a preradiation serum PSA level below 10 ng/ml, a Gleason score of 6 or less, and a current PSA level that is less than 10 ng/ml. In addition to the restaging procedures, it is also recommended that candidates for salvage surgery undergo preoperative cystoscopy, examination under anesthesia, transrectal ultrasonography with seminal vesicle biopsies, and either barium enema or colonoscopy to assess the transverse colon as a potential conduit if necessary.

## Results

Results following salvage radical prostatectomy are given in **Table 2–7**. Salvage radical prostatectomy has been used successfully to eradicate locally recurrent cancer after definitive radiotherapy.[97–106] In a series of 39 patients, Rogers et al. reported an overall nonprogression rate of 55% at 5 years.[97] Salvage radical prostatectomy after full-dose radiation therapy is a technically challenging operation that is associated with more complications than primary radical prostatectomy.

## Complications

Complications seem to be related to final pathologic stage following salvage radical prostatectomy **(Table 2–8)**. Complications such as urinary incontinence, bladder neck contracture, and rectal and ureteral injury are more frequent after salvage radical prostatectomy than reported in contemporary series of primary radical prostatectomy.[97] The incidence of rectal injury during salvage prostatectomy ranges from 0% to 20%. Postoperative incontinence can be expected in 15% to 60% of patients following salvage prostatectomy. Clinical understaging of patients with radioresistant prostate cancer is common, with only 20% to 40% of tumors being organ-confined on final pathologic staging.

## CRYOTHERAPY FOR PROSTATE CANCER

Cryosurgery involves the destruction of prostatic tissue by in situ freezing and devitalization of malignant tissue. It is not a new technique, but one that has engendered a renewed interest because of percutane-

TABLE 2–8

## COMPLICATIONS AND FINAL PATHOLOGIC STAGE FOLLOWING SALVAGE RADICAL PROSTATECTOMY

| SERIES | n | RECTAL INJURIES (%) | INCONTINENCE (%) | ORGAN-CONFINED (%) | NOT ORGAN-CONFINED (%) |
|---|---|---|---|---|---|
| Link and Freiha, 1991[103] | 14 | 0 | 55 | 36 | 64 |
| Zincke, 1992[104] | 32 | 6 | 27 | 34 | 66 |
| Stein et al, 1992[105] | 13 | 8 | 15 | 38 | 62 |
| Ahlering et al, 1992[100] | 11 | 0 | 64 | 36 | 64 |
| Pontes et al, 1993[99] | 43 | 9 | 30 | 30 | 70 |
| Brenner et al, 1994[106] | 10 | N/A | N/A | 30 | 70 |
| Rogers et al, 1995[97] | 39 | 15 | 58 | 20 | 80 |

ous probe placement and improvements in imaging and cryotechnology.[107, 108] At Columbia, cryosurgery is offered to patients who have failed radiotherapy with local recurrence, clinical stage T3 disease, significant comorbidity, or preference for cryotherapy.

## Advantages and Disadvantages

A potential advantage is that cryotherapy may be delivered through thin probes that are placed percutaneously, sparing the patient a large surgical procedure. In addition, cryotherapy may be used repeatedly, in combination with or following other therapies, to treat prostate cancer. The potential disadvantage is that it may be very difficult to reliably freeze the entire prostate and kill all viable tumor cells while avoiding significant damage to surrounding structures such as the urinary sphincters, neurovascular bundles, and rectum. In addition, there is a significant learning curve in mastering this technique.

## Techniques

**Figure 2–28:** Modern techniques of cryoablation of the prostate. Cryoablation is a minimally invasive procedure that is usually performed under regional anesthesia in the operating room. With the patient in the lithotomy position, a suprapubic tube is placed, under cystoscopic visualization. An urethral warming device is placed to facilitate urethral visualization by TRUS as well as to circulate warm water through the urethra in order to minimize damage during the freezing process. A, Cryoprobes are introduced percutaneously into the prostate through the perineum with the assistance of TRUS. At Columbia, freezing is accomplished by circulation through the cryoprobes with argon gas. Careful monitoring of the freezing process is provided by TRUS, and one or two freeze-thaw cycles may be used. Recent advances using thermocouple devices allow for accurate temperature monitoring in and around the prostate. These probes allow for increased cell killing as well as decreased damage to the anterior rectal wall and urethral sphincter. B, Transverse ultrasound image showing the position of the sheaths and temperature probes.

The usual hospital stay is 1 day. Most patients experience gross hematuria, some degree of perineal and scrotal swelling, and ecchymosis during the first 24 hours. The suprapubic tube is used to drain the bladder until adequate spontaneous voiding occurs through the urethra, generally 5 to 14 days after the procedure. Follow-up care should include inquiry into complications such as sexual dysfunction and incontinence, serial PSA measurements, digital rectal examinations, and TRUS. Sextant biopsies using TRUS may provide the best assessment of residual viable tumor cells. Repeat cryotherapy could be performed if residual tumor is noted, or the patient may proceed to other forms of therapy.

## Results

**Figure 2–29:** Histologic findings following prostate cryosurgery. The prostatic epithelium and stroma undergo hemorrhagic necrosis, similar to ischemic injury, while the architectural framework of the gland remains and undergoes a reepithelialization from a transitional cell epithelium progenitol.[109] A, Before cryoablation. B, After cryoablation.

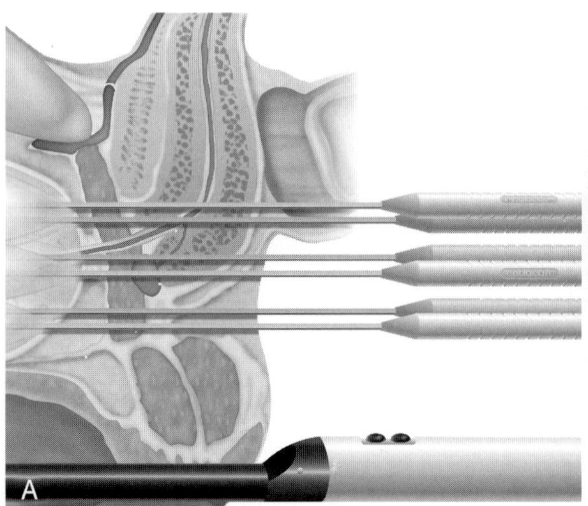
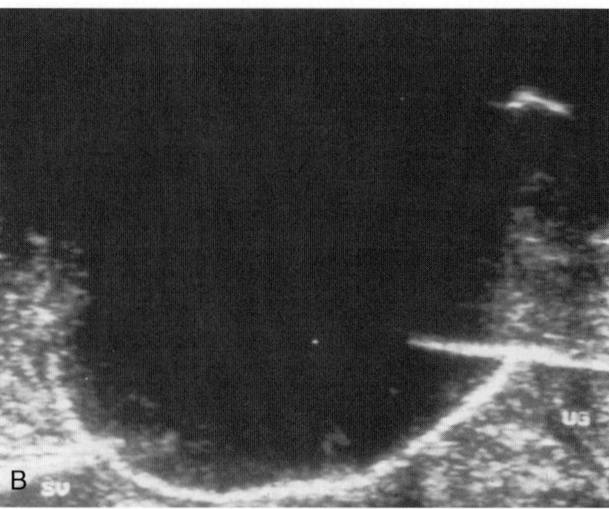

**Figure 2–28**

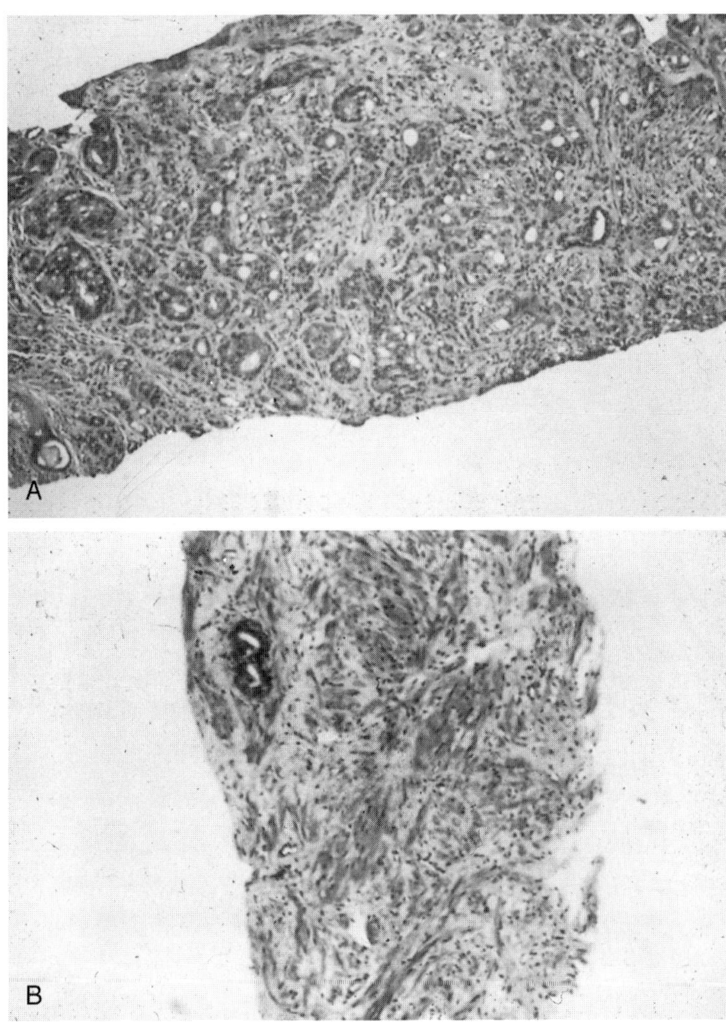


**Figure 2–29**

Results of cryotherapy of prostate cancer are measured by serum PSA and prostatic biopsies **(Table 2–9)**. Positive biopsy rates following cryosurgery of the prostate range from 3.0% to 14.6% for clinical stage T1–T2 tumors.[110-114] In a recent study of 176 patients who underwent 207 cryosurgical procedures for localized prostate cancer at the University of California at San Francisco, cryosurgery was associated with favorable serum PSA levels in 49% of patients 3 years after treatment. They reported a positive prostate biopsy rate after cryosurgery of 38%.[115] Cryosurgery is a re-emerging technique, and long-term data are still needed regarding the efficacy of this modality in the definitive management of patients with prostate cancer.

## TABLE 2–9

### RESULTS OF RADICAL PROSTATE CRYOSURGERY

| SERIES | n | FOLLOW-UP (MONTHS) | POSITIVE BIOPSY STAGE T1–T2 (%) | POSITIVE BIOPSY STAGE T3 (%) |
|---|---|---|---|---|
| Cohen, 1995[110] | 354 | 24 | 14.6* | — |
| Littrup and Sparschu, 1995[113] | 130 | N/A | 4.9 | 13 |
| Bahn et al, 1995[111] | 130 | 3–6 | 3.0 | N/A |
| Shinohara and Carroll, 1995[112] | 65 | 3 | 18.0* | — |
| Schimdt, 1996[114] | 137 | 24 | 8.0 | N/A |

*Includes stages T1–T3.

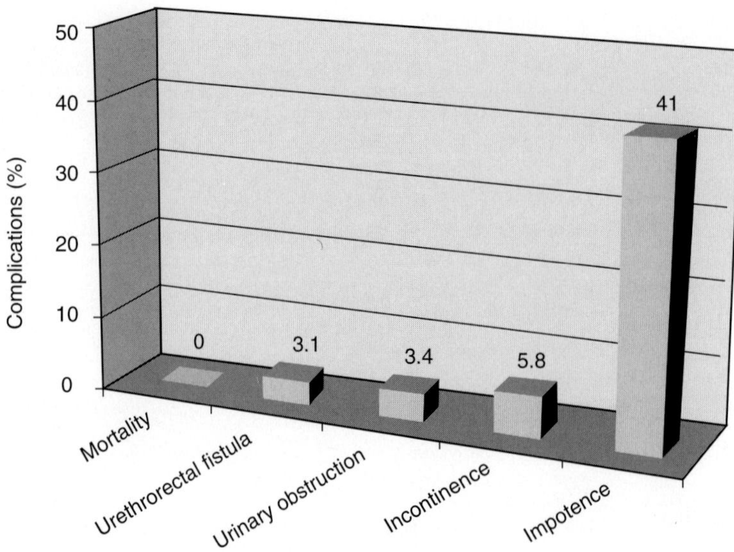


**Figure 2–30**

## Complications

**Figure 2–30:** Complications of TRUS-guided radical prostate cryosurgery. The rate of impotence is about 41.0% and the rate of incontinence is about 5.8%. Other complications include urethrorectal fistula and urinary obstruction. In a recent study assessing quality of life after salvage cryotherapy in over 100 patients, 72% reported some degree of incontinence, 85% who were potent before cryotherapy became impotent, and 26% had moderate to significant perineal pain. Incontinence, sloughing of tissue, and perineal pain were significantly reduced with a urethral warming catheter. Overall, satisfaction with cryotherapy was 33% in this setting.[116]

## REFERENCES

1. Young HH: Early diagnosis and radical cure of carcinoma of the prostate: Being a study of 40 cases and presentation of radical operation which was carried out in 4 cases. Bull Johns Hopkins Hosp 16:315, 1904.
2. Young HH: Conservative perineal prostatectomy: A presentation of new instruments and technique. JAMA 41:999, 1903.
3. Millen T: Retropubic prostatectomy: A new extravesical technique: Report on twenty cases. Lancet 2:693, 1945.
4. Memmelaar J: Total prostatovesiculectomy: Retropubic approach. J Urol 62:349, 1949.
5. Chute R: Radical retropubic prostatectomy for cancer. J Urol 71:347, 1954.
6. Campbell EW: Total prostatectomy with preliminary ligation of the vascular pedicle. J Urol 81:464, 1959.
7. Reiner WG, Walsh PC: An anatomic approach to the surgical management of the dorsal vein and Santorini's plexus during radical retropubic prostatectomy. J Urol 121:198, 1979.
8. Walsh PC, Donker, PJ: Impotence following radical prostatectomy: Insight into etiology and precaution. J Urol 128:492, 1982.
9. Walsh PC, Lepor H, Eggleston JC: Radical prostatectomy with preservation of sexual function: Anatomical and pathological considerations. Prostate 4:473, 1983.
10. Brendler CB, Walsh PC: The role of radical prostatectomy in the treatment of prostate cancer. CA Cancer J Clin 42:212, 1992.
11. Mettlin C, Jones GW, Murphy GP: Trends in prostate cancer care in the United States, 1974–1990: Observation from the patient care evaluation studies of the American College of Surgeons Commission on Cancer. CA Cancer J Clin 43:83, 1993.
12. Catalona WJ, Smith DS, Ratliff TL, et al: Measurement of prostate-specific antigen in serum as a screening test for prostate cancer. N Engl J Med 324:1156, 1991.
13. Catalona WJ, Smith DS, Ratliff TL, et al: Detection of organ-confined prostate cancer is increased through prostate specific antigen-based screening. JAMA 27:948, 1993.
14. Nadler RB, Andriole GL: Who is best benefited by radical prostatectomy? Urol Clin North Am 10:581, 1996.
15. Walsh PC, Quinlan, DM, Morton, RA, et al: Radical retropubic prostatectomy: Improved anastomosis and urinary continence. Urol Clin North Am 17:679, 1990.
16. Mettlin CJ, Murphy GP, McGinnis LS, et al: The National Cancer Data Base report on prostate cancer. Cancer 76:1104–1112, 1995.
17. Mettlin CJ, Murphy GP, Cunningham MP, et al: The National Cancer Data Base report on race, age, and region variations in prostate cancer treatment. Cancer 80:1261–1266, 1997.
18. Greenlee RT, Hill-Harmon MB, Murray T, et al: Cancer statistics, 2001. CA Cancer J Clin 51:1, 2001.
19. Pound CR, Partin AW, Epstein JI, et al: PSA following anatomical radical retropubic prostatectomy: Patterns of recurrence and cancer control. Urol Clin North Am 24:395, 1997.
20. Partin AW, Yoo J, Carter HB, et al: The use of prostate specific antigen, clinical stage and Gleason score to predict pathological stage in men with localized prostate cancer. J Urol 150:110, 1993.
21. Oesterling J: Prostate-specific antigen: A critical assessment of the most useful tumor marker for adenocarcinoma of the prostate. J Urol 145:907, 1991.
22. Olsson CA, Goluboff ET: Detection and treatment of prostate cancer: Perspective of the urologist. J Urol 152:1695, 1994.
23. Catalona WJ, Smith DS: 5-year tumor recurrence rates after anatomical radical retropubic prostatectomy for prostate cancer. J Urol 152:1837, 1994.
24. Ohori M, Goad JR, Wheelar TM, et al: Can radical prostatectomy alter the progression of poorly differentiated prostate cancer? J Urol 152:1843, 1994.
25. Trapasso JG, DeKernion JB, Smith RB, et al: The incidence and significance of detectable levels of serum prostate specific antigen after radical prostatectomy. J Urol 152:1821, 1994.
26. Zincke H, Oesterling JE, Blute ML, et al: Long-term (15 years) results after radical prostatectomy for clinically localized (stage T2c or lower) prostate cancer. J Urol 152:1850, 1994.

27. Rainwater LM, Segura JW: Technical considerations in radical retropubic prostatectomy: Blood loss after ligation of dorsal venous complex. J Urol 143:1163, 1990.

28. Kavoussi LR, Myers JA, Catalona WJ: Effect of temporary occlusion of hypogastric arteries on blood loss during radical retropubic prostatectomy. J Urol 146:362, 1991.

29. Frazier HA, Robertson JE, Paulson DF: Radical prostatectomy: The pros and cons of the perineal versus the retropubic approach. J Urol 147:888, 1992.

30. Leandri P, Rossignol G, Gautier J, et al: Radical retropubic prostatectomy: Morbidity and quality of life. Experience with 620 consecutive cases. J Urol 147:883, 1992.

31. Eastham JA, Scardino PT: Radical prostatectomy. In Walsh PC, Retik AB, Vaughn ED Jr, Wein AJ (eds): Campbell's Urology, 7th ed. Philadelphia, WB Saunders, 1998, pp 2547–2564.

32. Steiner MS, Morton RA, Walsh PC: Impact of anatomical radical prostatectomy on urinary continence. J Urol 145:512, 1991.

33. Catalona WJ, Basler JW: Return of erections and urinary continence following nerve sparing radical retropubic prostatectomy. J Urol 150:905, 1993.

34. Hautmann RE, Sauter TW, Wenderoth UK: Radical retropubic prostatectomy: Morbidity and urinary continence in 418 consecutive cases. Urology (suppl)43:47, 1994.

35. Geary ES, Dendinger TE, Freiha FS, et al: Incontinence and vesical neck strictures following radical retropubic prostatectomy. Urology 45:1000, 1995.

36. Eastham JA, Kattan MW, Rogers E, et al: Risk factors for urinary incontinence after radical prostatectomy. J Urol 156:1707, 1996.

37. Goluboff ET, Saidi JA, Mazer S, et al: Urinary continence after radical prostatectomy: The Columbia experience. J Urol 159:1276, 1998.

38. Fowler FJ Jr, Barry MJ, Lu-Yao G, et al: Effect of radical prostatectomy for prostate cancer on patient quality of life: Results from a Medicare survey. Urology 45:1007, 1995.

39. Murphy GP, Mettlin C, Menck H, et al: National patterns of prostate cancer treatment by radical prostatectomy: Results of a survey by the American College of Surgeons Committee on Cancer. J Urol 152:1817, 1994.

40. Litwin MS, Hays RD, Fink A, et al: Quality-of-life outcomes in men treated for localized prostate cancer. JAMA 273:129, 1995.

41. Quinlan DM, Epstein JI, Carter BS, et al: Sexual function following radical prostatectomy: Influence of preservation of neurovascular bundles. J Urol 145:998, 1991.

42. Catalona WJ: Surgical management of prostate cancer. Cancer 75:1903, 1995.

43. Pienta KJ, Esper PS: Risk factors for prostate cancer. Ann Intern Med 118:793, 1993.

44. Spitz MR, Currier RD, Fueger JJ, et al: Familial patterns of prostate cancer: A case control analysis. J Urol 146:1305, 1991.

45. Carter BS, Bova GS, Beaty TH, et al: Hereditary prostate cancer: Epidemiologic and clinical features. J Urol 150:797, 1993.

46. Carter BS, Beaty GS, Steinberg GD, et al: Mendelian inheritance of familial prostate cancer. Proc Natl Acad Sci 89:3367, 1992.

47. Whittemore AS, Kolonel LN, Wu AH, et al: Prostate cancer in relation to diet, physical activity, and body size in blacks, whites, and Asians in the United States and Canada. J Natl Cancer Inst 87:652, 1995.

48. Baquet CR, Horm JW, Gibbs T, et al: Socioeconomic factors and cancer incidence among blacks and whites. J Natl Cancer Inst 83:551, 1991.

49. Pienta KJ: Etiology, epidemiology, and prevention of the carcinoma of the prostate. In Walsh PC, Retik AB, Vaughn, ED Jr, Wein AJ (eds): Campbell's Urology, 7th ed. Philadelphia, WB Saunders, 1998, pp 2489–2496.

50. Smith DS, Catalona WJ: Nature of prostate cancer detected through prostate specific antigen based screening. J Urol 152:1732, 1994.

51. Epstein JI, Walsh PC, Brendler CB: Radical prostatectomy for impalpable prostate cancer: The Johns Hopkins experience with tumor found on transurethral resection (stages T1a and T1b) and on needle biopsy (stage T1c). J Urol 152:1721, 1994.

52. De la Taille A, Rubin MA, Bagiella E, et al: Can perineural invasion on prostate needle biopsy predict prostate specific antigen recurrence after radical prostatectomy? J Urol 162:103–106, 1999.

53. Douglas TH, Sesterhen IA, Moul JDN, et al: The significance of PSA detected, nonpalpable adenocarcinoma of the prostate (stage T1c). J Urol 153 (suppl):251A, 1995.

54. Chodak GW, Thisted RA, Gerber GS, et al: Results of conservative management of clinically localized prostate cancer. N Engl J Med 330:246, 1994.

55. Albertsen PC, Fryback DB, Storer BE, et al: Long-term survival among men with conservatively treated localized prostate cancer. JAMA 274:626, 1995.

56. Aus G, Hugosson J, Norlen L: Long-term survival and mortality in prostate cancer treated with noncurative intent. J Urol 154:460, 1995.

57. Cooner WH, Mosley BR, Rutherford DL Jr, et al: Prostate cancer detection in a clinical urological practice by ultrasonography, digital rectal examination, and prostate specific antigen. J Urol 143:1146, 1990.

58. Catalona WJ, Richie JP, Ahmann FR, et al: Comparison of digital rectal examination and serum prostate specific antigen in the early detection of prostate cancer: Results of a multicenter clinical trial of 6630 men. J Urol 151:1283, 1994.

59. Ellis WJ, Chetner MP, Preston SD, et al: Diagnosis of prostatic carcinoma: The yield of serum prostate specific antigen, digital rectal examination and transrectal ultrasonography. J Urol 52:1520, 1994.

60. Catalona WJ, Smith DS, Ornstein DK: Prostate cancer detection in men with serum PSA concentrations of 2.6 to 4.0 ng/ml and benign prostate examination: Enhancement of specificity with free PSA measurements. JAMA 277:1452, 1997.

61. Benson MC, Whang IS, Olsson CA, et al: Use of prostate specific antigen density to enhance predictive value of intermediate levels of serum prostate specific antigen. J Urol 147:817, 1992.

62. Carter HB, Pearson JD, Metter JE, et al: Longitudinal evaluation of prostate specific antigen levels in men with and without prostate disease. JAMA 267:2215, 1992.

63. Oesterling JE, Jacobsen SJ, Chute CG, et al: Serum prostate-specific antigen in a community-based population of healthy men: Establishment of age-specific reference ranges. JAMA 270:860, 1993.

64. McCormack RT, Rittenhouse HG, Finlay JA, et al: Molecular forms of prostate-specific antigen and the human kallikrein gene family: A new era. Urology 45:729, 1995.

65. Lilja H: Significance of different molecular forms of serum PSA: The free, non-complexed from of PSA versus that complexed to alpha-1-antichymotrypsin. Urol Clin North Am 20:681, 1993.

66. Stenman UH, Hakama M, Knekt P, et al: Serum concentrations of prostate specific antigen and its complex with $\alpha$-1-antichymotrypsin before diagnosis of prostate cancer. Lancet 344:1594, 1994.

67. McGregor B, Tulloch AG, Quinlan MF, et al: The role of bone scanning in the assessment of prostatic carcinoma. Br J Urol 50:178, 1978.

68. Rifkin MD, Zerhouni EA, Gatsonis CA, et al: Comparison of magnetic resonance imaging and ultrasonography in staging early prostate cancer: Results of a multi-institutional cooperative trial. N Engl J Med 323:621, 1990.

69. Tempany CMC, Rahmouni AD, Epstein JI, et al: Invasion of the neurovascular bundle by prostate cancer: Evaluation with MR imaging. Radiology 181:107, 1991.

70. Hodge KK, McNeal JE, Terris MK, et al: Random systematic versus directed ultrasound guided biopsy transrectal core biopsies of the prostate. J Urol 142:71, 1989.

71. Escew LA, Bare RL, McCullough DL: Systemic 5 region prostate biopsy is superior to sextant method for diagnosing carcinoma of the prostate. J Urol 157:199, 1997.

72. Levine MA, Ittman M, Melamed J, et al: Two consecutive sets of transrectal ultrasound guided sextant biopsies of the prostate for the detection of prostate cancer. J Urol 159:471, 1998.

73. Fleshner NE, Fair WR: Indications for transition zone biopsy in the detection of prostatic carcinoma. J Urol 158:556, 1997.

74. Lui PD, Terris MK, McNeal JE, et al: Indications for ultrasound guided transition zone biopsies in the detection of prostate cancer. J Urol 153:1000, 1995.

75. Partin AW, Kattan M, Subong ENP, et al: Combination of prostate-specific antigen, clinical stage, and Gleason score to predict pathological stage of localized prostate cancer. JAMA 277:1445, 1997.

76. Zincke H, Utz DC, Taylor WF: Bilateral pelvic lymphadenectomy and radical prostatectomy for clinical stage C prostate cancer: Role of adjuvant treatment for residual cancer and in disease progression. J Urol 135:1199, 1986.

77. Narayan P: Neoplasms of the prostate gland. In Tanagho EA, McAninch JW (eds): Smith's General Urology, 14th ed. Norwalk, CT, Appleton & Lange, 1995, pp 392–433.

78. Byar DP, Mostofi, FK, Veterans Administrative Cooperative Urologic Research Groups: Carcinoma of the prostate: Prognostic evaluation of certain pathologic features in 208 radical prostatectomies. Cancer 30:5, 1972.

79. Saitoh H, Hida M, Shimbo T, et al: Metastatic patterns of prostatic cancer: Correlation between sites and number of organs involved. Cancer 54:3078, 1984.

80. Cho KR, Epstein JI: Metastatic prostate carcinoma to supradiaphragmatic lymph nodes: A clinicopathologic and immunohistochemical study. Am J Surg Pathol 17:336, 1994.

81. Walsh PC: Anatomic radical retropubic prostatectomy. In Walsh PC, Retik AB, Vaughn ED Jr, Wein AJ (eds): Campbell's Urology, 7th ed. Philadelphia, WB Saunders, 1998, pp 2565–2588.

82. Ness PM, Walsh PC, Zahurak M, et al: Prostate cancer recurrence in radical surgery patients receiving autologous or homologous blood. Transfusion 32:31, 1992.

83. Gibbons RP: Radical perineal prostatectomy. In Walsh PC, Retik AB, Vaughn ED Jr, Wein AJ (eds): Campbell's Urology, 7th ed. Philadelphia, W.B. Saunders, 1998, pp 2589–2604.

84. Bluestein DL, Bostwick DG, Bergstralh EJ, et al: Eliminating the need for bilateral pelvic lymphadenectomy in select patients with prostate cancer. J Urol 151:1315, 1994.

85. Danella JF, deKernion J, Smith RB, et al: A contemporary incidence of lymph node metastases in prostate cancer: Implications for laparoscopic lymph node dissection. J Urol 149:1488, 1993.

86. Petros JA, Catalona WJ: Lower incidence of unsuspected lymph node metastases in 521 consecutive patients with clinically localized prostate cancer. J Urol 147:1574, 1992.

87. Andriole GL, Smith DS, Rao G, et al: Early complications of contemporary anatomical radical retropubic prostatectomy. J Urol 152:1858, 1994.

88. Litwiller SE, Djavan B, Klopukh BV, et al: Radical retropubic prostatectomy for localized carcinoma of the prostate in a large metropolitan hospital: Changing trends over a 10-year period (1984–1994). Urology 45:813, 1995.

89. Lerner SE, Blute ML, Lieber, MM, et al: Morbidity of contemporary radical retropubic prostatectomy for localized prostate cancer. Oncology 9:379, 1995.

90. Dillioglugil O, Leibmen BD, Leibman NS, et al: Risk factors for complications and morbidity after radical retropubic prostatectomy. J Urol 157:1760, 1997.

91. Foote J, Yun S, Leach GE: Postprostatectomy incontinence: Pathophysiology, evaluation, and management. Urol Clin North Am 18:229, 1991.

92. Goluboff ET, Chang DT, Olsson CA, et al: Urodynamics and the etiology of post-prostatectomy urinary incontinence: The initial Columbia experience. J Urol 156:1059, 1995.

93. Abi-Aas AS, MacFarlane MT, Stein A, et al: Detection of local recurrence after radical prostatectomy by prostate specific antigen and transrectal ultrasound. J Urol 147:952, 1992.

94. Paulson DF: Impact of radical prostatectomy in the management of clinically localized disease. J Urol 152:1826, 1994.

95. Takayama T, Krieger JN, True LD, et al: Recurrent prostate cancer despite undetectable prostate specific antigen. J Urol 148:1541, 1992.

96. Oefelein MG, Smith N, Carter M, et al: The incidence of prostate cancer progression with undetectable serum prostate specific antigen in a series of 394 radical prostatectomies. J Urol 154:2128, 1995.

97. Rogers E, Ohori M, Kassabian VS, et al: Salvage radical prostatectomy: Outcomes measured by serum prostate specific antigen levels. J Urol 153:104, 1995.

98. Lerner SE, Blute ML, Zincke H: Critical evaluation of salvage surgery for radiorecurrent/resistant prostate cancer. J Urol 154:1103, 1995.

99. Pontes JE, Montie J, Klein E, et al: Salvage surgery for radiation failure in prostate cancer. Cancer 71:976, 1993.

100. Ahlering TE, Lieskovsky G, Skinner DG: Salvage surgery plus androgen deprivation for radioresistant prostatic adenocarcinoma. J Urol 147:900, 1992.

101. Epstein JI, Pizov G, Walsh PC: Correlation of pathologic findings with progression after radical retropubic prostatectomy. Cancer 71:3582, 1993.

102. Cheng L, Sebo TJ, Slezak J, et al: Predictors of survival for prostate carcinoma patients treated with salvage radical prostatectomy after radiation therapy. Cancer 83:2164, 1998.

103. Link P, Freiha FS: Radical prostatectomy after definitive radiation therapy for prostate cancer. Urology 27:707, 1991.

104. Zincke H: Radical prostatectomy and exenterative procedures for local failure after radiotherapy with curative intent: Comparison of outcomes. J Urol 147:894, 1992.

105. Stein A, Smith RB, DeKernion JB. Salvage radical prostatectomy after failure of curative radiotherapy for adenocarcinoma of the prostate. Urology 40:197, 1992.

106. Brenner PC, Russo P, Wood DP, et al: Salvage radical prostatectomy in the management of locally recurrent prostate cancer after 125-I implantation. Br J Urol 75:44, 1994.

107. Gonder M, Soanes W, Shuman S: Cryosurgical treatment of the prostate. Invest Urol 3:372, 1966.

108. Onik GM, Cohan J, Reyes GD, et al: Transrectal ultrasound-guided ablation of the prostate. Cancer 72:1291, 1993.

109. Shabaik A, Wilson S, Bidair M, et al: Pathologic changes in prostate biopsies following cryoablation therapy of prostate carcinoma. J Urol Pathol 3:183, 1995.

110. Cohen JK: Cryosurgical ablation of the prostate: Patterns of failure and two year post treatment data compared to external beam radiation therapy. J Urol 153:503A, 1995.

111. Bahn DK, Lee F, Solomon MH, et al: Prostate cancer: Ultrasound guided percutaneous cryoablation: Work in progress. Radiology 194:551, 1995.

112. Shinohara K, Carroll PR: Improved results of cryosurgical ablation of the prostate. J Urol 153 (suppl):385A, 1995.

113. Littrup PJ, Sparschu RA: Transrectal ultrasound and prostate cancer risks: The "tailored" prostate biopsy. Cancer 75:1807, 1995.

114. Schmidt JD: Cryotherapy for Carcinoma of the Prostate. In Petrovidh Z, Baert L, Brady LW (eds): Carcinoma of the Prostate. Berlin, Springer Verlag, 1996, pp 347–354.

115. Koppie TM, Shinohara K, Grossfeld GD, et al: The efficacy of cryosurgical ablation of prostate cancer: The University of California, San Francisco experience. J Urol 162:427–432, 1999.

116. Perrotte P, Litwin MS, McGuire EJ, et al: Quality of life after salvage cryotherapy: The impact of treatment parameters. J Urol 162:398–402, 1999.

# 3

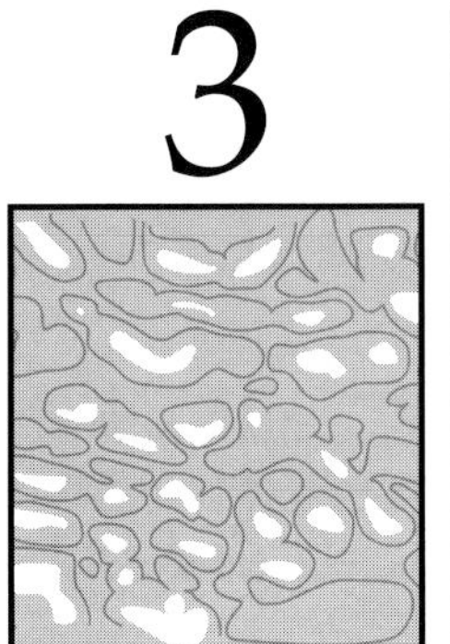

# Radiotherapy for Prostate Cancer

*Gary M. Freedman*

*Benjamin Movsas*

*Gerald E. Hanks*

Radiation therapy has been a national standard in the treatment of prostate cancer for the latter half of the twentieth century. External beam radiation is widely available throughout the United States, and good quality and outcomes have been reported from major academic centers to smaller community facilities. Radiation is an accepted option for the treatment of a wide range of patients, from the younger man to one of advanced age, from the healthy man to one with serious comorbidities, and from the man with the earliest of detectable tumors to one with locally advanced disease. These factors have all made radiation the most commonly used modality for treatment of prostate cancer in the United States.

Since 1990 there has been a dramatic increase in the diagnosis of early stage prostate cancer because of increased public awareness and the use of serum prostate-specific antigen (PSA) screening. This same period has seen the growth of radical prostatectomy because of advances in techniques that have lessened surgical morbidity for the younger patient. Although no well-designed prospective randomized comparison is available, careful retrospective comparisons of similarly matched patients demonstrate the equal outcomes in early stage disease between external beam radiation and radical prostatectomy. The choice to undergo radiation or surgery should be based on the patient's tumor characteristics, personal preference, willingness or suitability to undergo surgery, and thorough understanding of different potential side effects from the two modalities.

The introduction of the PSA test into clinical practice has revolutionized patient selection and follow-up after radiation. The pretreatment PSA measurement is now recognized as the most important prognostic factor for cancer control after radiation. In combination with clinical stage and histologic grade, the PSA identifies those patients who may be appropriately treated by radiation alone and those who may benefit from adjuvant therapy. The level of serum PSA after treatment has become an early sensitive marker for cure after radiation that is more accurate than traditional clinical and radiographic endpoints. PSA has also become an important tool for comparing patient outcomes following radiation or surgery.

Conformal therapy has been the most important advance in external beam radiation during the last decade. This process has permitted the safe delivery of higher doses of radiation to the tumor while increasing protection of normal tissue. As a result, patients treated with conformal techniques have improved cancer control and reduced unwanted side effects compared with those in patients undergoing conventional radiation. Although pioneered in a few centers of academic excellence, conformal radiotherapy is easily translatable to community radiation centers and should become the new national standard of care. Since 1990 there has also been a resurgence in the use of brachytherapy, or radiation implants, for prostate cancer. This renewed interest is due to technical advances in operative procedure, computer planning, and quality control. This use of radiation has become a promising alternative to prostatectomy or external beam radiation for carefully selected patients.

Radiation also plays a major role in the management of more advanced disease, as primary or adjuvant treatment. External beam radiation remains the standard potentially curative therapy for locally advanced disease. Several prospective randomized trials since 1990 have demonstrated the role of radiation used with adjuvant hormones in these patients. As an adjuvant therapy, radiation may be indicated for the patient at high risk for local recurrence after radical prostatectomy, or for the patient on systemic hormones with positive regional lymph nodes but no evidence of distant metastases. Finally, radiation continues to be an important palliative measure in the treatment of metastatic disease.

## BACKGROUND AND EPIDEMIOLOGY

**Figure 3–1:** This timeline charts the major advances over the past century in the clinical management of carcinoma of the prostate.[1–18]

**Figure 3–2:** Patterns of care for 251,416 patients with newly diagnosed prostate cancer in the United States between 1992 and 1994. This graph shows that radiation therapy is one of the two most common initial treatments for prostate cancer nationwide. During the decade from 1984 to 1994, radiation was the most common single modality used in the initial management of prostate cancer, varying from 27% to 31% of newly diagnosed patients.[19, 20] These reports by the American College of Surgeons Commission on Cancer, American Cancer Society, and the National Cancer Institute represent broad national data on the treatment of prostate cancer from diverse hospital settings, geographic regions, ethnic groups, and patient income levels. (Adapted from Mettlin CJ, Murphy GP, Cunningham MP, et al: The National Cancer Data Base report on race, age, and region variations in prostate cancer treatment. Cancer 80:1261–1266, 1997.)

## PATIENT SELECTION

**Figure 3–3:** Candidates for external beam radiation therapy. The Venn diagram illustrates the wide clinical range of patients who may be appropriately offered treatment with external beam radiation.

Although commonly understaged by clinical findings, prostate cancer that is pathologically organ-confined in a majority of cases includes patients with the combination of T1 through T2A* tumors, Gleason scores at or below 6, and PSA values at or below 10 ng/ml.[21] The choice of management of this favorable subgroup of patients is controversial, but accepted options for treatment generally include observation, radical prostatectomy, or radiation therapy.[22] Observation alone may be most appropriate for men of advanced age or poor health predicting a life expectancy less than 10 years or a low histologic tumor grade.[22–26] Surgery is the most common choice of treatment for younger, healthy men with early stage disease,[19, 20] but radiation is an equally acceptable option for these patients.[22, 27–30] External beam radiation is a more appropriate choice than surgery for men at higher risk for surgical complications because of age or comorbidities.

Locally advanced tumors extend outside the prostatic capsule and may involve the seminal vesicles or regional lymph nodes. The clinical characteristics that are associated with a high risk for these pathologic findings are tumors stage T2B* and higher, Gleason

---

*1997 American Joint Committee on Cancer Staging.[55]

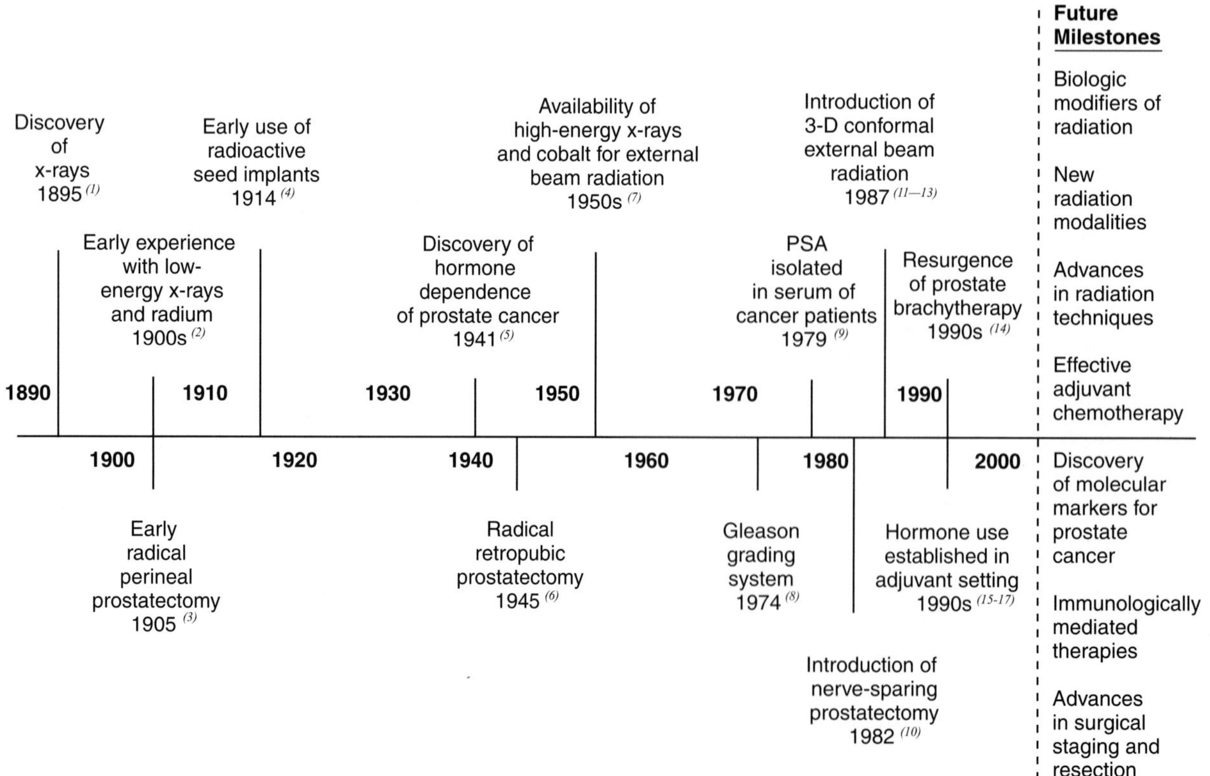


**Figure 3–1**

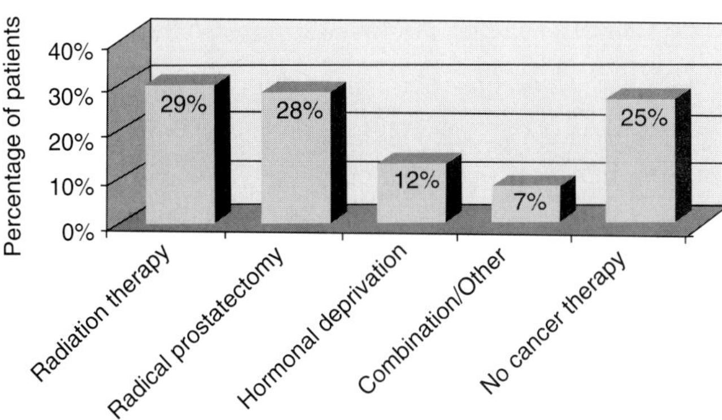


**Figure 3–2**

score 8 to 10, and PSA levels above 20 ng/ml.[21] External beam radiation, often in conjunction with hormone therapy, is the standard treatment for these patients.[15–18, 22, 29, 31–37] Radical prostatectomy is usually not recommended for these patients because of the high risk for extracapsular disease or lymph node metastases at surgery.[21, 38–41]

Radiation therapy is often used as an adjuvant therapy after prostatectomy for patients with pathologic features indicating a high risk of local recurrence or with a rising serum PSA after surgery.[42–50] For the patient with positive regional lymph nodes without distant metastatic disease, hormonal therapy has been commonly used alone as a palliative measure; however, there are subgroups of patients who may also benefit from the addition of local or regional radiation to hormones.[51–54] Radiation is the gold standard for palliating metastatic disease that is refractory to hormonal treatment.

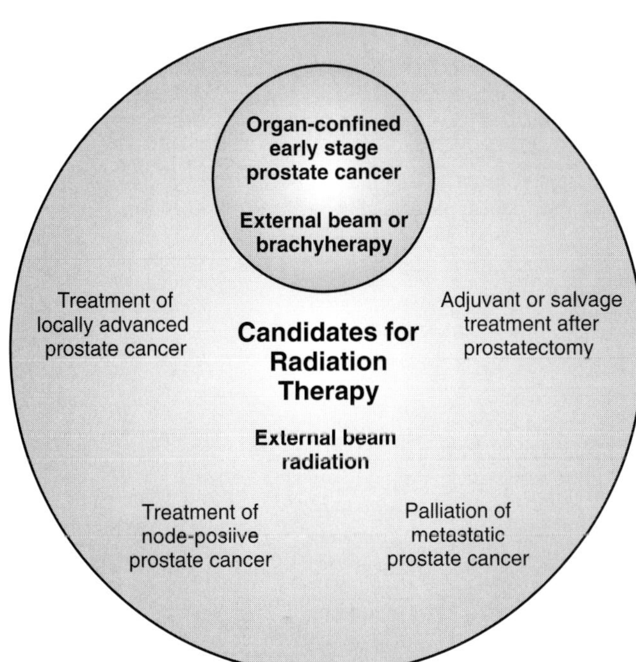


**Figure 3–3**

**Table 3–1:** In the evaluation of a patient prior to radiation therapy, several elements of the patient history and physical examination are particularly relevant to the radiation oncologist (Table 3–1). The baseline sexual, urinary, and gastrointestinal function of the patient should be documented prior to beginning treatment. Although previous pelvic radiation is an absolute contraindication to definitive treatment, inflammatory bowel disease or collagen vascular diseases are typically considered relative contraindications to radiation. The extent of local disease palpated during the digital rectal examination (DRE) is crucial for assigning a clinical stage.

Measurement of the serum PSA level has become an important part of the pretreatment staging of a patient prior to radiation. The serum PSA level plays an essential role in improving the accuracy of clinical staging in relation to the pathologic extent of disease.[21, 56] The level of serum PSA, or often the rate of rise between serial values, is the most important predictor of cancer control before radiation and the most accurate indicator of treatment failure after radiation.[34, 57–62]

Imaging tests including transrectal ultrasound (TRUS), computed tomography (CT), and magnetic res-

## TABLE 3–1

### EVALUATION OF A PATIENT PRIOR TO RADIATION THERAPY

Patient history
 Established baseline urinary, gastrointestinal, and sexual function
 Identify contraindications to radiation
Physical examination
 Digital rectal/prostate examination
 Stool Hemoccult test
Laboratory studies
 PSA
 Complete blood cell count
 Serum chemistries
 Liver function tests
 Alkaline phosphatase
Imaging studies
 Chest x-ray
 CT scan of abdomen and pelvis*
 Bone scan†
 *Optional*—Prostate ultrasound
 *Optional*—Prostate MRI
 *Investigational*—Bone marrow MRI‡
Pathologic examination
 Sextant prostate needle biopsy
  Scoring of major and minor Gleason patterns
  Identification of perineural invasion
 *Optional*—Pelvic lymph node dissection‡

*Recommended for radiation therapy planning; should be obtained with patient casted in the treatment position.

†May be deferred in asymptomatic patients with PSA levels <10 ng/ml.

‡Consider in patients with bulky tumors (T2B–T4), Gleason scores of 8 to 10, or PSA levels >20 ng/ml.

onance imaging (MRI) have been shown to be inaccurate in clinically staging the extent of disease at presentation.[63, 64] Any radiographically suspicious lymph node on CT should be confirmed pathologically by needle biopsy[22] or dissection. CT scans are most appropriately obtained with the patient in the treatment position for use during treatment planning for radiation therapy. MRI also may be useful during radiation planning in cases of uncertain clinical extracapsular extent of disease when it may modify the treatment portals or in cases of distorted pelvic anatomy. Bone scan can be reserved for patients with bone pain, those with PSA levels above 10 ng/ml, Gleason score of 8 or higher, or T3/T4 palpable tumors.[22, 65, 66] Bone marrow MRI may be useful for staging locally advanced disease or clarifying an equivocal bone scan in selected high-risk patients.[67]

A transrectal sextant biopsy of the prostate should be done in all patients, taking adequate cores from the apex, middle, and base of each lobe. Biopsies of the seminal vesicles may be considered if they appear clinically suspicious but are not routinely performed. The pathologic findings should be carefully reviewed for Gleason scoring and the presence of perineural invasion. A second review of the biopsy material by a pathologist specializing in adenocarcinoma of the pros-

tate will often result in clinically important changes in the initial Gleason scoring.[68]

The overwhelming majority of patients undergoing radiation therapy have unknown regional lymph node status. Imaging studies including CT, MRI, and ultrasound do not accurately determine pathologic lymph node status.[63, 64] For the individual with clinical risk factors for locally advanced disease, a negative lymph node dissection could influence the design of radiation portals and the decision to use adjuvant hormones. The pathologic nodal status is also valuable information for patient stratification in radiation therapy clinical trials and comparisons of outcomes between surgery and radiation. However, a lymph node dissection is rarely obtained prior to radiotherapy in clinical practice.

## CONFORMAL RADIATION TREATMENT PLANNING

**Figure 3–4:** Important elements of three-dimensional (3-D) conformal external beam radiation therapy. The process of delivering conformal external beam radiotherapy represents a concerted effort to enhance the therapeutic window by improving upon the cancer

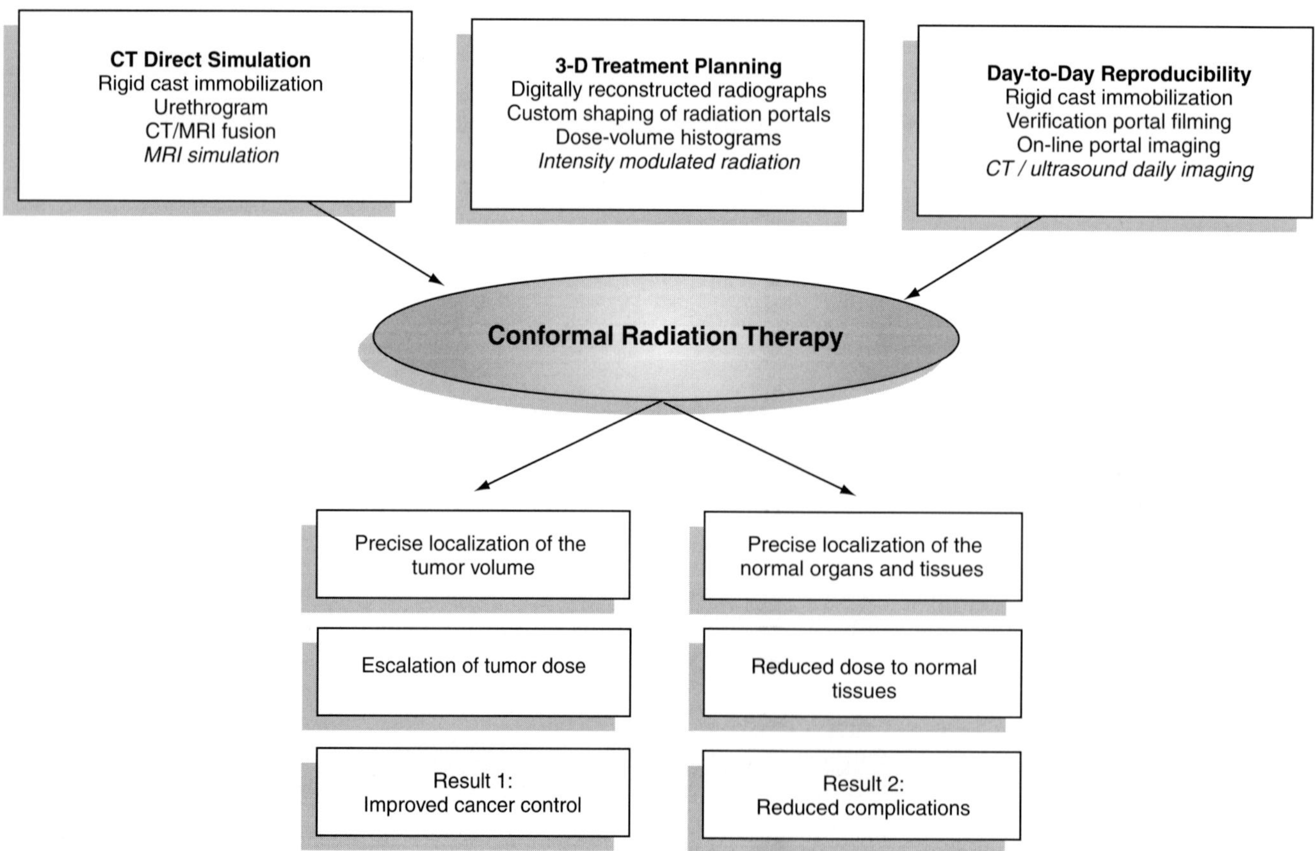


Figure 3–4

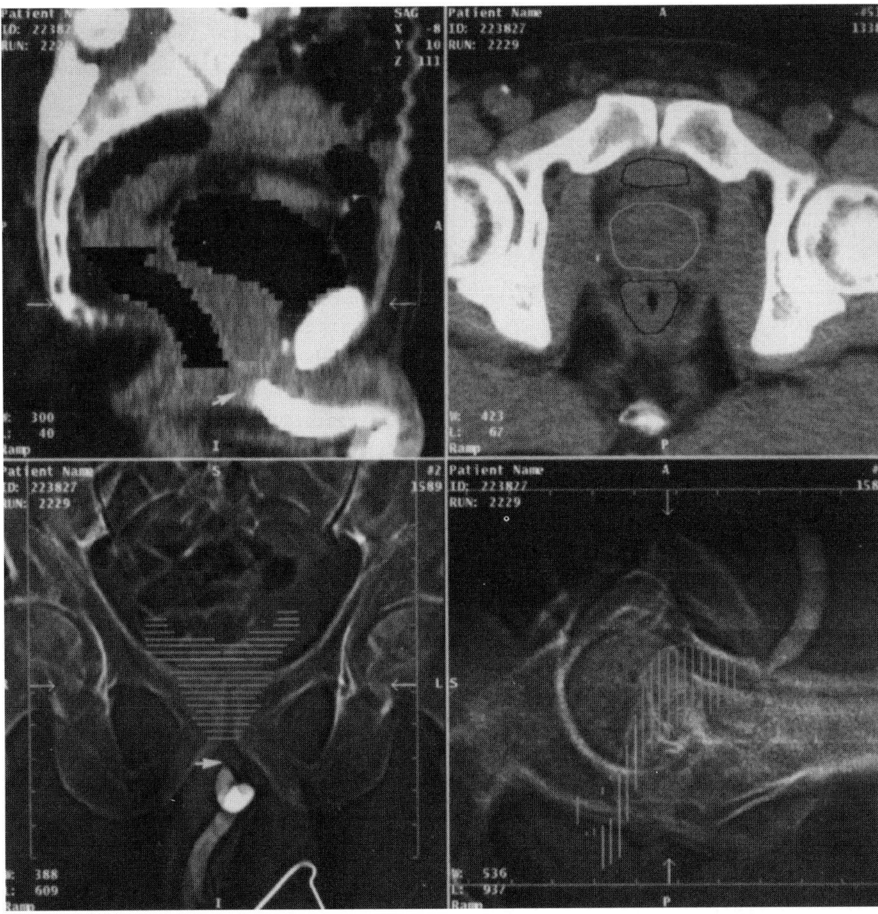

**Figure 3–5**

control and by reducing the morbidity associated with conventional radiation. The primary principles of conformal therapy are accurate identification of the radiation target in three dimensions, the custom shaping of treatment fields to cover the target yet minimize irradiation of nearby normal tissues, and the reproducible positioning and immobilization of the patient during radiation.

**Figure 3–5:** Computed tomographic (CT) simulation for conformal external beam radiation therapy. The purpose of radiation simulation is the accurate identification of the target volume as well as the neighboring normal organs in order to customize the treatment portals. This patient had a clinically organ-confined tumor, and therapy was designed to treat the prostate alone.

CT scan and urethrogram achieve the accurate localization of the prostate in conformal therapy. Conventional simulation in the past had used fluoroscopy, and the position of the prostate was determined indirectly by bony landmarks or contrast material in the bladder or rectum. This figure illustrates the information shown to the physician by the treatment planning computers during CT simulation. The upper right screen is a single axial CT scan image through the level of the prostate. The prostate and other pelvic structures are outlined into the computer by the physician on the axial CT scan slices. The left and right lower images integrate these contoured axial slices to show the target locations in anterior and lateral views. The upper left screen is a computerized reconstruction of a midline sagittal view.

The patient is immobilized during the CT scan in a custom body mold that will be used each day during treatment. Intravenous (IV) contrast medium may be used during the scan to improve the distinction between the base of the prostate and the bladder. A retrograde urethrogram is performed in all patients under sterile conditions during the CT simulation. The contrast material fills the urethra and forms a cone at the narrowing caused by the urogenital diaphragm (arrow in left upper and lower images). The combination of CT scanning with a urethrogram is more accurate in localizing the inferior position of the prostate than conventional simulation.[69] At the completion of simulation, the patient is marked with point-sized tattoos so that the position during simulation may be recreated daily on the actual treatment machine.

Fox Chase Cancer Center
PQ2000        2229
25-Jun-96 10:49
Patient Name
ID: 223827
length
width
DR Radiograph
Isocenter : p
Localized Iso
Mag.  : 1.09X
Gantry:    0.0°
Collim:   90.0°
Table : 360.0°
X  cm : 10.00
Y  cm : 10.00
Window   425
Level    223
Map      Ramp
A

Fox Chase Cancer Center
PQ2000        2229
25-Jun-96 10:49
Patient Name
ID: 223827
length
width
DR Radiograph
Isocenter : p
Localized Iso
Mag.  : 1.16X
Gantry:   90.0°
Collim:   90.0°
Table : 360.0°
X  cm : 10.00
Y  cm : 10.00
Window   425
Level    223
Map      Ramp
B

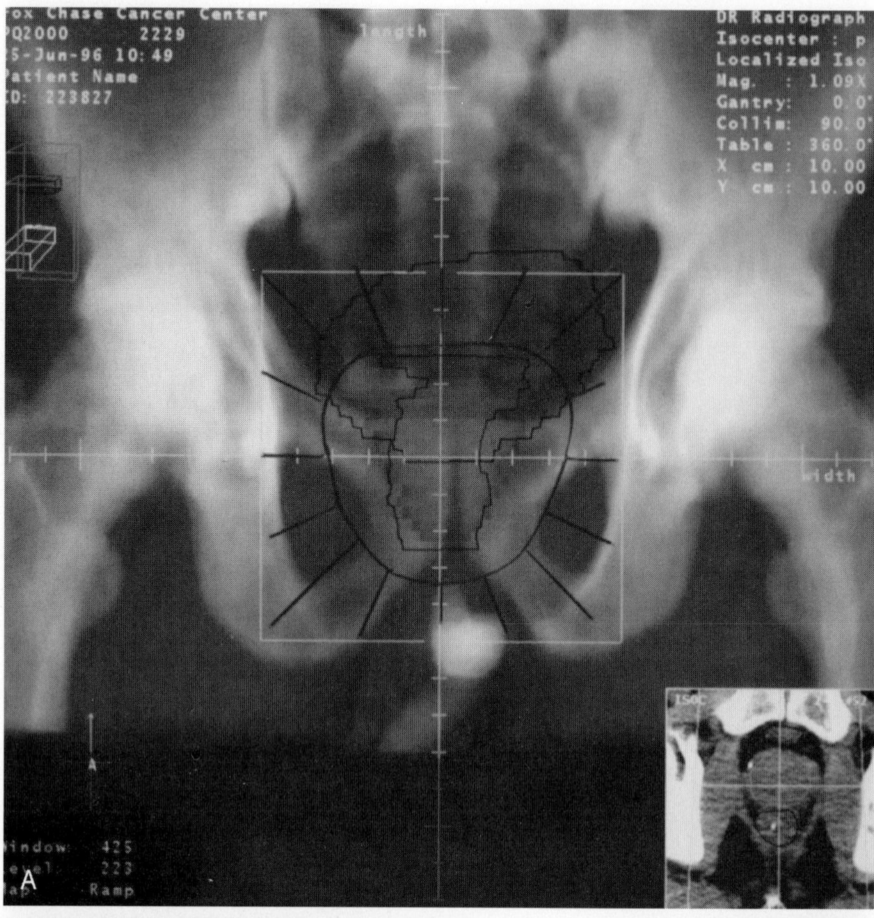

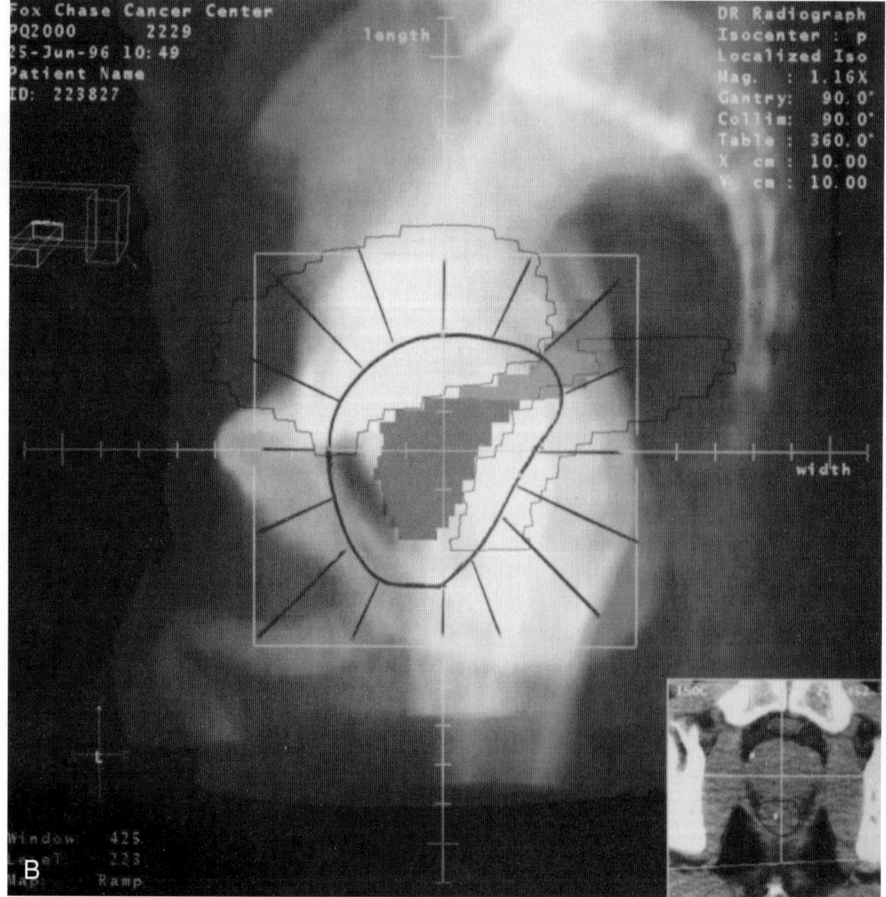

**Figure 3–6**

**Figure 3–6:** Two simulation films showing treatment portals for conformal external beam radiation therapy. The 3-D information from the planning CT scan obtained at simulation is digitally reconstructed to design the actual treatment portals. At Fox Chase Cancer Center, four or more beams are used each day of treatment to create a homogeneous dose distribution around the prostate—anterior, posterior, right and left lateral. *A* shows the final reconstructed radiograph of the anterior field, and *B* shows the lateral field. The crosshairs and box respectively indicate the center and the edges of the radiation portals. A custom contoured outline is then drawn (shown in black) around the prostate with a small margin in order to minimize the dose delivered to the neighboring tissues (rectum, bladder, and so on.)

**Figure 3–7:** Radiation dose distribution in a single axial plane through the level of the prostate. The dose delivered from each custom-shaped radiation portal is superimposed upon the patient's anatomy obtained during simulation. The planning target volume (PTV) of irradiation includes the prostate (outlined in black) plus a margin of safety for subclinical tumor extension or errors due to daily variations in patient position and prostate motion. Conformal radiation allows for smaller margins of error than conventional radiation because of improvements in accuracy of target identification and patient positioning. The result of employing tighter radiation portals during conformal therapy is reduced dosage to surrounding normal tissue and fewer side effects.

The rectangular outlines indicate percentages of the prescribed dose that will be given to all tissue within that respective contour. In this plan, the prescribed dose is given within the inner lines because this contour totally encompasses the target volume. This targeting ensures that the minimum dose to any part of the prostate is the prescribed dose; areas closer to the center of the prostate (including tumor) receive an even higher dose than this minimum dosage prescribed. In most cases, a homogeneous dose through the target can be achieved, with areas rarely receiving higher than 110% of the dose. In this plan, the dose to the rectal mucosa varies from 90% at the anterior wall (small white arrow) to only 50% at the posterior wall (large white arrow). This reduction in dosage for normal tissues with conformal techniques is important to reduce unwanted side effects.

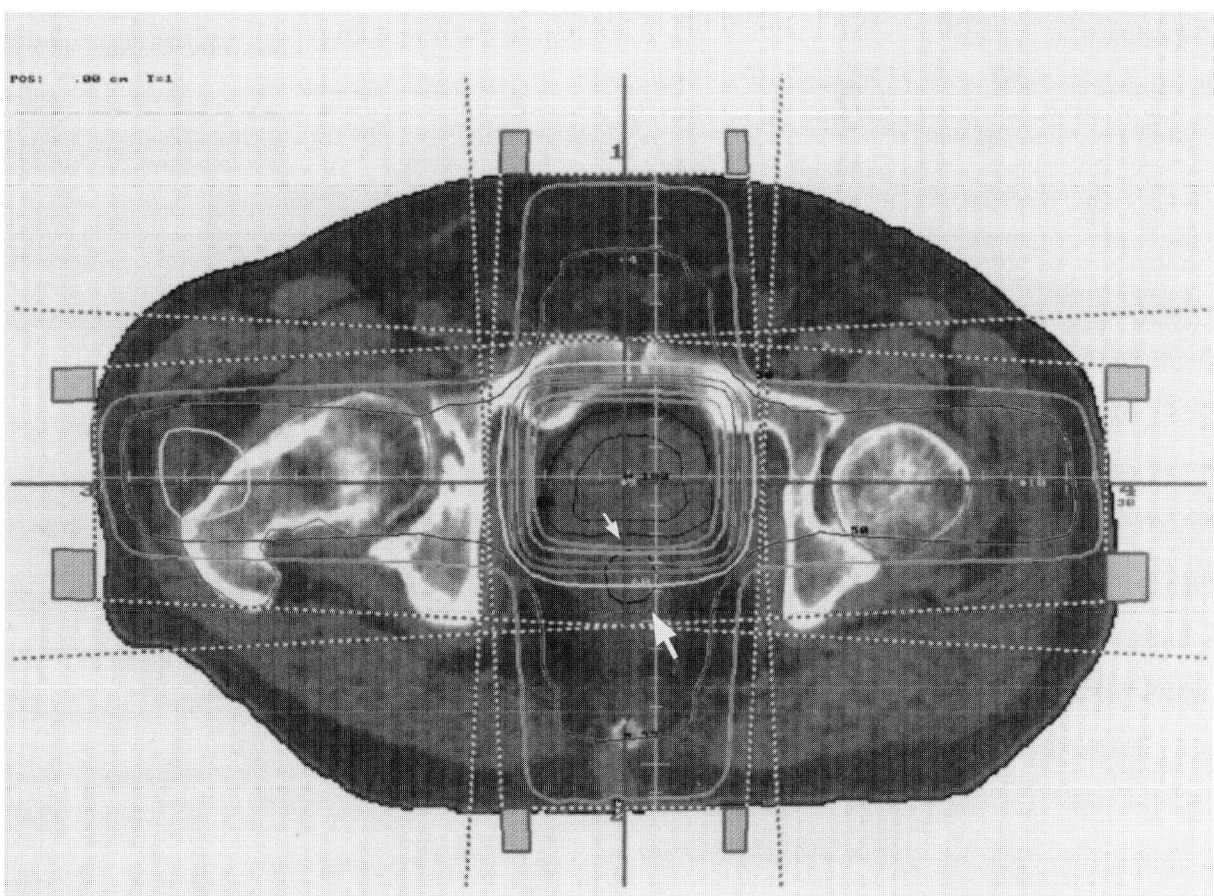


**Figure 3–7**

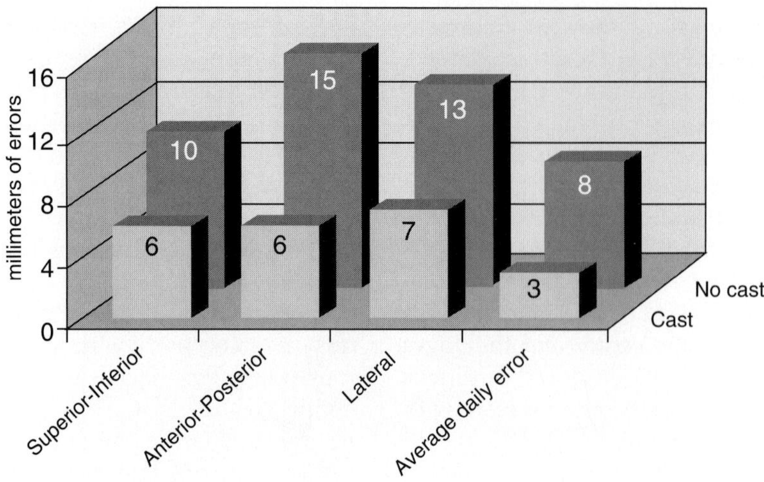



**Figure 3–8**

**Figure 3–8:** Reduction in daily set-up errors with rigid cast immobilization. The custom-made body mold or cast made for each patient is an important element of conformal therapy. The patient lies supine in the cast, which extends from the midthoracic spine to the thigh. It is essential that the patient be immobilized in this cast during the CT simulation as well as daily radiation treatments to minimize variations in organ location due to variable patient positioning. Using the cast during conformal therapy reduces average daily set-up error by 67% compared to not using the cast during conventional therapy.[12] This improved patient set-up accuracy allows the radiation oncologist to reduce the size of the radiation fields because less of a "safety" margin is needed around the prostate to ensure adequate coverage. This field reduction decreases the volume of nearby tissues and organs irradiated. (Adapted from Soffen EM, Hanks GE, Hwang CC, et al: Conformal static field therapy for low volume, low grade prostate cancer with rigid immobilization. Int J Radiat Oncol Biol Phys 20:141–146, 1991.)

**Figure 3–9:** Dose-volume histogram showing the dose reductions to the rectum achieved with conformal radiation portals. This graph shows the volume of rectum that receives any given percentage of the prescribed radiation dose. The upper curve was obtained with conventionally designed radiation portals, and the lower curve resulted from custom conformal contoured blocking in the same patients. The open white area between the two curves represents the reduction in dose given to a volume of that organ because of the conformal technique. On average, the conformal treatment lowers the dose to bladder by 14% and dose to the rectum by 12% over conventional corner-shaped blocking.[12] More important, the volume of each organ receiving the highest dose is substantially reduced. For example, the volume of rectum receiving over 80% of the prescribed dose is reduced from 35% to less than 10%. These reductions in irradiation of nearby normal organs due to conformal therapy are critical for reducing side effects for the patient. (Adapted from Soffen et al.[12])

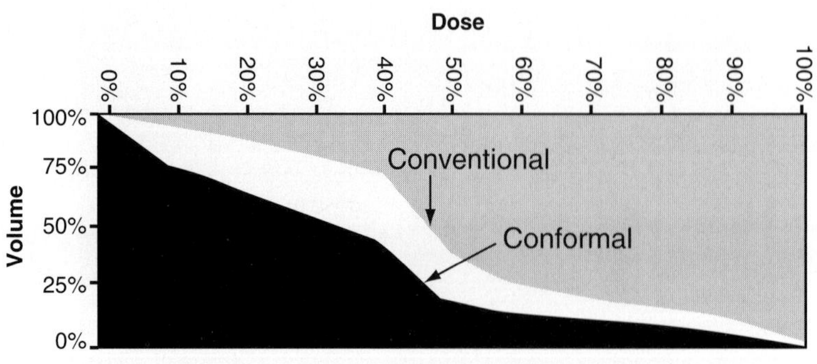



**Figure 3–9**

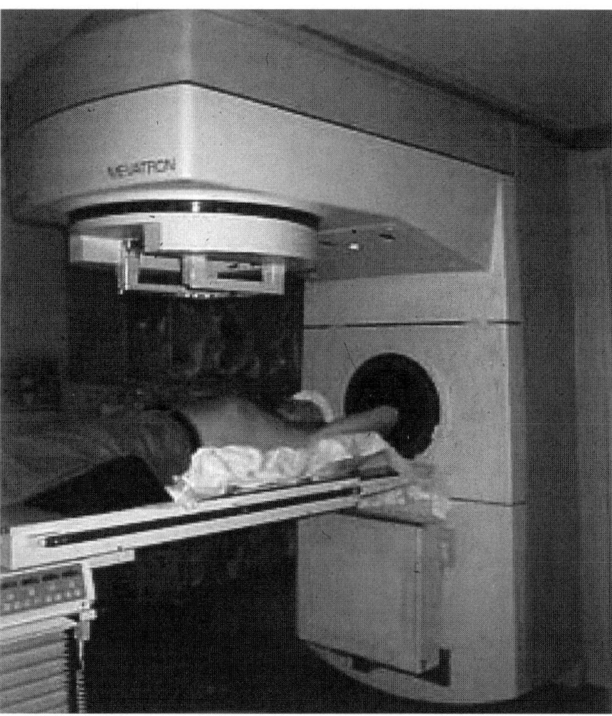

**Figure 3–10**

## RADIATION TREATMENT AND SIDE EFFECTS

**Figure 3–10:** Patient set-up for daily radiation treatment. The patient is set up on the table of the linear accelerator in a supine position within the custom-made cast every day of treatment. Fixed-position laser beams and the skin tattoos are used to properly position the patient in a reproducible manner. Once a week, films are taken of the radiation portals on the treatment machine to ensure that the patient is consistently positioned well and that the prescribed field sizes and blocks are used. Other methods of weekly quality control currently being investigated are on-line portal imaging, which replaces the hard-copy films with computer-enhanced images, and real-time portal imaging, which will allow physician monitoring of a beams-eye view during an actual radiation treatment. The most promising approach under investigation is daily CT scanning or ultrasound localization of the prostate prior to each treatment.[70] This is currently the most precise method under investigation to adjust conformal treatment fields on a daily basis to correct both for daily set-up variation of the patient and for prostate organ motion.

**Table 3–2:** Common side effects experienced during a course of external beam radiation are listed in Table 3–2. Radiation is delivered every day, Monday through Friday, usually for a period of 6 to 7 weeks. The radiation oncologist and a nurse will meet with each patient weekly throughout the course of treatment. These fre-quent visits ensure close monitoring of side effects and early intervention, if necessary. In the authors' experience, most men are able to continue their normal activities during external beam conformal radiation, including working, driving, light exercise, and sexual activity.

**TABLE 3–2**

**COMMON ACUTE SIDE EFFECTS AND THEIR MANAGEMENT DURING RADIATION THERAPY FOR PROSTATE CANCER**

| DIAGNOSIS | SYMPTOMS | MANAGEMENT |
| --- | --- | --- |
| *General* | | |
| Asthenia | Fatigue | Rest or decrease in vigorous activities |
| *Skin* | | |
| Dermatitis | Redness, dryness, itching, tanning | Emollients, steroid creams |
| *Urinary* | | |
| Cystourethritis | Frequency, urgency, dysuria, hematuria | Urinary analgesics or antispasmodics |
| Bladder outlet obstruction | Decreased stream strength, dribbling | Smooth muscle relaxants |
| *Gastrointestinal* | | |
| Enteritis | Cramping, diarrhea | Low-residue diet, antidiarrheals |
| Proctitis | Bleeding, pain | Analgesics, suppositories |

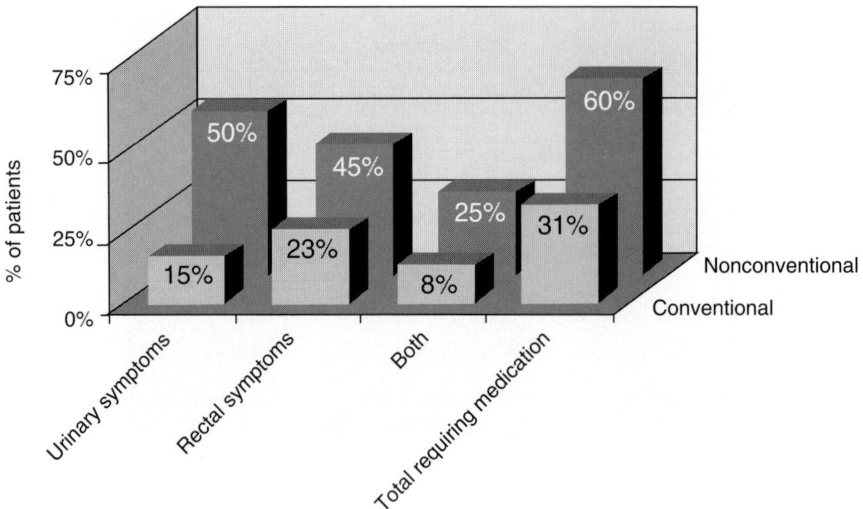


**Figure 3–11**

**Figure 3–11:** Reduction in acute morbidity rate due to treatment during conformal radiation. An analysis of side effects during treatment was conducted at Fox Chase Cancer Center in two cohorts of men. The adverse symptoms and medication use of 26 patients treated with conformal radiation techniques were compared to those of 20 patients treated with conventional methods. The patients treated with conformal techniques required significantly less medication for the palliation of acute bladder and rectal irritation during treatment. Other investigators have separately confirmed this clinically significant decrease in acute morbidity with conformal radiation techniques.[13, 71] (Adapted from Soffen et al.[72]).

**Table 3–3:** Series studying the frequency of incontinence following external beam irradiation for prostate cancer [73–80] are listed in Table 3–3. The majority of radiation series published during the past decade show the incidence of incontinence following external beam irradiation is less than 2%. Comparisons of incontinence across these studies should be approached cautiously because of marked differences in patient selec-

tion, technique of treatment, definition of incontinence, and method of data collection. Nonetheless, these low rates of incontinence following radiation are superior to the results generally observed following radical prostatectomy (2% to 43%).[73, 74, 81–85]

Urinary incontinence is a rare event (0.5%) following conformal external beam radiation at Fox Chase Cancer Center.[75] These excellent results were obtained using a strict definition of urinary incontinence of using pads one or more times per week, catheterization, or surgical intervention. Increased rates of incontinence after irradiation are associated with transurethral resection of the prostate prior to treatment[75, 78, 80] or altered radiation fractionation.[86] Although there is an increased incidence with aging alone, rates of incontinence following radiation remain low and not significantly increased for patients over the ages of 65 to 70.[73, 75, 76] However, a higher rate of incontinence has been reported after radical prostatectomy with increasing age.[73, 81, 85]

**Table 3–4:** Preservation of potency after external beam radiotherapy has been studied in many series.[15, 35, 73, 74, 76, 77, 87–92] Impotence related to age or comorbidity

## TABLE 3–3

### FREQUENCY OF INCONTINENCE AFTER EXTERNAL BEAM IRRADIATION FOR PROSTATE CANCER

| RADIATION SERIES | FOLLOW-UP (YEARS) | NO. PATIENTS | INCONTINENCE (%) | DEFINITION USED IN SERIES |
|---|---|---|---|---|
| Talcott et al.[73] | 1 crude | 113 | 5 | Use of pads |
| Lim et al.[74] | <1.5 median | 60 | 0 | Use of pads |
| Lee et al.[75] | 2.6 median | 758 | 0.5 | Use of pads |
| Jønler et al.[76] | 2.6 median | 90 | 11 | Use of pads daily |
| Crook et al.[77] | 2.8 mean | 192 | 2 | Use of pads |
| Green et al.[78] | 3 median | 241 | 4 | Not stated |
| Amdur et al.[79] | 5 minimum | 225 | 2 | Moderate complication |
| Perez et al.[80] | 6.5 median | 738 | 0.7 | Grade 2 complication |

## TABLE 3–4

### PRESERVATION OF POTENCY AFTER EXTERNAL BEAM RADIOTHERAPY

| RADIATION SERIES | FOLLOW-UP (YEARS) | NO. PATIENTS | POTENCY PRESERVATION (%) | DEFINITION USED IN SERIES |
|---|---|---|---|---|
| Talcott et al.[73] | 1 crude | 66 | 76 | Any erection within 4 weeks |
| Lim et al.[74] | <1.5 median | 46 | 46 | Adequate erections for intercourse |
| Chinn et al.[90] | 1.8 median | 60 | 62 | Adequate erections for intercourse |
| Helgason et al.[89] | 1.5–2 crude | 64 | 50 | Adequate erections for intercourse |
| Dicker et al.[88] | 2 actuarial | 318 | 72 | Adequate erections for intercourse |
| Nicolaou et al.[91] | 2.6 median | 45 | 73 | Adequate erections for intercourse |
| Jønler et al.[76] | 2.6 median | 68 | 63 | Full or partial erections |
| Crook et al.[77] | 2.8 mean | 192 | 65 | Adequate erections for intercourse |
| Mantz et al.[92] | 3 actuarial | 114 | 66 | Adequate erections for intercourse |
| Pilepich et al.[15] | 3.3 median | 102 | 72 | Sexual function |
| Shipley et al.[87] | 5 minimum | 29 | 45 | Full potency |
| Bagshaw et al.[35] | 9 actuarial | 576 | 50 | Any erection |

is a common finding in 18% to 48% of men prior to treatment in radiotherapy series.[35, 73, 76, 77, 88] For this reason, series reporting the preservation of sexual function after radiotherapy should limit the analysis to patients who were potent prior to treatment. Table 3–4 shows the results from a wide range of series consisting of both retrospective physician-collected data and patient-reported questionnaires. In men potent prior to radiation, 45% to 76% will have preservation of potency or sexual function after radiation. Similar to analyses of incontinence, comparisons of sexual function across retrospective studies are limited by wide variations in definition of potency, differences in patient selection and treatment techniques, and method of data collection. However, in general, these results after radiotherapy are superior to the reported incidence of potency preservation of 0% to 11% after radical prostatectomy, and are comparable to or better than rates of 35% to 76% reported within a similar period after the bilateral nerve-sparing procedure.[73, 82, 84, 93, 94]

Independently of pretreatment potency, age has been shown to significantly decrease the preservation of potency after surgery.[82, 84, 93, 94] In the surgical series from Johns Hopkins, the potency preservation rates declined from 75% for men in their 50s to only 25% for men older than 70.[94] However, in radiotherapy series, increasing age has not been correlated clearly with a higher rate of post-treatment potency.[90–92] Factors that have been reported to reduce potency after irradiation are marginal pretreatment potency, diabetes, cardiovascular disease, prior major urologic procedures, and use of adjuvant hormones.[88, 90, 92, 95]

**Figure 3–12:** Association between serious rectal complications and dose after definitive irradiation for prostate cancer. Schultheiss et al.[96] analyzed data on complications in 712 consecutive patients who received definitive radiation for prostate cancer at Fox Chase Cancer Center between 1986 and 1994. This graph shows that the incidence of serious rectal complication is strongly dependent upon the radiation dose delivered. Serious rectal complication was defined in this series as any proctitis or rectal bleeding after irradiation that required more than two coagulation procedures, hospitalization, or blood transfusion. Among 670 patients treated at Fox Chase Cancer Center between 1989 and 1993, the incidence of these serious rectal complications was 16 out of 670 (2.4%).[97] The actuarial rate at 3 years was 1.7% in patients receiving less than 74 Gy and 7% in patients receiving over 74 Gy ($p = 0.006$). The prognosis for treatment of these serious rectal complications is excellent—12 out of 16 patients (75%) were successfully managed with medication, coagulations, or blood transfusions without major surgery.[97] With later improvements in conformal shielding of the rectum, the rate of serious bleeding has decreased to fewer than 2% at doses of 75 to 76 Gy.[98] Similarly, low rates of serious rectal injury have been reported with 3-D conformal radiation elsewhere.[13, 99] (Adapted from Schultheiss TE, Lee WR, Hunt MA, et al: Late GI and GU complications in the treatment of prostate cancer. Int J Radiat Oncol Biol Phys 37:3–11, 1997.)

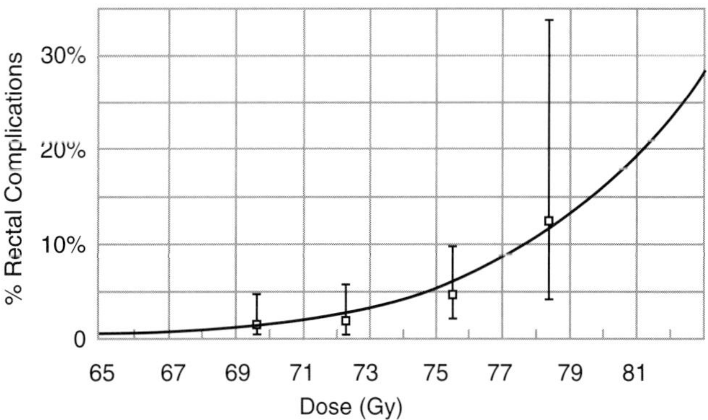


**Figure 3–12**

## RESULTS OF RADIATION THERAPY

**Figure 3–13:** Clinical versus biochemical assessment of cancer control after radiation therapy. The figure shows the freedom from cancer rates measured by clinical endpoints versus biochemical endpoints. The 453 patients are stratified by pretreatment PSA values. The graft depicts the 5-year results after treatment with external beam radiation therapy alone at Fox Chase Cancer Center. The biochemical freedom from disease (NED, no evidence of disease) relapse determined by serial PSA values after irradiation is a more accurate measure of cure than clinical assessment. This finding also has been demonstrated in other radiotherapy series[34, 37, 57, 61, 100] as well as in surgical series.[101, 102] Although after radical prostatectomy the PSA level should become undetectable, the value of PSA after radiation indicates that a cure of disease is controversial.[103] At Fox Chase Cancer Center, a patient is considered biochemically free of cancer if there is no clinical evidence for cancer recurrence and the PSA level is 1.5 ng/ml or less and is not rising on two successive measurements. (Adapted from Hanks GE, Corn BW, Lee WR, et al: External beam irradiation of prostate cancer. Conformal treatment techniques and outcomes for the 1990s. Cancer 75:1972–1977, 1995.)

**Figure 3–14:** Prognostic factors for biochemical freedom from disease after external beam radiation therapy. The serum PSA prior to treatment has been shown on multivariate analysis to be the most important prognostic factor for bNED control after irradiation for clinically local-regional prostate cancer.[58, 61, 105] Several other factors are of lesser importance than PSA but remain significant when weighing a patient's chance for cure after irradiation: PSA doubling time, Gleason score, palpation stage, use of conformal radiation technique, higher doses of irradiation, absence of perineural tumor invasion, and diploid tumor DNA.[62, 104, 106–109] Several factors have not been shown to be important predictors of bNED outcome after irradiation. Young age does not predict for worse bNED outcome after radia-

tion on univariate or multivariate analysis.[30] The American Joint Committee on Cancer stage,[55] when incorporating ultrasound or magnetic resonance imaging (MRI) to upstage tumors, is not significant compared to the stage by palpation of tumor alone.[106] The finding of over half of systematic biopsies to be positive does not provide further information than the pretreatment PSA alone.[110]

**Figure 3–15:** Disease control (bNED, biologically no evidence of disease) after definitive radiation for prostate cancer. The figure shows the survival free from clinical or biochemical disease recurrence of 455 consecutive patients treated by radiation therapy at Fox Chase Cancer Center. This series consists of all patients treated between 1988 and 1993 with tumors from T1 to T3, any Gleason score, and at least one known pretreatment PSA. Almost all had unknown regional lymph node status (NX) and all had no clinical evidence for distant metastases (M0). The actuarial rates of cure, defined as no clinical or biochemical evidence of cancer at last follow-up, are 61% at 5 years and 52% at 7 years after treatment.

Our results refute the claims made by Stamey et al. that only 20% of patients are cured within 5 years after radiotherapy.[111] The distribution of important prognostic factors in the patients from that series were unknown; however, in order to obtain the same poor results, we would need to select from our series only those patients with high pretreatment PSA, poorly differentiated tumors, and large bulky tumors. Investigators at the same institution as Stamey have independently reported that 38% of patients, twice the number reported by Stamey et al., were free of disease an average of 12.4 years after treatment.[112]

**Figure 3–16:** Improvement in biochemical disease-free survival (bNED) rate with conformal techniques of radiation. The outcome after external beam radiation alone has been carefully followed in all 603 patients treated at Fox Chase Cancer Center from December 1985 through December 1994. The figure shows that patients treated with conformal techniques of irradia-

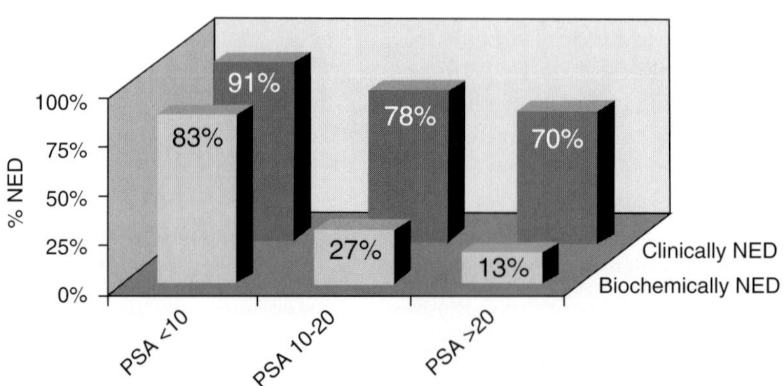


**Figure 3–13**

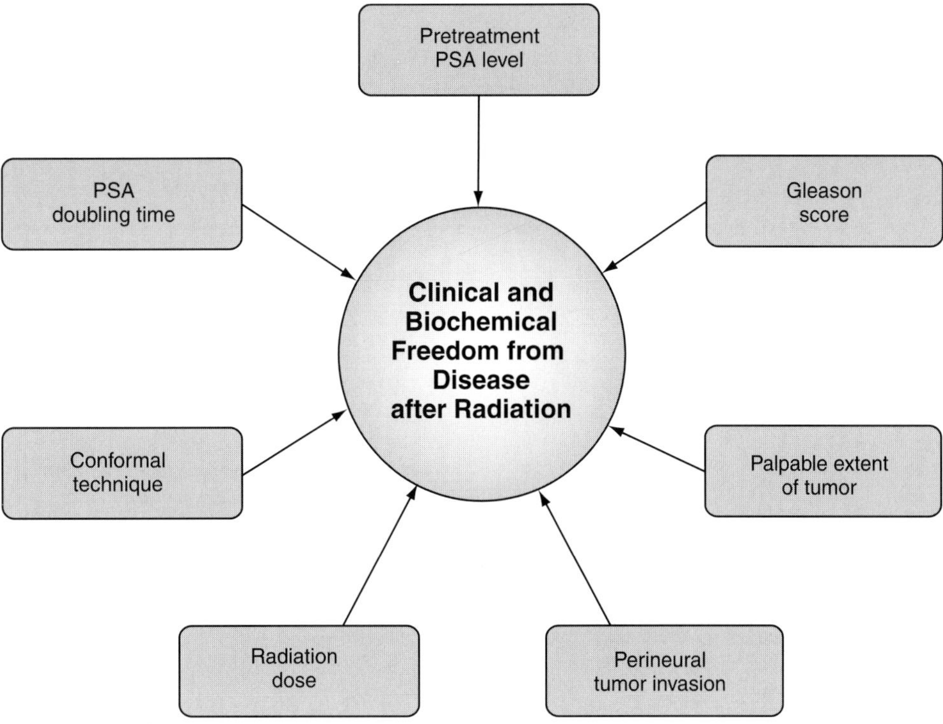



**Figure 3–14**

tion instituted after 1989 demonstrate a significant improvement in tumor control compared to patients treated with conventional techniques (p <0.0001). Recently, a randomized trial demonstrated that a modest dose increase (8 Gy) using conformal radiotherapy resulted in a significant improvement in tumor control for patients with a PSA level of more than 10 ng/ml.[113] In yet another study, this improved tumor control with conformal therapy continued to be significant at 5 years after radiation (independent of the pretreatment PSA, stage, or grade).[104]

## Early Organ-Confined Disease

**Table 3–5:** Several series have studied long-term survival rates for clinical stages T1 and T2 prostate cancer after conventional radiation.[29, 31, 33–37, 79, 114] The figures in Table 3–5 represent the long-term results of radiotherapy for clinically organ-confined disease from across the United States, both from well-respected single academic institutions and from national averages drawn from city- and community-based radiotherapy centers. After external beam radiotherapy for T1 tumors, the

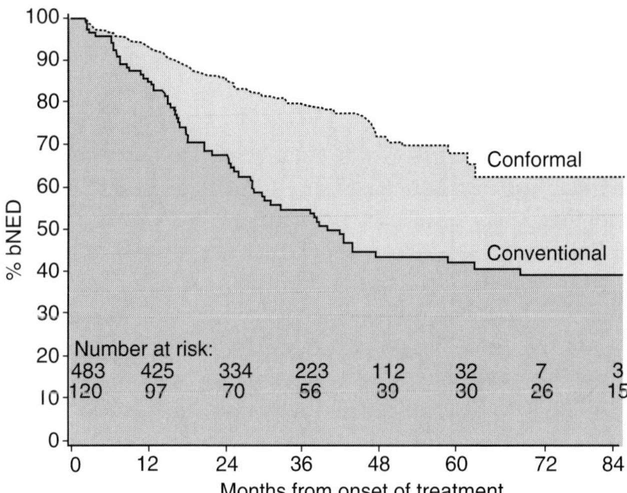



**Figure 3–15**                                                      **Figure 3–16**

## TABLE 3–5

## LONG-TERM SURVIVAL RATES FOR PROSTATE CANCER AFTER CONVENTIONAL RADIATION THERAPY

| RADIATION SERIES | NO. PATIENTS | CLINICAL STAGE | OVERALL SURVIVAL, % (DISEASE-FREE SURVIVAL, %) | | |
|---|---|---|---|---|---|
| | | | 5 years | 10 years | 15 years |
| Eastern Virginia Medical School[34] | 104 | T1b | — (82) | — (66) | — |
| | 72 | T2a | — (79) | — (57) | — |
| | 209 | T2b/c | — (73) | — (48) | — |
| LDS Hospital[33] | 20* | T1b-T2 | 85 (89)† | 60 (70)† | 40 (64)† |
| Massachusetts General Hospital[114] | 504 | T1-T2 | — | — (65)‡ | — |
| M.D. Anderson Cancer Center[29] | 104 | T1b | 83 (92)‡ | 79 (72)‡ | — |
| | 168 | T2 | 84 (82)‡ | 57 (59)‡ | 33 (59)‡ |
| Patterns of Care Study (1973)[31] | 60 | T1 | 84 (76) | 54 (53) | 41 (39) |
| | 312 | T2 | 74 (56) | 43 (27) | 22 (15) |
| Patterns of Care Study (1978)[31] | 116 | T1 | 85 (74) | 63 (52) | — |
| | 415 | T2 | 75 (53) | 46 (34) | — |
| Radiation Therapy Oncology Group[31] | 84 | T1 | 86 (—) | 64 (—) | — |
| Stanford University[35] | 96 | T1 | 95 (85)‡ | 73 (75)‡ | 50 (70)‡ |
| | 577 | T2 | 80 (70)‡ | 58 (50)‡ | 36 (38)‡ |
| University of Florida[79] | 27 | T1 | 74 (96)† | 69 (96)† | — |
| | 87 | T2 | 67 (72)† | 41 (44)† | — |
| Washington University[36] | 48 | T1b | 85 (78) | 70 (60) | — |
| | 252 | T2 | 82 (76) | 65 (56) | — |
| Yale University[37] | 165 | T1b-T2 | — (71)† | — (48)† | — |

*All pathologic node-negative patients.
†Numbers in parentheses are recurrence-free survival rates.
‡Numbers in parentheses are freedom from relapse rates.
*Note:*—indicates no data available.

overall survival rate at 10 years ranges from 54% to 79% and at 15 years it ranges from 41% to 50%. For T2 tumors, the results at 10 and 15 years are 41% to 65% and 22% to 36%, respectively. The clinical disease-free survival rate of these patients is generally 5% to 10% lower than the overall survival rate. Clinical assessment of disease-free survival underestimates that of the more sensitive PSA-based follow-up; using PSA, 35% to 72% of patients with T1 and 18% to 38% with T2 prostate cancers are alive and free of disease over 10 years after radiation therapy.[34, 112]

These excellent results were obtained despite many limitations in these early series. Patients were clinically staged in an era without pretreatment PSA level stratification, and the overwhelming majority had unknown pelvic lymph node status. The patients were generally unselected for age and comorbidities, with an average age of 65 to 70, as evidenced by up to 50% of the deaths at 10 to 15 years from other causes than prostate cancer.[31] In addition, the conventional radiotherapy techniques used in these studies should not be considered state of the art compared to conformal treatment in the 1990s.

**Figure 3–17:** bNED outcome after external beam radiation for early stage prostate cancer. This graph shows the importance of the pretreatment PSA values in clinically early stage prostate cancer treated by radiotherapy. These patients all had clinically organ-confined disease, tumor stages T1 through T2b, and well to

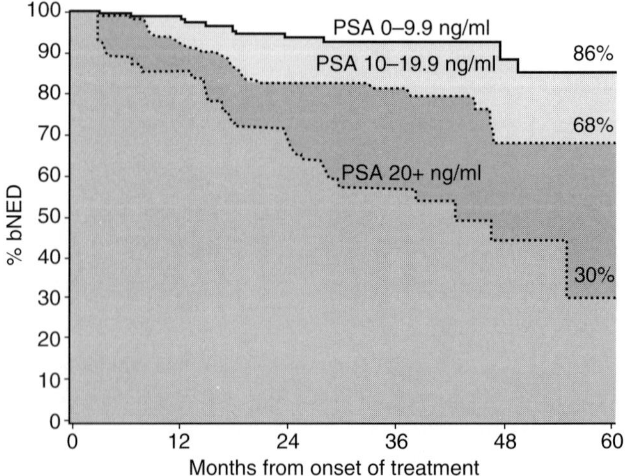


Figure 3–17

moderately differentiated tumors, with Gleason scores below 7. Five years after radiation, 86% of patients with pretreatment PSA values below 10 ng/ml have no clinical or biochemical evidence of disease. The bNED results decrease to 68% for pretreatment PSA values of 10 to 19.9 ng/ml and 30% for pretreatment PSA levels of 20 ng/ml or higher. This important ability of pretreatment PSA level to stratify patients into various groups at risk for failure after treatment has been confirmed both in radiotherapy[34, 58, 60] and surgical series.[101, 102]

**Table 3–6:** Table 3–6 gives the comparable bNED outcomes at 5 years for patients with clinical T1–T2 tumors and pretreatment PSA levels at 10 ng/ml or lower after treatment by radical prostatectomy or external beam radiation therapy.[60, 99, 101, 102, 115–118] Direct comparison of results after either radiation or surgery is complicated by differences in patient selection between modalities. Patients undergoing radiation are clinically staged, which commonly underestimates the risk of subclinical extracapsular disease or lymph node metastases compared to pathologic staging.[21,119] Imaging studies including CT, MRI, and ultrasound do not improve upon this inaccuracy in clinical staging.[63, 64] Patients treated with radiation therapy are also older on average than surgical patients.[19, 120] Based upon older age or medical contraindications to surgery, patients in radiation series could be expected to have worse overall survival rates when compared to healthy surgical patients. In addition, the Gleason scoring of prostate needle biopsies used in radiation series is significantly undergraded 23% to 41% of the time when compared to the final pathologic Gleason scores from radical prostatectomy specimens.[121]

The serum PSA level has improved the accuracy of clinical staging of patients when used in conjunction with the clinical tumor stage and grade.[21] This biochemical staging has enabled a more meaningful comparison of results between radiotherapy and surgical series. Despite the potential biases limiting comparisons across retrospective series, the results after radiation therapy have been shown to be comparable to surgery in similarly staged patients.[30, 33, 60, 99, 101, 102, 116–118, 122, 123] The figure shows the treatment outcomes for patients with early stage organ-confined disease, clinical stage T1-T2, and pretreatment PSA levels at 10 ng/ml or lower, from nationally respected academic institutions reporting the best results from either modality. The 5-year clinical and biochemical freedoms from disease are indistinguishable between the radiation and surgical series. Such data have led to consensus among both surgical and radiotherapy experts on the equivalency of these two treatments in this group of patients.[22, 27]

## TABLE 3–6

### TREATMENT OUTCOMES AFTER RADICAL PROSTATECTOMY OR EXTERNAL BEAM RADIATION

| | FOLLOW-UP MEDIAN (YEARS) | NO. PATIENTS | FIVE-YEAR bNED RATE (%) FOR GIVEN PRETREATMENT PSA LEVELS | | |
| --- | --- | --- | --- | --- | --- |
| | | | ≤ 4 ng/ml | 4–10 ng/ml | 0 ≤ 10 ng/ml |
| **Surgery Series** | | | | | |
| Cleveland Clinic[116] | 2.1 | 354 | 88 | 70 | 76 |
| Johns Hopkins[101] | 5† | 1018 | 94 | 82 | — |
| University of Pennsylvania[118] | 3.2 | 402‡§ | — | — | 85 |
| Washington University[102] | 4† | 1175* | 88–93 | 76 | — |
| **Radiation Series** | | | | | |
| Cleveland Clinic[116] | 1.8 | 253 | 100 | 65 | 75 |
| Fox Chase Cancer Center[115] | 3.3 | 185 | 89 | 83 | — |
| Joint Center for Radiation Therapy[118] | 3.2 | 225‡§ | — | — | 88 |
| MD Anderson[60] | 2.6 | 286 | 91 | 69 | — |
| Memorial Sloan-Kettering[117] | 3 | 167‡ | — | — | 85 |
| University of Michigan[99] | 3 | 133‡ | — | — | 75 |

*7-year results.
†Mean.
‡Gleason score ≤ 6.
§No T2b patients.
PSA = prostate-specific antigen; bNED = no biochemical evidence of cancer.

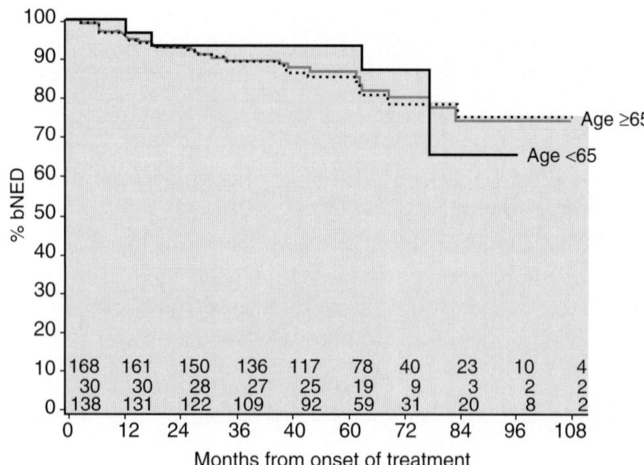

**Figure 3–18**

**Figure 3–18:** Radiation therapy for the younger patient with prostate cancer. The figure shows the clinical and PSA-based freedom from progression for 168 patients with clinically organ-confined disease and pretreatment PSA values at 10 ng/ml or lower treated by external beam radiotherapy at Fox Chase Cancer Center. There is no significant difference between the results within 8 years after treatment for men aged under 65 compared with men 65 and older. The comparable outcomes for patients under the age of 65 and older patients treated by radiotherapy have also been shown in other series.[28, 29, 116, 124] Radical prostatectomy has be-

come the more common choice of treatment for younger, healthy men with early stage prostate cancer.[19, 20, 120] The fact that younger men are more often candidates for surgery should not imply that they might not be equally well treated by radiation. The cancer control after radiation is the same as that of radical prostatectomy for similarly staged patients (see Table 3–6). The side effects of urinary continence and preservation of potency, which are especially important considerations for younger patients, are also comparable or superior after radiotherapy compared to the side effects of surgery (see Tables 3–3 and 3–4).

**Figure 3–19:** Ultrasound-guided transperineal radiation implant for early stage prostate cancer. Attempts to implant radioactive sources, or seeds, directly into the prostate for the treatment of cancer date back to the early part of this century. The goal of the implanted radiation is the same as conformal external beam therapy—the delivery of a high dose of radiation to the prostate while minimizing the dose to the nearby bladder and rectum. During the past few years, a renewed interest in prostate implantation has been generated by the development of modern transperineal implant techniques. These newer techniques are based on either intraoperative ultrasound guidance or preoperative CT-guided planning of seed placement. The implant remains a safe and less invasive procedure than radical prostatectomy and is a convenient form of radiation therapy when compared with 7 weeks of daily external beam treatment.

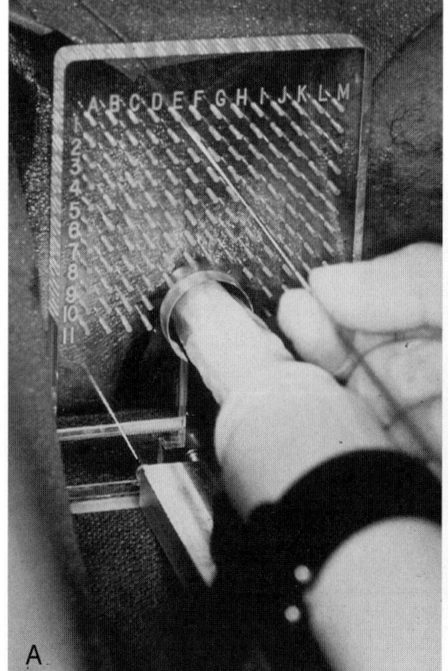


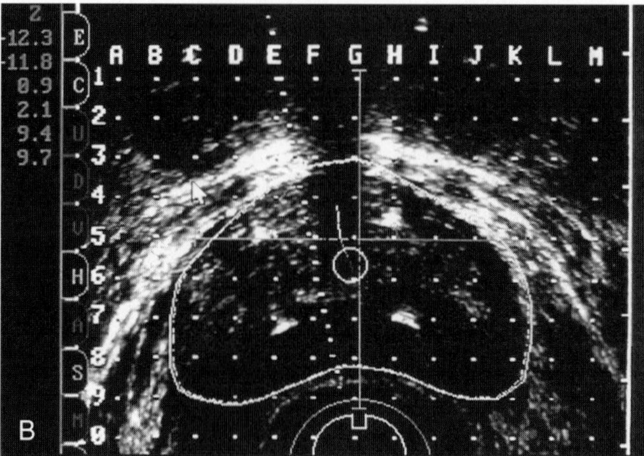


**Figure 3–19**

*A*, This patient is undergoing an ultrasound-guided transperineal implant procedure. The radioactive sources are placed into the prostate in a shielded operating suite while the patient is under general or spinal anesthesia. Hollow needles are guided through a sectored template through the perineal skin into the prostate. Using a transrectal ultrasound can optimize the position of the ends of these needles. The radiotherapist is able to use real-time ultrasound images (*B*) to guide the placement of each needle into its final position within the prostate. An optimal distribution will deliver uniform dose throughout the prostate while avoiding excess dose to the urethra and rectum. Urinary and rectal complications from poor placement are highly influenced by the experience and skill of the radiotherapist.

Table 3–7: Five-year results from modern radiotherapy implants for early stage prostate cancer are given in Table 3–7. The results during the 1980s using free-hand retropubic placement techniques of the radiation seeds were disappointing, with high rates of local failure from 17% to 52% for T2 tumors and 29% to 67% for T3 tumors between 5 and 10 years after the procedure.[125–128] Patients should be selected carefully before being offered the option of a radiation implant. The radioactive sources placed within the prostate deliver high doses within a small volume inside the gland itself; however, the dose will rapidly decrease to a subtherapeutic level within a short distance outside the prostatic capsule. The clinical tumor characteristics that select for patients with a low probability of extracapsular disease appropriate for implantation are tumor size T1–T2a, Gleason score 2 to 6, and PSA levels at 10 ng/ml or lower.[21] In addition, because the dose distribution from an implant becomes inhomogeneous over a large volume, implants may be contraindicated for very large prostate glands or bulky tumors. Table 3–7 provides data from recent implant series using modern techniques and shows that the early 5-year results in properly selected patients can be comparable to those achieved after radical prostatectomy or external beam radiation.[14, 118, 129–131]

## Locally Advanced Disease

Table 3–8: Table 3–8 gives the long-term survival rates of patients with T3 and T4 prostate cancer after conventional external beam radiation therapy.[29, 31–37, 79] Long-term results of treatment are available from well-respected academic institutions and national cooperative studies incorporating city- and community-based radiotherapy centers. The results for T3 prostate cancer after external beam radiation therapy show that 15% to 45% of patients will survive 10 years, and 13% to 31% will survive 15 years. Furthermore, the clinical

## TABLE 3–7

### FIVE-YEAR RESULTS OF RADIOTHERAPY IMPLANTS FOR EARLY STAGE PROSTATE CANCER

| | BLASKO ET AL.[14] | WALLNER ET AL.[129] | BEYER AND PRIESTLEY[130] | D'AMICO ET AL.[118] | STOREY ET AL.[131] |
|---|---|---|---|---|---|
| Total number of patients | 197 | 92 | 489 | 66 | 206 |
| Median follow-up (months) | 36 | 36 | 34 | 41 | 35 |
| **Five-Year bNED Survival Rate (%)** | | | | | |
| Clinical Stage | | | | | |
| T1a/b | 100 | — | 95 | n/a | — |
| T1c | 92 | — | n/a | — | — |
| T2a | 81–95 | — | 67–70 | — | — |
| T2b | n/a | — | 34 | — | — |
| Gleason score | | | | | |
| 2–4 | 93 | — | 85 | 83 | 65 |
| 5–6 | 92 | — | 62 | 60 | 66 |
| 7–10 | n/a | — | 30 | ≤15 | 41 |
| Pretreatment PSA levels | | | | | |
| <4 ng/ml | 98 | 100 | 93 | — | 84 |
| 4 ≤ 10 ng/ml | 90 | 80 | 72 | 86* | 72 |
| 10≤ 20 ng/ml | 89 | 45 | 42 | 35* | 51† |
| >20 ng/ml | 80 | 38 | 38 | ≤10* | — |

*Results for patients divided into low-, intermediate-, and high-risk subgroups based on pretreatment PSA levels, Gleason score, and T stage.
†PSA > 10 ng/ml.
n/a = not applicable.
*Note:* — indicates no data.

## TABLE 3–8

### LONG-TERM SURVIVAL RATES FOR PROSTATE CANCER AFTER CONVENTIONAL EXTERNAL BEAM RADIATION

| RADIATION SERIES | NO. PATIENTS | STAGE | OVERALL SURVIVAL, % (DISEASE-FREE SURVIVAL, %) 5 years | 10 years | 15 years |
|---|---|---|---|---|---|
| Committee on Radiation Therapy[32] | 372 | T3 | — (66) | — (38) | — (17) |
| Eastern Virginia Medical School[34] | 267 | T3 | — (47) | — (29) | — |
| LDS Hospital[33] | 15* | T3 | 67 (60)† | 40 (30)† | 15 (30)† |
| M.D. Anderson Cancer Center[29] | 602 | T3 | 74 (59)‡ | 45 (44)‡ | 31 (30)‡ |
| Patterns of Care Study (1973)[31] | 296 | T3/T4 | 56 (38) | 32 (26) | 23 (17) |
| Patterns of Care Study (1978)[31] | 197 | T3/T4 | 66 (45) | 33 (14) | — |
| Radiation Therapy Oncology Group[31] | 503 | T3/T4 | 70 (—) | 38 (—) | — |
| Stanford University[35] | 409 | T3 | 65 (45)‡ | 36 (28)‡ | 18 (20)‡ |
|  | 37 | T4 | 28 (22)‡ | 15 (16)‡ | 15 (16)‡ |
| University of Florida[79] | 111 | T3 | 73 (61)† | 38 (48)† | — |
| Washington University[36] | 412 | T3 | 65 (57) | 42 (38) | — |
| Yale University[37] | 120 | T3 | — (45)† | — (33)† | — |

*All pathologic node-negative patients.
†Numbers in parentheses are recurrence-free survival rates.
‡Numbers in parentheses are freedom from relapse rates.
*Note:*—indicates no data.

disease-free survival of these patients is 14% to 48% at 10 years and 16% to 30% at 15 years. Results for T4 prostate cancers are generally lower when separately reported in these series. When strict PSA-based follow-up is added to the clinical assessment, 11% to 22% of patients with T3–T4 prostate cancers are alive and free of disease over 10 years after radiation therapy.[34, 37, 112, 114] These survival results were obtained despite the likely inclusion of a significant number of node-positive patients during the pre-PSA era without pathologic staging. In addition, because the average age of these patients is 65 to 70 years at the time of radiation, approximately 50% of the deaths 10 to 15 years later are from other causes than prostate cancer.[31] Finally, it should again be noted that the conventional methods of radiotherapy used in these studies are no longer considered state of the art.

**Figure 3–20:** Five-year bNED outcome for patients with locally advanced disease treated by radiation therapy. The majority of patients with clinical features of palpable T2C disease or greater or a Gleason score from 8 to 10 have disease that pathologically extends outside the prostatic capsule.[21] This graph illustrates the 5-year bNED control for these patients who present with locally advanced prostate cancer. The pretreatment PSA level remains the most important prognostic factor for bNED outcome in these patients. This group has an overall higher rate of relapse compared to patients with organ-confined disease (see Fig. 3–17). However, the pretreatment PSA level is able to identify a subgroup, patients with PSA values below 10 ng/ml, which may do well after treatment with radiation alone—72% free of recurrence at 5 years. The majority of patients with these same locally advanced clinical features but with PSA levels of 10 ng/ml or higher have a biochemical recurrence within 5 years of radiation. This subgroup of patients are appropriate candidates for alternative treatment strategies to improve their cancer control compared with radiation alone.

**Figure 3–21:** Current strategies under investigation to improve tumor control for patients with locally advanced prostate cancer. The two most promising strategies for improving tumor control in patients with locally advanced disease are dose escalation and adjuvant hormone therapy.

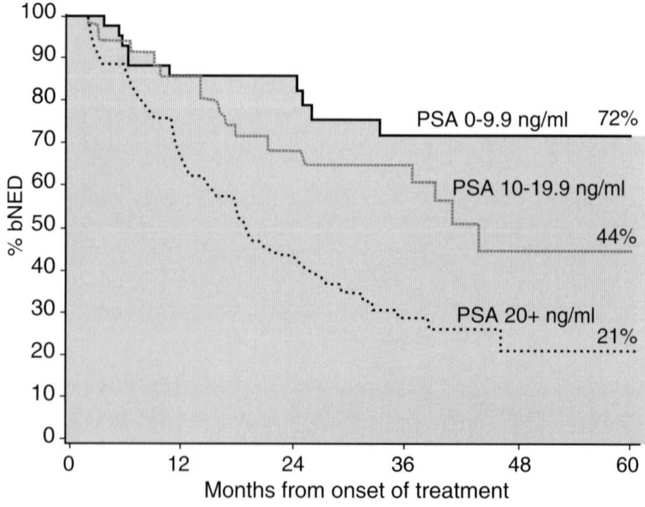


**Figure 3–20**

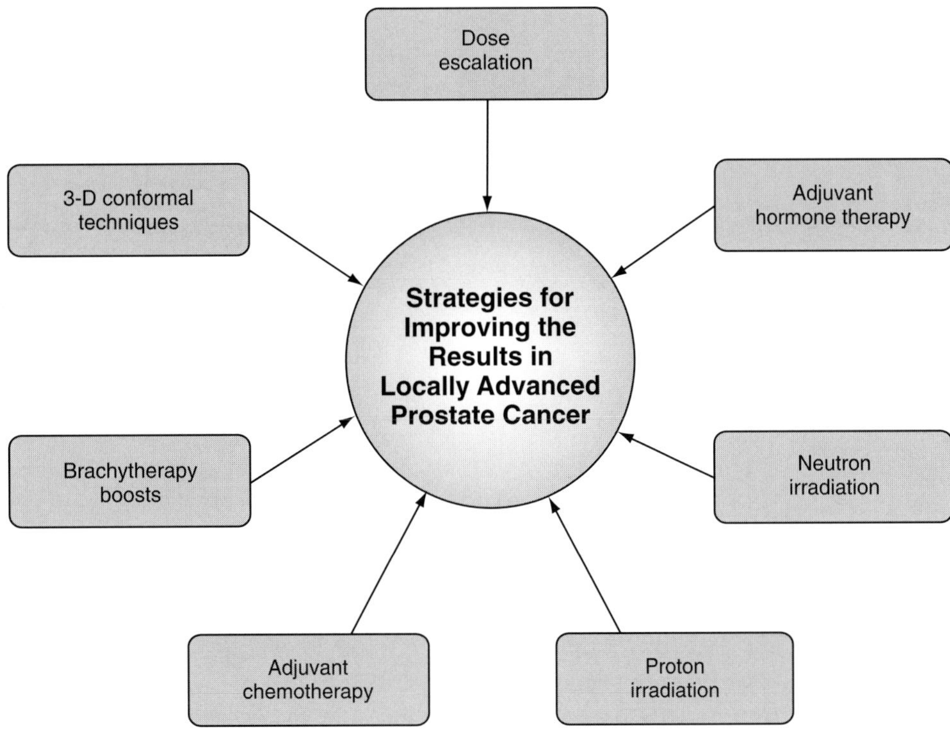


**Figure 3–21**

Dose escalation is based on the principle that higher doses of radiation may result in greater tumor kill. Locally advanced tumors, because of a greater volume of cancer cells, may require higher doses of radiation in order to approach the high rates of tumor control seen with low volume early stage disease. The escalation to these higher doses was dependent on the development of conformal external beam techniques so that the complications to nearby bladder and bowel would remain at acceptable levels. The use of an implant after pelvic external beam radiation to deliver higher doses to locally advanced tumors has also been reported with promising early results.[132, 133] A program for locally advanced tumors combining both of these strategies—conformal external beam radiation and ultrasound-guided temporary high-dose-rate interstitial implants—is now under development at Fox Chase Cancer Center. The use of androgen ablation in combination with external beam radiotherapy depends on the responsiveness of prostate cancer to hormonal manipulation. Several large, prospective randomized trials have demonstrated the efficacy of this treatment combination in locally advanced tumors compared to conventional irradiation alone.[15 17]

Radiation modalities other than conventional high-energy x-ray (also called photon) beams have been tested for the treatment of prostate cancer. Neutron radiation alone or combined with conventional photons have resulted in improved local-regional control compared to conventional photons alone in two separate randomized trials.[134, 135] Proton beam irradiation

combined with conventional photons has been reported with less promising results.[136] These radiation modalities are limited to only a few centers in the United States that have the financial resources for the modern equipment and technical support needed to safely conduct clinical trials.

**Figure 3–22:** Dose escalation: Improved biochemical disease control at 5 years with higher radiation doses. The figure illustrates how the biochemical rates of disease control in patients treated at Fox Chase Cancer Center vary by the given dose of external beam radiation. At 5 years after treatment, higher doses of irradiation have resulted in significantly improved patient outcomes. This benefit to escalating the radiation dose was observed in all three risk categories as defined by the pretreatment PSA levels (<10, 10 to 20, or 20+ ng/ml). The figure shows that patients with locally advanced disease and PSA between 10 and 20 ng/ml appear to have the greatest relative improvement with doses over 75 Gy to the prostate. Conformal radiation techniques are essential when these high doses of radiation are prescribed—normal tissue complications would be unacceptable with conventional radiation techniques at these doses. Additional studies are needed to assess the limits of conformal dose escalation and the durability of these improvements in cancer control. Furthermore, the subgroup of locally advanced patients that will most benefit from this strategy needs to be further defined. (Data from Pinover et al.[137] and Hanks et al.[109])

**Figure 3–23:** Adjuvant hormone therapy before and

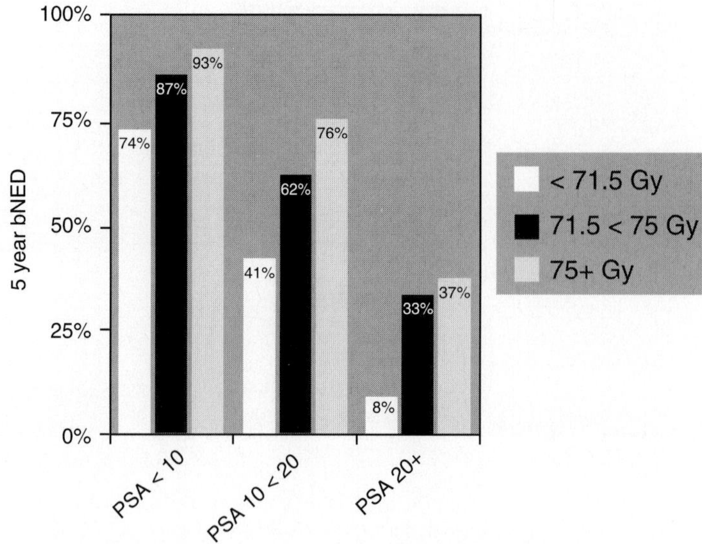



**Figure 3–22**

during radiotherapy for bulky locally advanced tumors: Results of RTOG 86–10. The Radiation Therapy Oncology Group recently reported the results of a large, prospective randomized trial testing the value of neoadjuvant hormone therapy in addition to radiation for bulky locally advanced disease.[15] All patients included in the trial had tumors clinically stage T2B or higher that were 25 cm$^2$ or greater on digital rectal examination. Regional nodes were reported positive in only 8% of the patients, most by clinical criteria, so the actual number with pathologically involved nodes was likely greater in this high-risk group of patients. The randomization was Zoladex (3.6 mg given subcutaneously every 4 weeks) and flutamide (250 mg given orally three times a day) 2 months before and during external beam radiation versus radiation alone. Irradiation consisted of conventional external beam tech-

niques and doses that were standard in the late 1980s—large pelvic fields to 45 ± 1 Gy plus a smaller prostate boost to a total dose of 65 to 70 Gy.

The 5-year actuarial results have been reported for the trial's 456 evaluable patients. The group receiving adjuvant hormones demonstrated a significant improvement in local progression (46% versus 71%, $p <$ 0.001) and progression-free survival (36% versus 15%, $p <$ 0.001) compared to radiation alone. A reduction in distant metastases with adjuvant hormones and radiation (34% versus 41%) did not reach statistical significance ($p = 0.09$), and there was no detectable difference in overall survival (62%, $p = 0.7$) between the two groups. There were no significant increases in major toxicities reported with the addition of adjuvant hormones to irradiation. (Adapted from Pilepich MV, Krall JM, Al-Sarraf M, et al: Androgen deprivation with radi-

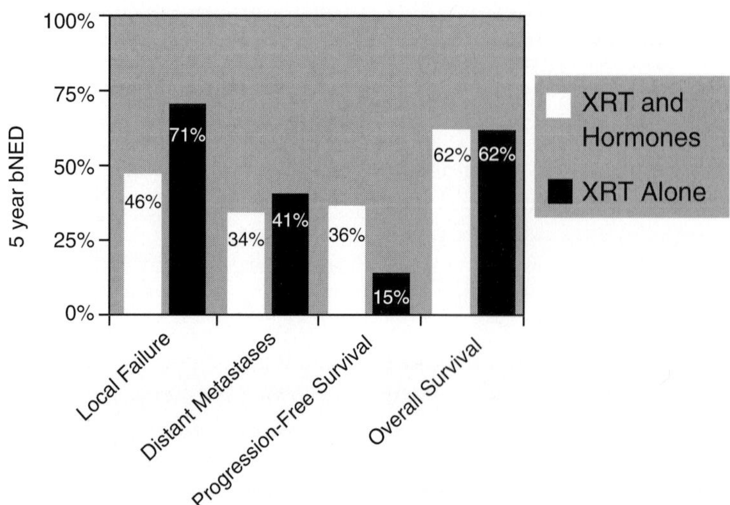



**Figure 3–23**

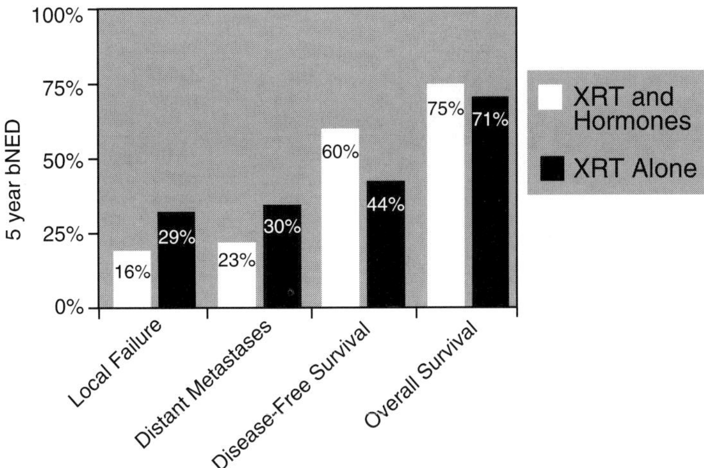


**Figure 3–24**

ation therapy compared with radiation therapy alone for locally advanced prostatic carcinoma: A randomized comparative trial of the Radiation Therapy Oncology Group. Urology 45:616–623, 1995.)

**Figure 3–24:** Adjuvant hormone therapy following radiotherapy for locally advanced prostate cancer: Results of RTOG 85–31. The Radiation Therapy Oncology Group has tested the value of postradiation adjuvant hormonal therapy for locally advanced patients at high risk for relapse.[16] The eligibility characteristics were clinical T3 tumor size, regional lymph node involvement (28% of patients, pathologically confirmed in two thirds), or positive seminal vesicles or surgical margins after prostatectomy (15% of patients). The radiotherapy protocol was similar to RTOG 86–10. The study prospectively randomized patients between immediate Zoladex (3.6 mg given subcutaneously every 4 weeks) for an indefinite period of time after completion of radiation versus starting hormones at the time of first relapse.

The 5-year actuarial results have been reported for the trial's 945 evaluable patients and are shown here.[16] The patients receiving immediate postradiation goserelin had significantly fewer local failures and distant failures. Moreover, these reductions in failures translated into a significantly better disease-free survival rate both by clinical and PSA-based criteria. A small difference in survival favoring the group with immediate hormone therapy did not reach statistical significance. However, the subgroup of patients with centrally reviewed poorly differentiated tumors (Gleason 8, 9, or 10) treated with hormones did show a statistically significant survival benefit at 5 years compared to the radiation alone arm (66% versus 55%, $p = 0.03$). The similar overall survival rate between the two groups taken as a whole at this early follow-up may be due to the high salvagability of patients failing observation with the late addition of goserelin—a sig-

nificant survival benefit for the whole group may become apparent with longer follow-up. (Adapted from Pilepich et al.[16])

**Figure 3–25:** Survival benefit with adjuvant hormone therapy during and after radiotherapy for locally advanced tumors: Results from the EORTC. Only one prospective randomized study has demonstrated an overall survival benefit to adjuvant hormonal therapy for locally advanced disease.[17] The EORTC analyzed 401 patients with high-grade or extracapsular disease randomized to receive radiotherapy alone or with adjuvant androgen therapy. In this study, goserelin was given during and after radiation for a total of 3 years (1 month of antiandrogen cyproterone acetate was given starting 1 week before goserelin).

The initial results were reported in the *New England Journal of Medicine* after a median follow-up of 45 months. Patients receiving hormones had an improved overall survival rate (Fig. 3–25A) compared with radiotherapy alone. Among 5-year survivors, the disease-free rate also improved (Fig. 3–25B) for patients receiving hormones. Updated results (with a median follow-up of 61 months) have recently been reported with 5-year local control rates of 79% versus 97% ($p < 0.001$), disease-free survival rates of 40% versus 75% ($p < 0.001$) and 5-year survival rates of 62% versus 78% ($p < 0.001$) all favoring combined modality treatment.[18]

In considering these prospective randomized trials for locally advanced disease, the optimal timing before, during, and after radiation for adjuvant hormones remains unclear. In addition, the optimal duration of adjuvant hormones has yet to be determined, but so far a benefit in survival has been seen only with a prolonged (3-year) course.[17] The RTOG has recently completed another prospective randomized trial (92–02) that was successful in accruing over 1500 patients with tumors at clinical stage T2C or higher. All patients received flutamide and Zoladex 2 months prior to and

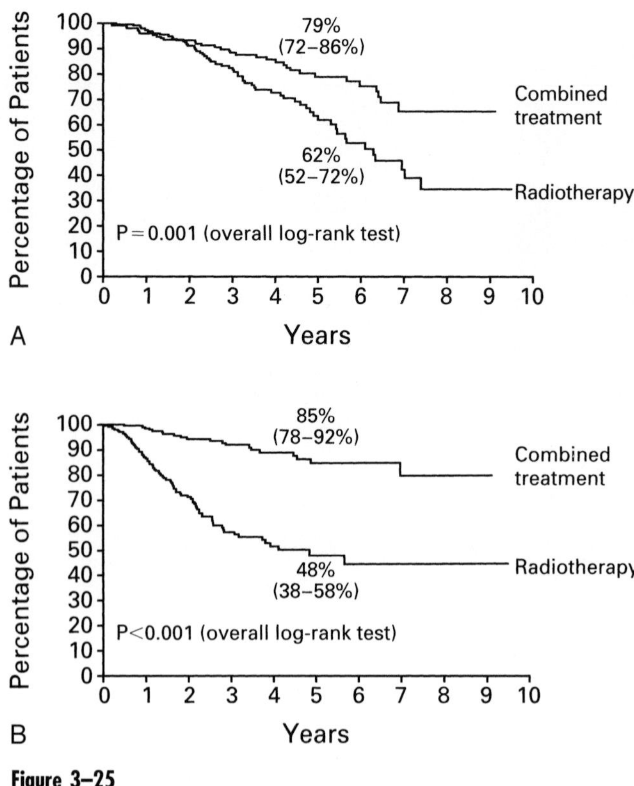

Figure 3–25

during radiation as in RTOG 86–10, and then were randomized to observation or adjuvant Zoladex as in RTOG 85–31 but limited to 2 years. The early results have confirmed improved disease-free survival, and higher overall survival in high-grade tumors, with the hormones given long-term compared to those given short-term. (From Bolla M, Gonzales D, Warde P, et al: Improved survival in patients with locally advanced prostate cancer treated with radiotherapy and goserelin. N Engl J Med 337:295–300, 1997. Copyright 1997 Massachusetts Medical Society.)

**Figure 3–26:** Improvement in 3-year biochemical freedom from disease for patients with locally ad-

vanced prostate cancer treated with external beam radiation and adjuvant hormone deprivation. The use of radiation and adjuvant hormones has been associated with an improvement in bNED outcome in patients with locally advanced disease at Fox Chase Cancer Center compared with radiation alone. The bNED outcomes are approximately 20 to 25% higher for patients with any one of these three characteristics treated with adjuvant hormones in addition to external beam radiation—patients with palpable tumor size T2B or T3, Gleason score 7 to 10, or pretreatment PSA levels over 15 ng/ml.[138] The greatest benefit in bNED control with adjuvant hormones was seen in those patients with all three of these clinical factors (69% versus 29%, $p = 0.003$). The use of adjuvant hormones is a strong independent prognostic factor for outcome on multivariate analysis. Longer observation of these patients will show whether the figures remain separated, suggesting an increase in cures with adjuvant hormones, or eventually meet, suggesting a delay in time to failure with adjuvant hormones. (Adapted from Anderson PR, Hanlon AL, Movsas B, et al: Prostate cancer patient subsets showing improved bNED control with adjuvant androgen deprivation. Int J Radiat Oncol Biol Phys 39:1025–1030, 1997.)

**Table 3–9:** Table 3–9 gives the 5- and 10-year survival rates in node-positive prostate cancer.[51–54, 139–143] Metastatic spread of disease to regional lymph nodes, even in the absence of clinical distant metastases, is usually an indicator of systemic disease at time of presentation. In pathologically confirmed node-positive patients, the risk of distant metastases is over 40% at 5 years and as high as 80% to 90% at 10 years. It is not unexpected that few are cured by surgery or radiation alone.[128, 140, 141, 144] However, half of the patients treated by hormonal therapy alone in the absence of local treatment experience a clinical local failure within 8 years.[143] Any potentially curative approach to treatment would need to address both the high risk of local and distant disease progression.

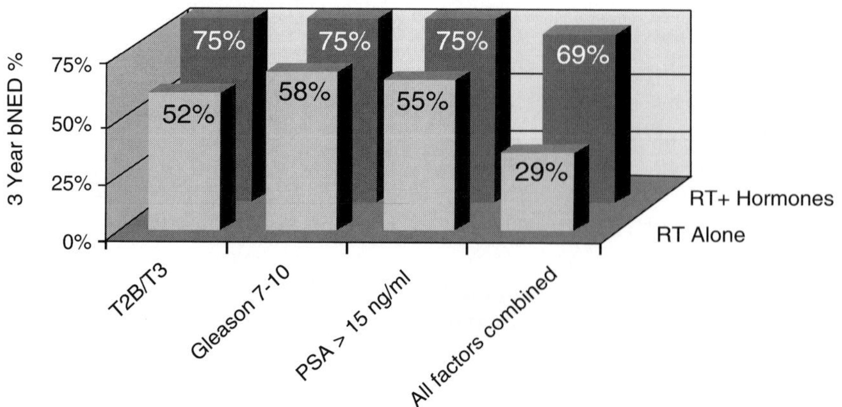


Figure 3–26

**TABLE 3–9**

## SURVIVAL RATES FOR NODE-POSITIVE PROSTATE CANCER

| | | OVERALL SURVIVAL (%) | | |
| SERIES | NO. OF PTS. | Radiation 5 yr/10 yr | Hormones 5 yr/10 yr | Radiation and Hormones 5 yr/10 yr |
| --- | --- | --- | --- | --- |
| Anscher and Prosnitz[139] | 24 | 29*/— | — | — |
| Gervasi et al.[140] | 152 | 65/32 | — | — |
| Hanks et al.[141] | 90 | 63/29 | — | — |
| Lawton et al.[142] | 56 | 76/33 | — | — |
| Zagars et al.[143] | 179 | — | 85/57† | — |
| Sands et al.[51] | 208 | — | 90‡/— | 100‡/— |
| Lawton et al.[52] | 173§ | 65/— | — | 73/— |
| Whittington et al.[53] | 71 | 0/— | — | 94/84† |
| Wiegel and Bressel[54] | 70 | — | — | 78/45 |

*5-year median follow-up.
†8-year result.
‡4-year result.
§Includes patients treated with prostatectomy.
*Note:* — indicates no data.

As shown in Table 3–9, long-term survival remains possible for many patients who present with node-positive prostate cancer. Several series have demonstrated promising results with the combination of radiation and androgen therapy for node-positive prostate cancer.[51–54] A randomized trial with a subgroup of 173 patients with positive nodes has been reported recently in the overall results from RTOG 85–31.[52] This trial included 173 randomized patients with pathologically confirmed positive regional lymph nodes to external beam radiation and immediate hormone therapy versus radiation and delayed androgen therapy only after relapse. The node-positive patients receiving radiation and hormones had an improvement in 5-year biochemical progression-free survival (55% versus 11%, $p = 0.0001$) and overall survival (73% versus 65%, $p$ value not significant). Further randomized studies are needed to establish whether there is an advantage in terms of quality of life or survival to early treatment with aggressive combined modality therapy for node-positive disease.

## PSA Failure after External Beam Radiation

**Figure 3–27:** Management of a PSA failure after external beam radiation therapy. Recurrence after external beam radiation is heralded by a rising PSA level in the absence of clinical disease in the vast majority of patients. The rate of failure in the prostate ranges from 8 to 48% for T1 to T3, NX, or N0 disease after radiation, depending on the initial PSA and stage of disease.[29,] [33, 34, 114] Routine prostate biopsies in the absence of a biochemical failure are not recommended—as many as one third of patients with positive prostate biopsies after radiation will convert to negative with 2 or more years of observation.[145] This change is likely due to inaccuracy in histologically separating viable tumor cells from lethally damaged cells after radiation. In addition, only a minority of patients with a positive biopsy will subsequently develop a local failure or have a symptomatic local failure in the absence of distant metastatic disease.[145] An isolated PSA failure may be appropriately managed with immediate androgen ablation, or delayed therapy until subsequent clinical failure.

Aggressive local salvage therapy after radiation may be indicated for a small subset of patients with a clinically isolated prostate-only failure. In this setting, radical prostatectomy or prostate brachytherapy have been associated with comparable rates of local control over 98%, and rates of 5-year bNED survival rates from 33% to 55%.[146–148] Prognostic factors include pathologically organ-confined recurrent disease (only known in surgical series), PSA level at time of salvage treatment below 10 ng/ml, and PSA response after the procedure. Serious perioperative complications after prostatectomy and subsequent incontinence are seen in half or more of patients previously irradiated.[146, 148] Brachytherapy has been reported to be better tolerated than prostatectomy in this setting with perioperative complications in one third and subsequent incontinence in 6% of patients.[147] Cryosurgery is presently under investigation and may be another option for local salvage of selected patients.

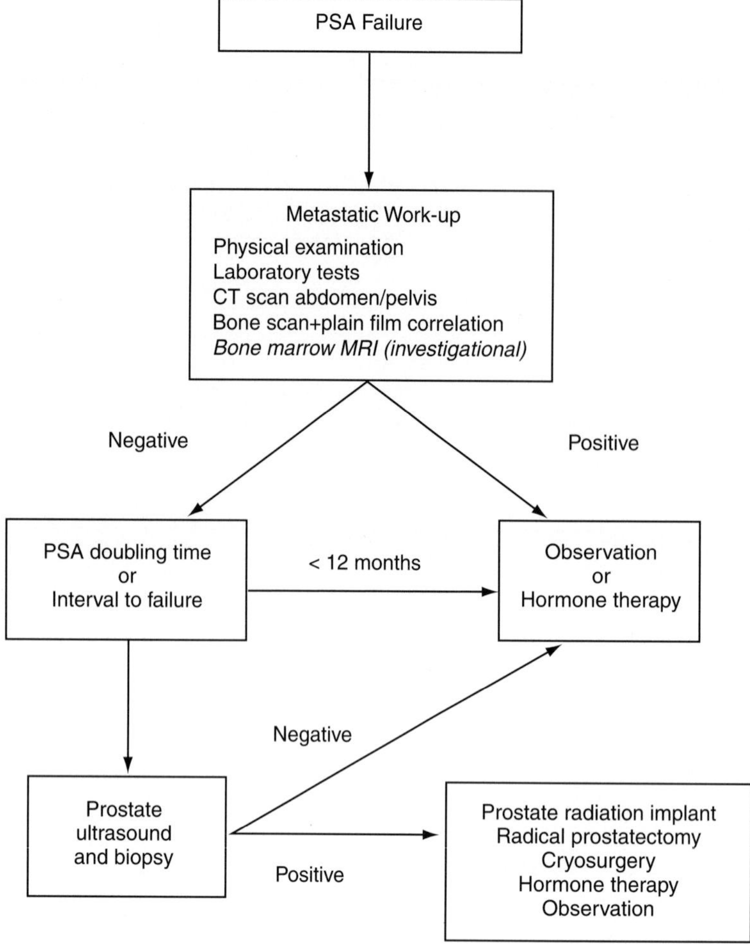


**Figure 3–27**

## POST-PROSTATECTOMY RADIATION THERAPY

**Figure 3–28:** Indications for adjuvant radiation after radical prostatectomy. Adjuvant pelvic radiation therapy is often used to treat residual microscopic disease in the pelvis after radical prostatectomy. Pathologic findings associated with an increased risk of local recurrence after radical prostatectomies are extracapsular tumor extension, positive surgical margins, and seminal vesicle invasion.[42, 44, 45, 47, 48] Radiation therapy can be used as an adjuvant to improve the local control of those patients who are at increased risk for pelvic failure after surgery. Adjuvant radiotherapy is also indicated for selected patients with a detectable PSA level after surgery, principally those in whom the PSA level and pathologic characteristics are suggestive of isolated local residual disease. Radiotherapy also may be used for the salvage treatment of palpable recurrence in the prostatic bed. A prospective randomized trial is under way to further assess the benefit of postprostatectomy radiation for pathologic stage C disease.

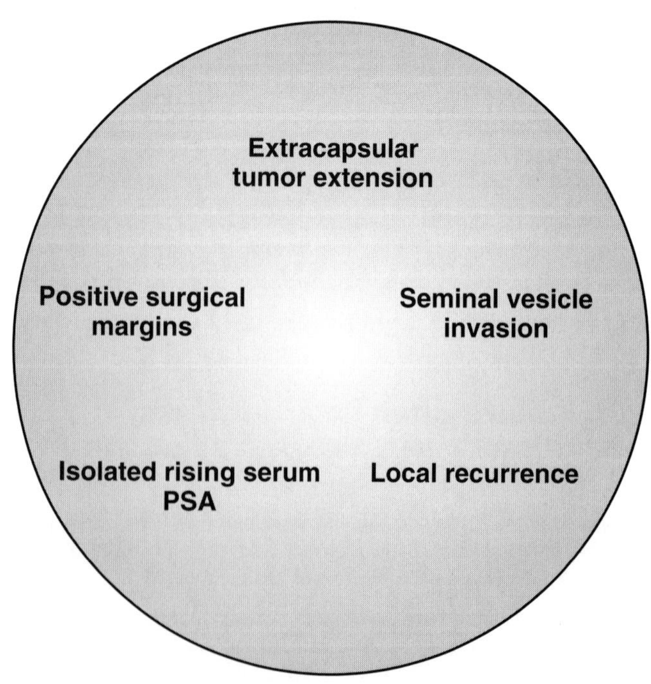


**Figure 3–28**

**TABLE 3–10**

**LOCAL CONTROL WITH ADJUVANT RADIATION AFTER PROSTATECTOMY FOR T3 PROSTATE CANCER**

| | | | LOCAL CONTROL | | | |
|---|---|---|---|---|---|---|
| AUTHOR | TREATMENT | NO. OF PTS. | 5 yrs | 10 yrs | 15 yrs | *p* value |
| Anscher et al.[47] | Prostatectomy | 113 | 80% | 60% | 53% | |
| | Prostatectomy + radiation | 46 | 96% | 92% | 82% | 0.0002 |
| Cheng et al.[45] | Prostatectomy | 660 | 84% | 68% | — | |
| | Prostatectomy + radiation | 131 | 100% | 86% | — | <0.05 |
| Meier et al.[44] | Prostatectomy | 39 | 85% | 69% | 48% | |
| | Prostatectomy + radiation | 19 | 94% | 94% | 94% | <0.05 |
| Schild et al.[48] | Prostatectomy | 228 | 83% | — | — | |
| | Prostatectomy + radiation | 60 | 100% | — | — | 0.02 |
| Shevlin et al.[42] | Prostatectomy | 31 | 80% | 72% | — | |
| | Prostatectomy + radiation | 16 | 100% | 100% | — | 0.03 |

*Note:* — indicates no data.

**Table 3–10:** Table 3–10 gives the improvement in local control with adjuvant radiation after prostatectomy for pathologic T3 prostate cancer.[42, 44, 45, 47, 48] The results from six series that retrospectively compare similar cohorts of patients treated at the same institution by radical prostatectomy with or without adjuvant radiation are shown. All patients had pathologic risk factors for recurrence after prostatectomy of extracapsular tumor extension, positive surgical margins, or seminal vesicle invasion. In those patients with pathologic T3–T4 disease after prostatectomy, adjuvant radiation was associated with significant reductions in the incidence of local recurrence that persist up to 15 years after surgery.

**Table 3–11:** PSA elevation after radical prostatectomy may indicate isolated local-regional or distant recurrence, depending on whether it develops slowly or quickly (Table 3–11). As is the case for patients treated by radiotherapy, the predominant first pattern of failure after radical prostatectomy has become an elevation of PSA in the absence of clinical or radiographic evidence pointing to the location of disease.[101, 102] The pathologic findings at surgery, time to PSA detection, and pattern of PSA level rise are used to identify those patients who are most likely to have isolated pelvic disease and those who have a component of subclinical distant metastases.[46, 149]

Adjuvant radiotherapy has high initial response rates in reducing the PSA level when detectable after surgery,[43, 46, 49, 50] and as discussed in Figure 3–28, radiation can reduce the risk of local failure in the tumor bed.[42, 44, 45, 47, 48] Both observations are presumably due to the sterilization of microscopic residual disease in the pelvis. Theoretically, by preventing subsequent seeding of distant metastases by isolated residual pelvic disease, adjuvant radiotherapy could result in an improvement in overall survival for these patients when compared to surgery alone. Some studies have shown this local control benefit may translate into a benefit in overall freedom from failure.[48, 150] However, most series have not demonstrated a reduction in distant metastases or improvement in overall survival with adjuvant radiotherapy.[42, 44, 45, 47, 48] Most of these studies have not had sufficient numbers of patients selected for high probability of isolated local residual disease to detect such a benefit. Therefore, the existence of a benefit to adjuvant radiotherapy for more than improving local control remains controversial.

## Palliation of Metastatic Disease

**Figure 3–29:** Palliation of prostate cancer metastatic to bone. Radiation therapy has an important role in

**TABLE 3–11**

**ISOLATED ELEVATED PSA LEVELS AFTER PROSTATECTOMY: COMPARISON OF LOCAL-REGIONAL AND DISTANT FAILURES**

| ISOLATED LOCAL-REGIONAL FAILURE | DISTANT +/− LOCAL-REGIONAL FAILURE |
|---|---|
| Slow rise of PSA | Rapid rise of PSA |
| Gleason score 2–7 | Gleason score 8–10 |
| Negative lymph nodes | Positive lymph nodes |
| Positive surgical margins | Negative surgical margins |
| No seminal vesicle invasion | Seminal vesicle invasion |
| PSA rise beyond 6 months | PSA rise within 6 months |

prostate cancer even in the setting of incurable metastatic disease. This figure shows a radiation portal for a patient treated with 2 weeks of palliative radiotherapy for symptomatic metastases to the thoracolumbar spine, causing pain and compression of the epidural space.

There are many indications for palliative radiation in prostate cancer. External beam radiation is the gold standard of treatment for painful bony metastases, with over 80% of patients reporting partial or complete relief of pain.[151] Treatment is also employed postoperatively for bony metastases causing pathologic fracture or impending fracture of a weight-bearing bone. Emergent radiotherapy is critical in the reversal or prevention of neurologic symptoms due to spinal cord compression by vertebral body metastases. Pathologic adenopathy may also cause pain or local obstruction that can be alleviated with palliative radiotherapy.

## REFERENCES

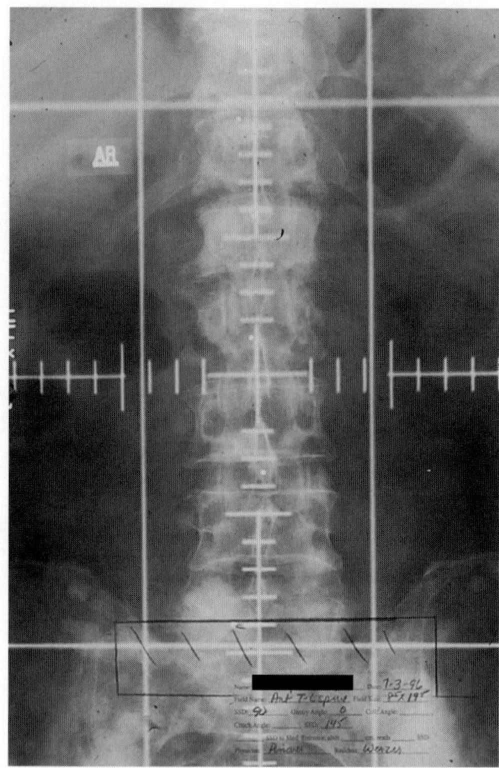

**Figure 3–29**



1. Roentgen WC: On a new kind of rays (preliminary communication). Translation of a paper read before the physikalische-medicinischen Gesellschaft of Würzburg on December 28, 1895. Br J Radiol 4:32, 1931.
2. Herbst RH, Polkey HJ: Prostatic malignancy. In Ballenger EG, Frontz WA, Hamer HG, et al (eds): History of Urology. Baltimore, Williams & Wilkins, 1933, pp 187–208.
3. Young HH: The early diagnosis and cure of cancer of the prostate: Being a study of 40 cases and presentation of a radical operation which was carried out in 4 cases. Bull Johns Hopkins Hosp 18:315–321, 1905.
4. Barringer BS: Radium in the treatment of carcinoma of the bladder and prostate. JAMA 68:1227, 1917.
5. Huggins C, Hodges CV: Studies on prostatic cancer. I. The effect of castration, of estrogens and of androgen injections on serum phosphatases in metastatic cancer of the prostate. Cancer Res 1:293–297, 1941.
6. Millin T: Retropubic prostatectomy, new extravesical technique: Report on 20 cases. Lancet 2:693–696, 1945.
7. Bagshaw MA, Kaplan HS, Sagerman RH: Linear accelerator supervoltage radiotherapy. VII. Carcinoma of the prostate. Radiology 85:121–129, 1965.
8. Gleason D, Mellinger G, Veterans Administration Cooperative Urological Research Group: Prediction of prognosis for prostatic carcinoma by combined histological grading and clinical staging. J Urol 111:58–64, 1974.
9. Papsidero LD, Wang MC, Valenzuela LA, et al: A prostate antigen in the sera of prostate cancer patients. Cancer Res 40:2428, 1980.
10. Walsh PC, Lepor H, Eggleston JC: Radical prostatectomy with preservation of sexual function: Anatomical and pathologic consideration. Prostate 4:473–485, 1983.
11. Ten Haken RK, Perez-Tamayo C, Tesser RJ, et al: Boost treatment of the prostate using shaped, fixed fields. Int J Radiat Oncol Biol Phys 16:193–200, 1989.
12. Soffen EM, Hanks GE, Hwang CC, et al: Conformal static field therapy for low volume, low grade prostate cancer with rigid immobilization. Int J Radiat Oncol Biol Phys 20:141–146, 1991.
13. Leibel SA, Heimann R, Kutcher GJ, et al: Three-dimensional conformal radiation therapy in locally advanced carcinoma of the prostate: Preliminary results of a phase I dose-escalation study. Int J Radiat Oncol Biol Phys 28:55–65, 1993.
14. Blasko JC, Wallner K, Grimm PD, et al: Prostate specific antigen based disease control following ultrasound guided 125iodine implantation for stage T1/T2 prostatic carcinoma. J Urol 154:1096–1099, 1995.
15. Pilepich MV, Krall JM, Al-Sarraf M, et al: Androgen deprivation with radiation therapy compared with radiation therapy alone for locally advanced prostatic carcinoma: A randomized comparative trial of the Radiation Therapy Oncology Group. Urology 45:616–623, 1995.
16. Pilepich MV, Caplan R, Byhardt RW, et al: Phase III trial of androgen supression using goserelin in unfavorable-prognosis carcinoma of the prostate treated with definitive radiotherapy: Report of RTOG Protocol 85–31. J Clin Oncol 15:1013–1021, 1997.
17. Bolla M, Gonzales D, Warde P, et al: Improved survival in patients with locally advanced prostate cancer treated with radiotherapy and goserelin. N Engl J Med 337:295–300, 1997.
18. Bolla M, Collete L, Gonzales D, et al: Long-term results of immediate adjuvant hormonal therapy with goserelin in patients with locally advanced prostate cancer treated with radiotherapy, a phase III EORTC Study. Int J Radiat Oncol Biol Phys 45:147, 1999.
19. Mettlin CJ, Murphy GP, McGinnis LS, et al: The National Cancer Data Base report on prostate cancer. Cancer 76:1104–1112, 1995.
20. Mettlin CJ, Murphy GP, Cunningham MP, et al: The National Cancer Data Base report on race, age, and region variations in prostate cancer treatment. Cancer 80:1261–1266, 1997.
21. Partin AW, Kattan MW, Subong ENP, et al: Combination of prostate-specific antigen, clinical stage, and Gleason score to predict pathological stage of localized prostate cancer: A multi-institutional update. JAMA 277:1445–1451, 1997.
22. Millikan R, Logothetis C: Update of the NCCN guidelines for treatment of prostate cancer. Oncology 11:180–193, 1997.
23. Jones GW: Prospective, conservative management of localized prostate cancer. Cancer 70:307–310, 1992.
24. Warner J, Whitmore WF Jr: Expectant management of clinically localized prostatic cancer. J Urol 152:1761–1765, 1994.
25. Johansson J, Holmberg L, Johansson S, et al: Fifteen-year survival in prostate cancer. A prospective, population-based study in Sweden. JAMA 277:467–471, 1997.
26. Albertsen PC, Hanley JA, Gleason DF, et al: Competing risk analysis of men aged 55 to 74 years at diagnosis managed conservatively for clinically localized prostate cancer. JAMA 280:975–980, 1998.
27. National Institutes of Health: Consensus development confer-

ence statement. Washington, DC, U.S. Government Printing Office 6, 1987.

28. Kaplan ID, Cox RS, Bagshaw MA: Radiotherapy for prostatic cancer: Patient selection and the impact of local control. Urology 43:634–639, 1994.

29. Zagars GK, von Eschenbach AC, Ayala AG: Prognostic factors in prostate cancer. Analysis of 874 patients treated with radiation therapy. Cancer 72:1709–1725, 1993.

30. Freedman GM, Hanlon AL, Lee WR, et al: Young patients with prostate cancer have an outcome justifying their treatment with external beam radiation. Int J Radiat Oncol Biol Phys 35:243–250, 1996.

31. Hanks GE, Krall JM, Hanlon AL, et al: Patterns of care and RTOG studies in prostate cancer: Long-term survival, hazard rate observations, and possibilities of cure. Int J Radiat Oncol Biol Phys 28:39–45, 1994.

32. del Regato JA, Trailins AH, Pittman DD: Twenty years follow-up of patients with inoperable cancer of the prostate (stage C) treated by radiotherapy: Report of a national cooperative study. Int J Radiat Oncol Biol Phys 26:197–201, 1993.

33. Lee RJ, Sause WT: Surgically staged patients with prostatic carcinoma treated with definitive radiotherapy: Fifteen-year results. Urology 43:640–644, 1994.

34. Kuban DA, El-Mahdi AM, Schellhammer PF: Prostate-specific antigen for pretreatment prediction and posttreatment evaluation of outcome after definitive irradiation for prostate cancer. Int J Radiat Oncol Biol Phys 32:307–316, 1995.

35. Bagshaw MA, Kaplan ID, Cox RC: Radiation therapy for localized disease. Cancer 71:939–952, 1993.

36. Perez CA, Lee HK, Georgiou A, et al: Technical and tumor-related factors affecting outcome of definitive irradiation for localized carcinoma of the prostate. Int J Radiat Oncol Biol Phys 26:581–591, 1993.

37. Rosenzweig KE, Morgan WR, Lytton B, et al: Prostate specific antigen following radiotherapy for local prostate cancer. J Urol 153:1561–1564, 1995.

38. Elder JS, Jewitt MJ, Walsh PC: Radical perineal prostatectomy for clinical stage B2 carcinoma of the prostate. J Urol 127:704–706, 1986.

39. Bigg SW, Kavoussi LR, Catalona WJ: Role of nerve-sparing radical prostatectomy for clinical stage B2 prostate cancer. J Urol 144:1420–1424, 1990.

40. Gibbons RP: Localized prostate carcinoma. Cancer 72:2865–2872, 1993.

41. Partin AW, Lee BR, Carmichael M, et al: Radical prostatectomy for high grade disease: A reevaluation 1994. J Urol 151:1583–1586, 1994.

42. Shevlin BE, Mittal BB, Brand WN, et al: The role of adjuvant irradiation following primary prostatectomy, based on histopathologic extent of tumor. Int J Radiat Oncol Biol Phys 16:1425–1430, 1989.

43. Lange PH, Lightner DJ, Medini E, et al: The effect of radiation therapy after radical prostatectomy in patients with elevated prostate specific antigen levels. J Urol 144:927–933, 1990.

44. Meier R, Mark R, St. Royal L, et al: Postoperative radiation therapy after radical prostatectomy for prostate carcinoma. Cancer 70:1960–1966, 1992.

45. Cheng WS, Frydenberg M, Bergstralh EJ, et al: Radical prostatectomy for pathologic stage C prostate cancer. Influence of pathologic variables and adjuvant treatment on disease outcome. Urology 42:283–291, 1993.

46. McCarthy JF, Catalona WJ, Hudson MA: Effect of radiation therapy on detectable serum prostate specific antigen levels following radical prostatectomy: Early versus delayed treatment. J Urol 151.1575–1578, 1994.

47. Anscher MS, Robertson CN, Prosnitz LR: Adjuvant radiotherapy for pathologic stage T3/4 adenocarcinoma of the prostate: Ten-year update. Int J Radiat Oncol Biol Phys 33:37–43, 1995.

48. Schild SE, Wong WW, Grado GL, et al: The results of radical retropublic prostatectomy and adjuvant therapy for pathologic stage C prostate cancer. Int J Radiat Oncol Biol Phys 34:535–541, 1996.

49. Wu JJ, King SC, Montana GS, et al: The efficacy of postprostatectomy radiotherapy in patients with an isolated elevation of serum prostate-specific antigen. Int J Radiat Oncol Biol Phys 32:317–323, 1995.

50. Schild SE, Buskirk SJ, Wong WW, et al: The use of radiotherapy for patients with isolated elevation of serum prostate specific antigen following radical prostatectomy. J Urol 156:1725–1729, 1996.

51. Sands ME, Pollack A, Zagars GK: Influence of radiotherapy on node-positive prostate cancer treated with androgen ablation. Int J Radiat Oncol Biol Phys 31:13–19, 1995.

52. Lawton CA, Winter K, Byhardt R, et al: Androgen supression plus radiation vs. radiation alone for patients with D1 (pN+) adenocarcinoma of the prostate (results based on a national prospective randomized trial, RTOG 85–31). Int J Radiat Oncol Biol Phys 38:931–939, 1997.

53. Whittington R, Malkowicz SB, Machtay M, et al: The use of combined radiation therapy and hormonal therapy in the management of lymph node-positive prostate cancer. Int J Radiat Oncol Biol Phys 39:673–680, 1997.

54. Wiegel T, Bressel M: Influence of the extent of nodal involvement on the outcome in stage D1 prostate cancer. Radiat Oncol Invest 2:144–151, 1994.

55. American Joint Committee on Cancer: Prostate. In Fleming ID, Cooper JS, Henson DE, et al (eds): AJCC Cancer Staging Manual, 5th ed. Philadelphia, Lippincott-Raven, 1997, pp 219–224.

56. Oesterling JE: Prostate specific antigen: Its role in the diagnosis and staging of prostate cancer. Cancer 75:1795–1804, 1995.

57. Kaplan ID, Cox RS, Bagshaw MA: Prostate specific antigen after external beam radiotherapy for prostatic cancer: Follow-up. J Urol 149:519–522, 1993.

58. Lee WR, Hanks GE, Schultheiss TE, et al: Localized prostate cancer treated by external-beam radiotherapy alone: Serum prostate-specific antigen-driven outcome analysis. J Clin Oncol 13:464–469, 1995.

59. Pisansky TM, Chan SS, Earle JD, et al: Prostate-specific antigen as a pre-therapy prognostic factor in patients treated with radiation therapy for clinically localized prostate cancer. J Clin Oncol 11:2158–2167, 1993.

60. Zagars GK, Pollack A: Radiation therapy for T1 and T2 prostate cancer: Prostate-specific antigen and disease outcome. Urology 45:476–483, 1995.

61. Zeitman AL, Coen JJ, Shipley WU: Radical radiation therapy in the management of prostatic adenocarcinoma: The initial prostate specific antigen value as a predictor of treatment outcome. J Urol 151:640–645, 1994.

62. Hanks GE, Hanlon AL, Lee WR, et al: Pretreatment prostate-specific antigen doubling times: Clinical utility of this predictor of prostate cancer behavior. Int J Radiat Oncol Biol Phys 34:549–553, 1996.

63. Rifkin MD, Zerhouni EA, Gatsonis CA, et al: Comparison of magnetic resonance and ultrasonography in staging early prostate cancer: Results of a multiinstitutional cooperative trial. N Engl J Med 323:621–626, 1990.

64. Hanks GE, Krall JM, Pilepich MV, et al: Comparison of pathologic and clinical evaluation of lymph nodes in prostate cancer: Implications of RTOG data for patient management and trial design and stratification. Int Radiat Oncol Biol Phys 23:293–298, 1992.

65. Chybowski FM, Larson Keller JJ, Bergstralh EJ, et al: Predicting radionuclide bone scan findings in patients with newly diagnosed, untreated prostate cancer: Prostate specific antigen is superior to all other clinical parameters. J Urol 145:313–318, 1991.

66. Vijayakumar V, Vijayakumar S, Quadri SF, et al: Can prostate-specific antigen levels predict bone scan evidence of metastases in newly diagnosed prostate cancer? Am J Clin Oncol 17:432–436, 1994.

67. Freedman GM, Negendank WG, Hudes GR, et al: Preliminary results of a bone marrow magnetic resonance imaging protocol for patients with high risk prostate cancer. Urology 54:118–123, 1999.

68. Wurzer JC, Al-Saleem TI, Hanlon AL, et al: Histopathologic review of prostate biopsies from patients referred to a comprehensive cancer center. Correlation of pathologic findings, analysis of cost, and impact on treatment. Cancer 83:753–759, 1998.

69. Algan Ö, Hanks GE, Shaer AH: Localization of the prostatic apex for radiation treatment planning. Int J Radiat Oncol Biol Phys 33:925–930, 1995.

70. Lattanzi J, McNeeley S, Pinover W, et al: A comparison of daily

CT localization to a daily ultrasound-based system in prostate cancer. Int J Radiat Oncol Biol Phys 43:719–725, 1999.

71. Sandler HM, Perez-Tamayo C, Ten Haken RK, et al: Dose escalation for stage C (T3) prostate cancer: Minimal rectal toxicity observed using conformal therapy. Radiother Oncol 23:53–54, 1992.

72. Soffen EM, Hanks GE, Hunt MA, et al: Conformal static field radiation therapy treatment of early prostate cancer versus non-conformal techniques: A reduction in acute morbidity. Int J Radiat Oncol Biol Phys 24:485–488, 1992.

73. Talcott JA, Rieker P, Clark JA, et al: Patient-reported symptoms after primary therapy for early prostate cancer: Results of a prospective cohort study. J Clin Oncol 16:275–283, 1998.

74. Lim AJ, Brandon AH, Fiedler J, et al: Quality of life: Radical prostatectomy versus radiation therapy for prostate cancer. J Urol 154:1420–1425, 1995.

75. Lee WR, Schultheiss TE, Hanlon AL, et al: Urinary incontinence following external beam radiotherapy for clinically localized prostate cancer. Urology 48:95–99, 1996.

76. Jønler M, Ritter MA, Brinkmann R, et al: Sequelae of definitive radiation therapy for prostate cancer localized to the pelvis. Urology 44:876–882, 1994.

77. Crook J, Esche B, Futter N: Effect of pelvic radiotherapy for prostate cancer on bowel, bladder, and sexual function: The patient's perspective. Urology 47:387–394, 1996.

78. Green N, Treible D, Wallack H: Prostate cancer: Post-irradiation incontinence. J Urol 144:307–309, 1990.

79. Amdur RJ, Parson JT, Fitzgerald LT, et al: Adenocarcinoma of the prostate treated with external-beam radiation therapy: 5 year minimum follow-up. Radiother Oncol 18:235–246, 1990.

80. Perez CA, Lee HK, Georgiou A, et al: Technical factors affecting morbidity in definitive irradiation for localized carcinoma of the prostate. Int J Radiat Oncol Biol Phys 28:811–819, 1994.

81. Steiner MS, Morton RA, Walsh PC: Impact of anatomical radical prostatectomy on urinary continence. J Urol 145:512, 1991.

82. Fowler FJ Jr, Barry MJ, Lu-Yao G, et al: Patient reported complications and followup treatment after radical prostatectomy. The national Medicare experience: 1988–1990. Urology 42:622–629, 1993.

83. Geary ES, Dendinger TE, Freiha FS, et al: Incontinence and vesical neck strictures following radical retropubic prostatectomy. Urology 45:1000–1006, 1995.

84. Catalona WJ: Surgical management of prostate cancer. Cancer 75:1903–1908, 1995.

85. Eastham JA, Kattan MW, Rogers E, et al: Risk factors for urinary incontinence after radical prostatectomy. J Urol 156:1707–1713, 1996.

86. Vanuytsel L, Ang KK, Vandenbussche L, et al: Radiotherapy in multiple fractions per day for prostatic carcinoma: Late complications. Int J Radiat Oncol Biol Phys 12:1589–1595, 1986.

87. Shipley WU, Zietman AL, Hanks GE, et al: Treatment related sequelae following external beam radiation for prostate cancer: A review with an update in patients with stages T1 and T2 tumor. J Urol 152:1799–1805, 1994.

88. Dicker AP, Zelefsky MJ, Leibel SA, et al: Risk factors for impotence in patients with carcinoma of the prostate treated with three-dimensional conformal radiation therapy. Int J Radiat Oncol Biol Phys 32:191, 1995 (abstract).

89. Helgason ÁR, Fredrikson M, Adolfsson J, et al: Decreased sexual capacity after external radiation therapy for prostate cancer impairs quality of life. Int J Radiat Oncol Biol Phys 32:33–39, 1995.

90. Chinn DM, Holland J, Crownover RL, et al: Potency following high-dose three-dimensional conformal radiotherapy and the impact of prior major urologic surgical procedures in patients treated for prostate cancer. Int J Radiat Oncol Biol Phys 33:15–22, 1995.

91. Nicolaou N, Bruner DW, Hanks GE, et al: Preservation of sexual function in young prostate cancer patients after radiation therapy: A positive factor in choice of a treatment modality. Int J Radiat Oncol Biol Phys 36:270, 1996 (abstract).

92. Mantz CA, Song P, Farhangi E, et al: Potency probability following conformal megavoltage radiotherapy using conventional doses for localized prostate cancer. Int J Radiat Oncol Biol Phys 37:551–557, 1997.

93. Geary ES, Dendinger TE, Freiha FS, et al: Nerve sparing radical prostatectomy: A different view. Urology 154:145–149, 1995.

94. Quinlan DM, Epstein JI, Carter BS, et al: Sexual function following radical prostatectomy: Influence of preservation of neurovascular bundles. J Urol 145:998, 1991.

95. Nicolaou N, Watkins-Bruner D, Hanlon A, et al: Preservation of sexual function and quality of life in younger prostate cancer patients after definitive radiation and androgen deprivation therapy: A pilot study. Proc Am Soc Clin Oncol 17:323a, 1998 (abstract).

96. Schultheiss TE, Lee WR, Hunt MA, et al: Late GI and GU complications in the treatment of prostate cancer. Int J Radiat Oncol Biol Phys 37:3–11, 1997.

97. Teshima T, Hanks GE, Peters RS, et al: Rectal bleeding after conformal 3D treatment of prostate cancer: Time to occurrence, response to treatment and duration of morbidity. Int J Radiat Oncol Biol Phys 39:77–83, 1997.

98. Lee WR, Hanks GE, Hanlon A, et al: Lateral rectal shielding reduces late rectal morbidity following high dose three-dimensional conformal radiation therapy for clinically localized prostate cancer: Further evidence for a significant dose effect. Int J Radiat Oncol Biol Phys 35:251–257, 1996.

99. Fukunaga-Johnson N, Sandler HM, McLaughlin PW, et al: Results of 3D conformal radiotherapy in the treatment of localized prostate cancer. Int J Radiat Oncol Biol Phys 38:311–317, 1997.

100. Zagars GK: Prostate-specific antigen as an outcome variable for T1 and T2 prostate cancer treated by radiation therapy. J Urol 152:1786–1791, 1994.

101. Pound CR, Partin AW, Epstein JI, et al: Prostate-specific antigen after anatomic radical retropubic prostatectomy. Patterns of recurrence and cancer control. Urol Clin North Am 24:395–405, 1997.

102. Catalona WJ, Smith DS: Cancer recurrence and survival rates after anatomic radical retropubic prostatectomy for prostate cancer: Intermediate-term results. J Urol 160:2428–2434, 1998.

103. American Society for Therapeutic Radiology and Oncology Consensus Panel: Consensus statement: Guidelines for PSA following radiation therapy. Int J Radiat Oncol Biol Phys 37:1035–1041, 1997.

104. Hanks GE, Corn BW, Lee WR, et al: External beam irradiation of prostate cancer. Conformal treatment techniques and outcomes for the 1990s. Cancer 75:1972–1977, 1995.

105. Zagars GK, von Eschenbach AC: Prostate-specific antigen: An important marker for prostate cancer treated by external beam radiotherapy. Cancer 72:538–548, 1993.

106. Pinover WH, Hanlon A, Lee WR, et al: Prostate carcinoma patients upstaged by imaging and treated with irradiation. Cancer 77:1334–1341, 1996.

107. Bonin SR, Hanlon AL, Lee WR, et al: Evidence of increased failure in the treatment of prostate carcinoma patients who have perineural invasion treated with three-dimensional conformal radiation therapy. Cancer 79:75–80, 1997.

108. Gauwitz MD, Pollack A, El-Naggar AK, et al: The prognostic significance of DNA ploidy in clinically localized prostate cancer treated with radiation therapy. Int J Radiat Oncol Biol Phys 28:821–828, 1994.

109. Hanks GE, Hanlon AL, Schultheiss TE, et al: Dose escalation with 3D conformal treatment: Five year outcomes, treatment optimization, and future directions. Int J Radiat Oncol Biol Phys 41:501–510, 1998.

110. Lee WR, Hanlon AL, Hanks GE: Systematic biopsies: Do they add prognostic information in men with clinically localized prostate cancer treated with radiation therapy alone? Radiology 198:439–442, 1996.

111. Stamey TA, Ferrari MK, Schmid H: The value of serial prostate specific antigen determinations 5 years after radiotherapy: Steeply increasing values characterize 80% of patients. J Urol 150:1856–1859, 1993.

112. Hancock SL, Cox RS, Bagshaw MA: Prostate specific antigen after radiotherapy for prostate cancer: A reevaluation of long-term biochemical control and the kinetics of recurrence in patients treated at Stanford University. J Urol 154:1412–1417, 1995.

113. Pollack A, Zagars GK, Smith LG, et al: Preliminary results of a randomized radiotherapy dose-escalation study comparing 70

Gy with 78 Gy for prostate cancer. J Clin Oncol 18:3904–3911, 2000.

114. Zietman AL, Coen JJ, Dallow KC, et al: The treatment of prostate cancer by conventional radiation therapy: An analysis of long-term outcome. Int J Radiat Oncol Biol Phys 32:287–292, 1995.

115. Hanks GE, Hanlon AL, Schultheiss TE, et al: Conformal external beam treatment of prostate cancer. Urology 50:87–92, 1997.

116. Keyser D, Kupelian PA, Zippe CD, et al: Stage T1-2 prostate cancer with pretreatment prostate-specific antigen level ≤ 10 ng/ml: Radiation therapy or surgery? Int J Radiat Oncol Biol Phys 38:723–729, 1997.

117. Zelefsky MJ, Leibel SA, Gaudin PB, et al: Dose escalation with three-dimensional conformal radiation therapy affects the outcome in prostate cancer. Int J Radiat Oncol Biol Phys 41:491–500, 1998.

118. D'Amico AV, Whittington R, Malkowicz SB, et al: Biochemical outcome after radical prostatectomy, external beam radiation therapy, or interstitial radiation therapy for clinically localized prostate cancer. JAMA 280:969–974, 1998.

119. Kleer E, Larson-Keller JJ, Zincke H, et al: Ability of preoperative prostate-specific antigen value to predict pathologic stage and DNA ploidy. Influence of clinical stage and tumor grade. Urology 41:207–216, 1993.

120. Harlan L, Brawley O, Pommerenke F, et al: Geographic, age, and racial variation in the treatment of local/regional carcinoma of the prostate. J Clin Oncol 13:93–100, 1995.

121. Johnstone PAS, Riffenburgh R, Saunders EL, et al: Grading inaccuracies in diagnostic biopsies revealing prostatic adenocarcinoma: Implications for definitive radiation therapy. Int J Radiat Oncol Biol Phys 32:479–482, 1995.

122. Hanks GE, Asbell S, Krall JM, et al: Outcome of lymph node dissection negative T1b, T2 (A-2, B) prostate cancer treated with external beam radiation therapy in RTOG 77–06. Int J Radiat Oncol Biol Phys 21:1099–1103, 1991.

123. Hanks GE: External beam radiation treatment for prostate cancer: Still the gold standard. Oncology 6:79–89, 1992.

124. Austin JP, Convery K: Age-race interaction in prostatic adenocarcinoma treated with external beam irradiation. Am J Clin Oncol 16:140–145, 1993.

125. Morton JD, Peschel RE: Iodine-125 implants versus external beam therapy for stages A2, B, and C prostate cancer. Int J Radiat Oncol Biol Phys 14:1153–1157, 1988.

126. Kuban DA, Anas EM, Schellhammer PF: I-125 interstitial implantation for prostate cancer: What have we learned 10 years later? Cancer 63:2415–2420, 1989.

127. Koprowski CD, Berkenstock KG, Borofski AM, et al: External beam irradiation versus 125 iodine implant in the definitive treatment of prostate carcinoma. Int J Radiat Oncol Biol Phys 21:955–960, 1991.

128. Leibel SA, Fuks Z, Zelefsky MJ, et al: The effects of local and regional treatment on the metastatic outcome in prostatic carcinoma with pelvic lymph node involvement. Int J Radiat Oncol Biol Phys 28:7–16, 1993.

129. Wallner K, Roy J, Harrison L: Tumor control and morbidity following transperineal iodine 125 implantation for stage T1/T2 prostatic carcinoma. J Clin Oncol 14:449–453, 1996.

130. Beyer DC, Priestley JB Jr: Biochemical disease-free survival following 125I prostate implantation. Int J Radiat Oncol Biol Phys 37:559–563, 1997.

131. Storey MR, Landgren RC, Cottone JL, et al: Transperineal 125 iodine implantation for treatment of clinically localized prostate cancer: 5-year tumor control and morbidity. Int J Radiat Oncol Biol Phys 43:565–570, 1999.

132. Dattoli M, Wallner K, Sorace R, et al: $^{103}$Pd brachytherapy and external beam irradiation for clinically localized, high risk prostatic carcinoma. Int J Radiat Oncol Biol Phys 35:875–879, 1996.

133. Stromberg J, Martinez A, Gonzales J, et al: Ultrasound-guided high dose rate conformal brachytherapy boost in prostate cancer: Treatment description and preliminary results of a phase I/II clinical trial. Int J Radiat Oncol Biol Phys 33:161–171, 1995.

134. Laramore GE, Krall JM, Thomas FJ, et al: Fast neutron radiotherapy for locally advanced prostate cancer. Final report of a Radiation Therapy Oncology Group randomized clinical trial. Am J Clin Oncol 16:164–167, 1993.

135. Russell KJ, Caplan RJ, Laramore GE, et al: Photon versus fast neutron external beam radiotherapy in the treatment of locally advanced prostate cancer: Results of a randomized prospective trial. Int J Radiat Oncol Biol Phys 28:47–54, 1994.

136. Shipley WU, Verhey LJ, Munzenrider JE, et al: Advanced prostate cancer: The results of a randomized comparative trial of high dose irradiation boosting with conformal protons compared with conventional dose irradiation using photons alone. Int J Radiat Oncol Biol Phys 32:3–12, 1995.

137. Pinover WH, Hanlon AL, Horwitz EM, et al: Defining the appropriate dose for prostate cancer patients with PSA < 10 ng/ml. Int J Radiat Oncol Biol Phys 42:142, 1998 (abstract).

138. Anderson PR, Hanlon AL, Movsas B, et al: Prostate cancer patient subsets showing improved bNED control with adjuvant androgen deprivation. Int J Radiat Oncol Biol Phys 39:1025–1030, 1997.

139. Anscher MS, Prosnitz LR: Prognostic significance of extent of nodal involvement in stage D1 prostate cancer treated with radiotherapy. Urology 39:39–43, 1992.

140. Gervasi LA, Mata J, Easley JD, et al: Prognostic significance of lymph nodal metastases in prostate cancer. J Urol 142:332–336, 1989.

141. Hanks GE, Buzydlowski J, Sause WT, et al: Ten-year outcomes for pathologic node-positive patients treated in RTOG 75–06. Int J Radiat Oncol Biol Phys 40:765–768, 1998.

142. Lawton CA, Cox JD, Glisch C, et al: Is long-term survival possible with external beam irradiation for stage D1 adenocarcinoma of the prostate? Cancer 69:2761–2766, 1992.

143. Zagars GK, Sands ME, Pollack A, et al: Early androgen ablation for stage D1 (N1 to N3, M0) prostate cancer: Prognostic variables and outcome. J Urol 151:1330–1333, 1994.

144. Sgrignioli AR, Walsh PC, Steinberg GD, et al: Prognostic factors in men with stage D1 prostate cancer: Identification of patients less likely to have prolonged survival after radical prostatectomy. J Urol 152:1077–1081, 1994.

145. Crook JM, Perry GA, Robertson S, et al: Routine prostate biopsies following radiotherapy for prostate cancer: Results for 226 patients. Urology 45:624–631, 1995.

146. Rogers E, Ohori M, Kassabian VS, et al: Salvage radical prostatectomy: Outcome measured by serum prostate specific antigen levels. J Urol 153:104–110, 1995.

147. Grado GL, Collins JM, Kriegshauser JS, et al: Salvage brachytherapy for localized prostate cancer after radiotherapy failure. Urology 53:2–10, 1999.

148. Pontes JE, Montie J, Klein E, et al: Salvage surgery for radiation failure in prostate cancer. Cancer 71:976–980, 1993.

149. Partin AW, Pearson JD, Landis PK, et al: Evaluation of serum prostate-specific antigen velocity after radical prostatectomy to distinguish local recurrence from distant metastasis. Urology 43:649–659, 1994.

150. Stein A, deKernion JB, Dorey F, et al: Adjuvant radiotherapy in patients post-radical prostatectomy with tumor extending through capsule or positive seminal vesicles. Urology 39:59–62, 1992.

151. Tong D, Gillick L, Hendrickson FR: The palliation of symptomatic osseous metastases. Cancer 50:893–899, 1982.

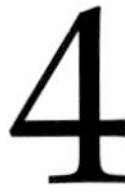

# 4

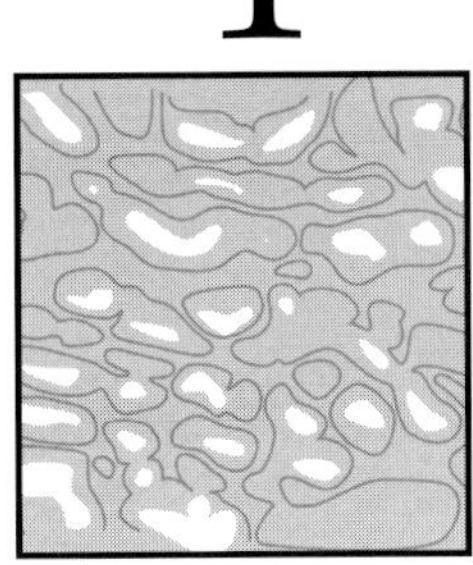

# Bladder and Other Urothelial Malignancies—Surgical Management

*Jürgen F. Linn*

*Sarel Halachmi*

*Mark P. Schoenberg*

Bladder cancer is one of the most common malignancies and therefore is an important public health problem. In the United States, approximately 53,200 new cases of bladder cancer were expected in the year 2000, and more than 12,000 individuals died from the disease.[1] The lifetime risk of developing bladder cancer has been estimated to be 2.8% for Caucasian men, 0.9% for African-American men, 1% for Caucasian women, and 0.6% for African-American women.[2]

The vast majority of bladder cancers are diagnosed as a result of the evaluation for painless hematuria. After cystoscopic inspection of the bladder, suspicious areas are transurethrally resected. In many cases, this approach is both diagnostic and therapeutic.

Ninety-five percent of bladder tumors diagnosed in North America and Europe are pathologically classified as transitional cell carcinomas (TCC). At the time of first diagnosis, more than 60% of TCC are superficial lesions that are confined to the mucosa or submucosa of the bladder. Even after complete transurethral resection (TUR) of all visible lesions, 50% to 70% of superficial bladder tumors recur, and up to 25% of these tumors progress in stage or grade.[3]

Controlled comparisons of intravesical chemotherapy for prophylaxis of recurrent superficial bladder cancer with thiotepa, doxorubicin, mitomycin C, and Epodyl have demonstrated a clear reduction in recurrence over the short term. Most of these agents fail to produce long-term cure of disease, however.[4] In a meta-analysis of seven series, patients treated with thiotepa, doxorubicin, or mitomycin C after TUR of tumor were compared with patients treated with surgery alone, and there was no evidence that intravesical chemotherapy reduced disease progression.[5] Comparisons of the different adjuvant intravesical treatments most often fail to demonstrate superiority of one agent over another, with the exception of immunotherapy with bacillus Calmette-Guérin (BCG). BCG appears to be superior to conventional intravesical chemotherapy in some but not all trials.[6–8] Moreover, some studies indicate that BCG immunotherapy, unlike chemotherapy, does reduce long-term tumor recurrence, progression, and mortality rate, especially in patients with carcinoma in situ (CIS) and high-grade superficial tumors.[7]

In patients with muscle invasive bladder cancer, a variety of therapeutic options are available. The appropriateness of each option is dependent upon the stage and grade of the tumor as well as the health and expected longevity of the patient. Complete removal of the bladder and prostate in the male and anterior exenteration (removal of the ovaries, fallopian tubes, uterus, bladder, and a portion of the anterior wall of the vagina) in females is the standard therapy for muscle invasive bladder cancer in the United States and in many other parts of the world. The development of continent urinary diversion and orthotopic bladder reconstruction in both male and female patients has increased patient acceptance of this form of therapy.

Long-term follow-up of patients with organ-confined bladder cancer after cystectomy has demonstrated disease-specific survival rates of 50% to 86%.[9]

Bladder preservation strategies that employ aggressive TUR combined with systemic chemotherapy and radiation therapy are under evaluation at many centers internationally.[10] Results from these trials are encouraging and suggest that bladder preservation may be possible in selected patients with invasive lesions, intercurrent medical problems that make radical surgery unsafe, or a strong desire to preserve the bladder. This topic is reviewed in detail in Chapter 5.

The use of neoadjuvant and adjuvant chemotherapy in the treatment of patients with bladder cancer remains controversial. Despite 10 years of clinical investigation, the exact role of adjuvant or neoadjuvant systemic chemotherapy combined with radical cystectomy in patients with invasive (T3–T4) bladder cancer remains unresolved.[11] Preliminary reports suggest that adjuvant and neoadjuvant therapy may be useful in a subset of patients with poor prognostic variables such as p53 mutation, although these observations need to be corroborated in controlled multicenter clinical trials.

This chapter provides an overview of bladder cancer diagnosis and surgical therapy directed by noninvasive radiographic imaging, endoscopic findings, and pathologic staging of disease.

**Figure 4–1:** Epidemiology. Bladder cancer is the fourth most common cancer found in American men and the eighth most common malignancy found in American women.[1] Differences in bladder cancer incidence by gender and among different ethnic groups is detailed in this diagram, which shows new cases per year per 100,000 population.

Generally speaking, bladder cancer is a disease of older, non-Hispanic, Caucasian men. In 1993, 82.3% of all reported cases involved patients who were 60 years of age or older. Approximately 73.5% of all patients were male, 92.1% were non-Hispanic Caucasian, and 78.1% were from the middle socioeconomic class.[2]

## RISK FACTORS FOR BLADDER CANCER

In 1895, the surgeon Rehn was the first to establish a relationship between bladder cancer and exposure to chemical dyes in the German textile industry.[12] More than 40 years later, animal experiments proved that 2-naphthylamine was the underlying cause of the tumors initially described by Rehn. Additional experiments demonstrated that other chemicals can contribute to bladder cancer development after occupation-related exposure. Most known bladder carcinogens are aromatic amines or their metabolites. Identification of specific carcinogens in the workplace has led to banning of the industrial use of 2-naphthylamine and benzidine.

The vast majority (94%) of bladder tumors are TCC. Benign lesions as well as nonepithelial cancers are extremely rare. Accurate histopathologic classification is important for clinical decision making.

Cigarette smoking has been strongly associated with the development of bladder cancer in several studies.[13] Smokers have a 2- to 10-fold increased risk of developing bladder malignancies. The mechanism of smoking-induced bladder cancer is most likely related to long-term exposure to high urinary concentrations of aromatic amines.

Inflammation of the bladder due to *Schistosoma haematobium* infection is closely related to the development of squamous cell bladder cancer.[14] Chronic cystitis due to urinary calculi, long-term indwelling catheters, or bladder diverticuli is less commonly associated with the development of squamous cell cancer of the bladder. For example, 80% of paraplegics have squamous cell metaplasia but only 5% develop squamous cell bladder cancer.

Other factors that can increase the risk of bladder cancer are long-term use of phenacetin, chemotherapy

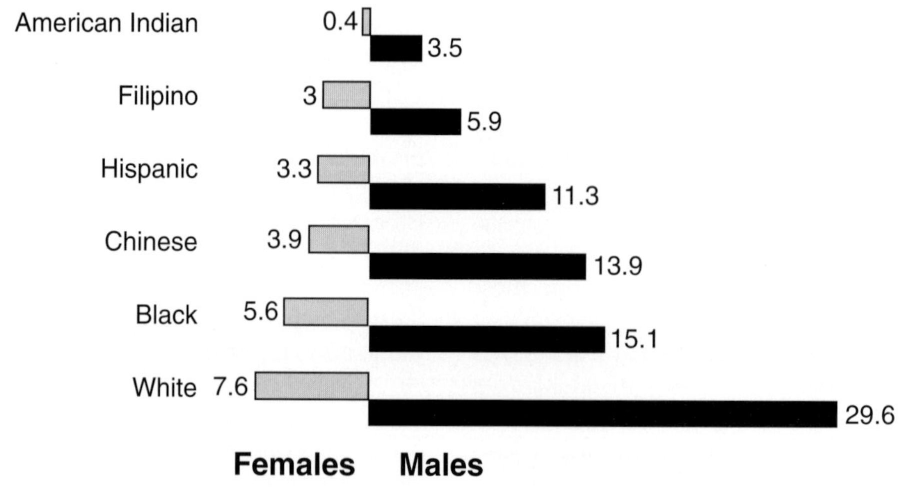


**Figure 4–1**    New cases per 100,000 population per year

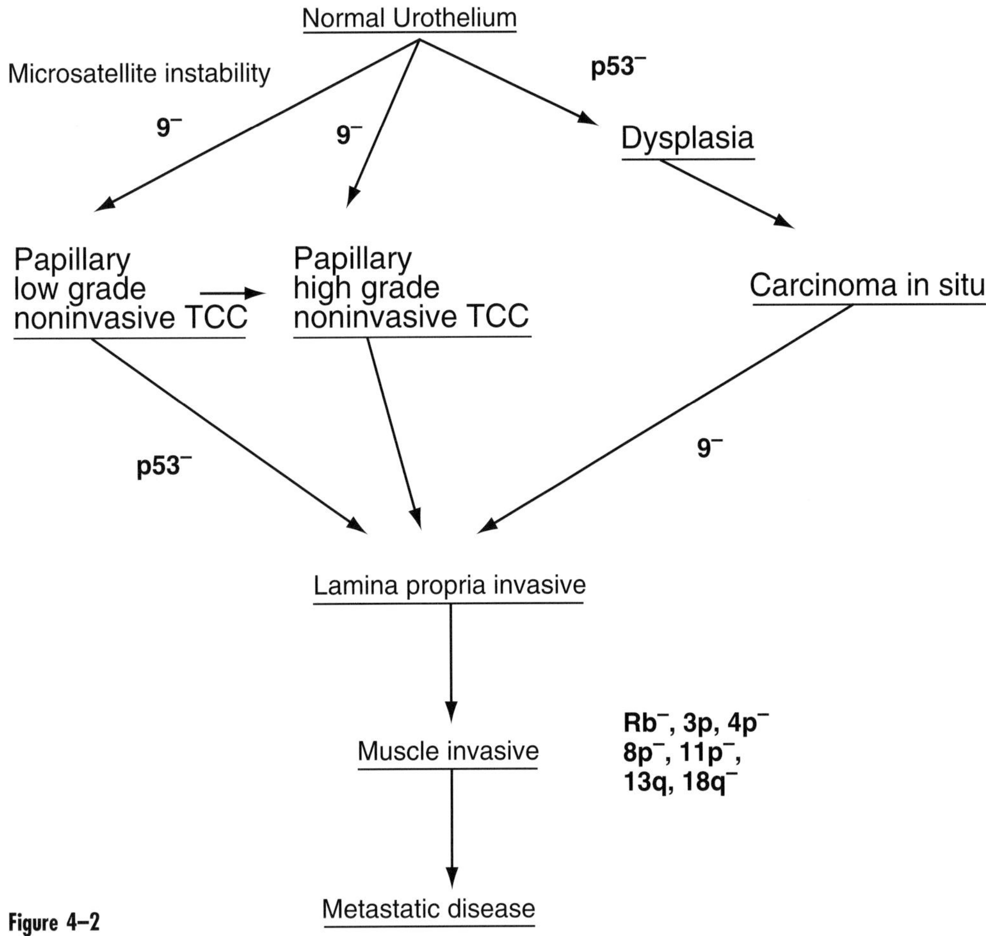


**Figure 4–2**

with cyclophosphamide, and pelvic radiation. The cyclophosphamide metabolite acrolein has been shown to be a potent bladder carcinogen.[15]

**Figure 4–2:** Molecular biology of bladder cancer. Recent genetic research has provided evidence that histologically and clinically distinct forms of bladder cancer are characterized by specific genetic alterations.[16] In superficial papillary transitional cell carcinomas (TCC), microsatellite instability at multiple loci on both the long and short arms of chromosome 9 is an early event in bladder carcinogenesis. Mutation of the p53 tumor suppressor gene on chromosomal arm 17p appears to be more common in invasive tumors. Loss of chromosomal arm 14q is a common abnormality associated with carcinoma in situ (CIS).

## STAGING OF BLADDER CANCER

For the 1997 American Joint Committee on Cancer (AJCC) Staging System, see Chapter 6. With the use of the additional prefix "p" for pathologic and "r" for resection, the stage of a given lesion can be described. TNM classification without a prefix means an assessment of tumor extent using clinical methods. The use of prefixes is very helpful because clinical staging does not always correlate with the results of histopathologic

examination, e.g., after radical cystectomy. Also, the exact differentiation between deep muscle invasion (T2b) and serosal penetration (T3a) can be difficult if the pathologist has only TUR specimens for evaluation.

**Figure 4–3:** The majority of patients (70%) with bladder cancer present with early stage, noninvasive disease. However, a significant percentage of patients with superficial tumors ultimately will progress to invasive

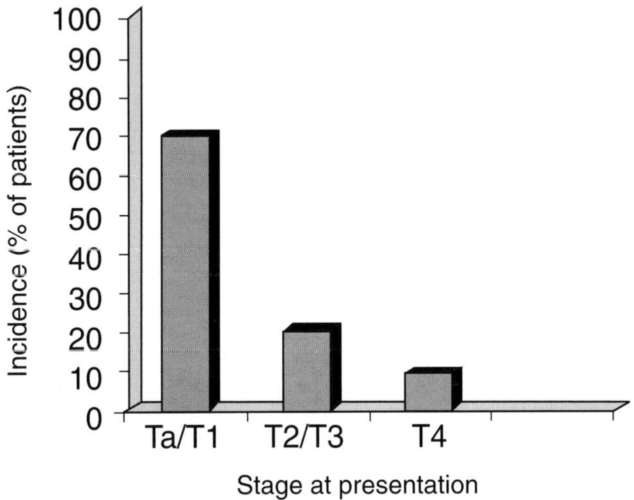


**Figure 4–3**

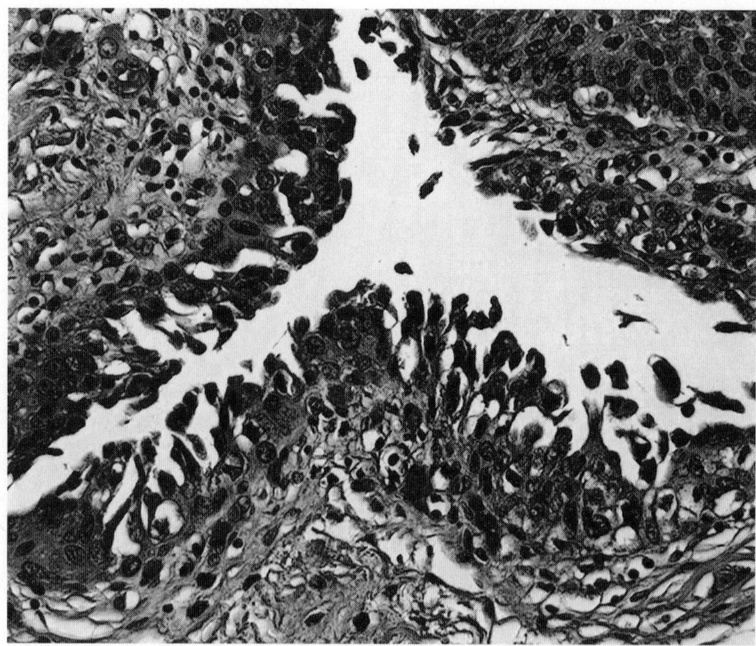

Figure 4–4

disease at a rate that varies from 40% for Ta to over 60% for T1.[3]

**Figure 4–4:** Histopathologically, carcinoma in situ (CIS) is characterized by poorly differentiated cells that are located within the urothelium. There is a marked variability in size of the nuclei, which appear hypercromatic and exhibit loss of polarity. Mitotic figures are more frequent. Carcinoma in situ may occur as an isolated lesion or may involve the bladder diffusely. Often CIS is not visible on cystoscopic examination. Clinical symptoms associated with CIS include urinary frequency, dysuria, and hematuria. The diagnosis of CIS is readily made by biopsy of the urothelium.

**Figure 4–5:** Bladder tumors are classified by a cytologic grading (G1 to G3). This histologic slide shows a well-differentiated G1 TCC with an increase in the number of cell layers, slight cytologic atypia, and rare mitotic figures.

**Figure 4–6:** Poorly differentiated tumors are designated as G3. Grade 3 tumors show focal high-grade atypia and frequent mitotic figures and are frequently muscle invasive.

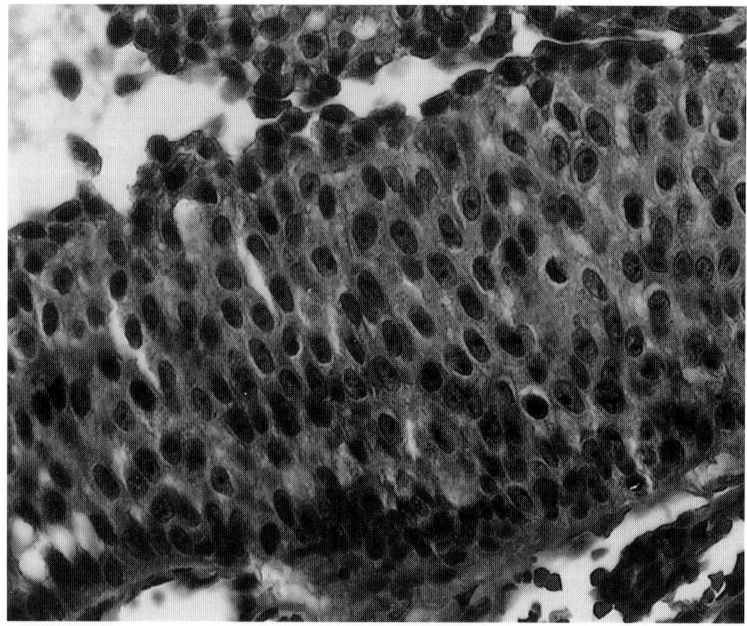

Figure 4–5

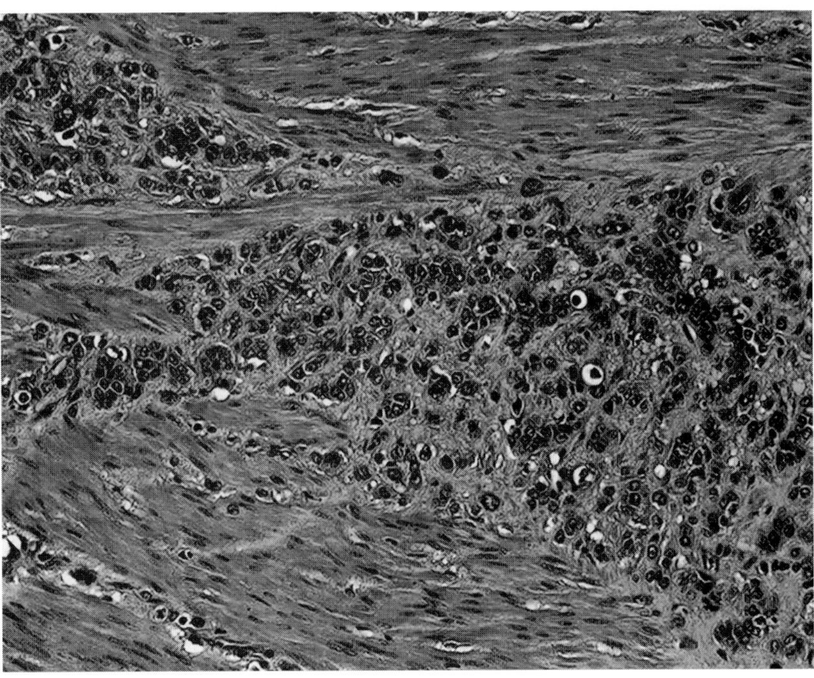

**Figure 4–6**

**Figures 4–7 (see Color Insert) and 4–8:** Superficial tumors of the bladder appear macroscopically as a flat papillary lawn or as exophytic cauliflower-like figures with a small stalk or vascular pedicle attached to the bladder wall. The microscopic architecture of the layers of the bladder wall remains unchanged even in exo-phytic growing tumors. There is no evidence for muscle infiltration with epithelial cells.

Figure 4–7 shows the cystoscopic view of a small papillary superficial bladder tumor. Figure 4–8 shows the corresponding histologic appearance, which demonstrates the noninvasive growth of the tumor.

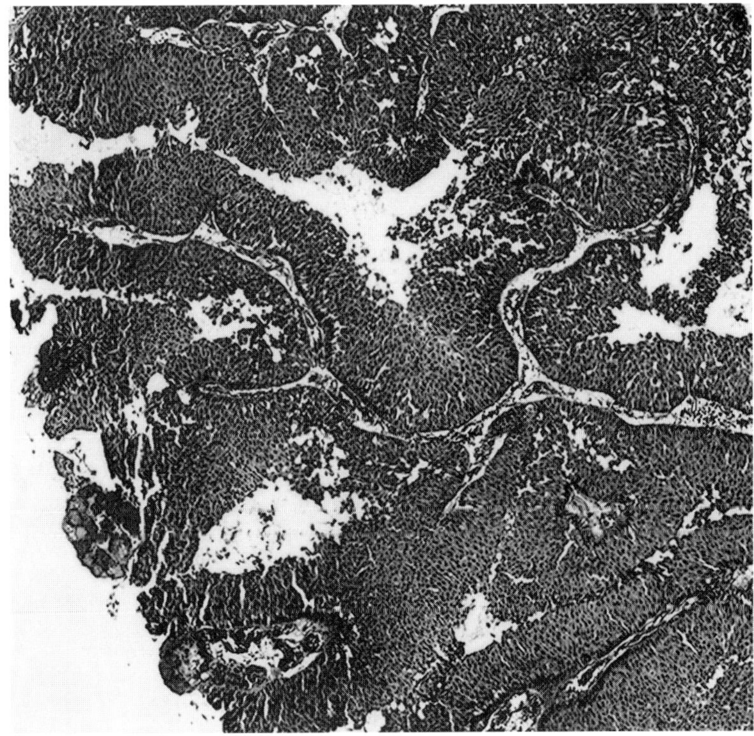

**Figure 4–8**

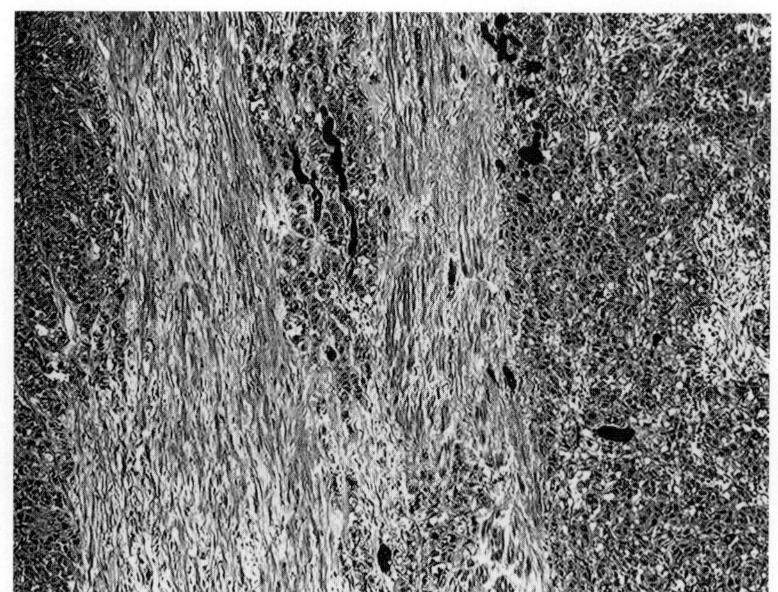

**Figure 4–10**

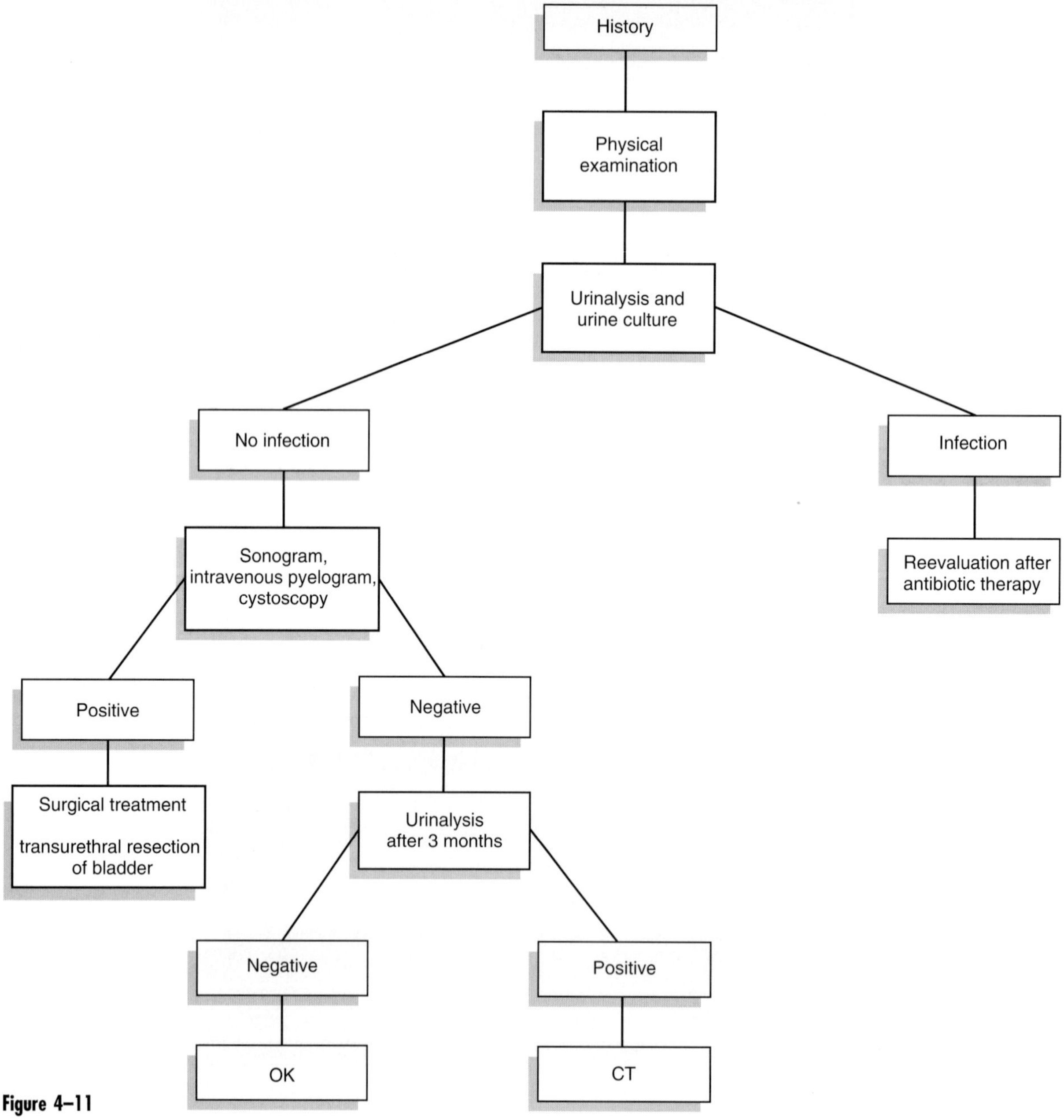

**Figure 4–11**

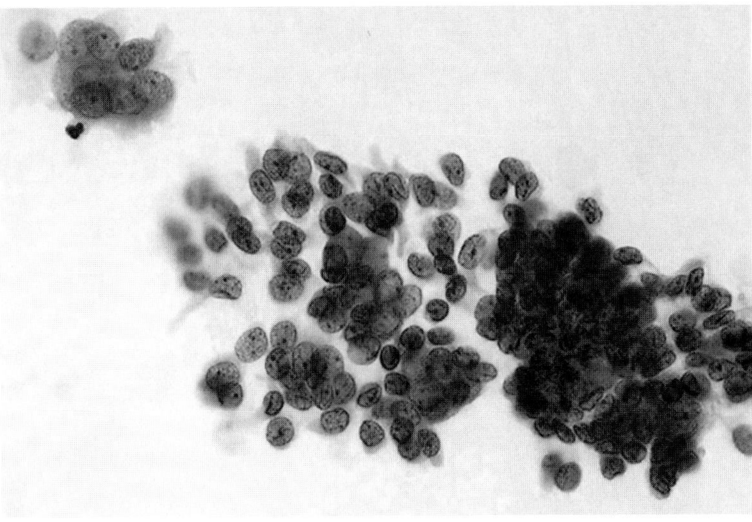

Figure 4–12

**Figures 4–9 (see Color Insert) and 4–10:** Invasive tumors by definition grow into the detrusor musculature, have a broad base, and are more likely to be nodular then exophytic. They often show superficial necrosis, edema, and inflammation of the surrounding tissue. Microscopically, nests of epithelial cells invade the muscle and sometimes the perivesical fat.

Figure 4–9 shows the cystoscopic view of a solid, highly malignant, infiltrating bladder tumor. Figure 4–10 shows the corresponding histologic appearance, which demonstrates extensive muscle invasion with tumor cells.

**Figure 4–11:** Differential diagnosis and work-up of gross hematuria. Hematuria is the antecedent complaint of most patients diagnosed with bladder cancer. Whereas initial hematuria is usually caused by disorders of the urethra or prostate and terminal hematuria indicates disorders of the trigone or bladder neck, total gross painless hematuria often signifies the presence of tumors of the bladder or the upper urinary tract. In contrast, painful hematuria is often caused by urinary calculi or infectious diseases. Asymptomatic microscopic hematuria can occur in 13% of the general population.[17] Although microscopic hematuria is often idiopathic, it may be a sign of any disease associated with gross hematuria. The work-up of patients with hematuria is demonstrated on this flow diagram.

**Figures 4–12 and 4–13:** Urinary cytologic examination can detect the presence of urothelial tumor cells. The overall specificity of standard Papanicolaoustained urine cytologic specimens ranges between 78% and 95%, with a sensitivity of about 70%.[18] However, low-grade carcinomas are difficult to differentiate from normal epithelium, making cytologic diagnosis more challenging.

Figure 4–12 (G1 bladder carcinoma) shows slight atypia of urothelial cells with somewhat prominent nuclei. Cell clusters may contain over eight cells, and

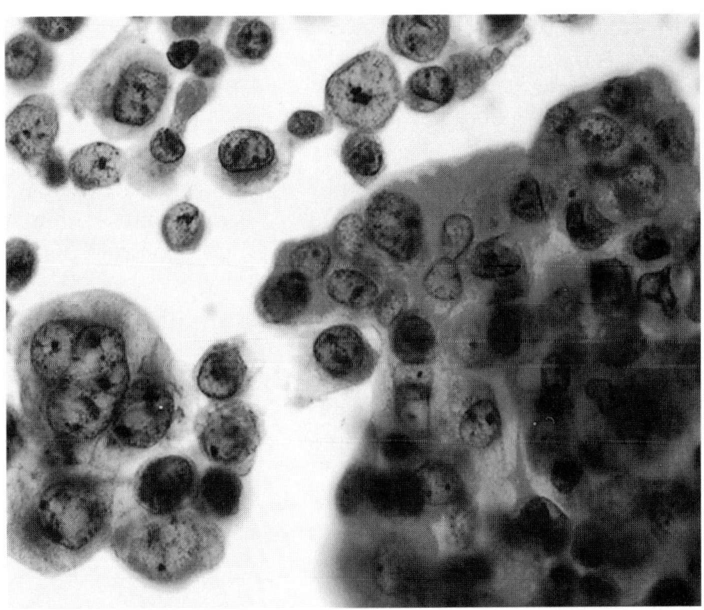

Figure 4–13

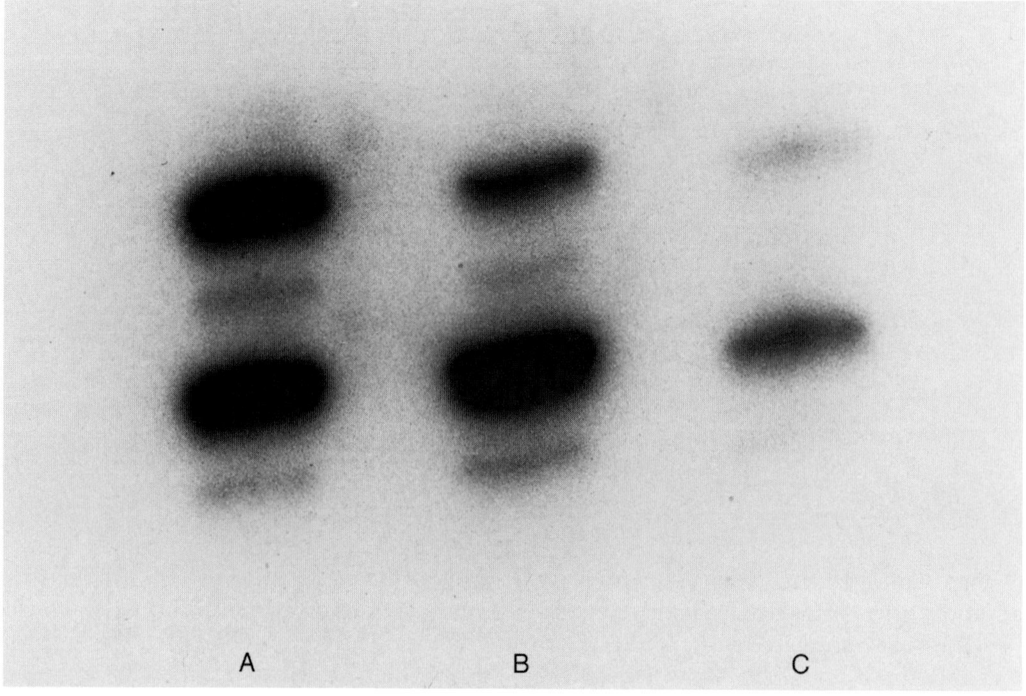



**Figure 4–14**

nuclear overlapping may be seen. Figure 4–13 (G3 bladder carcinoma) shows mostly single cells with large, very hyperchromatic nuclei. In rare cell clusters, nuclear overlapping is apparent, and giant cells can be found.

**Figure 4–14:** Molecular biologic techniques may soon enhance the detection of bladder cancer cells in voided urine specimens.[19] Using highly polymorphic microsatellite markers and the polymerase chain reaction (PCR), alterations in DNA structure characteristic of tumor cells such as loss of heterozygosity (LOH), or the appearance of new alleles (microsatellite instability) can be detected in up to 95% of all urine samples from patients with bladder tumors. Follow-up studies predict recurrent disease correctly in 9 of 10 cases.[20] Prospective clinical trials are currently being conducted to confirm these preliminary observations.

The autoradiogram demonstrates the electrophoretic separation of the PCR amplified marker D9S747. *A*, In the left lane, is nonmalignant control DNA (lymphocyte DNA). The two bands represent the maternal and paternal alleles in a normal heterozygote. *B*, In the middle lane, tumor DNA has been amplified and loss of material from the upper band is consistent with LOH. *C*, A similar finding is present in the far right lane in DNA from a urine specimen from the same patient.

**Figure 4–15:** The role of sonography in the detection of bladder cancer is controversial. This imaging modality is useful to noninvasively exclude upper tract

disease such as hydronephrosis, renal calculi, or renal masses. Transurethral sonography has been used in some centers to evaluate the depth of bladder wall penetration by invasive tumors. It is an invasive test, however, and is not widely available.[21] The resolution of transvesical sonography allows detection of tumors with a diameter of more than 1 cm. Even tumors large enough to be visualized by ultrasound lack definition of depth of tumor invasion into the bladder wall, extravesical tumor extension, and metastasis of regional lymph nodes. This figure shows a longitudinal ultrasound scan of the bladder with large exophytic mass.

**Figure 4–16:** This intravenous pyelogram (IVP) was performed in a patient with a large right-sided bladder tumor. The upper tracts are normal. The IVP remains the classic method for imaging the upper urinary tract. Although the study provides information about the bladder, only larger tumors are visible as filling defects. The major role of the IVP is in the assessment of the upper urinary tract. Tumors of the ureter and the renal pelvis that may not be detected by sonography, CT, or MRI examinations can often be found on IVP. IVP should be performed on a regular basis in patients with a history of urothelial malignancy because upper tract recurrences can occur in as many as 21% of these patients during long-term follow-up.[22]

**Figure 4–17:** *A*, The pelvic CT scan demonstrates the extent of the right-sided bladder tumor in the patient whose IVP is described in Figure 4–16. A Foley catheter

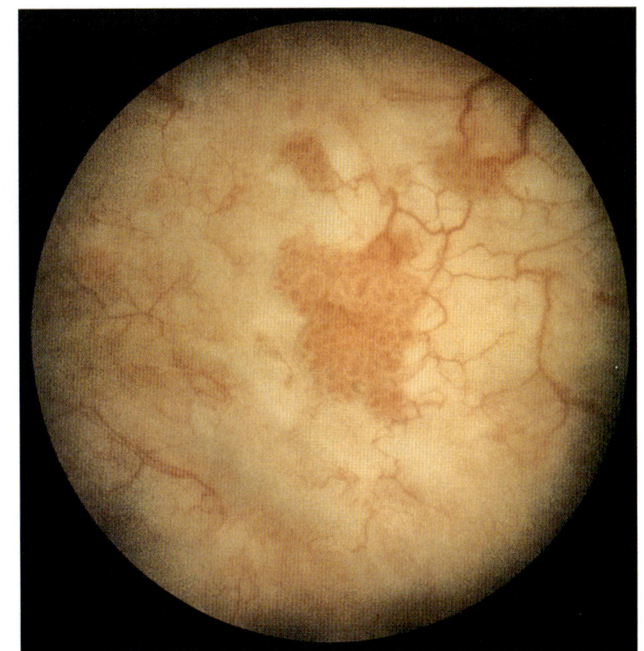

**FIGURE 4–7**

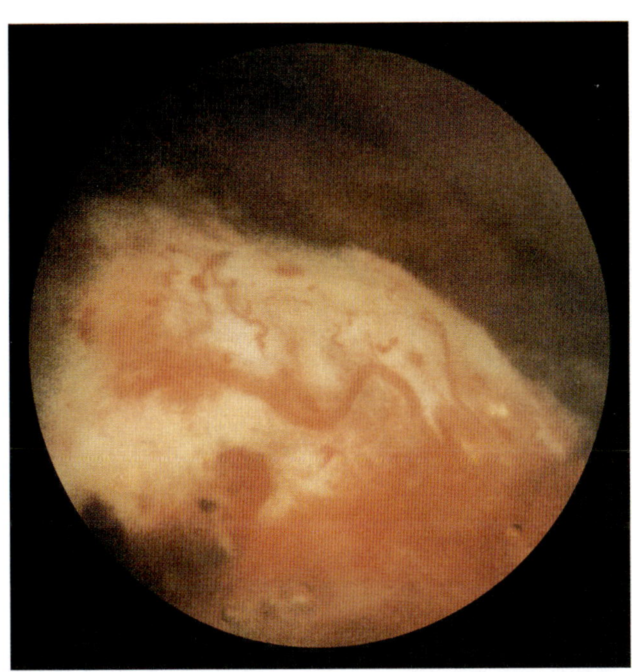

**FIGURE 4–9**

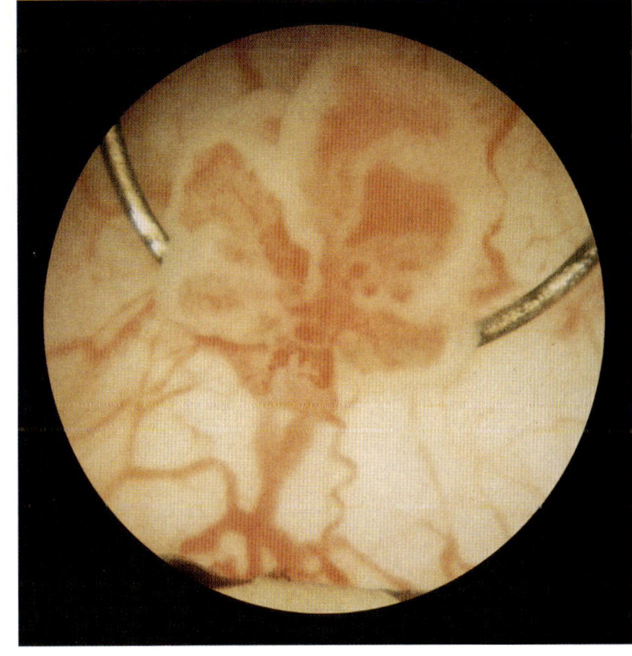

**FIGURE 4–20**

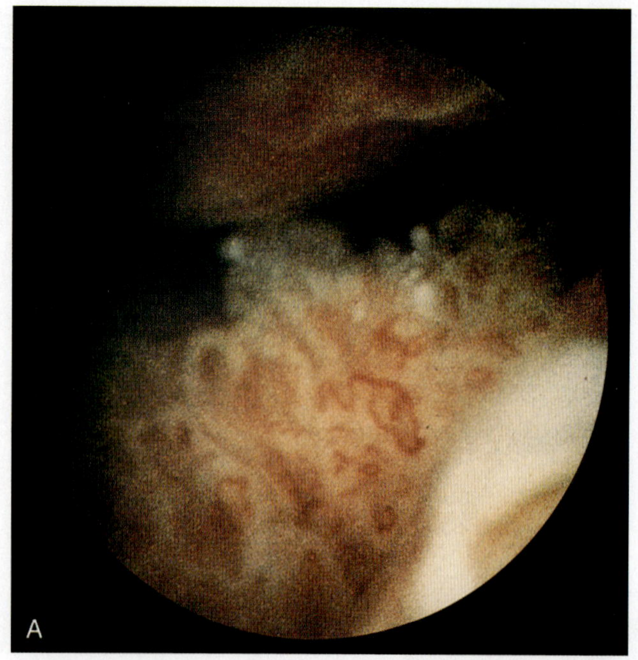

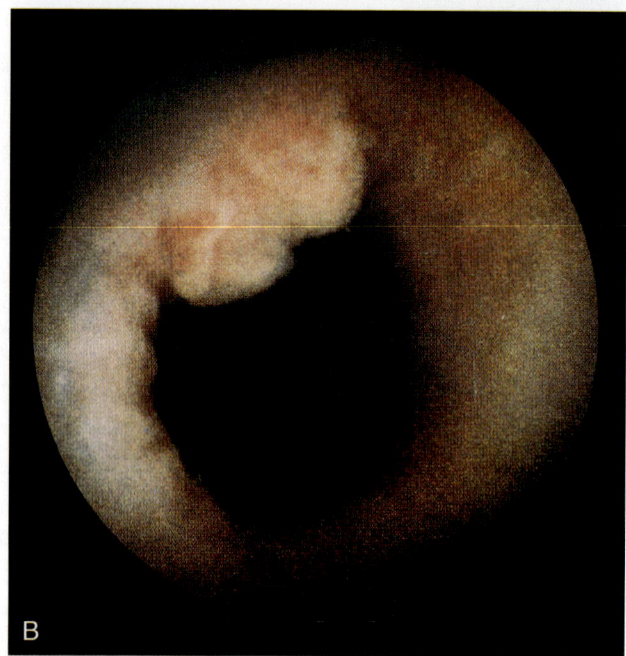

FIGURE 4–29 A & B

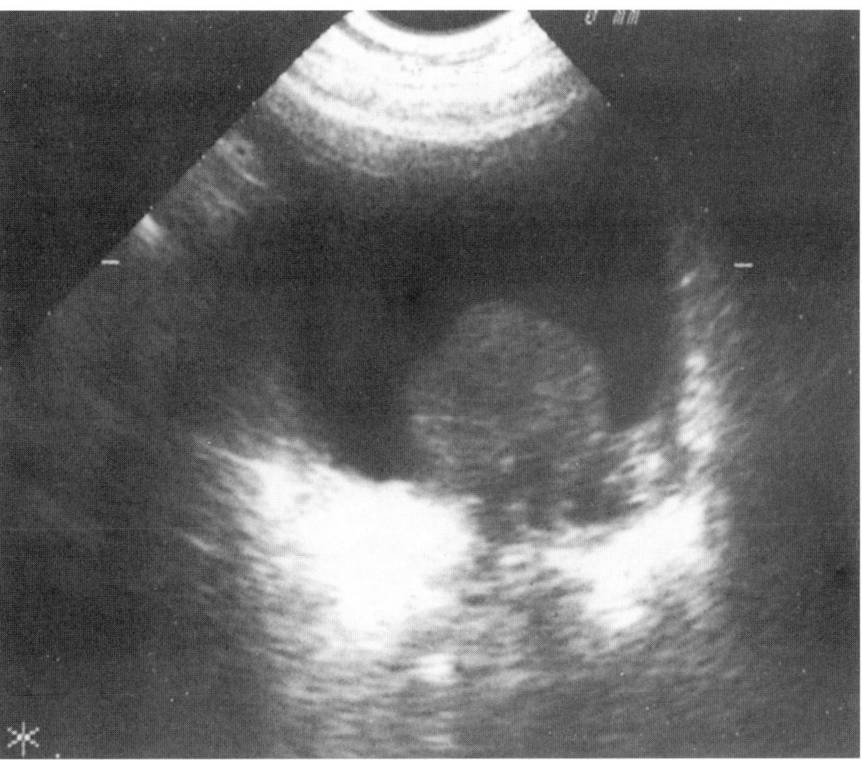

**Figure 4–15**

is seen adjacent to the bulging tumor mass in the anterolateral portion of the bladder.

Computed tomography (CT) has improved the clinical staging of patients with bladder cancer. CT examination is able to differentiate T3/T4 tumors from less invasive tumors in 80% of the cases (provided that the examination is performed before or at least 6 weeks after transurethral resection of the bladder). However, CT does not differentiate between superficial and intramural tumor (Ta to T2b). CT can also detect enlarged lymph nodes or metastasis, but the false-negative and false-positive rates are 15% to 40%. There are similar limitations in the assessment of small tumors less than 1 cm and carcinoma in situ by CT.

*B* and *C,* The MRI scans demonstrate $T_1$- and $T_2$-weighted images of a right-sided bladder tumor invading the wall adjacent to the trigone. Note the prominent seminal vesicles on the $T_2$-weighted image (*B*) and the dark tumor bulging at the base of the bladder. The tumor is bright on the $T_1$-weighted image (*C*) enhanced by intravenous injection of gadolinium.

MRI appears to be more accurate in the staging of bladder cancer than CT with particular respect to the evaluation of the bladder wall. It is superior to CT in defining the planes between the prostate and the bladder as well as the bladder and the vagina. It also seems to have superior sensitivity and specificity in the detection of lymph node metastases.

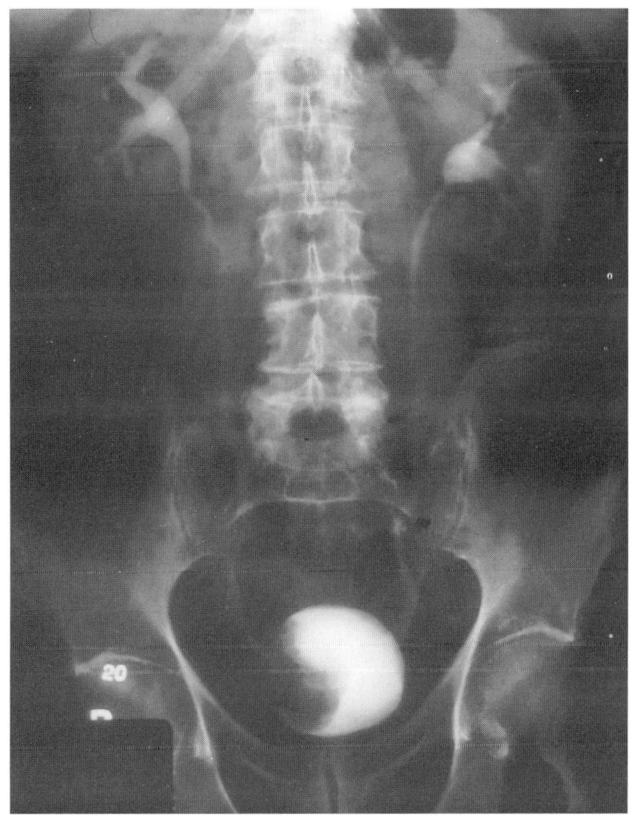

**Figure 4–16**

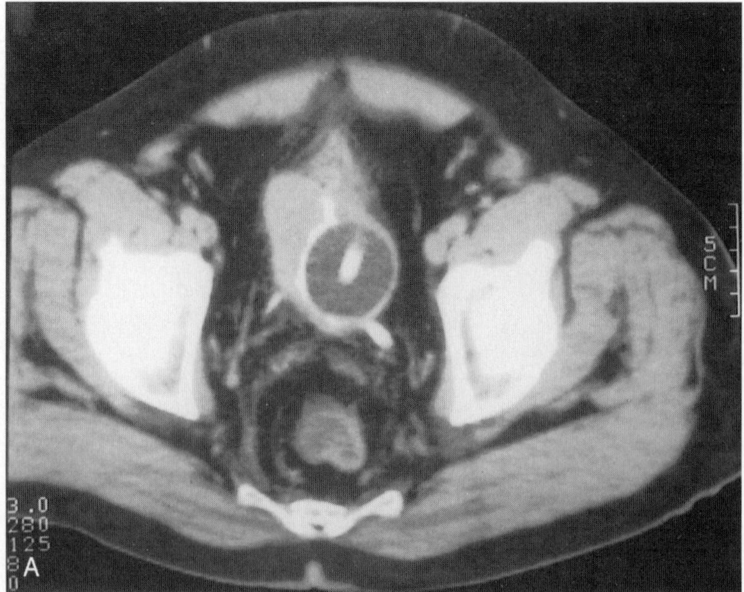

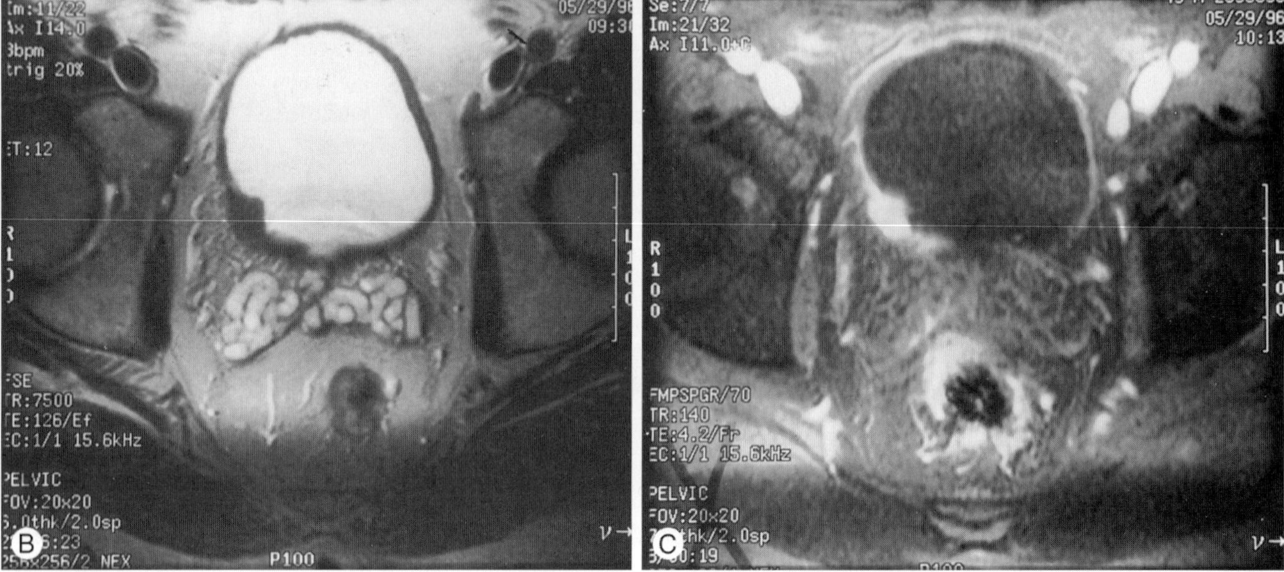

**Figure 4–17**

**Figure 4–18:** Cystoscopic examination is the gold standard for the diagnosis of bladder tumors. It allows the visualization of the tumor and characterization of its gross appearance. With the help of biopsies or transurethral resection, material for histopathologic examination can be obtained. This figure shows a cystoscope with a rigid sheath and its position in the bladder. The flexible cystoscope makes cystoscopy more tolerable for the patient.

**Figure 4–19:** It is useful to divide patients into three groups when planning therapy for bladder cancer: A low-risk superficial group, a high-risk superficial group, and a muscle invasive group. A TUR-B (transurethral resection of the bladder) should be performed at the beginning in all cases to confirm the diagnosis histologically. In case of superficial bladder cancer, the TUR can be both diagnostic and therapeutic. Instillation therapy has proved to be useful in prolonging the interval between recurrences; however, it does not definitively alter the risk of progression. Cystectomy remains the standard therapy in muscle invasive disease (staged higher than T1), and some clinicians recommend cystectomy for high-grade superficial disease that does not respond to aggressive local measures or for disease that is technically unmanageable endoscopically. Chapter 5 reviews the role of bladder conservation therapy using chemoradiation for muscle invasive disease. The benefit of adjuvant and neoadjuvant therapy in conjunction with exenterative surgery remains to be determined.

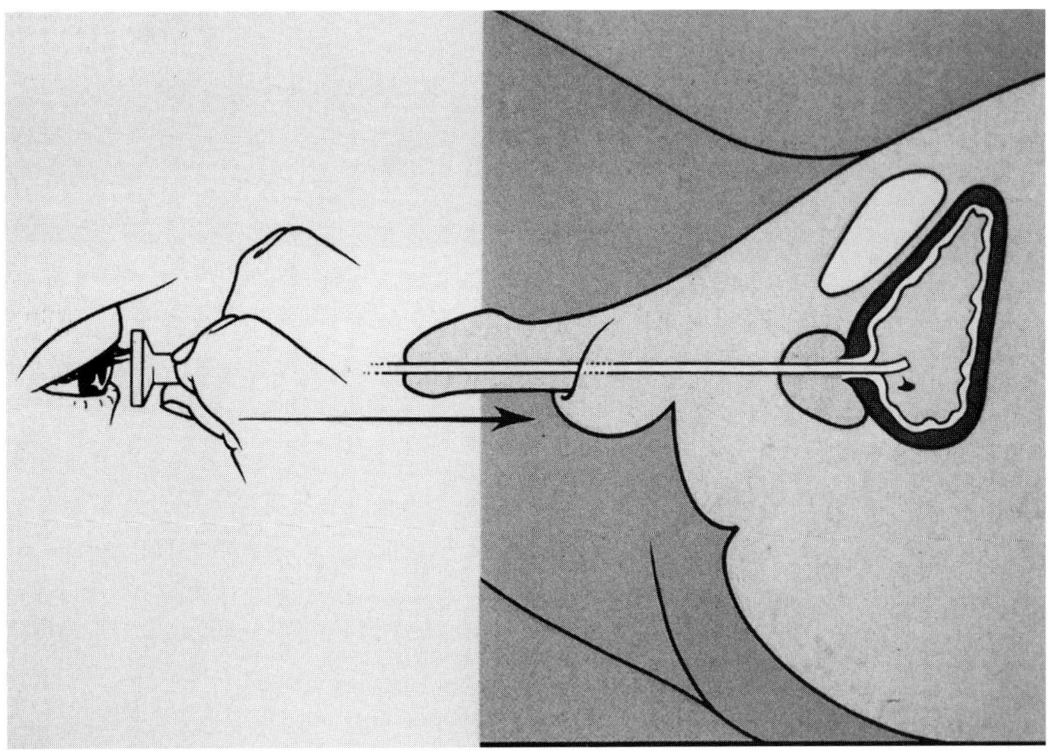

**Figure 4–18**

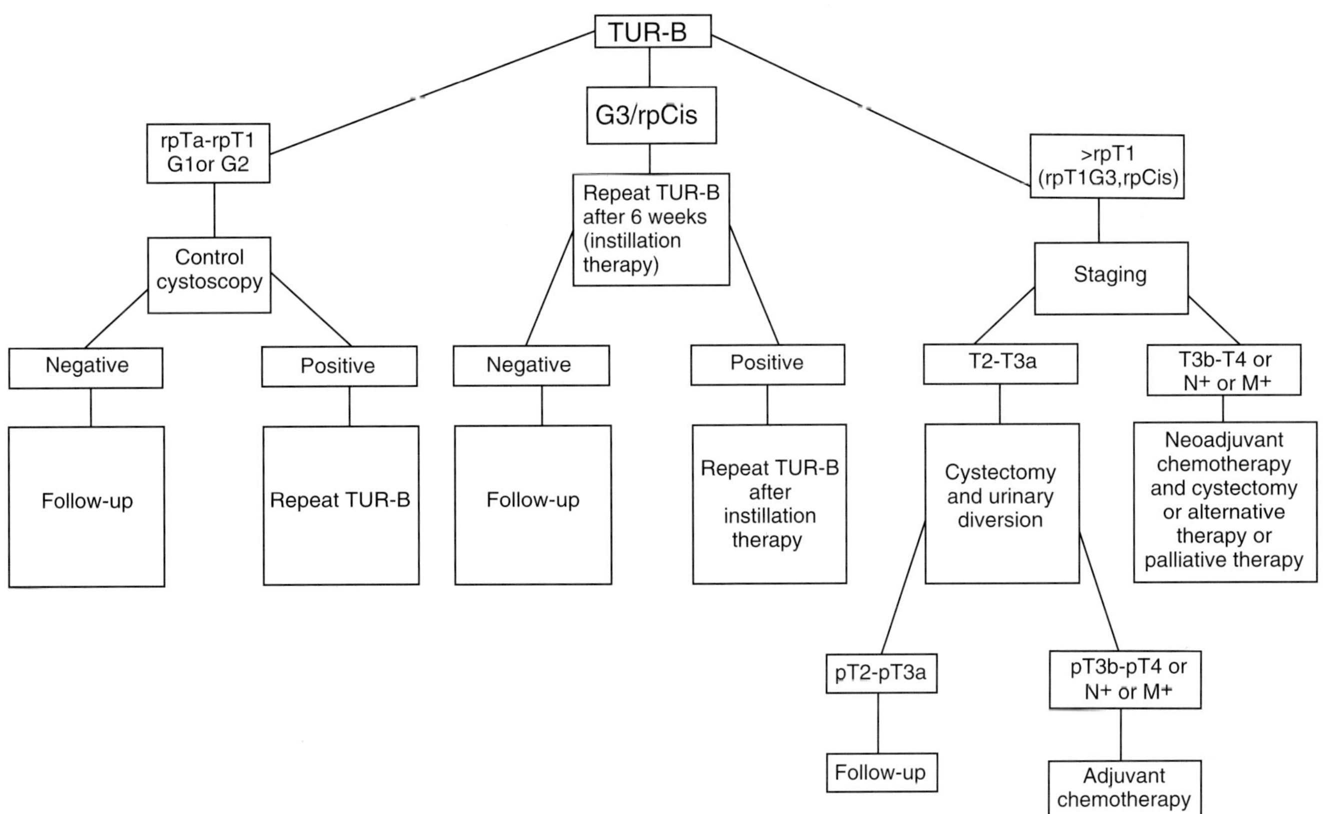


**Figure 4–19**

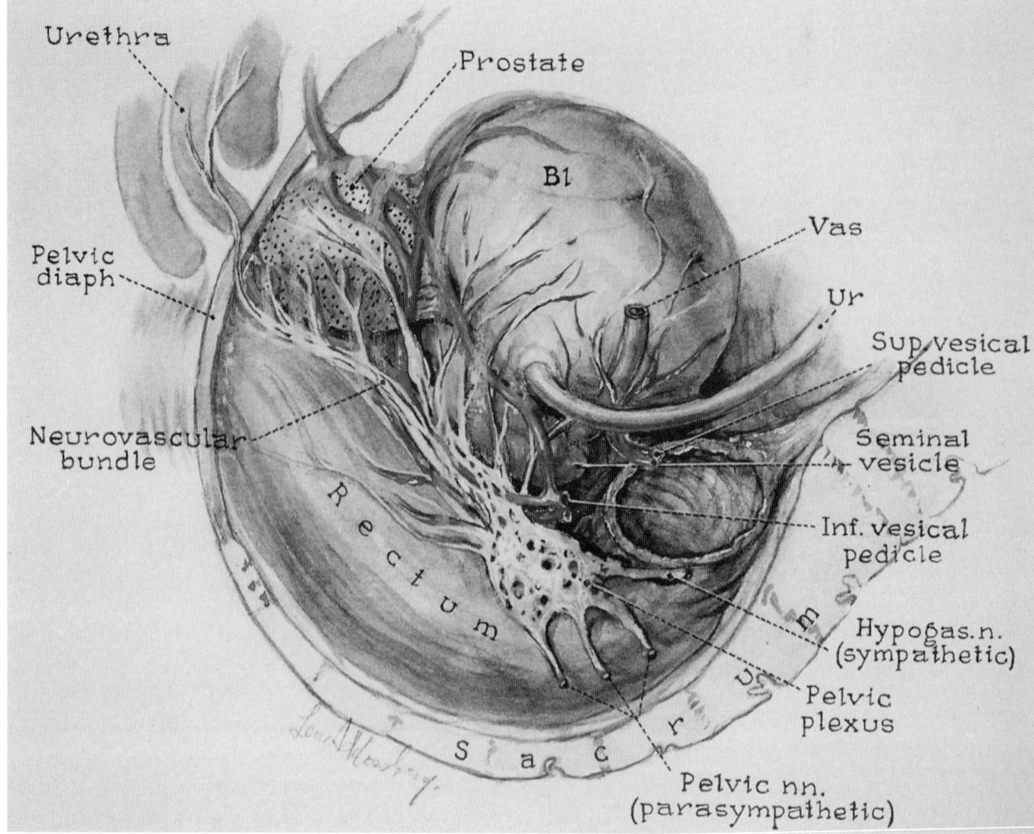


**Figure 4–21**

**Figure 4–20:** (See Color Insert.) Transurethral resection of bladder tumors. This figure shows a cystoscopic view of a bladder tumor and a TUR-loop behind the tumor. The loop can be powered with high-frequency electrical energy for cutting or cauterization of tissue. For TURB the surgeon draws the loop through the tumor. Afterward the tissue is rinsed out of the bladder through the sheath of the resectoscope. It is crucial that the surgeon obtain deep muscle biopsies at the time of TUR-B for both diagnosis and staging.

**Figure 4–21:** Radical cystectomy remains the gold standard for the treatment of muscle invasive bladder cancer.[23] Bladder conservation therapy is reviewed in the next chapter. Excellent 5-year disease-specific survival rates have been achieved at many centers when cystectomy has been employed to treat patients with

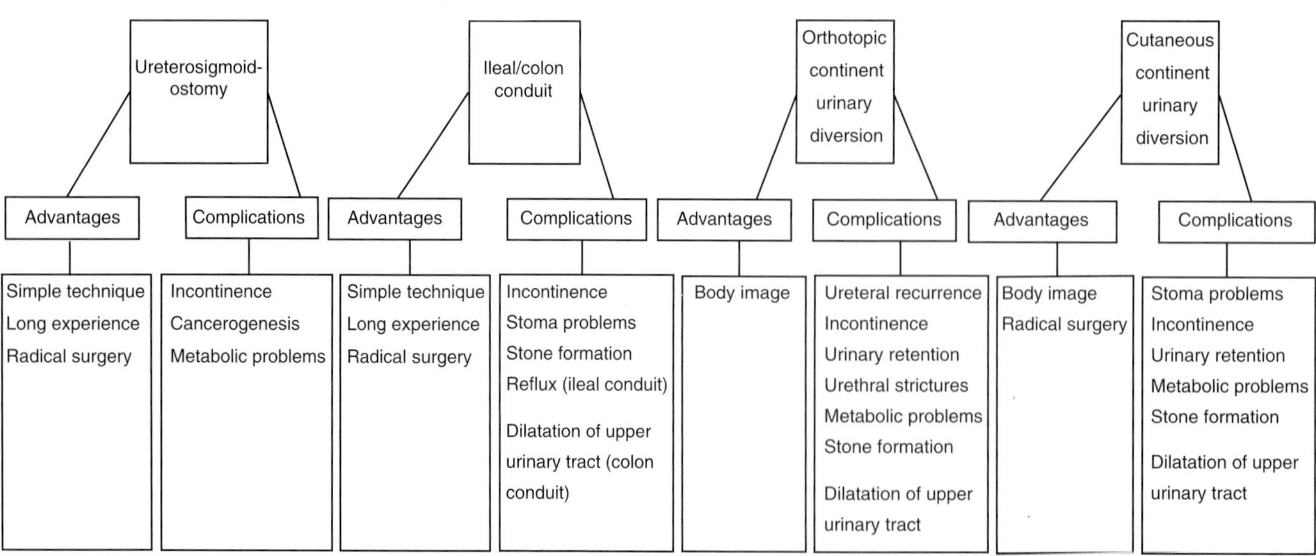


**Figure 4–22**

pT1 to pT2b disease. Death from metastasis is still a significant problem in patients with pT3–pT4 disease.[24] Continent diversion and orthotopic urinary tract reconstruction have made complete removal of the urinary bladder more acceptable to patients.[25, 26] Advances in nerve-sparing techniques have made preservation of sexual function possible in younger male patients treated by cystectomy.[27]

The figure shows a left lateral view of pelvic organs and neuroanatomy. The pelvic plexus and its branches that are important for sexual function are located retroperitoneally, lateral and posterior to the seminal vesicles. Thus, the seminal vesicle can be used as a landmark intraoperatively to avoid injury to the pelvic plexus when ligating the posterior pedicle.[27]

**Figure 4–22:** The decision to use one or another form of urinary tract reconstruction is made on the basis of the surgeon's experience and the patient's preference. Options are frequently dictated by anatomic considerations or intercurrent disease. An intensive discussion involving the urologist, the patient, possibly his relatives, and an enterostomal therapist should be part of the preoperative evaluation.

**Figure 4–23:** Although many new techniques for bladder replacement and urinary diversion are now being performed, the ileal conduit urinary diversion as described by Bricker[28] in 1950 remains the standard for urinary diversion internationally. The ileal loop has proved to be a procedure with a low morbidity rate and few complications. A patient with an ileal loop can maintain a favorable quality of life and preserve renal function.

For construction of an ileal loop a 10- to 12-cm segment of the ileum is selected, a standard bowel anastomosis reconstructs the continuity of the bowel, and the defect in the mesentery is closed (*A*). Ureteroileal anastomosis is then performed (*B*). *C*, The position of the ureteroileal anastomosis and the cutaneous stoma with two ureteral stents is shown here.

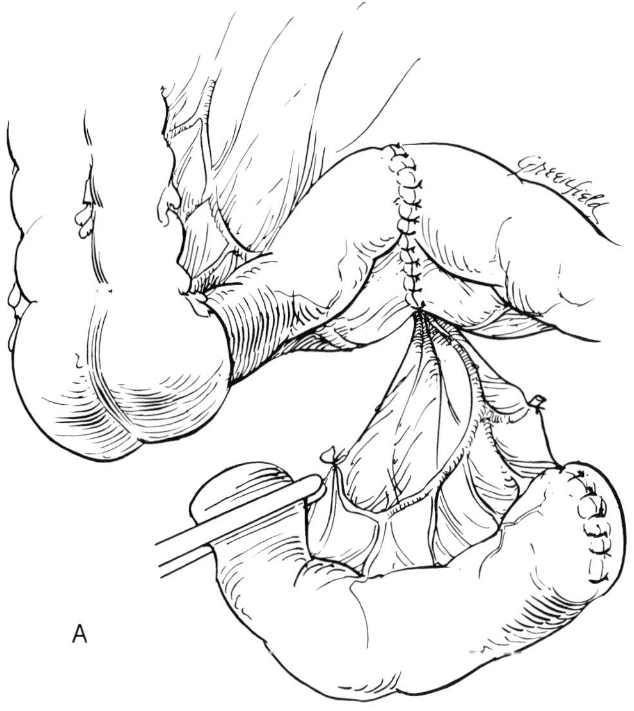

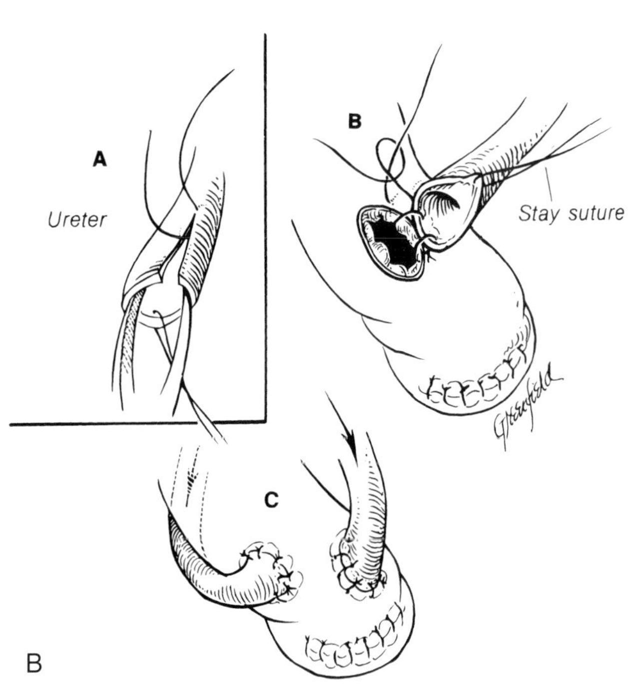


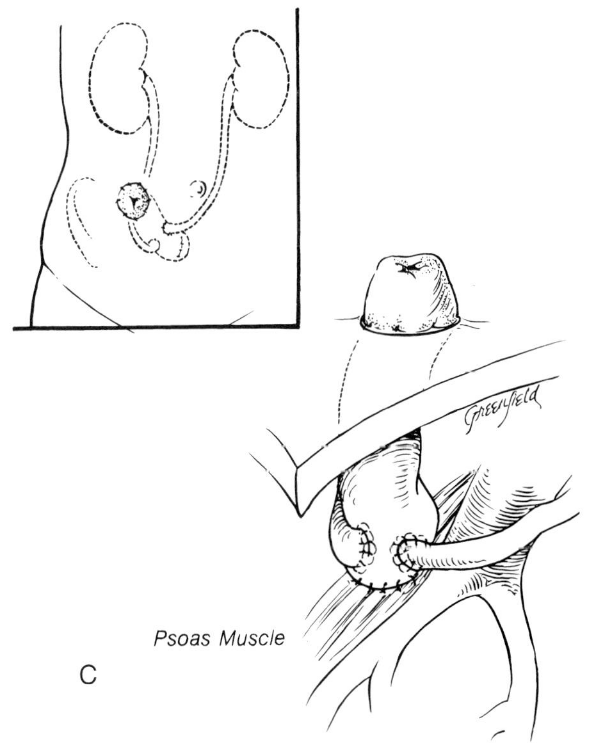


**Figure 4–23**

**Figure 4–24:** Orthotopic continent reservoirs have become popular in the last decade and rely upon meticulous dissection of the prostatic apex with preservation of the external urinary sphincter, as well as a watertight urethral anastomosis to the neobladder. The presence of tumor or cellular atypia in the prostatic urethra is a contraindication to orthotopic reconstruction. A variety of orthotopic continent diversions are performed. An example using right colon and ileum is shown.[29]

*A,* After standard or nerve-sparing cystectomy, ascending colon and terminal ileum are isolated on a

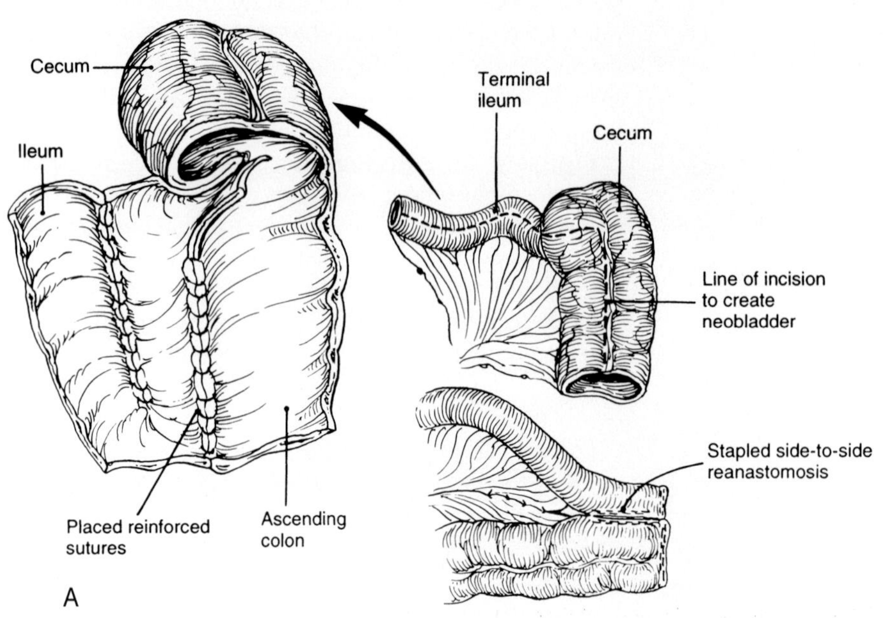


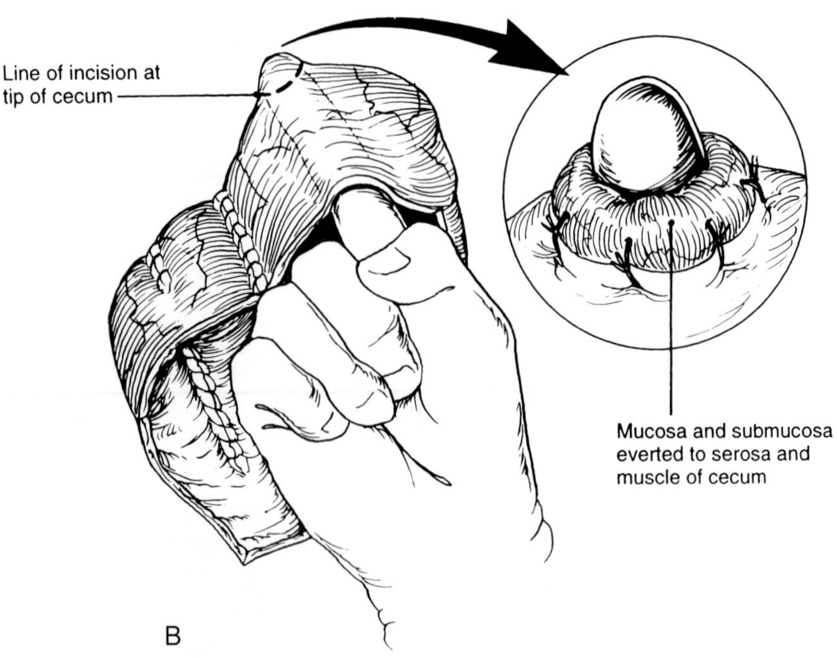


Figure 4–24

generous mesenteric pedicle. Intestinal integrity is reestablished by side-to-side bowel anastomosis. The detubularized segment of right colon and ileum is then refashioned into a sphere. *B,* At the most dependent portion of the cecum, a neobladder neck is created, permitting a direct urethral anastomosis. *C,* Antirefluxive ureter implantation is performed in the flap valve tunnel technique. *D,* After anastomosis between the buttonhole of the neobladder and the urethra the bowel segment is closed to a pouch.

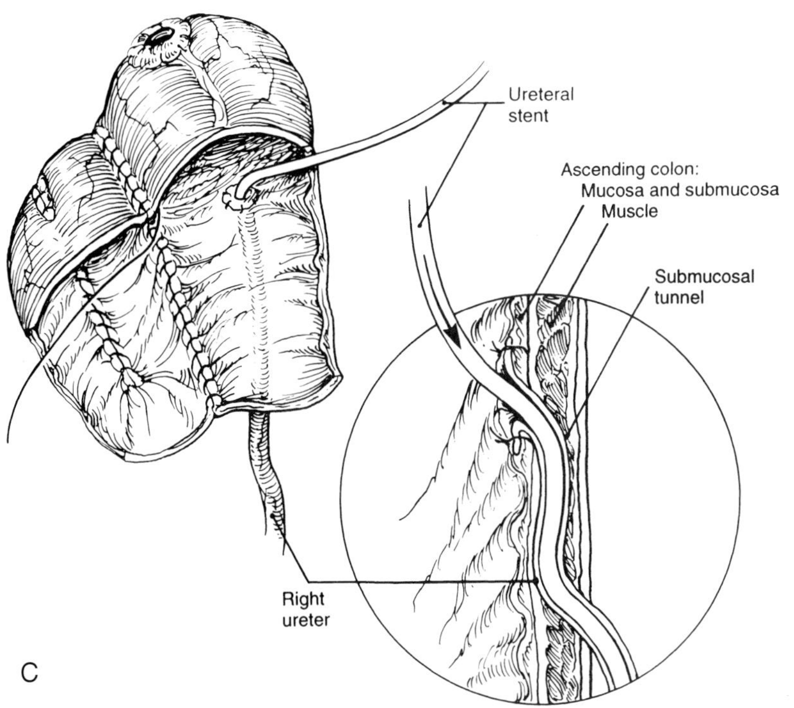


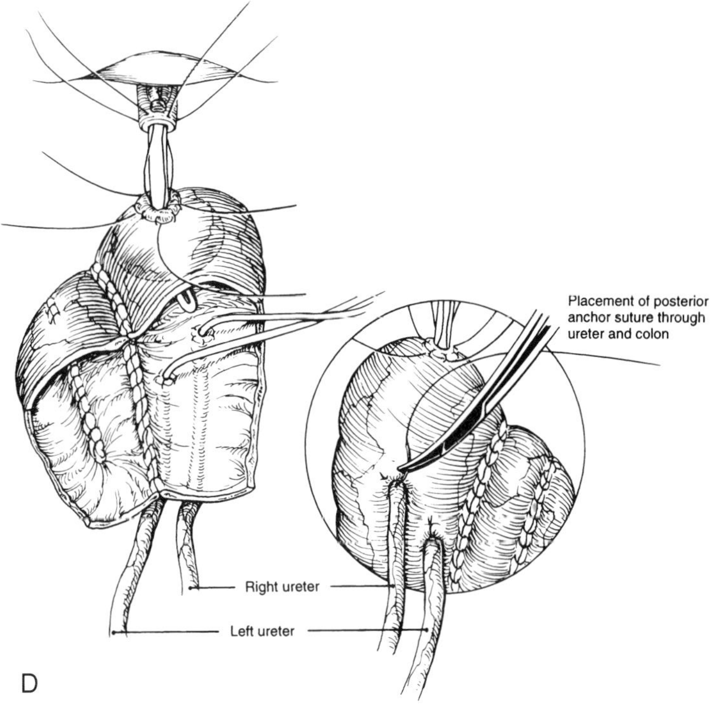


**Figure 4–24** *Continued*

**Figure 4–25:** The Mainz pouch technique is described here with a continent stoma to the umbilicus using the ascending colon and terminal ileum for the pouch and the appendix for the continence mechanism.[30]

*A*, Preparation of a pouch using terminal ileum and ascending colon. The last 4 cm of the cecal pole are not split at its antimesenteric tenia. The ureters are implanted at the aboral segment of the large bowel using antirefluxive techniques. *B*, After closure of the pouch a superficial incision of the intact tenia libera is performed at the cecal pole preserving the mucosal layer. *C*, The appendix is turned into the seromuscular slit and embedded by interrupted sutures. *D*, The continent appendix stoma can now be anastomosed to the umbilicus as a cosmetically and functionally ideal stoma outlet.

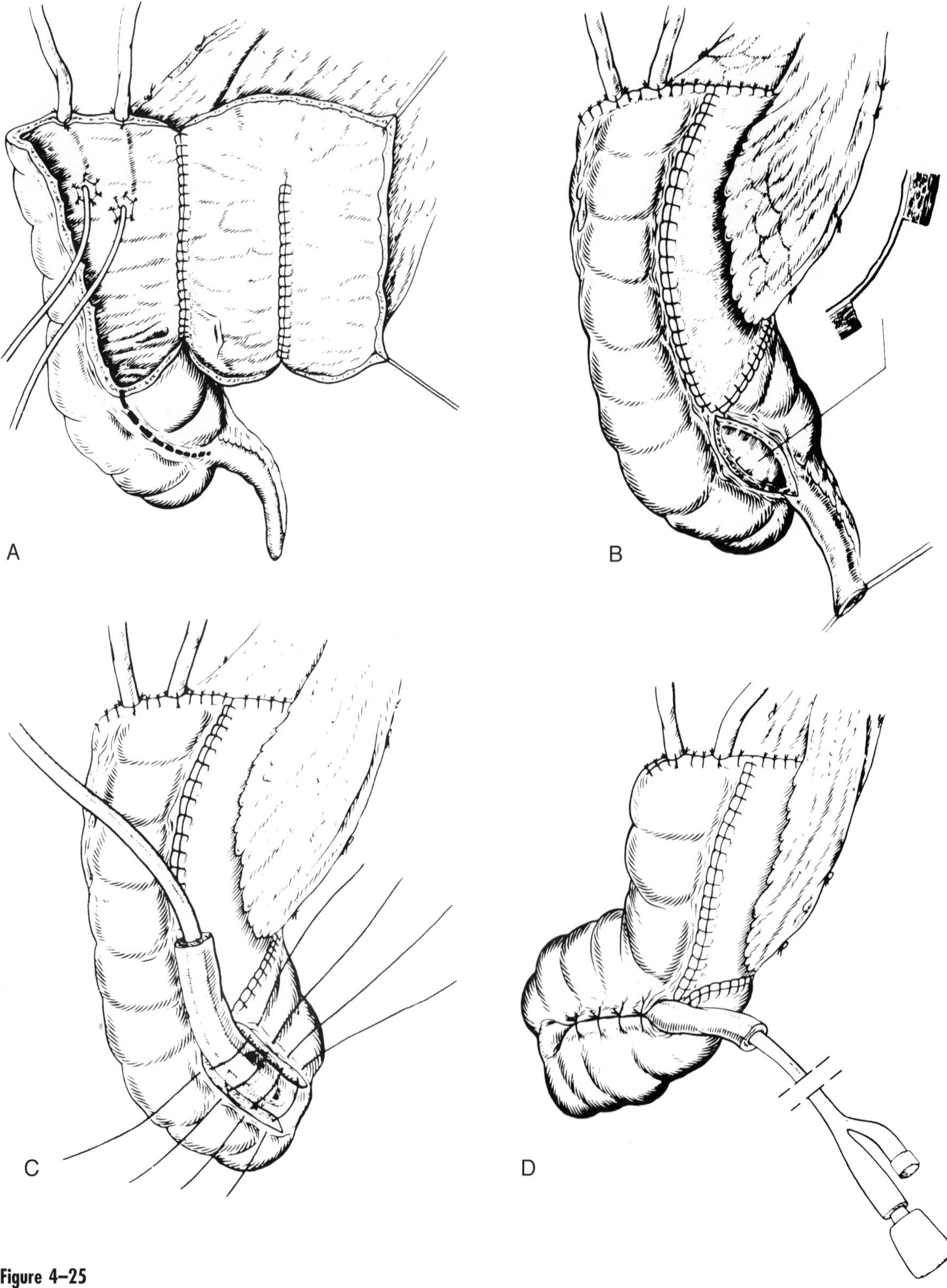

Figure 4–25

# UPPER URINARY TRACT TUMORS

**Figure 4–26:** Epidemiology, histopathology, and clinical features. Transitional cells line the renal pelvis and ureter. Tumors of the upper urinary tract are most commonly transitional cell carcinomas. About 2% of all patients with bladder cancer can be expected to develop upper urinary tract disease; however, 40% of patients with primary upper tract tumors develop subsequent bladder cancers later in the course of their disease.[31] The main symptoms of upper urinary tract tumors are gross hematuria (75%) and flank pain (30%).

Two-thirds of upper tract tumors occur in the renal pelvis, one third in the ureter. Of the ureteral tumors, 70% are located in the lower third of the ureter. The incidence of bilateral tumors is 2% to 3%.

**Figure 4–27:** Upper tract tumors are most frequently identified on IVP as radiolucent filling defects or obstructive lesions or, occasionally, because of nonvisualization of the collecting system. The IVP shows a radiolucent filling defect of the distal right ureter and the upper left infundibulum. A retrograde pyelogram combined with selective cytologic examination confirmed the diagnosis of an upper tract transitional cell carcinoma.

**Figure 4–28:** CT and MRI are helpful tools for the preoperative staging of upper tract tumors. The pelvic CT scan demonstrates a circular mass (*arrow*) within the lumen of the distal right ureter. Upon resection this mass was found to be a high-grade transitional cell carcinoma.

**Figure 4–29:** (See Color Insert.) Diagnostic ureterorenoscopy is indicated for direct vision evaluation of

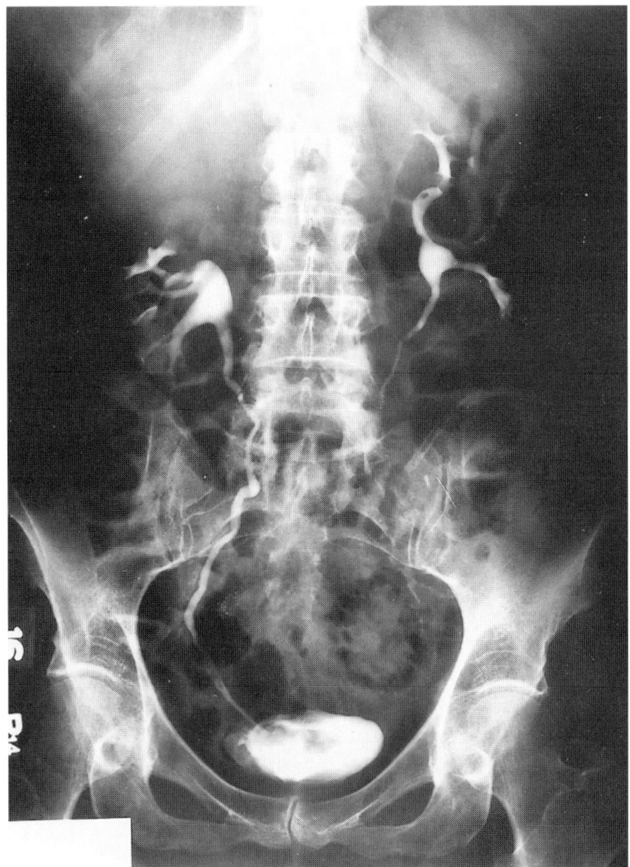

**Figure 4–27**

radiographic filling defects or obstruction, evaluation in case of bladder tumor at or near the ureteral orifices, and further evaluation of cystoscopically diagnosed upper tract hematuria. There might be an indication of ureterorenoscopic resection of small low-grade localized upper urinary tract tumors, especially in the patient with a solitary kidney or severe renal insufficiency. However, in patients with two functioning renal units, the role of conservative therapy is limited.

*A,* Ureterorenoscopic view of a large TCC extending throughout the renal pelvis and proximal ureter *B,* Ureterorenoscopic view of a TCC located at the ureteral pelvic junction.

**Figure 4–30:** In patients with organ-confined upper urinary tract tumors and normal contralateral renal function, nephroureterectomy with removal of a periureteral cuff of bladder tissue remains standard therapy. Removal of the complete ipsilateral renal unit and ureter is mandatory in light of the high rate of multifocality of upper tract tumors and the high rate of ureteral stump recurrence when upper tract TCC is treated by simple nephrectomy or partial ureterectomy.[32]

The technique of nephroureterectomy was first described by Reynes in 1902. After radical tumor nephrectomy using a flank or subcostal incision and deep

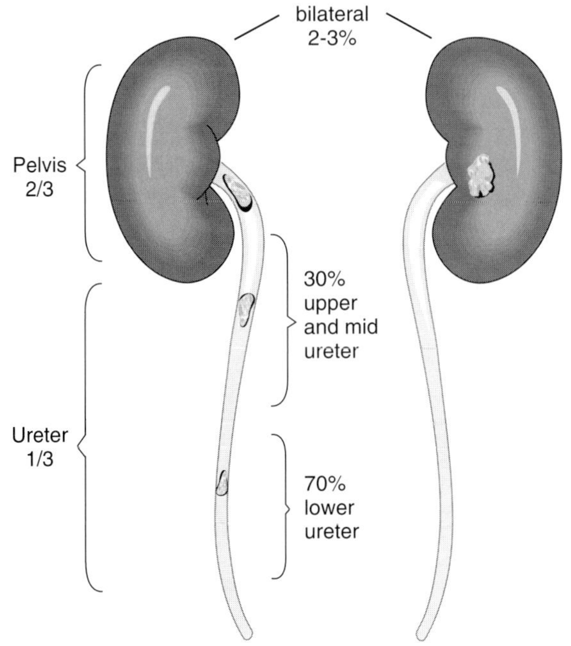



**Figure 4–26**

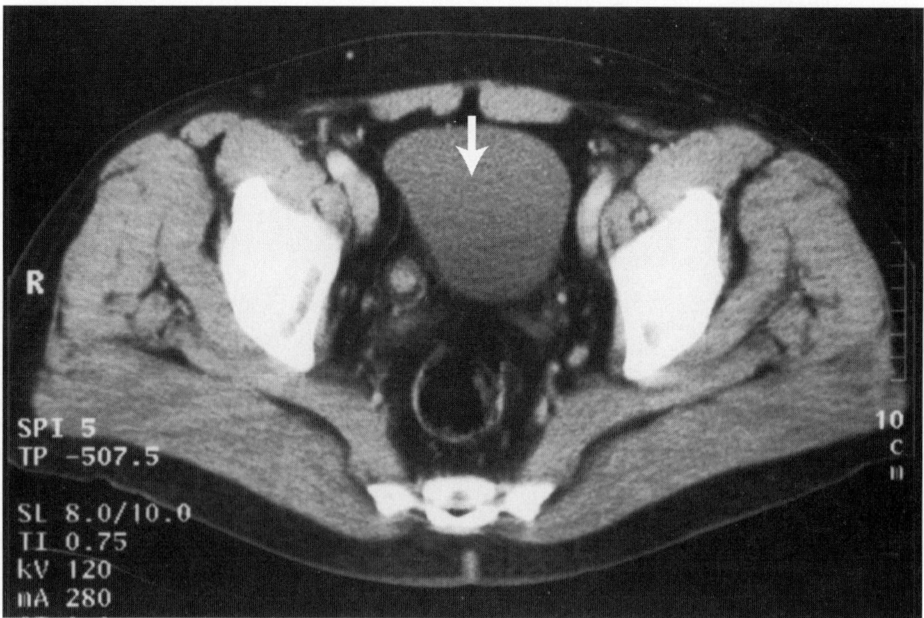

Figure 4–28

ligature of the ureter, the ureter stump, including 1 to 2 cm of normal bladder mucosa surrounding the ureteral orifice, is removed through a Gibson or midline incision.

The figure shows a ureterectomy with cuff of the bladder. For better visualization of the trigone and the contralateral ureter additionally an anterior cystostomy is performed.

### Acknowledgment

*The authors thank Angelo M. De Marzo and Jonathan I. Epstein for contributing the histologic images in this chapter.*

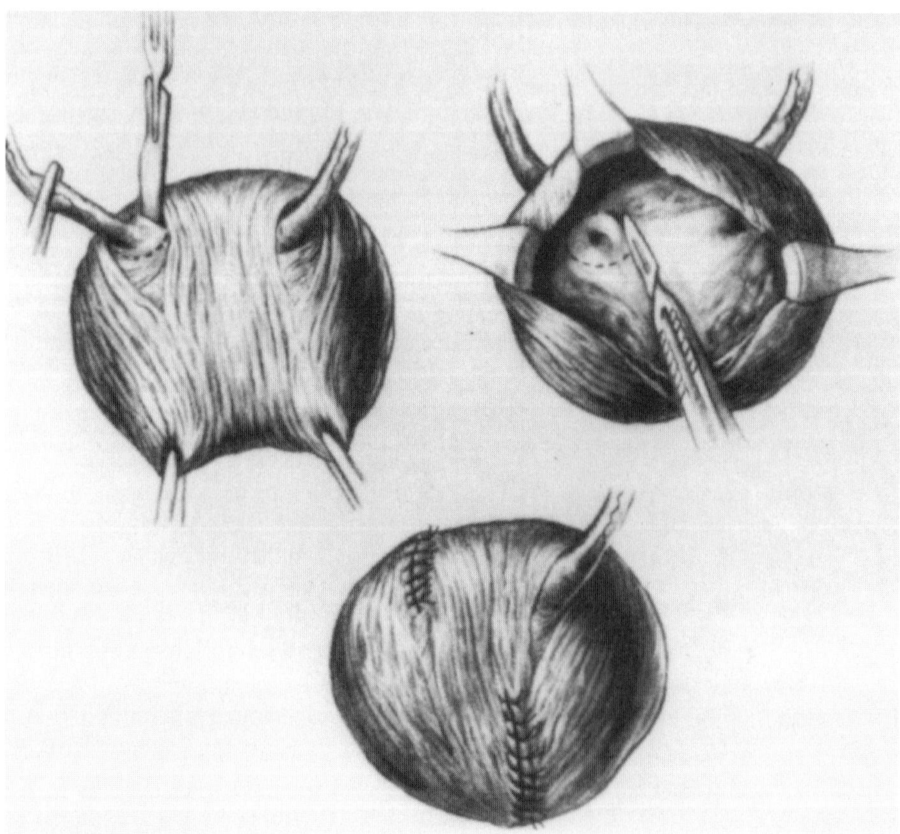

Figure 4–30

# REFERENCES

1. Greenlee RT, Murray T, Bolden S, Wingo PA: Cancer statistics. CA: Cancer J Clinicians 50(1):7–33, 2000.
2. Frades Y: Epidemiology of bladder cancer. In Vogelzang NJ, Scardino PT, Shipley WU, Coffey DS (eds): Comprehensive Textbook of Genitourinary Oncology. Baltimore, Williams & Wilkins, 1996, pp 298–304.
3. Rübben H, Lutzeier W, Fischer N, et al: Rheinisch Westfälische Technische Hochschule Aachen: Natural history and treatment of low and high risk superficial bladder tumors. J Urol 139:283–285, 1988.
4. Richie JP: Intravesical chemotherapy—Treatment selection, techniques and results. Urol Clin North Am 19:521–527, 1992.
5. Lamm DL: Long-term results of intravesical therapy for superficial bladder cancer. Urol Clin North Am 19:573–580, 1992.
6. Malmstrom P-U, Wijkstrom H, Lundholm C, et al: Five-year follow-up of a randomized prospective study comparing mitomycin C and bacillus Calmette-Guerin in patients with superficial bladder carcinoma. J Urol 161:1124–1127, 1999.
7. Lamm DL: BCG in perspective: Advances in the treatment of superficial bladder cancer. Eur Urol (suppl 1) 27:2–9, 1995.
8. Debryne FM, van der Meijden AP, Geboers AD, et al: BCG (RIVM) versus mitomycin intravesical therapy in superficial bladder cancer. First results of a randomized prospective trial. Urology (suppl 3) 31:20–25, 1988.
9. Lerner SP, Skinner DG: Radical cystectomy for bladder cancer. In Vogelzang NJ, Scardino PT, Shipley WU, Coffey DS (eds): Comprehensive Textbook of Genitourinary Oncology. Baltimore, Williams & Wilkins, 1996, pp 442–463.
10. Sternberg CN: Bladder-preserving treatments: Chemotherapy and conservative surgery. In Vogelzang NJ, Scardino PT, Shipley WU, Coffey DS (eds): Comprehensive Textbook of Genitourinary Oncology. Baltimore, Williams & Wilkins, 1996, pp 522–533.
11. Splinter TAW, Scher HI: Adjuvant and neoadjuvant chemotherapy for invasive (T3-T4) bladder cancer. In Vogelzang NJ, Scardino PT, Shipley WU, Coffey DS (eds): Comprehensive Textbook of Genitourinary Oncology. Baltimore, Williams & Wilkins, 1996, pp 464–471.
12. Rehn L: Blasengeschwülste bei Fuchsin-Arbeitern. Arch Klin Chir 50:588–600, 1895.
13. Hartge P, Silverman D, Hoover R, et al: Changing cigarette habits and bladder cancer risk: A case-control study. J Natl Cancer Inst 78:1119–1125, 1987.
14. El-Bolkainy MN, Mokhtar NM, Ghonhiem MA, Hussein MH: The impact of schistosomiasis on the pathology of bladder carcinoma. Cancer 48:2643–2648, 1981.
15. Travis LB, Curtis RE, Boice JD, Fraumeni JF Jr: Bladder cancer after chemotherapy for non-Hodgkin's lymphoma. N Engl J Med 321:544–545, 1989.
16. Gonzales-Zulueta M, Jones P: Molecular biology of bladder cancer. In Vogelzang NJ, Scardino PT, Shipley WU, Coffey DS (eds): Comprehensive Textbook of Genitourinary Oncology. Baltimore, Williams & Wilkins, 1996, pp 314–325.
17. Mohr DN, Offord KP, Owen RA, Melton J III: Asymptomatic microhematuria and urologic disease. A population based study. JAMA 256:224–229, 1986.
18. De Vogt HJ, Rathert P, Beyer-Boon ME: Urinary Cytology. New York, Springer Verlag, 1977.
19. Mao L, Schoenberg MP, Scicchitano M, et al: Molecular detection of primary bladder cancer by micro-satellite analysis. Science 271:659–662, 1996.
20. Steiner G, Schoenberg MP, Linn JF, Mao L, Sidransky D: Detection of bladder cancer recurrence by microsatellite analysis of urine. Nat Med 3:621–624, 1997.
21. Schulze S, Holm-Nielsen A, Mogensen P: Transurethral ultrasound scanning in the evaluation of invasive bladder cancer. Scand J Urol Nephrol 25:215–217, 1991.
22. Herr HW, Cookson MS, Soloway SM: Upper tract tumors in patients with primary bladder cancer followed for 15 years. J Urol 156:1286–1287, 1996.
23. Montie JE. Against bladder sparing. Surgery. J Urol 162:452–457, 1999.
24. Stöckle M, Meyenburg W, Wellek S, et al: Advanced bladder cancer (stage pT3b, pT4a, pN1 and pN2): Improved survival after radical cystectomy and 3 adjuvant cycles of chemotherapy. Results of a controlled prospective study. J Urol 148:302–306, 1992.
25. Boyd SD, Feinberg SM, Skinner DG, et al: Quality of life survey of urinary diversion patients: Comparison of ileal conduits versus continent Kock ileal reservoirs. J Urol 138:1386–1389, 1987.
26. Hart S, Skinner EC, Meyerowitz BE, et al: Quality of life after radical cystectomy for bladder cancer in patients with an ileal conduit, or cutaneous or urethral Kock pouch. J Urol 162:77–81, 1999.
27. Schlegel PN, Walsh PC: Neuroanatomical approach to radical cystoprostatectomy with preservation of sexual function. J Urol 138:1402–1406, 1987.
28. Bricker EM: Bladder substitution after pelvic evisceration. Surg Clin North Am 30:1511–1521, 1950.
29. Schoenberg MP, Marshall FF: The use of colon segments— Orthotopic ileocolic neobladder. Urol Clin North Am 32:55–63, 1995.
30. Thüroff JW, Alken P, Riedmiller H, et al: The Mainz pouch (mixed augmentation ileum and cecum) for bladder augmentation and continent urinary diversion. J Urol 136:17–26, 1986.
31. Mazeman E: Tumors of the upper urinary tract, calyces, renal pelvis and ureter. Eur Urol 2:120–126, 1976.
32. Charbit L, Gendreau MC, Mee S, Cukier J: Tumors of the upper urinary tract: 10 years of experience. J Urol 146:1243–1248, 1991.

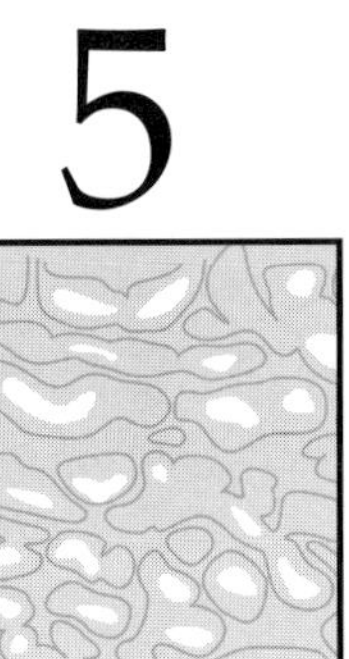

# 5

# Bladder Cancer: Radiotherapy and Chemotherapy

*Alan R. Schulsinger*

*Ramesh Vedula*

*Marvin Rotman*

*Gary Hudes*

## INTRODUCTION

Although cystectomy has been considered the standard treatment for muscle invasive urothelial carcinoma, the development of therapies that result in equivalent or better cancer control while at the same time preserving bladder function remains a worthwhile area of clinical research. Numerous chemotherapeutic agents have demonstrated significant antitumor activity in advanced transitional cell carcinomas that are beyond cure with surgery, and tumors of the urothelium are moderately radiosensitive. Neither chemotherapy nor radiotherapy alone as single modalities has curative potential for the majority of patients with locally advanced (nonresectable) disease. Thus, it was a logical step to combine these modalities and use them with aggressive transurethral resection (TUR) of the primary bladder tumor as an alternative to cystectomy for patients not deemed candidates for more aggressive surgery or for those desiring a potentially curative approach and bladder preservation.

Combined modality treatment with bladder preservation is an evolving field, fueled by advances in delivery of therapeutic radiation, identification of new active chemotherapeutic agents and combinations, and the accelerating pace of progress in cancer biology. There is increasing evidence that molecular markers, in addition to clinical parameters such as stage and grade, will prove valuable in predicting tumor progression and recurrence, and thus in optimizing treatment for individual patients. As described in this chapter, prime examples of molecular factors that may contribute to management of urothelial malignancy include p53 and retinoblastoma (pRb) proteins, and the functional status of two regulators of cell cycle progression at the G1 S boundary, p16$^{INK4a}$ and p21$^{waf1/cip-1}$.

As in many solid tumors, there remains an urgent need to identify effective systemic adjuvant or neoadjuvant therapy for patients at high risk for tumor dissemination. Based on the high response rates observed in metastatic disease, one might predict that such treatment should reduce the risk of tumor relapse following control of the primary tumor by surgery or radiotherapy, but it has been difficult to establish this benefit in randomized clinical trials. The challenge ahead will be to improve the design of clinical trials, selecting patients most likely to benefit from early systemic treatment (improved clinical staging, molecular markers), combined with more effective chemotherapy.

This chapter focuses on radiotherapy and systemic chemotherapy for the treatment of urothelial malignancy, including combined modality therapy for bladder preservation. The impact of molecular markers on the present and future management of urothelial malignancy is highlighted.

## RADIOTHERAPY

**Figure 5–1:** Radiotherapy in the management of bladder cancer. Radiotherapeutic management of bladder cancer comprises several clinical situations. Al-

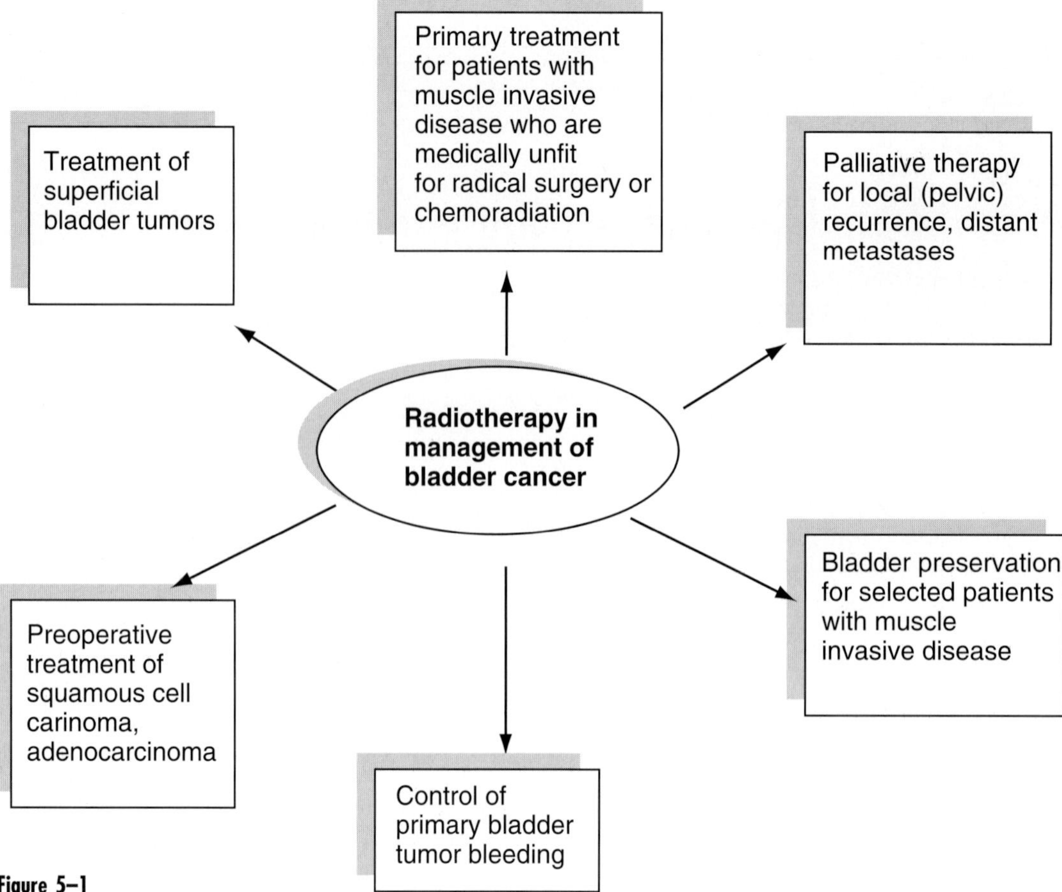


**Figure 5–1**

though they are not commonly used for superficial disease, brachytherapy or external beam radiotherapy or both have been used successfully as an alternative to intravesicle therapy.[1] In nontransitional cell histology such as squamous cell carcinoma and adenocarcinomas, preoperative radiation is typically administered prior to radical cystectomy in many centers. Combined with transurethral tumor resection (TUR) and chemotherapy, external beam radiotherapy is an established curative treatment strategy that permits bladder preservation for selected patients with muscle invasive transitional carcinoma. This combined modality approach also provides a therapeutic alternative for patients deemed medically unsuitable for radical cystectomy. Finally, radiotherapy (RT) is an essential tool for palliation of metastatic disease and recurrent tumor in the pelvis.

**Figure 5–2:** Clinical staging for radiotherapy of bladder cancer. After history and physical examination, cystoscopic examination and transurethral resection of the visible bladder tumor is attempted, with random biopsies of the surrounding normal-appearing urothelium. Bimanual examination under anesthesia is important to determine the size, consistency, and location of the tumor. A palpable tumor mass often indicates spread beyond the bladder wall ($\geq$T3) C, D. The extent of local infiltration into surrounding normal tissue is

assessed by determining whether the bladder tumor is freely mobile, tethered, or fixed. A bladder diagram showing the locations of all visible pathology and biopsies is completed at the time of cystoscopy.

**Figure 5–3:** Patient selection for definitive radiotherapy of bladder cancer: importance of T stage and initial transurethral surgery of the bladder (TURB). Most bladder-sparing strategies incorporate a maximum transurethral tumor resection (TURB) as the initial step. Together with clinical stage, the extent of initial TURB is an important predictor of complete response and survival following full-dose radiotherapy alone or with chemotherapy.[2–4] As illustrated here, survival rates following full-dose radiotherapy are highest for patients with no microscopic residual tumor following TURB (R0) and better for patients with visibly complete (only microscopic tumor residual) TURB (R1) compared with those with macroscopic tumor residual (R2) following initial TURB.[5]

Although a complete TURB alone may be curative for selected patients with single, small, superficially muscle invasive tumors (T2a) not associated with carcinoma in situ,[6,7] this procedure alone is inadequate for deeper or multifocal muscle invasive disease. The ability to perform at least a visibly complete TURB is related to the initial T stage, with rates of approximately 70% for T2 (nonpalpable) tumors and 40% for

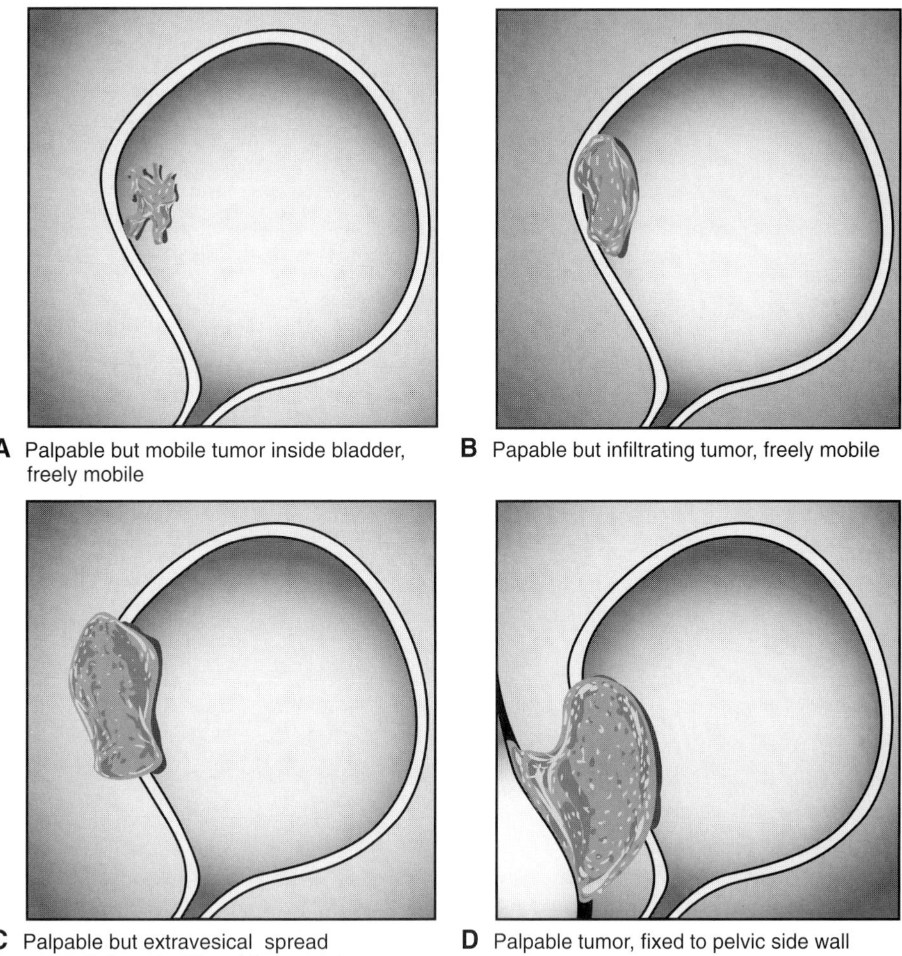



**Figure 5–2**

T3 (palpable) tumors.[3] As in the initial staging evaluation, bimanual examination following maximal TURB provides a more accurate picture of tumor extent and likelihood of complete response with treatment. (From Sauer R, Birkenhake S, Kühn R, et al: Efficacy of radiotherapy with platin derivatives compared to radiotherapy alone in organ-sparing treatment of bladder cancer. Int J Radiat Oncol Biol Phys 40(1):121, 1998.)

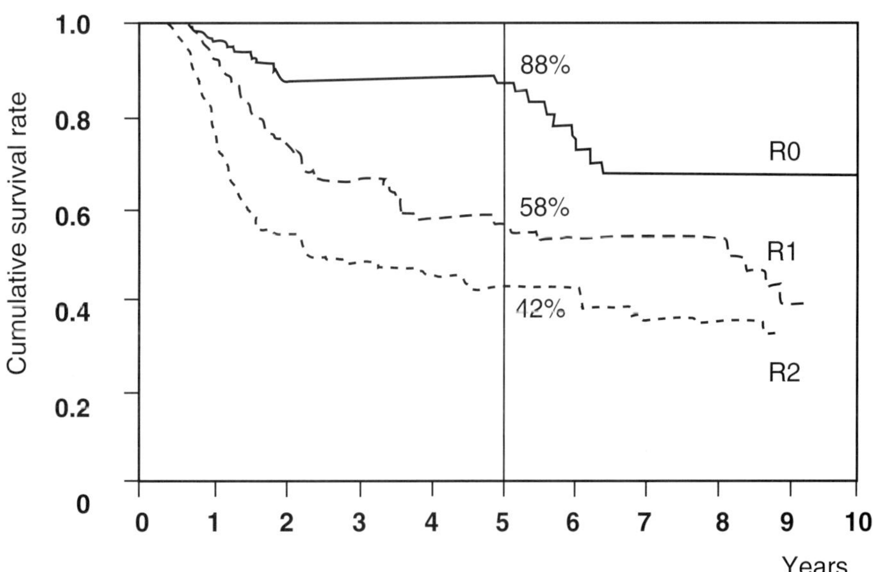



**Figure 5–3**

**Tables 5–1 and 5–2:** Clinical versus pathologic staging of bladder cancer. Analysis of radical cystectomy specimens shows that the pathologic tumor (P) stage is often higher or lower than the clinical T stage that is determined on the basis of TUR, bimanual examination, and imaging studies.[8–10] As shown in Table 5–1, the rate of understaging is especially high in patients with clinical T2 tumors. Cystectomy series indicate that 20% to 28% of all patients with muscle invasive bladder cancer have metastases to pelvic (regional) lymph nodes.[8–10] The majority of these patients will develop distant metastases. As shown in Table 5–2, risk of lymph node metastases increases with more advanced pathologic tumor (P) stage. Because of the inaccuracy of clinical staging methods, both overestimation and underestimation of tumor stage are inherent to nonoperative bladder-sparing strategies.

**Table 5–3:** Prognostic factors for survival following definitive radiotherapy for bladder cancer. Not all patients with muscle invasive tumors of the bladder are candidates for initial radiotherapy (or combined radiotherapy-chemotherapy). Tumor and patient characteristics that are predictive of complete response and survival include clinical stage (determined by TUR and bimanual examination under anesthesia), extent of residual tumor after TUR, ureteral obstruction (poor prognosis), tumor multiplicity and configuration, presence of diffuse carcinoma in situ, papillary versus solid or flat tumor surface morphology, and hemoglobin level.[2–4, 11–13] In multivariate analyses, lower pretreatment tumor stage (T2–T3A) and visibly complete TUR are independent predictors of favorable outcomes such as complete response (no residual bladder tumor) and survival with intact bladder.[4]

## TABLE 5–2

### INCIDENCE OF NODAL METASTASES ACCORDING TO PATHOLOGIC BLADDER TUMOR STAGE FOR 591 PATIENTS UNDERGOING RADICAL CYSTECTOMY WITH INTENT TO CURE

| PATHOLOGIC TUMOR STAGE | NO. OF PATIENTS | NO. (%) WITH POSITIVE NODES |
| --- | --- | --- |
| P0 | 37 | 0 (0) |
| PIS | 133 | 1 (.08%) |
| P1 | 52 | 7 (13) |
| P2 | 91 | 18 (20) |
| P3a | 70 | 17 (24) |
| P3b | 139 | 58 (42) |
| P4 | 69 | 31 (45) |
| Totals | 591 | 132 (22.3%) |

*Source:* Data from Lerner SP, Skinner DG, Lieskovsky G, et al: The rationale for en bloc pelvic lymph node dissection for bladder cancer patients with nodal metastases: Long-term results. J Urol 149:758–765, 1993.

## RADIOTHERAPY TECHNIQUES FOR BLADDER CANCER

**Figure 5–4:** Traditional technique for radiotherapy of bladder cancer. Traditional anterior (*A*) and lateral (*B*) fluoroscopic simulation films are used in the treatment of muscle invasive bladder cancer. Contrast material should be utilized to visualize the bladder. Initially, the entire bladder and the regional lymphatics are treated to a microscopic dose (approximately 40 to 45 Gy). Typically, patients are instructed to void prior to treatment in order to minimize the bladder volume during the initial portion of treatment. For planning of the

## TABLE 5–1

### STAGING ERROR OF PRIMARY TUMOR ACCORDING TO CLINICAL (T) VERSUS PATHOLOGIC (P) STAGE

| CLINICAL STAGE | NO. OF PATIENTS | UNDERSTAGED NO. (%) | OVERSTAGED NO. (%) | AGREEMENT NO. (%) |
| --- | --- | --- | --- | --- |
| T1 + Tis | 74 | 26 (35) | 12 (16) | 36 (49) |
| T2 | 87 | 48 (55) | 20 (23) | 19 (22) |
| T3 | 81 | 6 (8) | 31 (38) | 44 (54) |
| T4 | 19 | — | 2 (11) | 17 (89) |
| Totals | 261 | 80 (31) | 65 (25) | 116 (44) |

*Note:* Understaged-clinical stage less than pathologic stage; overstaged-clinical stage greater than pathologic stage; agreement-clinical stage equals pathologic stage.

*Source:* Pagano F, Bussi P, Galetti TP, et al: Results of contemporary radical cystectomy for invasive bladder cancer: A clinicopathological study with an emphasis on the adequacy of the tumor, nodes, and metastases classification. J Urol 145:45–50, 1991.

## TABLE 5–3

### RADIOTHERAPY OF BLADDER CANCER: FACTORS PREDICTIVE OF COMPLETE RESPONSE AND SURVIVAL WITH INTACT BLADDER

| FAVORABLE CHARACTERISTICS | UNFAVORABLE CHARACTERISTICS |
| --- | --- |
| Tumor stage T2, T3a | Tumor stage T3b, T4 |
| Absence of palpable bladder mass | Palpable mass present on bimanual examination |
| Absence of ureteral obstruction | Presence of ureteral obstruction |
| Visibly complete TUR | Visible tumor following TUR |
| Papillary histology | Solid/flat surface tumor histology |
| Hemoglobin ≥ 12 g/dl | Hemoglobin < 12 g/dl |
| Absence of diffuse carcinoma *in situ* | Presence of diffuse carcinoma *in situ* |

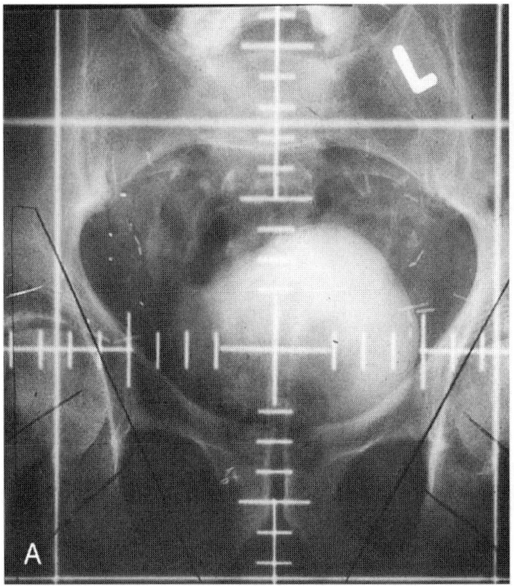
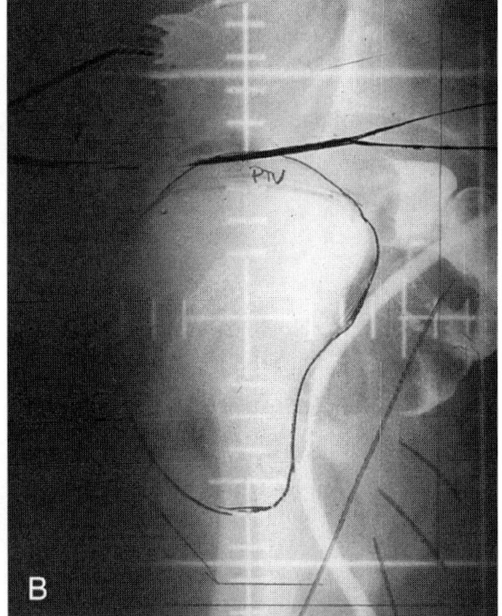

**Figure 5–4**

cone-down volume, care should be taken to spare a portion of normal bladder, if possible. For this purpose, patients should be treated with a full bladder for the cone-down portion of the treatment.

**Figure 5–5:** Anteroposterior (*A*) and lateral (*B*) views for fluoroscopic cone-down simulation films are shown here. This field is typically boosted for an additional 20 Gy for a total dose of 60 to 65 Gy to the tumor volume. A recent study has reported a significant correlation, on multivariate analysis, between total radiation dose (>57.5 Gy versus <57.5 Gy) and local control for bladder cancer.[13]

**Figure 5–6:** Recently, 3-D computed tomography (CT) guided treatment planning has been advocated for treatment of bladder cancer.[14] Standard simulation was reported to be inadequate for defining treatment volumes in 16% to 85% of patients. A recent study suggests that changes in bladder volume and shape related to bladder filling can result in clinically significant displacements of the target volume.[15] These volume changes are responsible for a target motion ranging from 3 to 15 mm with tumors located in the lateral and anterior walls. As expected, movement was most marked in the craniocaudal axis of the bladder dome. The authors suggest that a 2-cm margin around the tumor should compensate for the extreme volume changes during the boost treatment. This figure demonstrates use of CT simulation in the planning of the boost for bladder cancer. In this example, three noncoplanar radiation beams are utilized to conform the

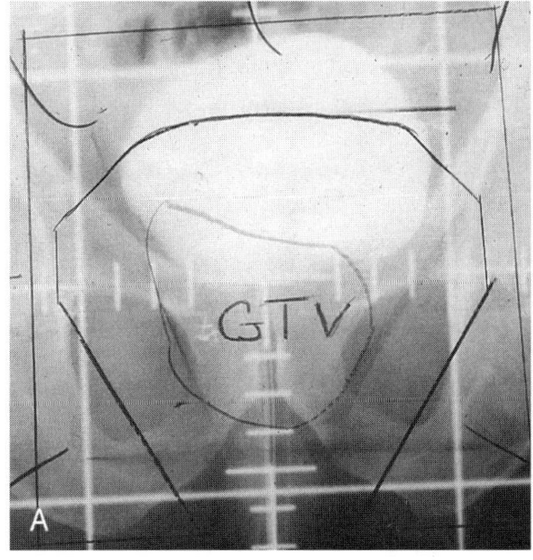
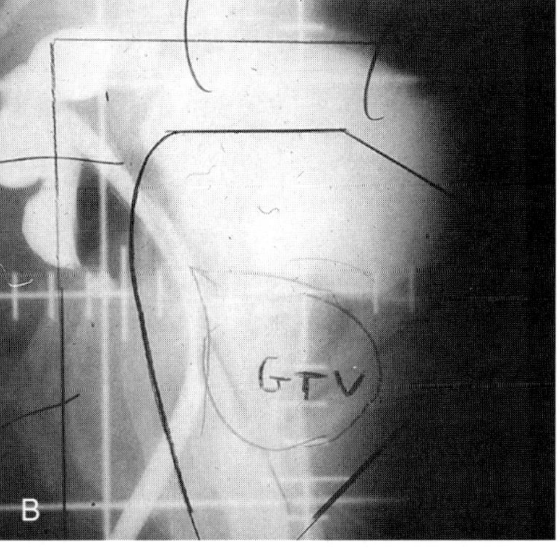

**Figure 5–5**

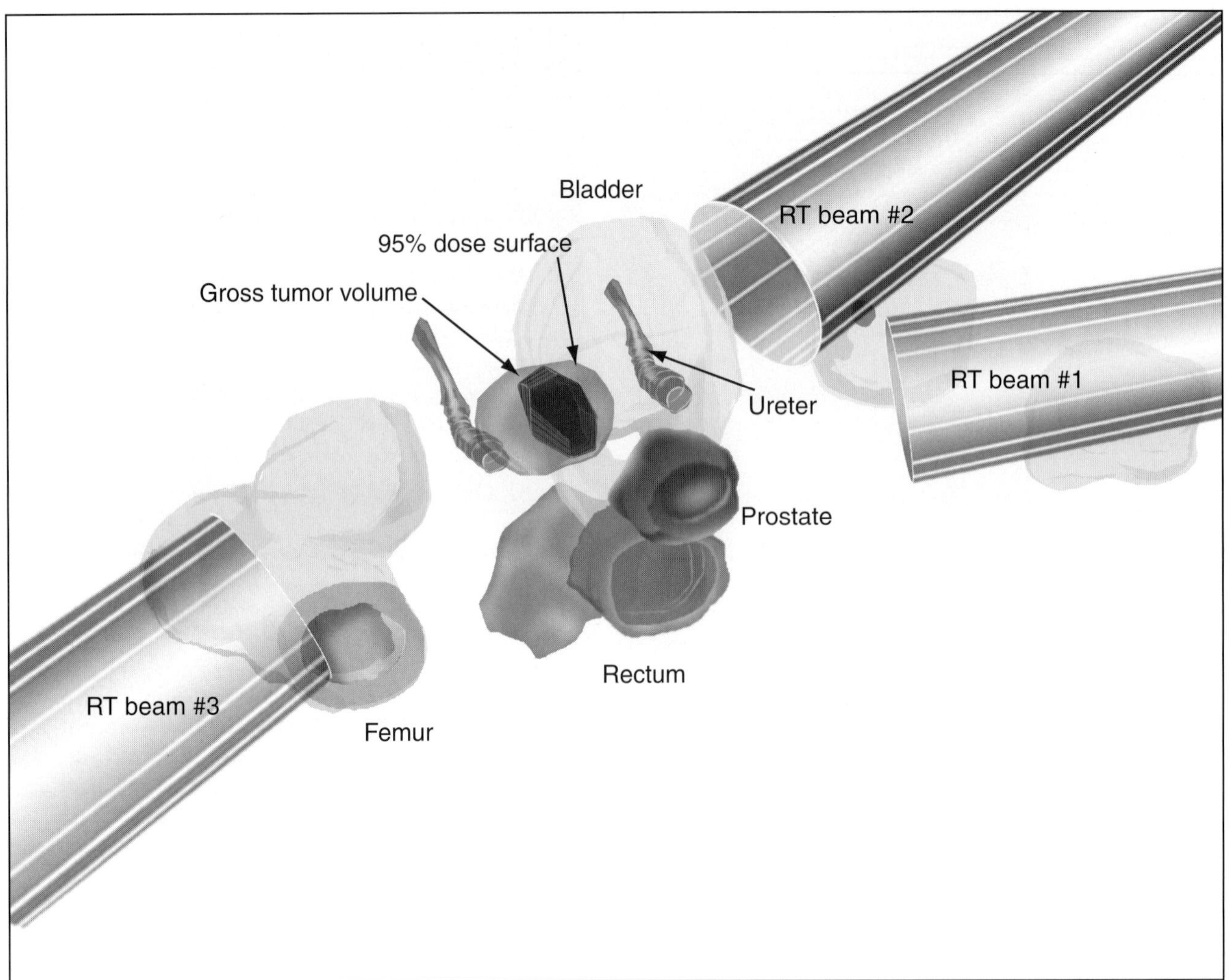


**Figure 5–6**

radiation dose cloud around the gross tumor volume. This technique is useful in precisely defining the target volume and sparing normal bladder from high radiation doses.

**Table 5–4:** Radiotherapy alone following TUR for muscle invasive bladder cancer: Results. Summarized in Table 5–4 are published results of TUR followed by radiotherapy in selected series of patients.[2, 12, 18–20] As seen in the table, cancer control outcomes are generally superior for patients with T2 tumors. Variability in the results may be explained by differences in patient selection, staging evaluation, extent of TUR prior to radiation, timing and extent of response evaluation, and other factors, including treatment techniques.

Among the endpoints used to evaluate radiotherapy and other bladder-sparing therapies are complete response in the bladder (defined as no visible or microscopic evidence of tumor on posttherapy cystoscopy with biopsies and cytology), lack of development of distant metastases, tumor recurrence (both superficial and muscle invasive) in the bladder, local control, overall survival, and survival with the bladder intact. In all series, complete response following radiotherapy is the strongest independent predictor of 5-year survival. In addition to measures of cancer control, function of the retained bladder and other aspects of quality of life are important outcomes relevant to bladder-sparing treatments.

**Figure 5–7:** Radiotherapy and chemotherapy as single modality treatments can each produce tumor regression in patients with muscle invasive transitional cell carcinoma, and each modality is very effective against smaller tumors confined to the bladder. The aims of combining chemotherapy and radiation are to produce an additive or greater local effect against the primary bladder tumor and to eradicate systemic metastases.

As shown in Figure 5–7, most bladder preservation protocols employ concomitant chemotherapy (cisplatin or 5-FU) with radiation therapy after a maximum TURB. After receiving a radiation dose of approximately 40 Gy, patients are typically evaluated by cystoscopy, bladder biopsies, and urine cytology. Patients achieving a complete response receive additional che-

## TABLE 5–4

### RESULTS OF RADIOTHERAPY FOLLOWING TRANSURETHRAL RESECTION FOR MUSCLE INVASIVE BLADDER CANCER

| AUTHOR[†] | T STAGES | NO. OF PATIENTS | COMPLETE RESPONSE RATE (%) | OVERALL 5-YEAR SURVIVAL RATE (%) |
|---|---|---|---|---|
| Shipley[2] | T2/T3 | 37 | NR | 45 |
|  | T4 | 18 | NR | 9 |
| **Total** |  | **55** | **NR** | **31** |
| Gospodarowicz[12] | T2 | 42 | 71 | 59† |
|  | T3A | 26 | 58 | 52 |
|  | T3B | 41 | 39 | 29.7 |
|  | T4A | 6 | 50 | 50 |
|  | T4B | 6 | 0 | 16 |
| **Total** |  | **121** |  | **31.6** |
| Duncan[16] | T1 | 174 | 48 | 64 |
|  | T2 | 248 | 49 | 46 |
|  | T3 | 272 | 41 | 31 |
|  | T4 | 53 | 49 | 21 |
| **Total** |  | **747** | **45.9** | **43.5** |
| Greven[17] | T1 | 35 | 26‡ | 39 |
|  | T2 | 35 | 36 | 59 |
|  | T3 | 36 | 18 | 10 |
|  | T4 | 7 | 0 | 0 |
| **Total** |  | **113** | **27** | **34** |
| Smaaland[18] | T2 | 35 | 69 | 26 |
|  | T3/T4 | 111 | 36 | 10 |
| **Total** |  | **146** | **44** | **14** |

*Superscript numbers correspond to references at the end of this chapter.

†Cause-specific survival rate.

‡Local control rate; complete response rate not given.

motherapy and radiotherapy to a total of 65 Gy. Nonresponding patients and those with only partial response (including positive urine cytologic findings only) go on to immediate cystectomy.

**Table 5–5:** Results of combined TUR + chemotherapy + radiation for bladder cancer. Although results of combined modality treatment suggest higher rates of complete response and 5-year survival compared with those of radiotherapy alone, these advantages have not been established in randomized trials. The 5-year survival rates for combined TUR, chemotherapy, and radiation are similar to those reported for radical cystectomy, and a functional bladder is preserved in approximately 40% of patients.[3, 19–23]

The "ideal" candidate for bladder preservation has primary clinical stage T2 tumor, no associated ureteral obstruction, visibly complete TUR, and a complete response after induction of chemoradiation based on endoscopic evaluation, including biopsy and cytology. A recent study found that bladder cancers with a high apoptotic index (AI) and high Ki-67 index were significantly associated with improved complete response (CR) and local control rates following chemoradiation for bladder preservation.[24] The p53 and *bcl*-2 expressions were not found to be important predictors. When the AI and Ki-67 indices were combined, the association with initial CR ($p < 0.001$), local control ($p = 0.0002$), and cancer-specific survival with preserved bladder ($p = 0.008$) was highly significant.

Bladder-preserving trimodality treatment should be administered by dedicated multidisciplinary teams.[25] Patients who elect this approach must undergo lifelong close follow-up, including regular cystoscopy and bi-

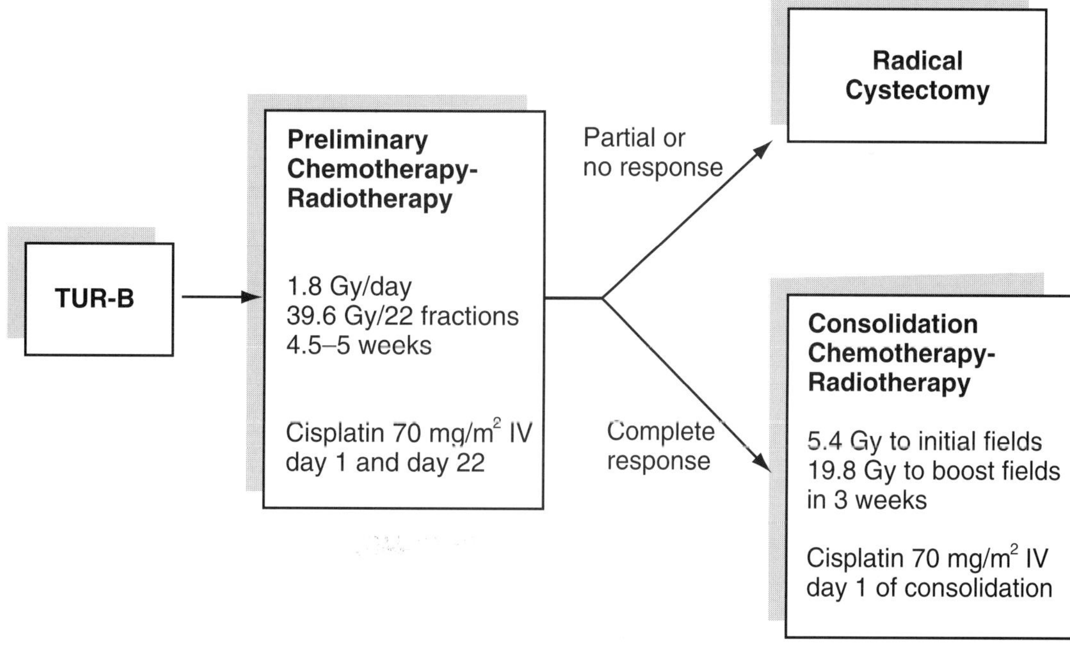


**Figure 5–7**

**TABLE 5–5**

## RESULTS OF CONCURRENT CHEMORADIATION FOR BLADDER CANCER

| | TREATMENT | | | NO. OF PATIENTS | | | | | |
| AUTHOR | Chemotherapy | Tumor Radiation Dose (cGy) | MEDIAN FOLLOW-UP | Total Enrolled | Completed Therapy | Complete Response | Alive with Bladder | Distant Metastases | SURVIVAL |
|---|---|---|---|---|---|---|---|---|---|
| Shipley[19] | Cisplatin* | 6480 | 24 mo | 70 | 62 | 49 (70%) | 36 (51%) | NA | 50%, 2.5 yr |
| Tester[20] | Cisplatin | 6000 | 36 mo | 49† | 42 | 28 (65%) | 22 (42%) | 18 (42%) | 64%, 3 yr |
| Housset[21] | Cisplatin + 5-FU | 4400, bid split course | 27 mo‡ | 54 | 51 | 40 (74%) | 19/22 (86%)§ | 16 (30%) | 62%, 3 yr |
| Dunst[3] | Cisplatin | 5000 | 18 mo | 67 | 67 | 45 (67%) | NG | NG | 66%, 3 yr |
| Russell[22] | 5-FU | 6600 | 18 mo | 40 | 34 | 24 (70.5%) | 18 (45%) | 18% | 64%, 45 mo |
| Rotman[23] | 5-FU | 6000–6500 | 38 mo | 20 | 20 | 14 (70%) | NG | 39% | 38%, 5 yr |

*Cisplatin given concurrently and following radiotherapy; all but five patients had residual tumor in bladder prior to chemoradiation.
†42 evaluable, all with residual bladder tumor prior to chemoradiation.
‡18 of 40 complete responders elected immediate cystectomy.
§Mean follow-up.
NG = not given.

opsy, so that cystectomy can be performed as early as possible for muscle infiltrating recurrence. In addition to recurrent muscle invasive disease, patients retaining the bladder remain at lifelong risk for development of new superficial tumors.

**Figure 5–8:** Chemoradiation schema at SUNY Health Science Center, Brooklyn. Between 1980 and 1993, 22 evaluable patients with biopsy-proved transitional cell carcinoma of the urinary bladder were treated with irradiation and continuous infusion of 5-FU (CCIC) at SUNY HSCB. Twenty-one of these patients had muscle invasive disease (T2 = 7 patients; T3/T4 = 14). This group of patients was referred because of medical inoperability, technical inoperability (locally advanced disease), or refusal of radical surgery by the patient.

As shown here, 5-fluorouracil (5-FU) was administered as a 120-hour continuous infusion at a rate of 25 mg/kg/day. Treatment was initiated either on weeks 1, 4, and 7 or 2, 5, and 8 of external beam radiation treatment. Five patients received a single bolus injection of mitomycin C (10 mg/m²) on day 1 of external beam radiation therapy. Results, which are summa-

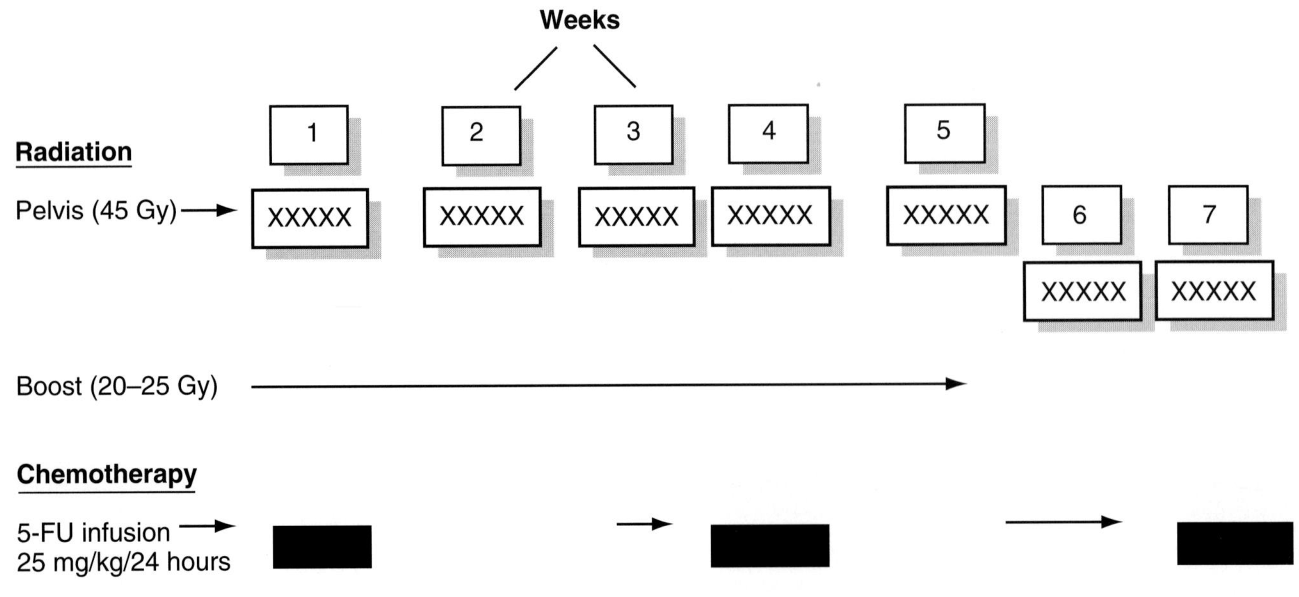


**Figure 5–8**

**TABLE 5–6**

## RESULTS OF NEOADJUVANT CISPLATIN-BASED CHEMOTHERAPY AND CONCURRENT CHEMORADIATION FOR BLADDER CANCER

| AUTHOR | NEOADJUVANT CHEMOTHERAPY | TUMOR RADIATION DOSE (cGy) | MEDIAN FOLLOW-UP | TOTAL COMPLETED TREATMENT/TOTAL ENROLLED | COMPLETE RESPONSE (%) | ALIVE WITH BLADDER (%) | WITH DISTANT METASTASES (%) | ACTUARIAL SURVIVAL |
|---|---|---|---|---|---|---|---|---|
| Kaufman[26] | CMV | 6480 | 48 mo | 42/53 | 53% | 31% | 42% | 53%, 4 yrs. |
| Tester[27] | CMV | 6480 | 52 mo | 85/91 | 80% | 44% | 22% | 62%, 4 yrs. |
| Given[28] | CMV or MVAC | 6480 | 60 mo | 49* | 62% | 18% | NG | 39%, 5 yrs. |
| Shipley[29] | CMV versus | 6480 | 60 mo | 49/61 (80%) | 61% | 36% | 33% | 48%, 5 yrs. |
|  | None | 6480 | 60 mo | 58/62 (94%) | 55% | 40% | 39% | 49%, 5 yrs. |

*94 patients entered, 90 completed chemotherapy, 49 elected RT and completed treatment.
NG = not given.

rized in Table 5–5, demonstrated complete response in 70% of patients and 38% alive at 5 years.[23]

**Table 5–6:** Neoadjuvant cisplatin-based chemotherapy and concurrent chemoradiation for bladder cancer. Uncontrolled studies suggested that the addition of two to four cycles of neoadjuvant cisplatin-based chemotherapy prior to concurrent cisplatin and radiation improved outcomes over those of chemoradiation alone.[26–28] However, as summarized in this table, a multicenter randomized trial showed that the addition of two cycles of neoadjuvant CMV (methotrexate, cisplatin, and vinblastine) chemotherapy was more toxic than chemoradiation alone, did not provide better local or distant control of tumor, and did not improve overall survival for patients with muscle invasive bladder cancer.[29] Longer follow-up indicates that patients remain at risk for muscle invasive and superficial disease recurrence beyond 5 years.[28]

## CHEMOTHERAPY OF BLADDER CANCER

**Figure 5–9:** There are several settings in which systemic chemotherapy is used for treatment of bladder cancer and other urothelial malignancies. Beyond its conventional role in the control and palliation of metastatic disease, chemotherapy has been used increasingly in combination with TURB and radiotherapy for patients with muscle invasive tumors who desire bladder-sparing treatment, or who are considered unfit for radical surgery. Radiation-sensitizing and additive antitumor effects are exploited when chemotherapy is administered concurrently with radiotherapy. Eradication of clinically undetectable distant metastases is an important objective of chemotherapy when administered before (neoadjuvant) or after (adjuvant) definitive surgery or radiotherapy of muscle invasive bladder tumor. Chemotherapy has been employed as the initial modality for patients with locally advanced (T4b), unresectable tumors or regional nodal metastases. Patients so treated may become candidates for potentially curative surgical resection of residual masses if there has been a substantial reduction of tumor volume in response to chemotherapy.[30]

**Table 5–7:** Activity of selected chemotherapeutic agents in advanced bladder cancer. Transitional cell carcinoma of the bladder is a chemotherapy-sensitive tumor. Summarized in Table 5–7 are rates of objective response for patients with metastatic bladder cancer treated with older, single cytotoxic agents.

**Table 5–8:** Selected combination chemotherapy regimens in advanced urothelial tumors, results of nonrandomized trials. Summarized in Table 5–8 are results of phase I and II trials of combination chemotherapy for patients with metastatic bladder cancer. Although objective response rates are usually greater for combination therapies than for single agents, toxicity to normal host tissues increases significantly. Regimens incorporating cisplatin and methotrexate such as MVAC (methotrexate + vinblastine + Adriamycin + cisplatin) and CMV (cisplatin + methotrexate + vinblastine) have been most commonly used. Because these regimens routinely produce severe toxicity, the support of a dedicated oncology team and good communication between the treatment staff and patient are essential. In other trials, addition of hematologic growth factors allowed only a slight increase of MVAC dose intensity and was not sufficient to augment response or survival compared with the standard doses.[32–42]

**Table 5–9:** Selected combination chemotherapy regimens in advanced urothelial tumors, results from ran-

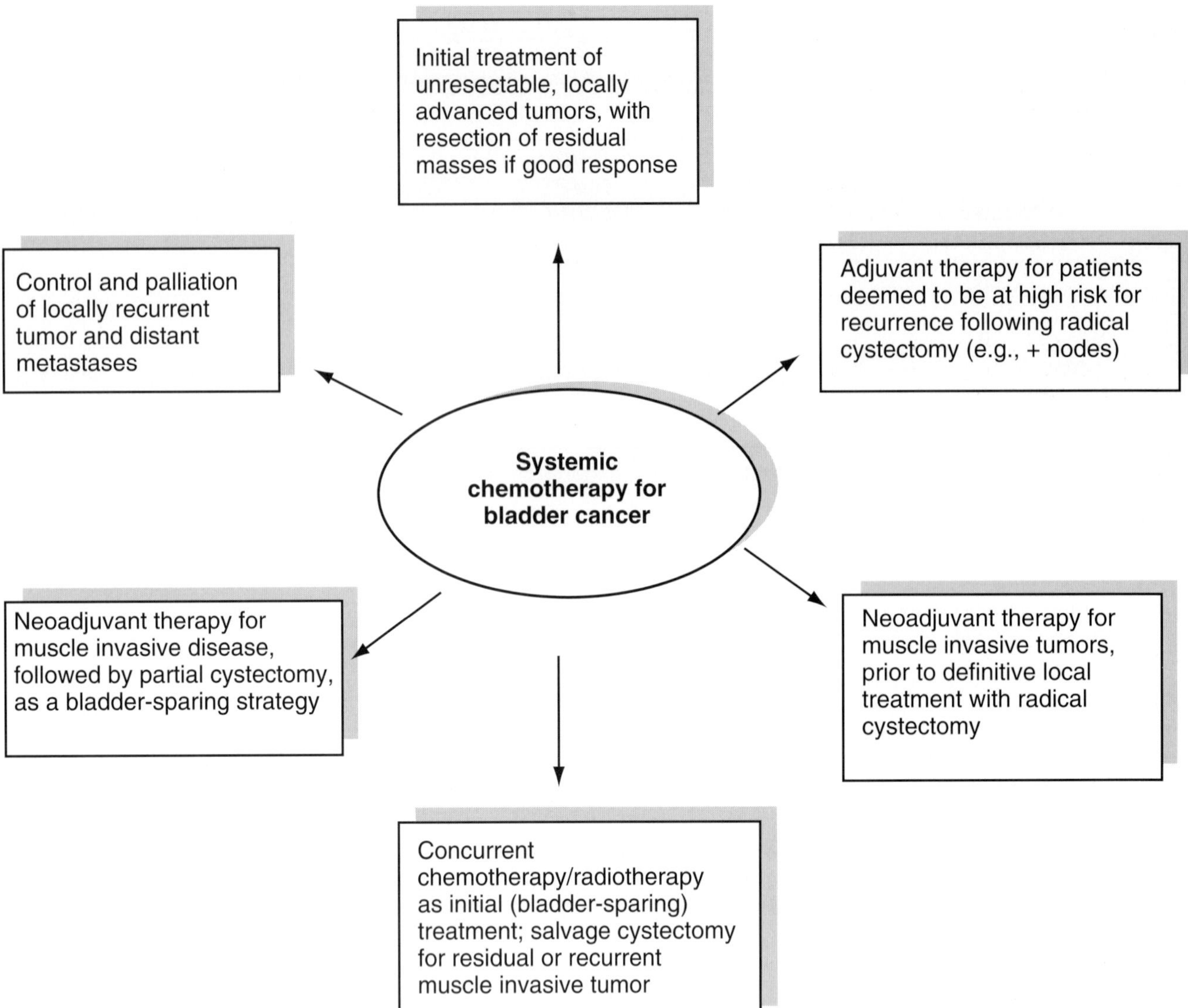


Figure 5–9

## TABLE 5–7

### ACTIVITY OF SELECTED CHEMOTHERAPEUTIC AGENTS IN ADVANCED BLADDER CANCER

| AGENT | NO. OF PATIENTS | PR + CR* (%) (95% CONFIDENCE INTERVAL) |
|---|---|---|
| Cisplatin | 320 | 30 (25–35) |
| Methotrexate | 236 | 29 (23–38) |
| Carboplatin | 41 | 21 (6–50) |
| Doxorubicin | 248 | 17 (12–23) |
| Vinblastine | 38 | 16 (4–28) |
| 5-Fluorouracil | 105 | 15 (12–19) |
| Vincristine | 42 | 14 (3–25) |
| Mitomycin C | 42 | 13 (3–23) |
| Cyclophosphamide | 26 | 7 (0–17) |

*PR = partial response rate; CR = complete response rate.
*Source:* Adapted from Yaguda A: Chemotherapy of urothelial tract tumors. Cancer 60:574–585, 1987.

domized trials. An international phase III trial has demonstrated superior activity for the four-drug MVAC combination compared with cisplatin alone, both in terms of response and survival. However, greater toxicity was produced by MVAC, and fewer than 5% of patients survived for 5 years, thus highlighting the limitations of chemotherapy for metastatic disease. In other randomized trials, MVAC was shown to be superior to the three-drug combination of cyclophosphamide, doxorubicin, and cisplatin (CISCA). The CMV combination (cisplatin, methotrexate, and vinblastine) has proved more effective than the same regimen without cisplatin (MV). More recently, in a large international phase III trial, the two-drug combination of cisplatin plus gemcitabine produced a similar response rate and survival as the four-drug MVAC regimen, with less mucositis and fewer neutropenic complications.[47a] Although toxic, MVAC remains the standard against which new combinations should be tested.

**SELECTED COMBINATION CHEMOTHERAPY REGIMENS IN ADVANCED UROTHELIAL TUMORS: RESULTS OF NONRANDOMIZED TRIALS**

| AGENTS | NO. OF PATIENTS | PR (%) | CR (%) | PR + CR (%) (95% CONFIDENCE LIMITS) | MEDIAN SURVIVAL (MONTHS) |
|---|---|---|---|---|---|
| Methotrexate + cisplatin*[32] | 47 | 21 | 21 | 42 (28–56) | NR |
| Cisplatin + methotrexate + vinblastine (CMV)*[33] | 60† | 14 | 14 | 56 (42–70) | < 11 |
| Methotrexate + cisplatin + vinblastine + doxorubicin (MVAC)[34] | 121 | 46 | 26 | 72 (64–80) | NR |
| Methotrexate + cisplatin + paclitaxel‡[35] | 25 | 10 | 0 | 40 (22–61) | NR |
| Cisplatin + paclitaxel*[36] | 29 | 52 | 10 | 62 (44–80) | NR |
| Carboplatin + paclitaxel[37] | 33 | 39 | 12 | 51 (34–68) | 8.5 |
| Ifosfamide + paclitaxel + cisplatin[38] | 30 | 57 | 20 | 77 (60–92) | 18.3 |
| Vinblastine + ifosfamide + gallium nitrate*[39] | 45 | 14 | 6 | 44 (30–60) | 10 |
| Cyclophosphamide + doxorubicin + cisplatin (MDA)[40] | 97 | 28 | 36 | 64 (54–74) | 10 |
| Gemcitabine + cisplatin*[41] | 28 | 36 | 21 | 57 (37–76) | 13.2 |
| Cisplatin + docetaxel[42] | 25 | 32 | 28 | 60 (39–79) | 13.6 |

*Denotes data from multi-institutional, cooperative group trials.
†Includes 50 patients evaluable for response.
‡After failure of cisplatin-based chemotherapy.
Superscript numbers correspond to references at the end of the chapter. NR = not reported.




**SELECTED COMBINATION CHEMOTHERAPY REGIMENS IN ADVANCED UROTHELIAL TUMORS: RESULTS FROM RANDOMIZED TRIALS**

| TREATMENT ARMS | NO. OF PATIENTS | PR (%) | CR (%) | PR + CR (%) (95% CI) | MEDIAN SURVIVAL (MONTHS) |
|---|---|---|---|---|---|
| Cisplatin + methotrexate vs. | 53 | 36 | 9 | 45 (31–58) | 8.7 |
| Cisplatin[43] | 55 | 22 | 9 | 31 (19–43) | 7.2 |
| MVAC vs. | 120 | 25 | 14 | 39 (30–48) | 12.5 |
| Cisplatin[44] | 126 | 9 | 3 | 12 (6–18) | 8.2 |
| MVAC vs. | 54 | 35 | 30 | 65 (52–77) | 14.5 |
| CISCA[45] | 48 | 25 | 21 | 46 (32–62) | 11 |
| Cisplatin vs. | 48 | 15 | 2 | 17 (6–28) | 6.0 |
| Cyclophosphamide + doxorubicin + cisplatin[46] | 45 | 11 | 22 | 33 (19–47) | 7.3 |
| Methotrexate + vinblastine vs. | 106* | 12 | 7 | 19 (11–27) | 4.5 |
| Cisplatin + methotrexate + vinblastine[47] | 108† | 36 | 10 | 46 (36–56) | 7.0 |
| Cisplatin + gemcitibine vs. | 203 | 37.2 | 12.2 | 49 (42–56) | 13.8 |
| MVAC[47a] | 202 | 33.8 | 11.9 | 46 (39–53) | 14.8 |

CISCA = cyclophosphamide 650 mg/m$^2$ day 1, doxorubicin 50 mg/m$^2$ and cisplatin 100 mg/m$^2$ day 2; MVAC = methotrexate 30 mg/m$^2$ days 1, 15, 22, vinblastine 3 mg/m$^2$ days 2, 15, 22, doxorubicin 30 mg/m$^2$ day 2, and cisplatin 70 mg/m$^2$ day 2.
*Includes 93 patients evaluable for response.
†Includes 88 patients evaluable for response.

## TABLE 5–10

## ANTITUMOR ACTIVITY OF NEWER AGENTS IN UROTHELIAL MALIGNANCY

| AGENT | NO. OF PATIENTS | PR | CR | PR + CR (%) | 95% CI |
|---|---|---|---|---|---|
| Paclitaxel[48] | 26 | 4 | 7 | 42 | 23–63 |
| Gemcitabine[49–51] | 91 | 16 | 8 | 26 | 17–35 |
| Ifosfamide*[52] | 47 | 6 | 4 | 21 | 11–36 |
| Trimetrexate*[53] | 48 | 7 | 1 | 17 | 7–30 |
| Gallium nitrate*[54] | 23 | 3 | 1 | 17 | 2–33 |
| Docetaxel*[55] | 30 | 4 | 0 | 13 | 4–31 |

*Activity as second-line treatment following platinum-based first-line chemotherapy.

Superscripts indicate references at the end of this chapter.

**Table 5–10:** Antitumor activity of newer agents in urothelial malignancy. Although combination chemotherapy is superior to single-agent treatment of advanced and metastatic bladder cancer, cure and prolonged survival occur only rarely, and only in favorable-prognosis patients (see Fig. 5–10). Further progress will depend on the identification of newer, more effective drugs and their integration into more active combinations. Undergoing evaluation are novel combination therapies that incorporate newer agents such as paclitaxel, ifosfamide, and gemcitabine. More than ever, progress in the systemic therapy of bladder cancer will depend on the commitment of physicians and patients to participation in well-designed, randomized clinical trials. Only through such trials will it be possible to recognize real advances in treatment.

**Figure 5–10:** By correlating survival with patient and tumor characteristics before chemotherapy, models have been derived that predict survival durations for specific subgroups of patients with recurrent or metastatic bladder cancer following treatment with chemotherapy. Although such models are expected to change as treatment improves and better prognostic factors are identified, they provide a rational basis for stratifying patients for randomized trials and for interpreting results of uncontrolled trials. For bladder cancer, the models (shown here) reported by Bajorin et al.[56] and Saxman et al.[57] based on MVAC chemotherapy are similar in that the major determinants of survival are performance status and presence or absence of visceral (lung, liver, bone) metastases. In addition to living longer, patients in the most favorable prognostic category (with no risk factors) with Karnofsky performance scores of 80 or above and no visceral metastases have a greater likelihood of objective tumor regression following platinum-based chemotherapy. (From Bajorin DF, Dodd PM, Mazundar M, et al: Long term survival in metastatic transitional-cell carcinoma and prognostic

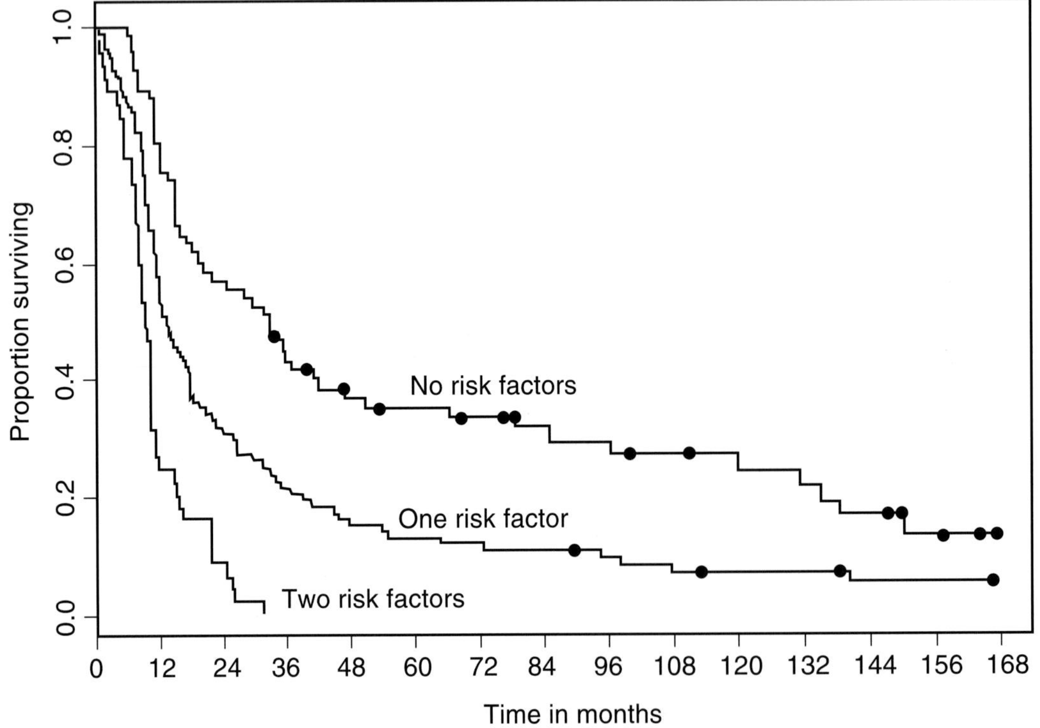


**Figure 5–10**

## TABLE 5–11

## RANDOMIZED TRIALS OF ADJUVANT AND NEOADJUVANT CHEMOTHERAPY FOR PATIENTS WITH MUSCLE INFILTRATING BLADDER CANCER

| AUTHOR | TIMING OF CHEMOTHERAPY | NO. OF PATIENTS | CHEMOTHERAPY ARM | RESULTS |
|---|---|---|---|---|
| Skinner[58] | Adjuvant | 91 | Cisplatin-based versus no therapy | Delay in time to progression for treatment group |
| Freiha[59] | Adjuvant | 50 | Immediate versus delayed (at recurrence) CMV | Delay in time to progression favoring immediate chemotherapy; no survival advantage |
| Stökle[60] | Adjuvant | 49 | MVEC versus no therapy (patients not offered chemotherapy at relapse) | Delay in recurrence favoring chemotherapy; survival advantage for chemotherapy |
| Nordic-1[61] | Neoadjuvant | 325 | Cisplatin + doxorubicin | No difference in survival overall; chemotherapy improved survival for subgroup with T3-T4a tumors |
| MRC-EORTC Intercontinental Trial[62] | Neoadjuvant | 976 | CMV | No difference in survival or time to progression |
| RTOG[29] | Neoadjuvant | 123 | CMV | No difference in survival |
| U.S. Intergroup[63] | Neoadjuvant | 317 | MVAC | Survival advantage for chemotherapy group |
| Bassi[64] | Neoadjuvant | 206 | MVAC | No difference in survival |

Superscript numbers represent references at the end of this chapter. CMV = cisplatin, methotrexate, and vinblastine. MVEC = methotrexate, vinblastine, epirubicin, and cisplatin. MVAC = methotrexate, vinblastine, doxorubicin, and cisplatin.

factors predicting outcome of therapy. J Clin Oncol 17(10):3178, 1999.)

**Table 5–11:** Adjuvant and neoadjuvant chemotherapy for muscle-invasive bladder cancer. Approximately 50% of patients with deep muscle invasion and locally advanced tumors have tumor recurrence with distant metastases, usually within 2 years of surgery or external beam radiotherapy. Systemic treatment administered either before (neoadjuvant) or following (adjuvant) radiotherapy or surgery would seem logical to eradicate distant micrometastatic disease. The efficacy of combination chemotherapy in patients with locally advanced or metastatic bladder cancer, particularly in those who have minimal or no symptoms, good functional status, and limited extent of tumor, supports this strategy. However, as shown in Table 5–11, proof that adjuvant or neoadjuvant chemotherapy actually leads to improved survival for patients with bladder cancer has been elusive. The results of three small adjuvant chemotherapy trials utilizing MVAC or similar chemotherapy indicate that time to recurrence may be significantly prolonged for patients with pathologically staged, unfavorable (T3b–T4 and N+) tumors. A U.S. intergroup trial has shown an advantage in survival for patients receiving three cycles of MVAC therapy prior to radical cystectomy for muscle invasive tumors.

**Figure 5–11:** The EORTC-MRC neoadjuvant chemotherapy trial. The challenge of defining the role of systemic chemotherapy in patients with muscle infiltrating tumors is exemplified by a large, well-designed international cooperative group study of patients with T2 or G3, T3 or T4a, N0–X, M0 transitional cell carcinomas of the bladder treated with curative cystectomy or full-dose external beam radiotherapy. The patients were randomly assigned to receive three cycles of CMV (cisplatin, methotrexate, and vinblastine with folinic acid rescue) chemotherapy (491 patients) or no chemotherapy (485 patients) before surgery or radiotherapy.[62] In patients who underwent cystectomy, the proportion with histologic complete response (no residual tumor in the bladder) was 32.5% among those who received chemotherapy compared with 12.3% in the group without chemotherapy. Overall, 50% of patients were alive at 3 years. Despite a higher complete response (CR) proportion in the bladder for the chemotherapy treated patients, the difference in survival at 3 years was only 5.5% (55.5% for the chemotherapy group versus 50% for the no chemotherapy group. The overall survival distributions (A) reveal a nonsignificant difference by log-rank test. The metastasis-free survival distribution (B) favored the chemotherapy group, with a 21% decrease in risk of developing metastasis that reached

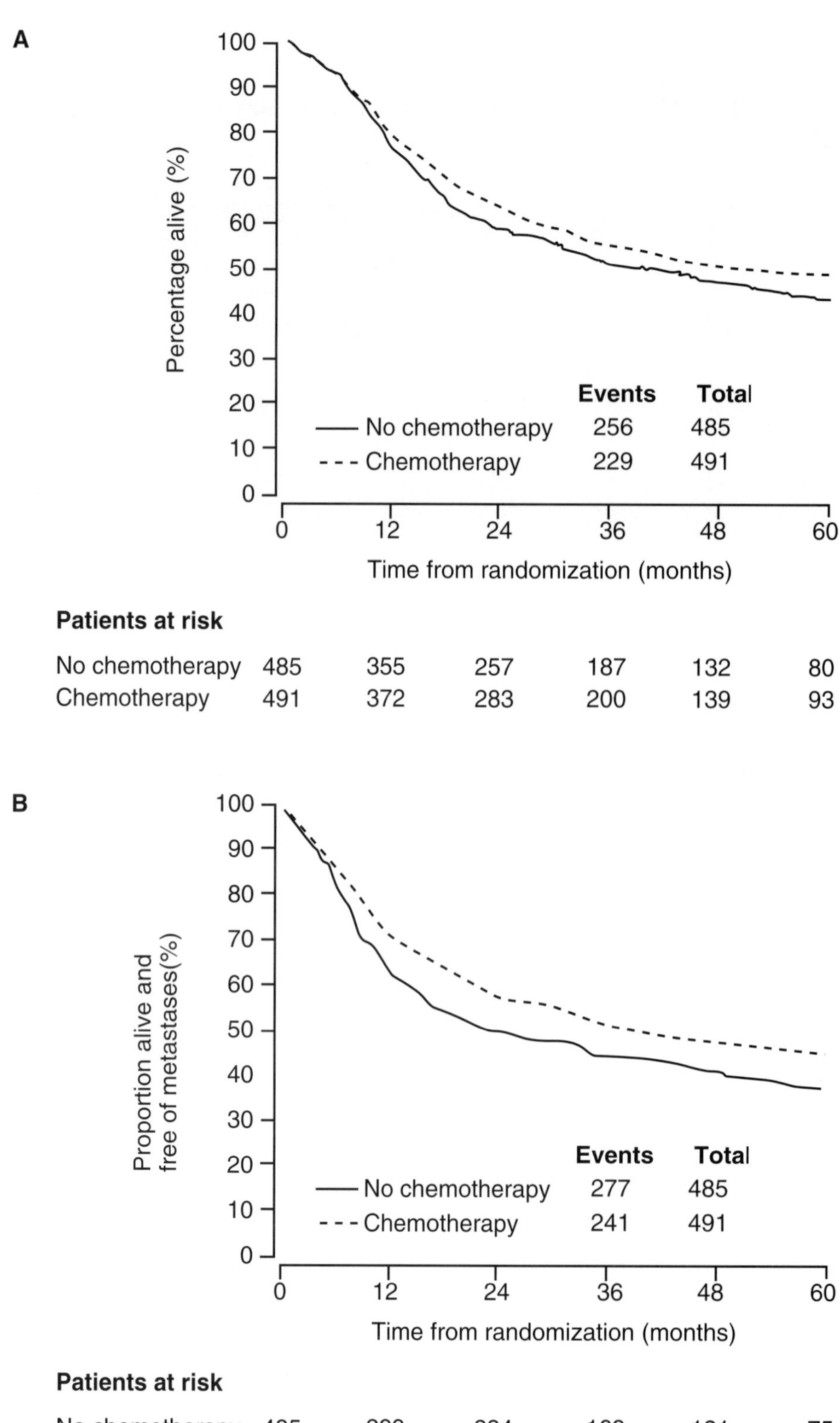



**Figure 5–11**

statistical significance ($p = 0.007$). There was no evidence of a difference in local control when surgically treated or radiotherapy treated patients were compared. Subgroup analysis of surgically and radiotherapy treated patients revealed similar effects of chemotherapy in both groups. (From International Collaboration of Trialists: Neoadjuvant cisplatin, methotrexate, and vinblastine chemotherapy for muscle invasive bladder cancer: a randomized controlled trial. Lancet 354:533–540, 1999.)

## TABLE 5–12

## UNCONTROLLED TRIALS OF NEOADJUVANT MVAC OR CMV THERAPY FOR BLADDER CANCER

| AUTHOR | NO. OF PATIENTS | TUMOR STAGE | CHEMOTHERAPY | NO. (%) PATHOLOGICALLY STAGED (PARTIAL OR RADICAL CYSTECTOMY) | POST-CHEMOTHERAPY CLINICAL DOWNSTAGING | NO. (%) NON-CYSTECTOMY PATIENTS ALIVE WITH INTACT BLADDER | MEDIAN FOLLOW-UP (Months) | OVERALL SURVIVAL RATE |
|---|---|---|---|---|---|---|---|---|
| Herr[65] | 71 | T2–T4 | MVAC | 46 (66%) P0 in 11, PIS-4 P1-1, $\geq$ P2 – 30 | 61%, T0 in 48%, TIS in 13% | 20 (28%) | 24 | 58% |
| Vogelzang[66] | 29 | T2–4N0-2M0 (72% T2–T3a) | MVAC | ND | 20/29 (69%) T0 in 9 (31%) | — | 57 | 71% |
| Sternberg[67] | 46 | T2-T4N0M0 (58% T2–T3a) | MVAC | 28, 16 (57%) 6 (21%) CR | 31/40 (78%) T0 in 50% | 16/46 (35%) | 33 | 70% |
| Maffezini[68] | 39 | T3–T4 5 N+ | CMV (no TURB prior to chemotherapy) | 23/39 (59%) 10% P0 | 23/39 (59%) T0 in 15% | All cystectomy | 12 | NA |
| Stroughi[69] | 36 | T2–T4 | MVAC | ND | T0 in 14 (47%) | 6/36 (17%) | 78 | 53% |

MVAC = methotrexate + vinblastine + adriamycin (doxorubicin) + cisplatin; CMV = cisplatin + vinblastine + methotrexate; ND = not done.

**Table 5–12:** Neoadjuvant chemotherapy and bladder preservation. Eradication of micrometastases and increased survival times have appropriately been considered important goals of neoadjuvant chemotherapy. In addition, downstaging of the primary bladder tumor suggests that bladder preservation may also be considered an important benefit of chemotherapy. Similar to radiotherapy, primary chemotherapy for patients with muscle invasive tumors may result in bladder preservation for selected patients if repeat clinical staging documents complete response or downstaging to superficial disease (<T2) only. Approximately 10% to 15% of patients who were considered complete responders by clinical restaging (including TUR and cytology) following neoadjuvant chemotherapy have residual tumor in the cystectomy specimen.[65]

Partial cystectomy (with pathologic restaging and resection of residual tumor or scar) and radiotherapy are other bladder-preserving options following neoadjuvant chemotherapy. Representative results of this approach are shown in Table 5–12.[65–69] Most series include patients managed with a variety of approaches, depending on the response to neoadjuvant chemotherapy. Although patients with residual muscle infiltrating disease are usually offered radical cystectomy, those who attain CR after chemotherapy have been managed with partial cystectomy, radiotherapy, or observation alone. The collective experience suggests that the probability of complete response to chemotherapy is greatest for patients with less invasive (T2) tumors, and that survival is poor for patients with residual muscle infiltrating tumor (>T1) following chemotherapy.[70]

**Figure 5–12:** Neoadjuvant chemotherapy and partial cystectomy for bladder cancer. These CT scans are those of a patient who presented with hematuria and subsequently was found to have high-grade, muscle invasive TCC arising in a bladder diverticulum and obstructing the left ureter. In the scan, the pretreatment tumor mass appears to extend beyond the bladder (A). After four courses of methotrexate + vinblastine + doxorubicin + cisplatin (MVAC), the mass regressed completely and the diverticulum became apparent (B). Cystoscopy and urine cytologic examination revealed no evidence of tumor (clinical CR). The patient underwent operative staging with bladder biopsies, partial cystectomy, and resection of the diverticulum. All specimens were negative for tumor. The patient remains tumor free 4 years after partial cystectomy.

**Figure 5–13:** Adjuvant chemotherapy trials and molecular markers. Clinical trials of adjuvant chemotherapy in pathologically staged patients following cystectomy may increase the likelihood of demonstrating significant survival improvement with chemotherapy. The next generation of bladder cancer trials will incorporate molecular markers such as tumor pRb, p53, and p21[cip1/waf-1] status, which may predict tumor behavior and prognosis.[71, 72] Data from the University of Southern California (USC) radical cystectomy experience in 185 cases, which are shown in the Figure, illustrate the potential of pRb and p53 status in determining prognosis. As shown here, patients with mutated or altered p53 (p53alt) and those with altered pRb (pRbalt) had a greater rate of tumor recurrence (A) and death (B) following cystectomy. Patients with alter-

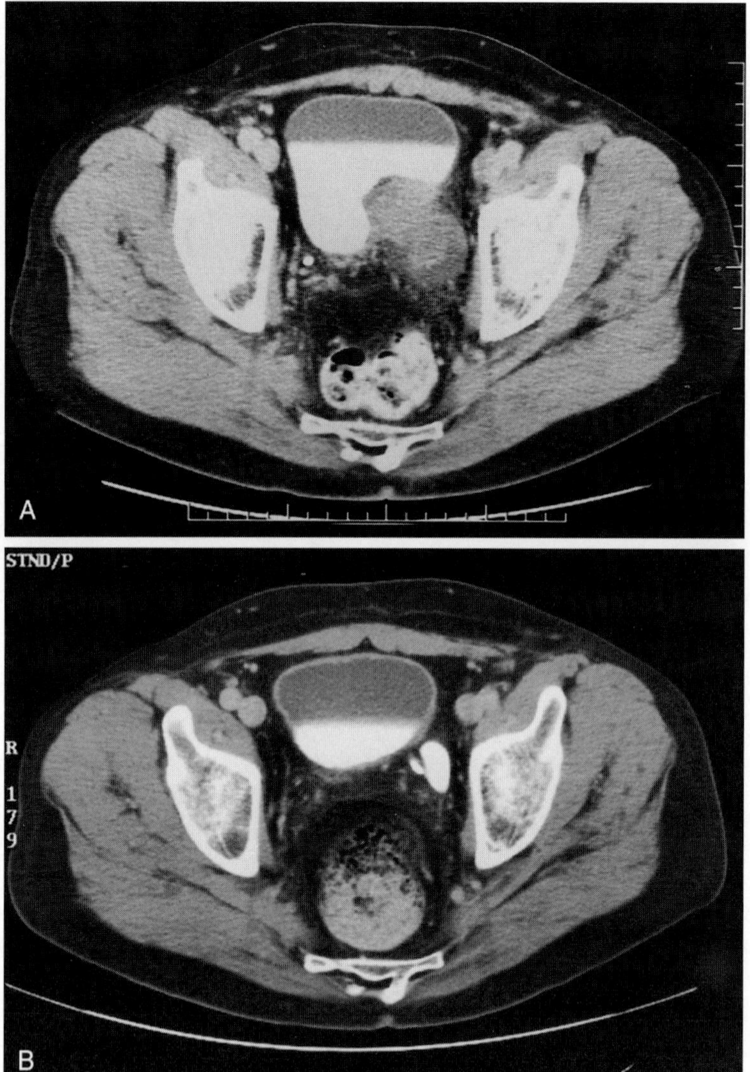

Figure 5–12

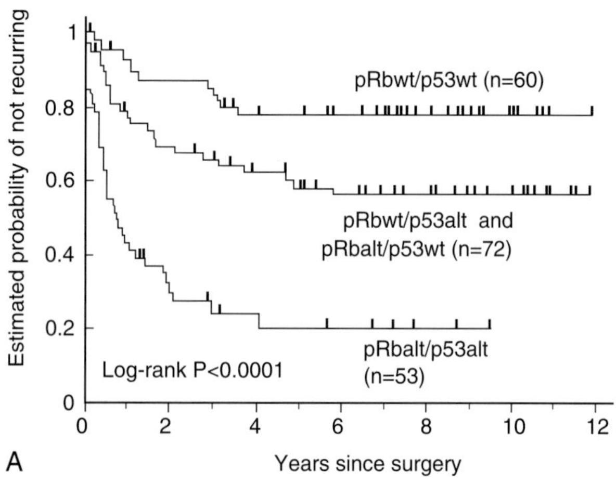


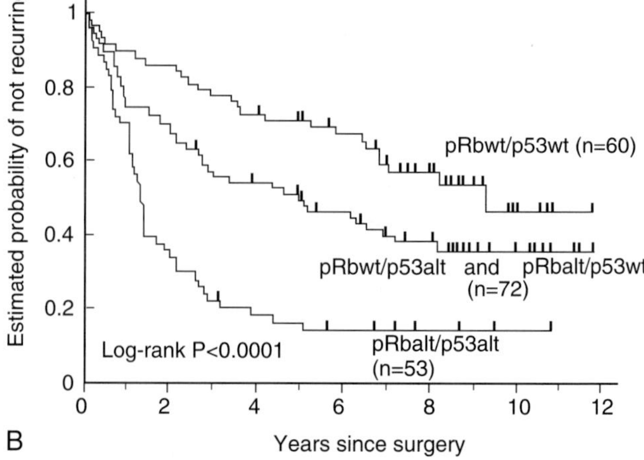


Figure 5–13

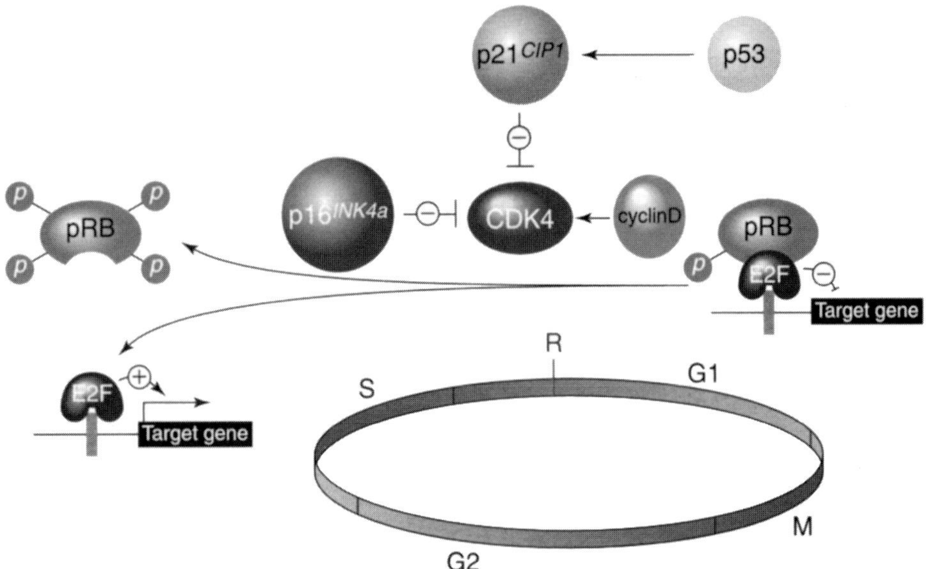


**Figure 5–14**

ations in both pRb and p53 had a higher rate of tumor recurrence and death than those with alterations in only one of these proteins.[71] The need for effective chemotherapy is greatest for these patients. In a provocative retrospective analysis,[73] patients with tumors that harbored altered p53 seemed more likely to benefit from chemotherapy than those with wild-type p53, a hypothesis that will be tested prospectively in a clinical trial.

**Figure 5–14:** Cell cycle regulation: molecular determinants of tumor progression and recurrence of bladder cancer. Tumor growth is dependent on rates of cell proliferation and cell death (apoptosis). The cell cycle describes sequential periods of time that cells spend in a resting ("nonproliferating") phase (G0-G1), in synthesizing new DNA (S-phase) and in preparing for and undergoing cell division or mitosis (G2-M). A number of proteins regulate transitions between the phases of the cell cycle. Particularly relevant to bladder cancer, the retinoblastoma protein (pRb) is an important regulator of the transition between G1 and the S phase, which is the initial commitment to cell proliferation. pRb and several other key proteins including p53, p21[cip1/waf-1], and p16[INK4A]/p19[ARF] serve as "brakes" to the cell cycle machinery at a specific restriction (R) point. They restrain G1–S phase transition and cell proliferation, opposing the actions of cyclins and cyclin-dependent kinases (CDKs), which are families of proteins that drive cell proliferation by releasing the "breaking" function of pRb. CDK proteins such as CDK4 are activated when complexed with a cyclin molecule. The cyclin-CDK complex phosphorylates pRb, resulting in the release from Rb of E2F-1 and related transcription factors, which promote transcription of genes required for DNA synthesis and cell proliferation.[74]

This schematic illustrates the actions and interactions of several key proteins of the pRb pathway. Induction of p21[cip1/waf-1] is one mechanism by which p53 can orchestrate Rb-mediated cell-cycle arrest. Loss of any of these growth-suppressing proteins through deletion, gene mutation or inactivation can contribute to the malignant phenotype and more aggressive tumor behavior. (From Chin L, Pomerantz J, DePinho RA: The INK4a/ARF tumor suppressor: one gene—two products—two pathways. Trends Biochem Sci 23:291–296, 1998.)

**Figure 5–15:** Growth factor signaling pathways. Growth-promoting signals (endocrine and paracrine growth factors) can originate from outside the cell or can be produced by the cancer cell itself, resulting in autocrine growth. Cell contact with surrounding stromal cells (and noncellular components) may also influence survival and proliferation through signaling pathways.

Growth factors act through binding to intracellular or membrane receptors. Members of a large family of growth factor receptors span the cell membrane with extracellular, transmembrane, and cytoplasmic (intracellular) domains. Because the cytoplasmic domains possess intrinsic tyrosine kinase activity, these receptors are known as receptor tyrosine kinases (RTKs). RTKs such as the platelet-derived growth factor receptor (PDGF-r), epidermal growth factor receptor (EGF-r), and insulin-like growth factor receptor are activated by binding to the appropriate growth factor (ligand). Growth factor binding to extracellular domains induces receptor dimerization, which in turn alters the conformation of the receptor cytoplasmic domains and increases the intrinsic tyrosine kinase activity.

Activated RTKs phosphorylate tyrosines within the receptor (autophosphorylation) and on other intracellu-

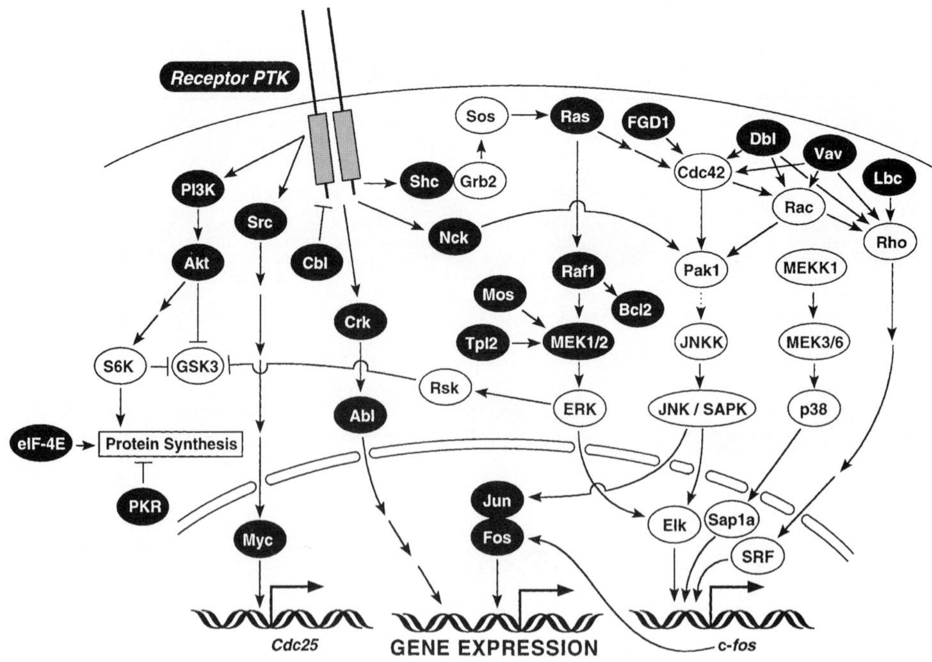



**Figure 5–15**

lar proteins that are recognized on the basis of specific amino acid sequences. Conversely, autophosphorylation of RTKs leads to their recognition by adaptor or "docking" proteins that transmit the membrane signal to more distal members of the signaling cascade.[75] Ultimately, growth factor signaling reaches the nucleus, culminating in transcription of genes that regulate cell growth and survival. A partial schematic of several signaling routes linking the cell membrane to the nucleus is shown in Figure 5–15. (From Hunter T: Oncoprotein networks. Cell 88:333–346, 1997.)

RTKs can act as oncogenes and can transform cells through gene amplification—an increase of gene copy number that increases the amount of functioning receptor protein. Alternatively, mutations in the protein coding region of the gene can produce receptors that have persistently high tyrosine kinase activity, even in the absence of growth factor binding. Although gene amplification is rare, increased EGF-r expression has been observed in transitional carcinomas of the bladder and has been associated with more aggressive behavior and poor prognosis.[76–78] Inhibition of EGF-r tyrosine kinase activity with antibodies[79] and small molecule kinase inhibitors[80] is a rapidly developing therapeutic strategy with potential application in bladder cancer.

**Figure 5–16:** Restoration of p53 function as potential therapy for bladder cancer. Losses of pRb and p53 tumor suppressor functions are common in transitional cell carcinomas of the bladder and are associated with tumor progression. Loss of p53 function occurs commonly through a combination of gene deletion, whereby one copy of the p53 gene is lost, followed by

mutation of the remaining p53 allele. The majority of p53 gene mutations are missense mutations that code for proteins with unstable folding (conformation) and loss of DNA binding. Loss of DNA binding prevents p53 from activating transcription of p21 and other genes involved in restraining cell growth (Fig. 5–14). As demonstrated by Foster and colleagues,[82] restoration or repair of nonfunctioning tumor suppressor proteins such as p53 would be an attractive therapeutic strategy in bladder cancer and other solid tumors.

In the protein immunoblots shown in Figure 5–16, treatment of Saos-2 tumor cells with the small synthetic molecule CP-31398 stabilized mutant p53 conformation and restored DNA binding properties that are characteristic of normal p53. The drug-stabilized mutant proteins shown in the figure (top bands) gain the ability to activate transcription of a relevant downstream gene,

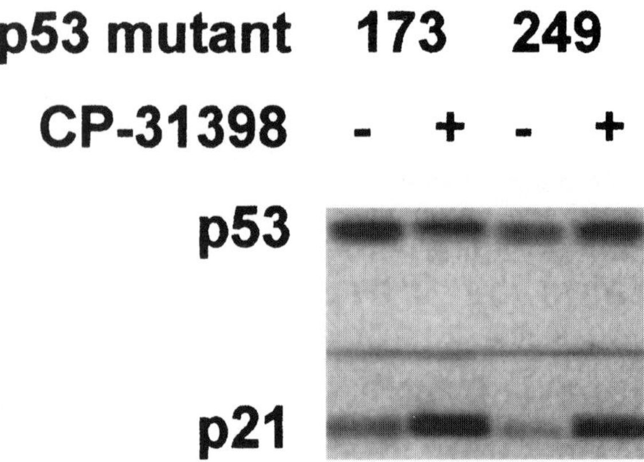



**Figure 5–16**

p21$^{\text{waf-1/cip1}}$ (lower bands). Saos-2 tumor cells were transfected to produce stable clones capable of expression position 173 or 249 mutant p53 proteins. The proteins expressed from position 173 or 249 mutant p53 proteins are shown in the ($-$) lanes, and proteins from the same cells treated with CP-31398 are shown in the ($+$) lanes. Although the total amount of p53 is unchanged in each ($-$)/($+$) pair, it can be seen that CP-31398 treatment elevates levels (increased band intensity) of p21. In vivo treatment of small human tumor xenografts with naturally mutated p53 using the same drug inhibited tumor growth.[81] Pharmacologic repair of mutant, "conformationally challenged" proteins such as p53 is an interesting approach with therapeutic potential in bladder cancer and other diseases. (From Foster BA, Coffey HA, Morin MJ, Rastinejad F: Pharmacological rescue of mutant p53 conformation and function. Science 286:2507, 1999. Copyright 1999 by the American Association for the Advancement of Science.)

## REFERENCES


1. Vander Werf A, Messing BHP, Hop WCG: Carcinoma of the urinary bladder (categories T1NXM0) treated by either radium implant or by transurethral resection only. Int J Radiat Oncol Biol Phys 7:299, 1981.
2. Shipley WU, Prout GR, Kaufman SD, Perrone TL: Invasive bladder carcinoma: The importance of initial transurethral surgery and other significant prognostic factors for improved survival with full-dose irradiation. Cancer 60:514 520, 1987.
3. Dunst J, Sauer R, Schrott KM, et al: Organ-sparing treatment of advanced bladder cancer: A 10-year experience. Int J Radiat Oncol Biol Phys 30(2):261–266, 1994.
4. Pollack A, Zagars GK, Swanson DA: Muscle-invasive bladder cancer treated with external beam radiotherapy: Prognostic factors. Int J Radiat Oncol Biol Phys 30:267–277, 1994.
5. Sauer R, Birkenhake S, Kühn R, et al: Efficacy of radiochemotherapy with platinum derivatives compared to radiotherapy alone in organ-sparing treatment of bladder cancer. Int J Radiat Oncol Biol Phys 40(1):121–127, 1998.
6. Solsona E, Iborra I, Ricós JV, et al: Feasibility of transurethral resection for muscle-infiltrating carcinoma of the bladder: Prospective study. J Urol 147:1513–1515, 1992.
7. Herr HW: Conservative treatment of muscle-infiltrating bladder cancer: Prospective experience. J Urol 138:1162, 1987.
8. Pagano F, Bassi P, Galetti TP, et al: Results of contemporary radical cystectomy for invasive bladder cancer: A clinicopathological study with an emphasis on the inadequacy of the tumor, nodes and metastases classification. J Urol 145:45–50, 1991.
9. Vieweg J, Geschwend JE, Herr HW, Fair W: Pelvic lymph node dissection can be curative in patients with node positive bladder cancer. J Urol 161:449–454, 1999.
10. Lerner SP, Skinner DG, Lieskovsky G, et al: The rationale for en bloc pelvic lymph node dissection for bladder cancer patients with nodal metastases: Long-term results. J Urol 149:758 765, 1993.
11. Fung CY, Shipley WU, Young RH, et al: Prognostic factors in invasive bladder carcinoma in a prospective trial of preoperative adjuvant chemotherapy and radiotherapy. J Clin Oncol 9(9):1533–1542, 1991.
12. Gospodarowicz MK, Hawkins NV, Rawlings GA, et al: Radical radiotherapy for muscle invasive transitional cell carcinoma of the bladder: Failure analysis. J Urol 142:1448–1454, 1989.
13. Moonen L, Voet HVD, DeNijs R, et al: Muscle-invasive bladder cancer treated with external beam radiation: Influence of total dose, overall treatment time, and treatment interruption on local control. Int J Radiat Oncol Biol Phys 42(3):525–530, 1998.
14. Larsen LE, Engelholm SA: The value of 3-dimensional radiotherapy planning in advanced carcinoma of the urinary bladder based on computed tomography. Acta Oncol 33:655–659, 1994.
15. Miralbell R, Nouet P, Rouzaud M, et al: Radiotherapy of bladder cancer: Relevance of bladder volume changes in planning boost treatment. Int J Radiat Oncol Biol Phys 41(4):741–746, 1998.
16. Duncan W, Quilty PM: The results of a series of 963 patients with transitional cell carcinoma of the bladder primarily treated by radical megavoltage x-ray therapy. Radiother Oncol 7:299–310, 1986.
17. Greven KM, Solin L, Hanks GE: Prognostic factors in patients with bladder carcinoma treated with definitive irradiation. Cancer 65:908–912, 1990.
18. Smaaland R, Aksley A, Tonder B, et al: Radical radiation treatment of invasive and locally advanced bladder carcinoma in elderly patients. Br J Urol 67:61–69, 1991.
19. Shipley WU, Prout Jr GR, Einstein AB, et al: Treatment of invasive bladder cancer by cisplatin and radiation in patients unsuited for surgery. JAMA 258(7):931–935, 1987.
20. Tester W, Porter A, Asbell S, et al: Combined modality program with possible organ preservation for invasive bladder carcinoma: Results of RTOG protocol 85-12. Int J Radiat Oncol Biol Phys 25(5):783–790, 1993.
21. Housset M, Maulard C, Chretien Y, et al: Combined radiation and chemotherapy for invasive transitional-cell carcinoma of the bladder: A prospective study. J Clin Oncol 11:2150–2157, 1993.
22. Russell KJ, Boilau MA, Higano C, et al: Combined 5-fluorouracil and irradiation for transitional cell carcinoma of the urinary bladder. Int J Radiat Oncol Biol Phys 19:693–699, 1990.
23. Rotman M, Aziz H, Porrazzo M, et al: Treatment of advanced transitional cell carcinoma of the bladder with irradiation and concomitant 5-FU infusion. Int J Radiat Oncol Biol Phys 18:1131–1136, 1990.
24. Rodel C, Grabenhauer GG, Rode F, et al: Apoptosis, p53, BCL-2, and Ki-67 in invasive bladder carcinoma: Possible predictors for response to radiochemotherapy and successful bladder preservation. Int J Radiat Oncol Biol Phys 46:1213–1221, 2000.
25. Shipley W, Kaufman D, Heney N, et al: An update of combined modality therapy for patients with muscle invading bladder cancer using selective bladder preservation or cystectomy. J Urol 162:445–451, 1999.
26. Kaufman DS, Shipley WU, Griffin PP, et al: Selective bladder preservation by combination treatment of invasive bladder cancer. N Engl J Med 329(19):1377–1382, 1993.
27. Tester W, Caplan R, Heaney J, et al: Neoadjuvant combined modality program with selective organ preservation for invasive bladder cancer: Results of Radiation Therapy Oncology Group Phase II trial 8802. J Clin Oncol 14:119–126, 1996.
28. Given RW, Parsons JT, McCarley D, Wajsman Z: Bladder-sparing multimodality treatment of muscle-invasive bladder cancer: A five year follow-up. Urology 46:499–505, 1995.
29. Shipley WU, Winter KA, Kaufman DS, et al: Phase III trial of neoadjuvant chemotherapy in patients with invasive bladder cancer treated with selective bladder preservation by combined radiation therapy and chemotherapy: Initial results of Radiation Therapy Oncology Group 89-03. J Clin Oncol 16(11):3576–3583, 1998.
30. Dodd PA, McCaffrey JA, Herr H, et al: Outcome of postchemotherapy surgery after treatment with methotrexate, vinblastine, doxorubicin, and cisplatin in patients with unresectable or metastatic transitional cell carcinoma. J Clin Oncol 17:2546–2552, 1999.
31. Yagoda A: Chemotherapy of urothelial tract tumors. Cancer 60:574–585, 1987.
32. Stoter G, Splinter TAW, Child JA, et al (European Organization for Research on Treatment of Cancer Genito-urinary Group): Combination chemotherapy with cisplatin and methotrexate in advanced transitional cell cancer of the bladder. J Urol 137:663–667, 1987.
33. Harker WG, Meyers FJ, Freiha FS, et al: Cisplatin, methotrexate and vinblastine (CMV): An effective chemotherapy regimen for metastatic transitional cell carcinoma of the urinary tract. A Northern California Oncology Group Study. J Clin Oncol 3(11):1463–1470, 1985.

34. Sternberg CN, Yagoda A, Scher HI, et al: Methotrexate, vinblastine, doxorubicin and cisplatin for advanced transitional cell carcinoma of the urothelium: Efficacy and patterns of response and relapse. Cancer 64:2448–2458, 1989.

35. Tu S-M, Hossan E, Amato R, Kilbourn R, Logothetis CJ: Paclitaxel, cisplatin and methotrexate combination chemotherapy is active in the treatment of refractory urothelial alignancies. J Urol 154:1719–1722, 1995.

36. Dreicer R, Manola J, Roth B, et al: Phase II study of cisplatin and paclitaxel in advanced carcinoma of the urothelium: An Eastern Cooperative Oncology Group Study. J Clin Oncol 18:1058–1061, 2000.

37. Vaughn DJ, Malkowicz SB, Zoltick B, et al: Paclitaxel plus carboplatin in advanced carcinoma of the urothelium: An active and tolerable outpatient regimen. J Clin Oncol 16(1):255–260, 1998.

38. Bajorin DF, McCaffrey JA, Hilton S, et al: Treatment of patients with transitional-cell carcinoma of the urothelial tract with ifosfamide, paclitaxel and cisplatin: A phase II trial. J Clin Oncol 16(8):2722–2727, 1998.

39. Dreicer R, Propert KJ, Roth BJ, et al: Vinblastine, ifosfamide and gallium nitrate—An active new regimen in patients with advanced carcinoma of the urothelium. Cancer 79(1):110–114, 1997.

40. Logothetis CJ, Dexeus FH, Chong C, et al: Cisplatin, cyclophosphamide and doxorubicin chemotherapy for unresectable urothelial tumors: The M.D. Anderson Experience. J Urol 141:33–37, 1989.

41. Moore MJ, Winquist EW, Murray N, et al: Gemcitabine plus cisplatin, an active regimen in advanced urothelial cancer: A phase II trial of the National Cancer Institute of Canada Clinical Trials Group. J Clin Oncol 17(9):2876–2881, 1999.

42. Sengelov L, Kamby C, Lund B, Engelholm SA: Docetaxel and cisplatin in metastatic urothelial cancer: A phase II study. J Clin Oncol 16(10):3392–3397, 1998.

43. Hillcoat BL, Raghavan D, Matthews J, et al: A randomized trial of cisplatin versus cisplatin plus methotrexate in advanced cancer of the urothelial tract. J Clin Oncol 7(6):706–709, 1989.

44. Loehrer PJ Sr, Einhorn LH, Elson PJ, et al: A randomized comparison of cisplatin alone or in combination with methotrexate, vinblastine and doxorubicin in patients with metastatic urothelial carcinoma: A Cooperative Group Study. J Clin Oncol 10(7):1066–1073, 1992.

45. Logothetis CJ, Dexeus FH, Finn L, et al: A prospective randomized trial comparing MVAC and CISCA chemotherapy for patients with metastatic urothelial tumors. J Clin Oncol 8(6):1050–1055, 1990.

46. Khandekar JD, Elson PJ, DeWys WD, et al: Comparative activity and toxicity of cis-diamminedichloroplatinum (DDP) and a combination of doxorubicin, cyclophosphamide and DDP in disseminated transitional cell carcinomas of the urinary tract. J Clin Oncol 3(4):539–545, 1985.

47. Mead GM, Russell M, Clark P, et al: A randomized trial comparing methotrexate and vinblastine (MV) with cisplatin, methotrexate and vinblastine (CMV) in advanced transitional cell carcinoma: Results and a report on prognostic factors in a Medical Research Council study. Br J Cancer 78(8):1067–1075, 1998.

47a. von der Maase H, Hansen SW, Roberts JT, et al: Gemcitabine and cisplatin versus vinblastine, doxorubicin, and cisplatin in advanced or metastatic bladder cancer: Results of a large, randomized, multinational multicenter phase III study. J Clin Onc 17:3068–3077, 2000.

48. Roth BJ, Dreicer R, Einhorn LH, et al: Significant activity of paclitaxel in advanced transitional-cell carcinoma of the urothelium: A phase II trial of the Eastern Cooperative Oncology Group. J Clin Oncol 12:2264–2270, 1994.

49. Pollera CF, Ceribelli A, Crecco M, Calabresi F. Weekly gemcitabine in advanced bladder cancer: A preliminary report from a Phase I study. Ann Oncol 5:182–184, 1994.

50. Moore MJ, Tannock IF, Ernst DS, et al: Gemcitabine: A promising new agent in the treatment of advanced urothelial cancer. J Clin Oncol 15:3441–3445, 1997.

51. Stadler WM, Kuzel T, Roth B, et al: Phase II study of single-agent gemcitabine in previously untreated patients with metastatic urothelial cancer. J Clin Oncol 15(11):3394–3398, 1997.

52. Witte RS, Elson P, Bono B, et al: Eastern Cooperative Oncology Group Phase II trial of ifosfamide in the treatment of previously treated advanced urothelial carcinoma. J Clin Oncol 15(2):589–593, 1997.

53. Witte RS, Elson P, Khandakar J, Trump DL. An Eastern Cooperative Oncology Group Phase II trial of trimetrexate in the treatment of advanced urothelial carcinoma. Cancer 73:688–691, 1994.

54. Seidman AD, Scher HI, Heinemann MH, et al: Continuous infusion gallium nitrate for patients with advanced refractory urothelial tract tumors. Cancer 68:1561–1565, 1991.

55. McCaffrey JA, Hilton S, Mazumdar M, et al: Phase II trial of docetaxel in patients with advanced or metastatic transitional-cell carcinoma. J Clin Oncol 15(5):1853–1857, 1997.

56. Bajorin DF, Dodd PM, Mazumdar M, et al: Long-term survival in metastatic transitional-cell carcinoma and prognostic factors predicting outcome of therapy. J Clin Oncol 17(10):3173–3181, 1999.

57. Saxman SB, Propert KJ, Einhorn LH, et al: Long-term follow-up of a phase III intergroup study of cisplatin alone or in combination with methotrexate, vinblastine, and doxorubicin in patients with metastatic urothelial carcinoma: A cooperative group study. J Clin Oncol 15:2564–2569, 1997.

58. Skinner DG, Daniels JR, Russell CA, et al: The role of adjuvant chemotherapy following cystectomy for invasive bladder cancer: A prospective comparative trial. J Urol 145:459–467, 1991.

59. Freiha F, Reese J, Torti FM: A randomized trial of radical cystectomy versus radical cystectomy plus cisplatin, vinblastine, and methotrexate chemotherapy for muscle invasive bladder cancer. J Urol 155:495–500, 1996.

60. Stökle M, Meyenburg W, Wellek S, et al: Adjuvant polychemotherapy of nonorgan-confined bladder cancer after radical cystectomy revisited: Long-term results of a controlled prospective study and further clinical experience. J Urol 153:47–52, 1995.

61. Malmstrom P, Rintala E, Wahlqvist R, et al: Five-year follow-up of a prospective trial of radical cystectomy and neoadjuvant chemotherapy: Nordic Cystectomy Trial I. J Urol 155:1903–1906, 1996.

62. International Collaboration of Trialists, MRC Advanced Bladder Cancer Working Party, EORTC Genito-Urinary Group, Australian Bladder Cancer Study Group, National Cancer Institute of Canada Clinical Trials Group, Finnbladder, Norwegian Bladder Cancer Study Group, and Club Urologico Español de Tratamiento Oncologico (CUETO) Group: Neoadjuvant cisplatin, methotrexate, and vinblastine chemotherapy for muscle-invasive bladder cancer: a randomized controlled trial. Lancet 354:533–540, 1999.

63. Natale RB, Grossman HB, Blumenstein B, et al: SWOG 8710 (Int-0080): Randomized phase III trial of neoadjuvant MVAC + cystectomy versus cystectomy alone in patients with locally advanced bladder cancer. Proc Am Soc Clin Oncol 20:2a (abstr no. 3), 2001.

64. Bassi P, Pappagalio GL, Sperandio P, et al: Neoadjuvant M-VAC chemotherapy of invasive bladder cancer: Results of a multicenter phase III trial. J Urol 161(s):264, 1999 (abstract 1021).

65. Herr HW, Bajorin DF, Scher HI: Neoadjuvant chemotherapy and bladder-sparing surgery for invasive bladder cancer: Ten-year outcome. J Clin Oncol 16:1298–1301, 1998.

66. Vogelzang NJ, Moormeier JA, Awan AM, et al: Methotrexate, vinblastine, doxorubicin and cisplatin followed by radiotherapy or surgery for muscle invasive bladder cancer: The University of Chicago Experience. J Urol 149:753–757, 1993.

67. Sternberg CN, Arena MG, Calabresi F, et al: Neoadjuvant M-VAC (methotrexate, vinblastine, doxorubicin and cisplatin) for infiltrating transitional cell carcinoma of the bladder. Cancer 72(6):1975–1982, 1993.

68. Maffezini M, Torelli T, Villa E, et al: Systemic preoperative chemotherapy with cisplatin, methotrexate and vinblastine for locally advanced bladder cancer: local tumor response and early follow-up results. J Urol 145:741–743, 1991.

69. Stroughi M, Simon SD: Primary methotrexate, vinblastine, doxorubicin and cisplatin chemotherapy and bladder preservation in locally invasive bladder cancer: A 5-year follow-up. J Urol 151:593, 1994.

70. Splinter TAW, Scher HI, Denis L, et al (with European Organization for Research on Treatment of Cancer-Genitourinary Group): The prognostic value of the pathological response to combination chemotherapy before cystectomy in patients with invasive bladder cancer. J Urol 147:606–608, 1992.

71. Cote RJ, Dunn MD, Chatterjee SJ, et al: Elevated and absent pRb

expression is associated with bladder cancer progression and has cooperative effects with p53. Cancer Res 58:1090–1094, 1998.

72. Stein JP, Ginsberg DA, Grossfeld GD, et al: Effect of p21$^{WAF1/CIP1}$ expression on tumor progression in bladder cancer. J Natl Cancer Inst 90(14):1072–1079, 1998.

73. Cote RJ, Esrig D, Groshen S, et al: p53 and treatment of bladder cancer. Nature 385:123–124, 1997.

74. Dyson N: The regulation of E2F by pRB-family proteins. Gene Dev 12:2245–2262, 1998.

75. Chin L, Pomerantz J, DePinho RA: The INKa/ARF tumor suppressor: One gene—two products—two pathways. Trends Biochem Sci 23:291–296, 1998.

76. Hunter T: Oncoprotein networks. Cell 88:333–346, 1997.

77. Sauter G, Haley J, Chew K, et al: Epidermal-growth-factor-receptor expression is associated with rapid tumor proliferation in bladder cancer. Int J Cancer 57:508–514, 1994.

78. Nguyen PL, Swanson PE, Jaszcz W, et al: Expression of epidermal growth factor receptor in invasive transitional cell carcinoma of the urinary bladder. Am J Clin Pathol 101(2):166–176, 1994.

79. Neal DE, Sharples L, Smith K, et al: The epidermal growth factor receptor and the prognosis of bladder cancer. Cancer 65:1619–1625, 1990.

80. Baselga J, Phister D, Cooper MR, et al: Phase I studies of anti-epidermal growth factor receptor chimeric antibody C225 alone and in combination with cisplatin. J Clin Oncol 18:904–914, 2000.

81. Kris M, Ranson M, Ferry D, et al: Phase I study of oral ZD1839, a novel inhibitor of epidermal growth factor receptor tyrosine kinase (EGFR-TK): Evidence of good tolerability and activity. Clin Cancer Res 5(suppl):3749s, 1999.

82. Foster BA, Coffey HA, Morin MJ, Rastinejad F: Pharmacological rescue of mutant p53 conformation and function. Science 286:2507–2510, 1999.

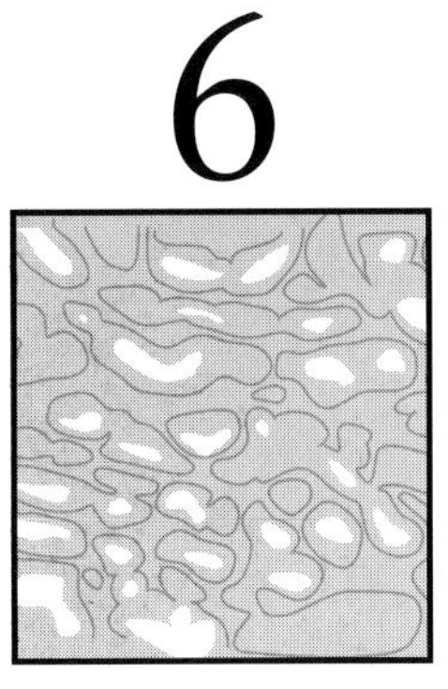

# 6

# Pathology and Staging of Genitourinary Cancer

*F. K. Mostofi*

*C. J. Davis, Jr.*

*I. A. Sesterhenn*

## INTRODUCTION

The purpose of this chapter is to present an overview of the pathologic features of malignancies of the prostate, bladder, kidney, and testis. Most of the illustrations are reproduced in the Color Section: Figures 6–1 through 6–14, 6–16 through 6–30, 6–32 through 6–41, and 6–43 through 6–53. Each section in the chapter starts with color images of that group of tumors, accompanied by a brief description of each figure. The focus of the ensuing text is a description of those light microscopic findings that establish the diagnosis, including comments on immunohistochemistry as indicated. With each of these organs, the recently revised classification of the World Health Organization (WHO) is discussed, and the TNM staging classification is provided. Although this chapter deals mainly with genitourinary malignancies, it also includes a number of benign tumors that commonly present problems in the differential diagnosis, such as renal adenomas, angiomyolipomas, and testicular stromal tumors (most of which are benign).

## TUMORS OF THE PROSTATE

### Staging Systems

Two different clinical staging systems are used: the ABCD system is used in a number of clinics in the United States, and the TNM system has been proposed by the International Union Against Cancer (UICC) and adopted by the American Joint Committee on Cancer (AJCC).

American stage A is applied to prostate carcinoma (PCa) found in tissues removed for benign enlargement of the prostate; stage B describes tumors confined to the prostate; stage C refers to tumors that have extended outside the prostate; and stage D refers to metastatic tumors. Each category is further subdivided into levels 1, 2, and 3. In essence, these levels describe clinical estimates of the local status of the tumor.

The TNM staging of PCa has been recently revised. The primary tumor is categorized as T1, T2, T3, and T4 based on the local extent of the tumor, and each category is subdivided into two or three subcategories. In the TNM system, pathologic stages follow the clinical stages, but are distinguished by the letter "P" (Fig. 6–15).

Prostate cancer is staged according to primary tumor (T), clinical (T), pathologic (pT) descriptions:

| | |
|---|---|
| pTX | Primary tumor cannot be assessed (TX) |
| pT0 | No evidence of primary tumor |
| pT1 | Clinically unapparent tumor, not palpable or visible by imaging (T1) |
| pT1a | Tumor an incidental histologic finding in 5% or less of tissue resected (T1a) |
| pT1b | Tumor an incidental histologic finding in more than 5% of tissue resected (T1b) |
| pT1c | Tumor identified by needle biopsy (e.g., because of elevated serum PSA) (T1c) |
| pT2 | Tumor confined within the prostate (T2) |
| pT2a | Tumor involves one lobe (T2a) |
| pT2b | Tumor involves both lobes (T2b) |

T1a
T1b
T = pT
≤ 5%
> 5%
T2a
T2a
T = pT
T2b
pT2b
T3a
pT3a
T3a
pT3a
T3b
pT3b
T4
pT4

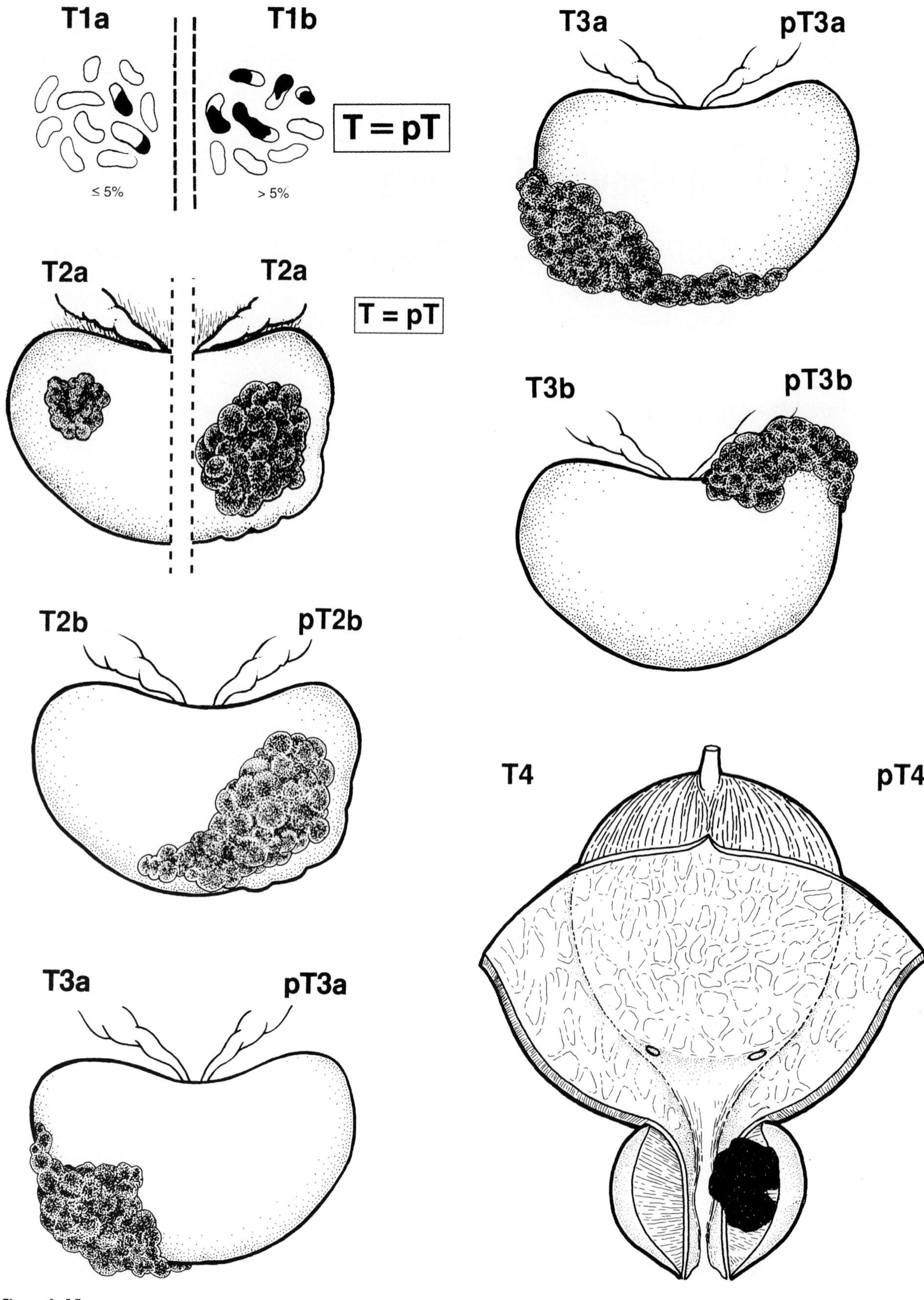

Figure 6–15

pT3    Tumor extends through the prostate capsule

pT3a    Extracapsular extension (unilateral or bilateral) (T3a)

pT3b    Tumor invades seminal vesicle(s) (T3b)

pT4    Tumor is fixed or invades adjacent structures other than seminal vesicles: bladder neck, external sphincter, rectum, levator muscles, or pelvic wall (T4)

In this classification, lymph node metastasis is indicated by N and distant metastasis by M, and pathologic designations are pN and pM.

## Histologic Features

Of the several different concepts of zonal anatomy of the prostate, the most popular at present is that of McNeal, who divides the prostate into anterior fibromuscular, transition, central, and peripheral zones. The transition zone is difficult to identify with certainty in the prostate that is the seat of hyperplasia or carcinoma. It has long been recognized that hyperplasia develops in the inner or periurethral portion of the gland and carcinoma in the outer portion.

Histologically, the prostate consists of tubuloalveolar glands opening into the prostatic urethra via ducts. Five basic cell types are seen in the prostate:

1. The prostatic acinar or secretory cells account for the majority of epithelial elements. These cells produce prostatic enzymes.

2. The basal cells surround, to a variable extent, the secretory cells and are located at the basement membrane. These stem cells differentiate into secretory cells, but they may transform to squamous, transitional, or mucous epithelium. Whereas basal cells do not produce prostatic enzymes, they react positively with high-molecular-weight keratin.

3. Transitional epithelium is found in the excretory ducts surrounding the urethra and prostatic urethra.

4. Paracrine-endocrine cells may be present as part of secretory, basal, or transitional cells. These cells produce a number of peptides, the most common of which are serotonin, calcitonin, bombesin-like peptides, and somatostatin. Although the precise function of these cells is unknown, they may be important for growth, differentiation, and secretory regulation of the gland.

5. The fifth cell type consists of stromal elements—fibrous and smooth muscle cells. Estimates of the proportion of prostate occupied by stroma varies from 30% to 70%, but the amount of stroma differs in the various regions of the prostate. It is most prominent in the anterior portion.

Any of these cells can participate in hyperplasia and neoplasia.

The periphery of the prostate is formed by a predominantly concentric layer of fibromuscular stroma followed by a layer of fibrofatty tissue referred to as "capsule." The most common malignant tumor of the prostate is prostatic acinar carcinoma, which accounts for more than 95% of all prostate cancers.

## Criteria for Pathologic Diagnosis

The diagnosis of prostatic carcinoma is based on the finding of nuclear anaplasia, abnormal glandular morphology, and an invasive pattern of stromal dispersion, in any combination. Except in high-grade tumors, one must usually depend on prominent nucleoli to recognize nuclear anaplasia. Abnormal glandular morphology may be in the form of darker cytoplasm with marked acinar size and shape variation and irregular contours or a cribriform growth pattern, poorly formed glands, or no glands. Malignant glands may have one or several cell layers, but there should be no obvious peripheral layer of flat or ovoid basal cells. Rarely, a diagnosis of prostatic carcinoma (PCa) can be based solely on a pattern of stromal dispersion if it takes the form of widespread infiltration between benign elements or invasion of perineural, lymphatic, or vascular spaces. In all suspicious lesions, we prefer to identify nucleoli, which represent a more objective feature than glandular shapes and location.

The minimum criterion for diagnosis of carcinoma is finding any of these three features: altered architecture, invasive growth pattern, and/or nuclear anaplasia. The presence of large nucleoli is the most important criterion for diagnosis of prostate carcinoma. Three lesions are often misdiagnosed as prostate carcinoma: atrophy, basal cell hyperplasia, and involutional changes in the seminal vesicle. In atrophy the acini are lined by a layer of cells, but the cells are small and have little or no cytoplasm. The nuclei are small and hyperchromatic. In basal cell hyperplasia, the change may be seen in single or multiple acini. The acini may be in lobules or diffuse. In all categories the cells are elongated uniformly, with occasional maturation to secretory cells. The nests have a regular outline. In involutional changes of the seminal vesicles, the mucosal foldings mimic closely packed acini of carcinoma. The lining cells have large hyperchromatic nuclei and are confined to the luminal layer.

### Cell Types
### Histologic Classification of Epithelial Tumors

Benign
   Papillary adenoma

Precursor Lesion
   Prostatic intraepithelial neoplasia
Malignant
   Adenocarcinoma (carcinoma)
   Variants of adenocarcinoma
   Urothelial (transitional cell) carcinoma
   Squamous cell carcinoma
   Basal cell carcinoma
   Small cell carcinoma
   Undifferentiated carcinoma
Nonepithelial Tumors
Hematopoietic and Lymphoid Tumors
Unclassified Tumors
Treatment Effects

## Precursor Lesions

Epithelial and glandular abnormalities in cancer-bearing prostates have been known for a long time and have various designations. These abnormalities generally fall into two categories: (1) those in which there is anaplasia of intra-acinar secretory epithelium and (2) those in which there is new gland formation. These two distinct categories are often confused.

The first category has been variously described as precancerous lesions, hyperplasia with malignant change, carcinoma in situ, dysplasia, intraductal or ductal acinar dysplasia with three grades, preneoplastic prostates, large acinar atypical hyperplasia, or prostatic intraepithelial neoplasia (PIN) with three grades. At an international conference sponsored by the American Cancer Society, the results of which were reported by Drago,[18] it was recommended that the term dysplasia be dropped and prostatic intraepithelial neoplasia be used for these lesions, which are then distinguished as high and low grade.

Because the histologic diagnosis of low-grade PIN, or PIN 1, is rather subjective, and interobserver reproducibility that identifies this category is poor, the diagnosis of PIN is restricted here to lesions with nuclear abnormalities similar to grade II and grade III prostatic acinar carcinoma. Hyperplasia exhibiting borderline nuclear atypia is reported here as atypical hyperplasia.

PIN has a characteristic appearance. The area stands out as a group of pre-existing, generally large acini or ducts that are more cellular than the adjacent hyperplastic glands. The cells are usually large. There is generally intra-acinar growth of cells, resulting in piling up of the epithelium. Occasionally, however, the lining cells may be one or two layers in thickness.

The nuclei are large and may vary in shape. They are vacuolated and contain one or more large nucleoli. Viewed by themselves, the cells are indistinguishable from nuclear grade 2 or 3 PCa, but in PIN, by definition, the changes are confined to the acini or ducts. The basal layer may be continuous or discontinuous.

PIN, as thus defined, is closely related to PCa. Kovi and colleagues[34] reported that in patients under the age of 60, PIN was associated with PCa in 87%, whereas in patients over the age of 60, the association between PIN and PCa and PIN and hyperplasia is about equal. Also, they reported that PIN is detected about 5 years before the appearance of carcinoma.

In most cases, the immunopathologic reactions of PIN are identical to the accompanying PCa. The proliferation rate of the PIN, as determined by $^3$H thymidine and the study of argyrophilic nucleolar organizing regions (AGNORs), shows that PIN is close to PCa. These observations suggest that PIN, as defined here, is the preinvasive stage of some PCa. However, the natural history of PIN has not been established. If PIN is present in a biopsy or transurethral resection (TUR), the pathologist must study additional sections and all available tissue for the existence of possible PCa, and the urologist must be alerted that the patient may have PCa elsewhere or may develop PCa.

The second category, which has been variously described as atypical hyperplasia, atypical adenomatous hyperplasia, or adenosis, has been regarded by some observers as premalignant. However, there is no evidence to support this view. The authors classify these glandular proliferations as microacinar hyperplasia.

Here the term "atypical glands" is preferred to refer to aggregates of small glands lined by a single layer of cells (i.e., an absence of the basal cell layer). In such cases, the differential diagnosis is small acinar PCa or microacinar hyperplasia. When the glands are closely aggregated with no suggestion of stromal dispersion, which characterizes infiltrating PCa, and the individual cells are completely normal in appearance, we classify it as microacinar hyperplasia. When there is any doubt as to whether either of the two features (invasive dispersion or nuclear anaplasia) is present, the lesion is classified as atypical glands.

## Variants of Growth Patterns

Most prostate carcinomas form glands, which manifest one or more of the following patterns. Frequently more than one growth pattern is seen in an individual case. *Acinar*: An invasive carcinoma composed of secretory cells showing a variable degree of nuclear anaplasia devoid of basal cells and forming acini. They are simple in structure and without convolutions. Rarely, the acini are very small. *Cribriform*: Large acinar tumor in which the neoplastic cells show bridging across the lumen without intervening stroma. This is categorized as moderately differentiated tumor. *Fused gland*: Groups of acini are packed closely together without intervening stroma. Tumors showing fused gland patterns are categorized as poorly differentiated tumors. These differ from cribriform glands in that they are more cellular and are irregular in peripheral contour. At low power, the volume of the cells exceeds that of the luminal spaces. *Small cell carcinoma*: This is a malignant tumor identical to small cell carcinoma of the lung. Prostatic carcinoma may also be demonstrated, and without this element, metastatic disease must be considered, as well as extension from a primary bladder small cell carcinoma. *Undifferentiated carcinoma*: A malignant tumor that is too poorly differentiated to be placed in any other category.

## Grading Systems

The diagnosis of carcinoma should include grading. At least 30 grading systems have been proposed but were found to be unsatisfactory by other investigators. At present, four systems are in use.

The Gleason system recognizes a primary and secondary pattern, and in each, five types of patterns. The sum of the two constitutes the grade. Three other systems (described below) are based on nuclear anaplasia and differentiation.

The second system is the World Health Organization/Mostofi system, based on the degrees of nuclear anaplasia and differentiation.

### Degrees of Nuclear Anaplasia

**Mild Anaplasia.** The nuclei are fairly uniform with minimal variation in size and shape. They are very similar to those of benign glands with minimal discernible anaplastic features. This is the category in which the diagnosis of carcinoma is based on glandular morphology or invasive stromal dispersion.

**Moderate Anaplasia.** The characteristic feature of moderate nuclear anaplasia is the presence of many prominent nucleoli, readily seen on medium power and/or moderate variation in size or shape of nuclei.

**Marked Anaplasia.** The nuclei show marked variation in size and shape. They may be hyperchromatic, but more often they are vesicular, irregularly shaped, and two to three times larger than adjacent benign nuclei. Mitotic figures are, generally speaking, rare in carcinoma of the prostate, but with marked anaplasia they may be numerous and even abnormal.

In arriving at a WHO grade, the three degrees of anaplasia are counted as I, II, and III.

### Degrees of Glandular Differentiation

The WHO grading system regards the tumors that form small and large glands as well differentiated and those that are cribriform as moderately differentiated. Poorly differentiated tumors show little or no gland formation. In arriving at the WHO grade, degrees of differentiation are listed as follows:

1. All of the tumor is composed of well-differentiated elements.

2. The tumor is composed of at least some moderately differentiated elements. Well-differentiated elements may or may not be present, but no poorly differentiated elements are present.

3. The tumor has poorly differentiated elements, but these are estimated to comprise less than 15 percent of the tumor.

4. The tumor has poorly differentiated elements that are estimated to comprise between 16 and 25 percent of the tumor.

5. The tumor has poorly differentiated elements that are estimated to comprise over 26 percent of the tumor.

The WHO grade of the tumor is the sum of the anaplasia differentiation values. For example: If the nuclear grade is II and histologic grade is 3, the WHO grade is 5. If nuclear grade is III and histologic grade is 5, the WHO grade is 8. The third system is that of Gaeta et al.,[24] who found correlation between the two parameters (nuclear grade and glandular differentiation). They based the final grade on the worst of the two. The fourth system is that of Brawn[7] who proposed a grading system based on differentiation alone.

## Multicentricity

In a study of 208 total prostatectomy specimens, Byar and Mostofi[8] called attention to the multicentricity of PCa. Often, four or five separate foci of PCa may be seen in a prostate. These observations have been confirmed by many reports.

## Volume

It has long been recognized that small tumors are less likely to invade and metastasize than are large tumors. In fact, clinical staging of cancers is almost entirely based on the size of the tumor. McNeal[38] has reported that PCa less than 4 ml in volume appeared to correlate with protection from extensive capsule penetration, positive surgical margins, seminal vesicle invasion, and lymph node metastases. Conversely, PCa larger than 12 ml in size were nearly a homogeneous group in which all of the adverse determinations tended to be positive.

## Special Types of Carcinoma

**Endometrioid Carcinoma.** Melicow and Tannenbaum[12] described two categories of endometrioid PCa. In one, the glands are lined by tall columnar epithelium with vacuolated cytoplasm and single or double layers of nuclei. In the other, the cells are cuboidal and often piled up, and the cytoplasm is granular. Because the tumors originally described were said to occur in the utricle, which is of müllerian origin, and they were typically papillary, the lesion was designated as endometrioid PCa. These lesions represent the papillary growth variant of prostatic acinar carcinoma.

**Mucinous Adenocarcinoma.** Some luminal mucin is present in many PCa types, but rarely, the tumor may consist entirely of mucinous adenocarcinoma, raising the possibility of secondary carcinoma. The true nature of the lesion can be readily identified by prostatic acid phosphatase (PAP) and prostate-specific antigen (PSA), both of which are positive.

**Transitional and Squamous Cell Carcinoma.** Rarely, a prostatic biopsy may reveal a transitional or squamous cell carcinoma. Before such cell types can be accepted as a primary PCa, a clinically undetected carcinoma in situ or an infiltrating carcinoma of the bladder neck should be ruled out. Such tumors have a tendency to grow along the prostatic ducts from the prostatic urethra deep into the posterior lobe; they may be mistaken initially for a PCa.

**Basal Cell Carcinoma.** A rare variant of carcinoma is derived from basal cells, and histologically, it shows the typical pattern of basal cell hyperplasia, plus solid sheets of poorly differentiated cells with mitoses and tumor necrosis. There may be focal areas of squamous, transitional, and acinar differentiation. If these features are equivocal, recognition of basal cell carcinoma can be made by extraprostatic invasion by the tumor.

**Small Cell Neuroendocrine Carcinoma.** *(Oat Cell carcinoma).* This is a malignant tumor identical to small cell carcinoma of the lung. Prostatic carcinoma may also be demonstrated, and lacking this element, metastatic disease must be considered, as well as extension from a primary bladder small cell carcinoma.

**Undifferentiated Carcinoma.** This is a malignant tumor that is too poorly differentiated to be placed in any other category.

**Adenoid Cystic Carcinoma.** Most, if not all, the reported cases of adenoid cystic carcinoma are variants of basal cell hyperplasia. If there is no anaplasia of cells, but there is associated basal cell hyperplasia and the lesion is intraprostatic, then the lesion is not adenoid cystic carcinoma. To date, we have not seen a true case of adenoid cystic PCa.

## Paracrine-Endocrine Tumors

Mention has already been made of paracrine-endocrine cells. A prostatic tumor may show a few endocrine cells or may consist entirely of carcinoid cells or small oat cell–like tumors. These tumors are capable of producing endocrine and many other substances. Neuroendocrine substances demonstrated in PCa cells are serotonin, neuron-specific enolase, chromogranin, thyroid-stimulating hormone, adrenocorticotropic hormone, calcitonin, and others. In all such cases, PAP and PSA levels are valuable to determine prostatic origin of the tumor. Recognition of neuroendocrine cells may be clinically important, because resistance to treatment may be due to the presence of these cells. It should be noted that neuroendocrine activity is not limited to oat cell tumors but may be present in secretory cells.

Cohen and colleagues[11] have reported that of 22 stage B patients, 4 died of the disease, and 3 of those 4 were positive for neuroendocrine cells. Of 20 stage C patients, 5 died of the disease, and all 5 were positive for neuroendocrine cells. Of 48 patients with stage D disease, 37 died of tumors; 34 of them were positive for neuroendocrine cells. These investigators claimed that this prognostic factor was significantly superior to the Gleason system.

Recent reports indicate that the presence of paracrine-endocrine cells is of significance only in patients with low Gleason score, whereas other reports do not find any correlation.

## Immunopathology

Prostatic acid phosphatase (PAP) is a secretory enzyme with a molecular weight of 100,000 and several isomers. Whereas some investigators have found no cross-reactivity between isoenzymes of PAP and acid phosphatases of other organs, others have reported cross-reactivity.

Prostate-specific antigen (PSA) is an enzyme of 33,000 to 34,000 daltons with several isomers. The isomer identified has a pI of 6.9. PSA has proteolytic activity and belongs to the serine proteases. Its proteolytic activity is similar to chymotrypsin and trypsin. Clinically, PSA occurs in free and complex forms. The complex form consists of PSA bound to alpha-1 antichymotrypsin and protein C inhibitor. Low free PSA concentrations and total PSA are more likely to be seen in prostatic carcinoma than in benign conditions.

PAP and PSA are present in secretory cells of normal and hyperplastic prostates, including those lining prostatic ducts and prostatic urethra. Basal cells and transitional cells and squamous epithelium are negative for both enzymes. In normal and hyperplastic prostates, the reaction of both enzymes is identical, with all secretory cells positive for both.

In carcinomas, the expression of PAP and PSA is not necessarily related to the nuclear grade or differentiation. In general, well-differentiated carcinomas show both enzymes in most of the tumor cells, but with variable intensity. In moderately and poorly differentiated carcinoma, the reaction patterns of both enzymes may be similar or show marked differences. Either enzyme may be more strongly positive or completely negative. In our experience, in poorly differentiated carcinomas, PSA is less likely to be expressed than PAP.

**Special Types.** Papillary (endometrioid) prostatic carcinoma, mucinous carcinoma, and the rare cystadenocarcinoma are all positive for both enzymes. Transitional cell, squamous cell, and basal cell carcinomas are negative for both. Metastatic tumors often reflect the staining pattern of the primary tumor. Metastases of poorly differentiated carcinomas may show different staining patterns in different metastatic sites, reflecting the heterogeneous cell population of the primary.

Endocrine cells of the prostate react positive for PAP and PSA, as do endocrine cells in prostatic acinar carcinomas. They are usually positive for chromogranin and serotonin. However, carcinoids, particularly rectal carcinoid, will show a positive reaction for PAP, but not for PSA. Endocrine cells involving the bladder and urethra are positive for PAP and not for PSA.

Both irradiated and hormonally treated carcinomas still express prostatic enzymes in tumor cells showing treatment effect; therefore, these reactions are very helpful in identifying residual tumor.

## Treatment Effects

### Radiation

When the prostate is irradiated, it may be difficult to distinguish residual carcinoma cells from altered benign prostatic elements. The former often exhibit balloon degeneration and cytoplasmic vacuolization while the pattern of growth (single glands, fused glands, no glands) remains about what it was before treatment. The benign prostate shows a loss or reduction of the tall columnar secretory cells, and the original tubuloalveolar glands are reduced to narrow channels or solid cords lined mainly with atypical, often bizarre, basal cells. They may also show squamous metaplasia. Residual tumor cells retain PAP and PSA reactivity; this will identify the neoplastic cells on H&E (hematoxylin and eosin) sections. The question of tumor cell viability is often raised and is usually difficult to answer; thus, it may be more useful to comment on the presence or absence of any tumor cells devoid of radiation change.

### Estrogen Therapy

As with radiation, the tumor cells retain PSA and PAP activity. Tumor cell nuclei become small and pyknotic, with loss of nucleoli. Cytoplasmic swelling with rupture of cell membranes leads to several nuclei within the same cleared space. The benign prostate shows atrophy of glandular epithelium as well as squamous

metaplasia of the ducts. On rare occasions, prostatic carcinoma apparently undergoes squamous metaplasia in this setting, leading to squamous carcinoma.

### Antiandrogen Therapy

Benign elements of the prostate become atrophic, and the basal cells become unusually prominent and are sometimes associated with squamous islands. Residual tumor cells may exist only as smudged, ghost cells within the stroma. Some tumor glands show loss of cell membranes, reduction of cell size, and crowding of nuclei.

## TUMORS OF THE BLADDER

## Staging

Pathologic stage is based on the depth of local extension in the bladder wall. TNM classification has recently been revised (Fig. 6–31).

| | |
|---|---|
| pTX | Primary tumor cannot be assessed |
| pT0 | No evidence of primary tumor |
| pTa | Papillary tumor confined to mucosa; no infiltration of lamina propria |
| pTis | Nonpapillary, noninfiltrating tumor confined to mucosa—carcinoma in situ |
| pT1 | Tumor invades subepithelial connective tissue |
| pT2 | Tumor invades muscle |

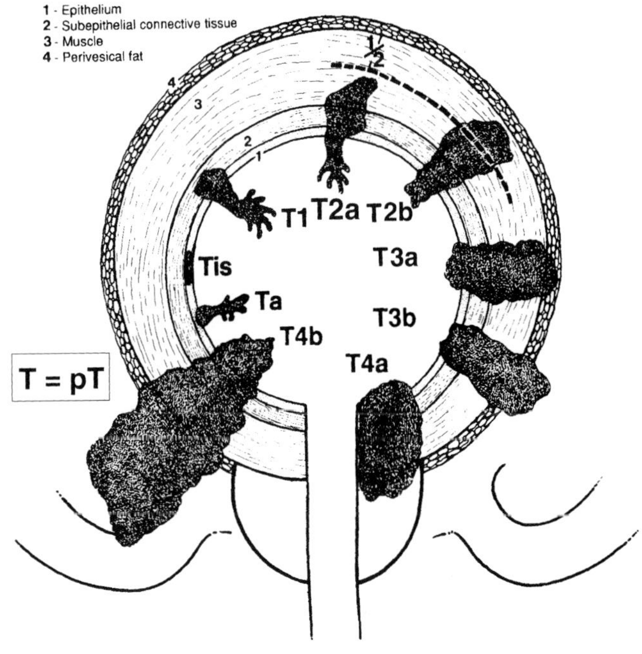


**Figure 6–31**

pT2a     Tumor invades superficial muscle (inner half)

pT2b     Tumor invades deep muscle (outer half)

pT3      Tumor invades perivesical tissue

pT3a     Microscopically

pT3b     Macroscopically (extravesical mass)

pT4      Tumor invades any of the following: prostate, uterus, vagina, pelvic wall, abdominal wall

pT4a     Tumor invades prostate or uterus or vagina

pT4b     Tumor invades pelvic wall or abdominal wall

Regional lymph nodes are designated by N.

NX      Regional lymph nodes cannot be assessed

N0      No regional lymph node metastasis

N1      Metastasis in a single lymph node 2 cm or less in greatest dimension

N2      Metastasis in a single lymph node more than 2 cm, but not more than 5 cm in greatest dimensions, or multiple lymph nodes. None more than 5 cm in greatest dimension

N3      Metastasis in the lymph node more than 5 cm in greatest dimension

Distant metastasis is indicated by M.

MX      Distant metastasis cannot be assessed

M0      No distant metastasis

M1      Distant metastasis

## Histologic Features

The normal urinary bladder is lined with transitional epithelium, more correctly called urothelium. The thickness of the epithelial layer depends on whether the bladder is empty or full or distended. In its collapsed state, the epithelium is five to seven layers thick; in the distended state it is two to three cell layers. The luminal surface is lined with large umbrella cells. The configuration of these cells varies from flat to cuboidal, depending on distention or contraction of the bladder. They cover the intermediate and basal layers of transition epithelial cells. The epithelial layer rests on a thin, delicate basement membrane.

The lamina propria (sometimes called submucosa) consists of loose fibrovascular tissue that contains irregularly sized muscle bundles referred to as muscularis mucosae. The muscularis propria is arbitrarily divided into superficial and deep layers. The muscularis is surrounded by a layer of fibroadipose tissue, and all but the anterior surface is covered by peritoneum.

## CHARACTERIZATION OF CARCINOMA OF THE BLADDER

### Pattern of Growth

Papillary (70%)
Papillary and infiltrating (20%)
Infiltrating (10%)
Nonpapillary and noninfiltrating, such as carcinoma in situ (1%)

### Histologic Features

Urothelial carcinoma (90%)
Squamous carcinoma (7%) (in Africa and the Middle East it is 80% to 90%)
Adenocarcinoma (2%)
Undifferentiated carcinoma (1%)
Mixtures; most commonly transitional and squamous or glandular carcinoma

### Grades

I    Slight but definite anaplasia, orderly architecture
II   Moderate anaplasia, predominant disorder of architecture
III  Marked anaplasia, architectural chaos

### Mode of Spread

Implantation
Broad front
Tentacular
Lymphatic
Blood vessels

---

With few exceptions, grade I papillary carcinomas are initially noninvasive or invade only the lamina propria. About half of grade II carcinomas are initially invasive of lamina propria and later invade superficial muscle. The invasive tumors usually originate as invasive neoplasms but may develop in a papillary carcinoma. It must be emphasized that lymphatic and vascular invasion occurs in 7% to 10% of these papillary tumors.

## Clinical Course

The rate of recurrence is higher in grade II tumors. Multiple or large tumors have a higher risk of recurrence than do single or small tumors; 46% recur in 5 years, 65% in 10 years, and 81% in 15 years.

Although the tumors recur, they tend to remain essentially localized; only 20% progress to infiltrating tumors, but it is possible that even some of these started as papillary and infiltrating tumors. About 10% invade lymphatics, and 17% metastasize.

The course of these tumors, as of all bladder tumors, is complicated by multicentricity, aggressive potential of the cell, existence of preneoplastic changes and carcinoma in situ (CIS) elsewhere in the bladder, and iatrogenic seeding that may occur when the tumor is resected transurethrally.

# Papillary Noninfiltrating Epithelial Tumors

## Benign Tumors

### Urothelial (Transitional Cell) Papilloma

This papillary tumor has a delicate fibrovascular stroma covered by urothelium indistinguishable from that of the normal bladder. The lesion is characterized by discrete papillary fronds, with occasional branching in some cases, but without fusion. The stroma may show some edema or inflammatory cells, the epithelium has no atypia, and umbrella cells are prominent.

---

## CLASSIFICATION OF EPITHELIAL TUMORS

### Epithelial Tumors of the Bladder

#### Benign

Urothelial (transitional cell) papilloma
Urothelial (transitional cell) papilloma, inverted type
Squamous cell papilloma
Villous adenoma

#### Papillary Urothelial (Transitional Cell) Neoplasm of Low Malignant Potential

#### Malignant

Urothelial (transitional cell) carcinoma
Papillary urothelial (transitional cell) carcinoma
Infiltrating urothelial (transitional cell) carcinoma
Carcinoma in situ
Atypia and dysplasia
Variants of urothelial (transitional cell) carcinoma
Squamous cell carcinoma
Verrucous carcinoma
Adenocarcinoma
Urachal carcinoma
Clear cell adenocarcinoma
Small cell carcinoma
Undifferentiated carcinoma

### Nonepithelial Tumors

### Miscellaneous Tumors

Paraganglioma
Hematopoietic and lymphoid neoplasms
Carcinosarcoma
Malignant melanoma

---

Mitoses are rare and, if present, are basal in location and not abnormal. These tumors are rare, usually isolated, quite small, and typically seen in patients under the age of 50.

### Urothelial (Transitional Cell) Papilloma, Inverted Type

A tumor with the characteristics of a transitional cell papilloma but with an endophytic rather than an exophytic growth pattern. Most of these are solitary, pedunculated, or sessile and located in the bladder neck or trigone. The surface is covered by a continuous layer of epithelium that is histologically normal or slightly attenuated. Invaginations from the surface extend into the stroma to form a maze-like proliferation of anastomosing cords of transitional epithelium. The epithelium is normal, with some spindling in the center of the cords. Some will show squamous areas, and a few have glandular foci with goblet cells. Widely scattered neuroendocrine cells may be present. Mitoses are rare and usually absent. Some tumors show features of both papilloma and inverted papilloma. As defined here, they are without malignant potential but must be distinguished from low-grade carcinomas with a largely inverted growth pattern. These carcinomas lack the maze-like pattern and exhibit instead lobules or plates of solid epithelial masses and usually surface papillations.

### Squamous Cell Papilloma

Squamous cell papilloma is characterized by a bland proliferation of squamous epithelium, usually having the cytologic features of condyloma acuminatum identical to that seen in other sites. Condylomas are distinguished from other squamous cell papillomas by the presence of koilocytes and the demonstrable human papillomavirus (HPV) subtypes 6/11. Most are associated with urethral condylomas or follow long-standing cystostomy or indwelling catheter. Extensive acanthosis with deep, pushing margins typical of verrucous carcinoma is lacking.

### Villous Adenoma

This is a benign neoplasm in which papillary fronds covered by colonic-type glandular epithelium project into the lumen of the bladder or urachus. Tall, pseudostratified, colonic-type epithelium lines villous or tubulovillous fronds identical to villous adenomas of the large bowel. Nuclei are dark, elongated, and basal in location. Prominent nucleoli or stromal invasion indicates malignant change. As with other forms of glandular metaplasia, there is a malignant potential.

## Papillary Urothelial (Transitional Cell) Neoplasm of Low Malignant Potential

This new category is defined as a papillary tumor of urothelium that resembles the typical papilloma but shows an increased cellular proliferation, exceeding six cell layers in thickness. Although the counting of cell layers is an approximation, these papillary tumors clearly exceed in thickness that of normal bladder epithelium. The pattern gives the impression of predominant order with minimal or no variation of architectural and nuclear features. Mitoses are infrequent and usually have a basal location. Umbrella cells are present and may not be prominent. As with papillomas and low-grade papillary carcinomas, these cells may show a prominent inverted growth pattern.

This lesion does not progress to carcinoma in the overwhelming majority of cases. However, these patients have an increased risk of developing new papillary lesions, which occasionally are of higher grade and capable of malignant progression.

This category includes many of the grade I papillary carcinomas of the 1973 WHO classification and grade I papillary urothelial tumors of European classifications.

## Malignant Tumors

### Urothelial (Transitional Cell) Carcinoma

This category refers to any malignant epithelial tumor of the bladder consisting entirely, partly, or focally of anaplastic urothelium (transitional epithelium). The basic elements in the diagnosis of urothelial carcinoma are growth pattern, nuclear grade, and tumor stage. The growth patterns are papillary, infiltrating, in situ, and any combination.

Unlike the papillomas and papillary neoplasms of low malignant potential, papillary urothelial (transitional cell) carcinomas show architectural disorder and nuclear atypia of variable degree, which is graded on a scale of I to III, because the rate of progression differs significantly with each of the three grades. In tumors with variable histologic features, the tumor is graded according to the highest grade area, although it has not been established whether minute foci of high-grade tumor impact on the prognosis.

The epithelium of grade I urothelial carcinomas has an overall orderly appearance but with easily recognizable variations of architectural and cytologic features. In contrast to the papillary urothelial neoplasms of low malignant potential, it is easy to recognize variations of nuclear polarity, size, shape, and chromatin. Mitoses are infrequent but may occur at any level of the epithelium, usually the basal third. Fronds should be evaluated when sectioned lengthwise through the core or when sectioned at right angles away from the base. Otherwise, there may be a misleading impression of increased cellularity and mitoses or loss of polarity.

The grade I papillary urothelial carcinomas described here correspond to some of those previously called grade I in the 1973 WHO classification. They also correspond to low-grade urothelial carcinomas and to grade 2A carcinomas in many European centers.

Grade II tumors exhibit an intermediate degree of abnormality. They are distinguished from grade I by a predominantly disordered architectural pattern but with retention of some elements of organization, e.g., polarity and nuclear uniformity. These elements are not seen in grade III. These features are unchanged from the previous WHO grade II carcinomas and correspond to grade 2B tumors in much of Europe. In the low-grade/high-grade scheme, they are included with the high-grade lesions.

Grade III tumors present an overall impression of complete disorder or chaos, with absence of polarity and, commonly, loss of superficial cells, marked variation of all nuclear parameters, and usually numerous irregularly distributed mitoses. The grade III carcinomas are identical to the grade III lesions of the 1973 WHO classification and correspond to the grade III tumors of European centers and to high-grade tumors of other centers.

With increasing grade, epithelial thickness may be variable owing to increasing loss of cellular cohesion. With few exceptions, grade I papillary carcinomas are initially noninvasive or invade only the lamina propria. About half of grade II carcinomas are initially invasive of lamina propria, and later invade superficial muscle. The invasive tumors usually originate as invasive neoplasms but may develop in a papillary carcinoma. It must be emphasized that lymphatic and vascular invasion occurs in 7% to 10% of these papillary tumors.

### Infiltrating and Metastatic Tumors

Invasive tumors are defined as those that have invaded the lamina propria, muscularis, perivesical fibroadipose tissue, the prostate, uterus, cervix, vagina, or pelvic or abdominal wall.

At the time of the initial examination, 24% of bladder tumors showed muscle invasion; 12% had further extension.

Most of the tumors are urothelial. In contrast to papillary tumors and tumors that are papillary and infiltrating, invasive carcinomas have foci of squamous and glandular structures or spindle cells. About one fourth are undifferentiated. The tumors are mostly grade III but may be grade II or even, rarely, grade I.

The distinction between lamina propria invasion and tangential sections through surface epithelium or von Brunn nests can be difficult but is important. With noninvasive lesions, the basement membrane preserves a smooth, regular contour that differs from the irregular contours of invasive aggregates. Thin-walled vessels often line basement membranes of noninvasive nests. With invasive lesions, the character of the adjacent stroma often differs from that seen in other areas, e.g., fibrosis, sclerosis, and retraction artifacts. The last type frequently is mistaken for lymphatic or vascular invasion. When the space contains no blood or lymphocytes or obvious endothelial cell lining, it likely represents shrinkage artifact.

The lamina propria may contain smooth muscle fibers that are usually thin and discontinuous and is referred to as the muscularis mucosa. It should not be confused with thick fascicles of the muscularis propria. The former are found approximately in the mid lamina propria, parallel to the surface and often associated with prominent vessels.

In papillary and infiltrating tumors, the depth of penetration of the muscularis is more superficial than in sessile nodular tumors. Also, the mode of infiltration is usually different. In the former the infiltration is usually along a broad front, whereas in invasive tumors the infiltration is more often tentacular; both subjacent and lateral invasion may be seen in this group. Vascular and lymphatic invasion is found in more superficially invasive tumors half as often as in more deeply invasive tumors.

### Variants of Urothelial (Transitional Cell) Carcinoma

Four variants will be discussed. *Urothelial (transitional cell)* carcinoma with squamous and/or glandular metaplasia or anaplasia is applied to tumors that, in addition to transitional cell elements, have benign squamous or glandular cells or carcinomas of these cells. These should be listed in the diagnosis.

*Spindle cell carcinoma (sarcomatoid carcinoma)* refers to transitional or squamous carcinomas that contain spindle cell elements. These mimic various sarcomas, but the epithelial nature is demonstrable with cytokeratin or epithelial membrane antigen.

*Osteoclast variant* refers to transitional or squamous carcinomas that are associated with cells in the stroma that resemble osteoclasts. These are graded without respect to giant cells.

*Urothelial carcinoma with ectopic placental glycoprotein production* applies to urothelial carcinomas that produce trophoblastic hormones, usually β-hCG (human chorionic gonadotropin). These high-grade lesions have bizarre mononuclear or multinuclear cells that resemble syncytiotrophoblasts, but unlike choriocarcinoma, immunoreactivity is not confined to the giant cells but is also present in small cells.

Other variants consist of micropapillary, nested, microcystic, and hepatoid variants.

## Nonpapillary Noninfiltrating Flat Lesions

There are two categories of carcinoma in situ (CIS): (1) those seen in association with clinical carcinoma of bladder that may be found simultaneously with initial diagnosis of carcinoma or sequentially during follow-up of the patients treated for carcinoma of the bladder, and (2) those that occur initially and de novo.

In most instances, positive cytologic findings lead to the diagnosis of CIS. Not infrequently, however, the biopsy may show no epithelial layer but congestion, or only a single layer of cells or anaplasia of von Brunn nests. If the cells show anaplasia, the lesion should be diagnosed as CIS.

There has been much confusion about the pathologic definition and diagnoses of flat lesions. Some centers have limited the diagnosis of carcinoma in situ to only high-grade anaplastic changes involving the full thickness of the epithelium and label other abnormalities as dysplasia. WHO defined carcinoma in situ as anaplasia of surface epithelium or von Brunn nests but confined to the epithelial layer.

The cells are usually large and pleomorphic, but they may be small. The nuclei are enlarged hyperchromatic and irregularly shaped. The chromatin is coarse, with or without prominent nuclei, mitotic figures, often abnormal and present at any level.

Several growth patterns of CIS are recognized. In the first the entire thickness of the mucosa is involved, and the growth may be generalized or localized. In the second form the neoplastic change may be confined to the basal layers of the epithelium, pushing up the normal mucosa and eventually sloughing off the benign surface epithelium, leaving two layers of neoplastic cells. The third form has a pagetoid appearance with clusters of distinct malignant epithelial cells scattered amidst apparently benign epithelium. A fourth form is neoplasia involving the surface layers with the subjacent epithelium appearing benign. Whether these represent variable manifestations of the response of the epithelium to carcinogenesis or indicate intraepithelial spread of CIS has not been resolved.

Carcinoma in situ may involve not only the surface layer but also von Brunn nests, cystitis cystica, and nephrogenic adenoma. These changes may be seen in tissues with denuded or intact surface epithelium, but recognition of abnormalities is important in denuded areas.

Most CIS consists of transitional epithelium. A few examples may be squamous, and because many of these are well differentiated, the diagnosis of CIS may be difficult; however, slight to moderate anaplasia should be looked for. The diagnosis of in situ adenocarcinoma is often difficult, because these are usually well-differentiated neoplasms.

In summary, the diagnosis of CIS is limited to flat lesions, and CIS lesions are defined as showing varying degrees of anaplasia that may or may not involve the entire thickness of the epithelial layer. A second category of preinvasive lesion is designated atypia/dysplasia to apply to urothelium that is not normal, but the cytologic and architectural alterations are insufficient to warrant a diagnosis of carcinoma in situ.

## Nontransitional Cell Carcinoma

Transitional cell carcinomas constitute 90% of all carcinomas of the bladder. About 7% of tumors consist of squamous cell carcinoma, 2% are adenocarcinomas, and 1% are undifferentiated carcinomas. These cell types may be seen in pure form, but frequently squamous, glandular, and tubular areas are seen in transitional cell carcinomas.

Squamous cell tumors may be squamous papilloma (very rare) or squamous cell carcinoma: Two categories of carcinoma are recognized—the nonbilharzial and the bilharzial. The former is seen in the Western hemisphere and constitutes about 7% of bladder tumors. It is most often associated with long-standing chronic infection, vesical calculi, vesical diverticuli, chronic Foley catheter use, and cyclophosphamide treatment. Grossly, the tumors are bulky, often with ulceration and necrosis. The diagnosis of squamous cell carcinoma should be restricted to tumors that are purely squamous. The squamous cell carcinoma associated with bilharzial infection is the most common tumor seen in Egypt, parts of Africa, and the Middle East, where *Schistosoma haematobium* is prevalent. It constitutes about 60% to 80% of bladder tumors. Most, if not all, of these tumors are well differentiated, but by the time they are seen by a urologic surgeon, they typically show invasion of muscle, and over two thirds of these tumors have extended beyond the bladder. These tumors are deeply infiltrating, but tend to remain well differentiated and confined to the bladder.

Pure adenocarcinomas constitute about 2% of bladder tumors. They may be primary vesical, which includes those seen in exstrophy, urachal, and clear cell type, or they may be metastatic.

Primary vesical adenocarcinomas are usually preceded by a long history of cystitis, mucin in the urine, and cystitis glandularis. In the early stages, primary vesical adenocarcinomas are often difficult to diagnose because the biopsy may consist only of benign-appearing columnar mucus-producing epithelium or lakes of mucin. Invariably, there is associated glandular cystitis. Unless invasion can be demonstrated, it is impossible to diagnose malignancy. Histologically, the tumor may resemble colonic carcinoma with tall columnar, mucus-producing epithelium or a signet ring. The behavior of primary vesical adenocarcinoma is roughly that of infiltrating transitional cell carcinoma.

Urachal adenocarcinomas are confined to the dome or the anterior wall. They are primarily and principally intramural, with secondary involvement of the mucosa. The proper management of these tumors must take into account the space of Retzius and the anterior abdominal wall. Carcinoembryonic antigen is elevated in these patients.

Clear cell adenocarcinoma, also referred to as mesonephric or tubular adenocarcinoma, consists of tubular structures lined with cuboidal or flattened epithelium. The tumor may involve the entire thickness of the bladder and may be the malignant counterpart of nephrogenic adenoma. The bladder is frequently involved in adenocarcinomas that are primary in the cervix, uterus, prostate, and colon, but it is rare to have such metastatic tumors be initially manifested with bladder symptoms.

Undifferentiated carcinoma of the bladder is very rare. Instead of transitional, squamous, or glandular elements, the cells are primitive and undifferentiated. Histologically, the cells may be small or large. The small cell variant often shows paracrine-endocrine differentiation. The spindle cell variety simulates sarcoma. In these cases keratin and epithelial membrane antigen stains are positive. Such carcinomas may show areas of squamous differentiation.

## Carcinomas of More Than One Cell Type

In many bladder tumors, especially infiltrating and recurrent carcinomas, more than one cell type may be seen. Most commonly, it is transitional cell carcinoma with either squamous or glandular or tubular areas. Sometimes designated as metaplastic tumors, the less common element may have either a benign or malignant appearance. At other times, especially in older patients, there are spindle or undifferentiated elements, but many of these tumors will show some glandular or squamous differentiation. The pleomorphic cell population is simply indicative of the potentialities of vesical epithelium.

## Nonepithelial Tumors

Benign tumors include leiomyoma, neurofibroma, and hemangioma.

Malignant polypoid rhabdomyosarcoma (sarcoma botryoides) is the most common malignant tumor. Tumors of skeletal muscle are the most common in children and young adults. Several cell types are involved: round, spindle with or without cross striations, spider web cells, rhabdomyoblasts, and giant cells.

Leiomyosarcoma is characterized by interlacing bands of smooth muscle cell.

To make the diagnosis of carcinosarcoma, there must be two definite elements: carcinoma and sarcoma (osteosarcoma, chondrosarcoma, rhabdosarcoma, or fibrosarcoma).

# TUMORS OF THE KIDNEY

## Staging

TNM classification for renal carcinoma has recently been revised (Fig. 6–42).

Primary tumor is classified as pT.

pTX    Primary tumor cannot be assessed

pT0    No evidence of primary tumor

pT1    Tumor 7.0 cm or less in greatest dimension, limited to the kidney

pT2    Tumor more than 7.0 cm in greatest dimension, limited to the kidney

pT3    Tumor extends into major veins or invades adrenal gland or perinephric tissues but not beyond Gerota's fascia

pT3a   Tumor invades adrenal gland or perinephric tissues but not beyond Gerota's fascia

pT3b   Tumor grossly extends into renal vein(s) or vena cava below diaphragm

pT3c   Tumor grossly extends into vena cava above diaphragm

pT4    Tumor invades beyond Gerota's fascia

Regional lymph nodes are designated by pN.

pNX    Regional lymph nodes cannot be assessed

pN0    No regional lymph node metastasis

pN1    Metastasis in a single regional lymph node

pN2    Metastasis in more than one regional lymph node

Distant metastasis is indicated by M.

pMX    Distant metastasis cannot be assessed

pM0    No distant metastasis

pM1    Distant metastasis

Carcinomas of the renal pelvis, ureter, and urethra are classified as urothelial carcinoma. Staging of pelvic and ureteral tumors is indicated here:

Primary tumor (pT):

pTX    Primary tumor cannot be assessed

pT0    No evidence of primary tumor

pTa    Noninvasive papillary carcinoma

pTis   Carcinoma in situ

pT1    Tumor invades subepithelial connective tissue

pT2    Tumor invades muscularis

pT3    (Renal pelvis) Tumor invades beyond muscularis into peripelvic fat or renal parenchyma

pT4    Tumor invades adjacent organs or through the kidney into perinephric fat

Regional lymph nodes (N):

pNX    Regional lymph nodes cannot be assessed

pN0    No regional lymph node metastasis

pN1    Metastasis in a single regional lymph node 2 cm or less in greatest dimension

pN2    Metastasis in a single lymph node more than 2 cm but not more than 5 cm in greatest dimension

pN3    Metastasis in a lymph node more than 5 cm in greatest dimension

Distant metastasis (M):

pMX    Distant metastasis cannot be assessed

pM0    No distant metastasis

pM1    Distant metastasis

## Adenomas

### Papillary and Tubulopapillary Adenoma

Careful sectioning of kidneys at autopsy reveals that 7% to 22% of patients have one or more cortical adenomas. These tumors are seen almost exclusively in patients over age 40 and chiefly in males (about 3:1). Studies have also shown that they are increased in smokers and in renal vascular disease. The great majority are found as small white or gray nodules less than 2 cm in diameter, but a few are larger and may be cystic. The common cortical adenoma is almost always a very small lesion, and it is composed of cells with small, uniform nuclei, without nucleoli, and with very little cytoplasm. When these reach 1 to 2 cm in size, the cellular features of carcinoma are usually apparent: nucleoli or more abundant cytoplasm. Lesions smaller than 5 mm will almost always be classified as adenoma unless they have clear cells. Any clear cell tumor, regardless of size, is renal cell carcinoma.

### Oncocytic Adenoma (Oncocytoma)

These tumors are well circumscribed, occasionally have a capsule, and are usually described as mahogany or brown—similar to the adjacent cortex. There usually is a central scar, but the gross pathologic picture can be confusing. Those with microcystic histologic features will often appear as bloody tumors; at other times there may be far more scar tissue than tumor, so it will not be a brown specimen. Some have been over 20 cm but most are 3 to 6 cm. It may be the only benign tumor (in adults) that is more common in males, excluding the cortical adenomas. In most of the cases the cells are quite small and arranged into rounded or ovoid aggregations, which are densely packed at the periphery and more sparse centrally, where the scar

T1
pT1
T3a
T3a
Gerota fascia
Perinephric fat
T = pT
≤ 7 cm
T3b
pT3b
T3c
pT3c
pT2
T2
> 7 cm
T4
pT4
Gerota fascia
Perinephric fat

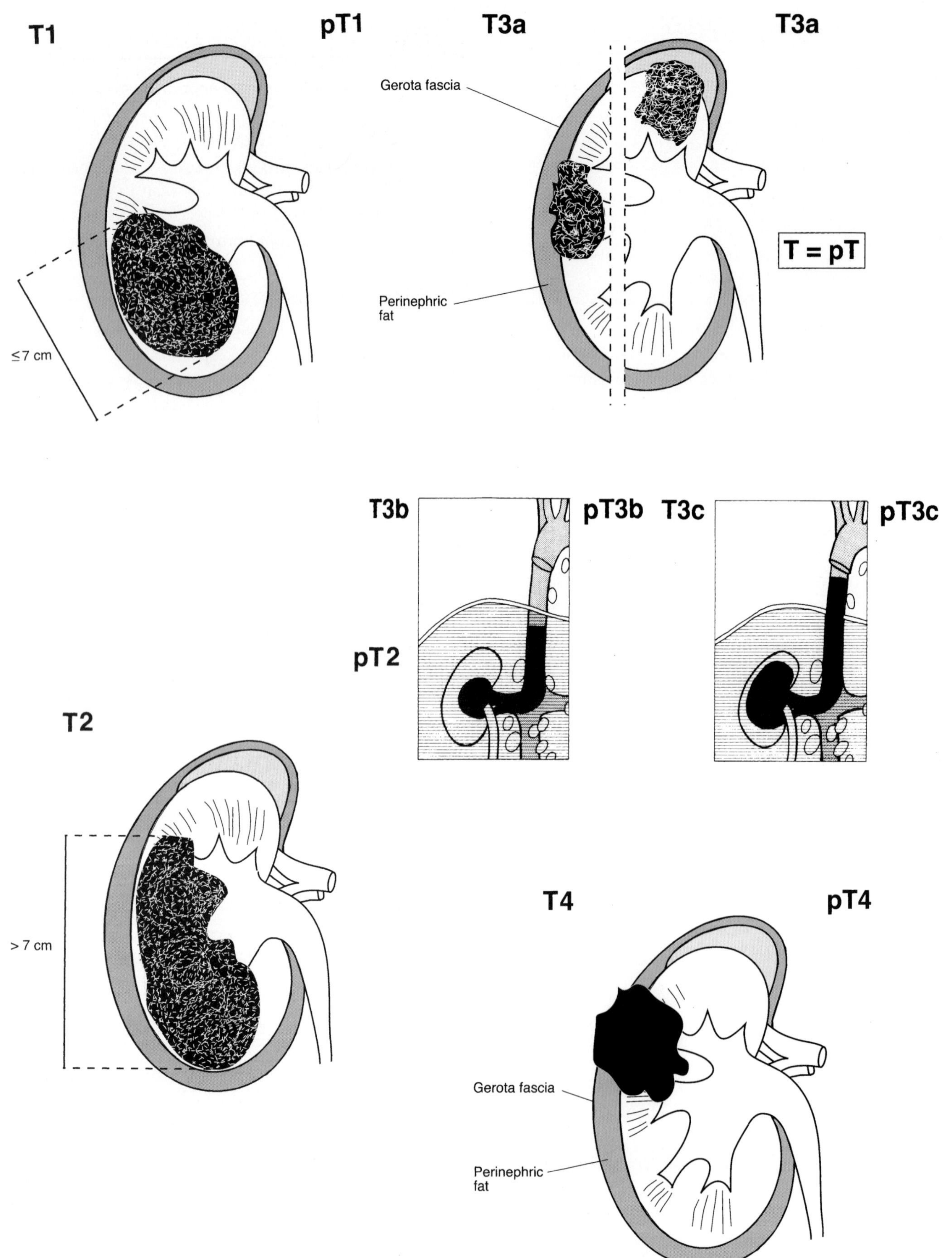

Figure 6–42

# $P$rostate

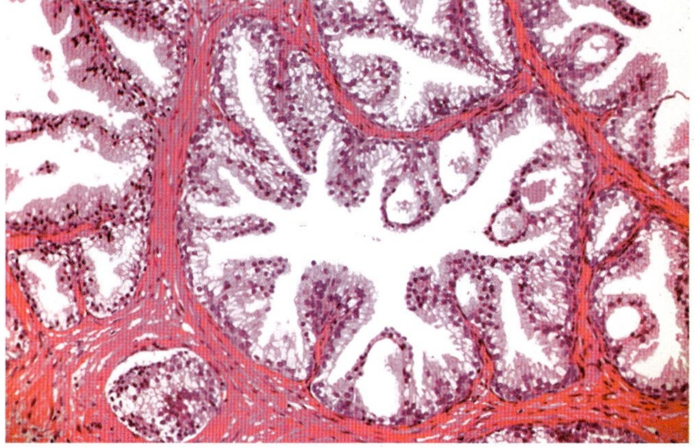

**FIGURE 6–1.** Benign prostatic hyperplasia. Large gland with papillary formation and lined by secretory and basal cells.

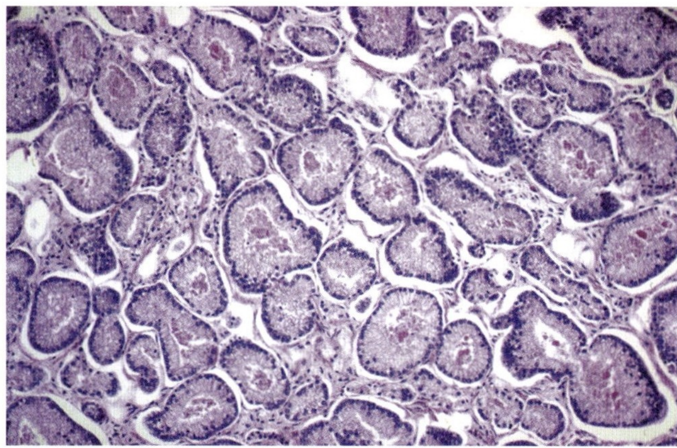

**FIGURE 6–4.** Large acinar well-differentiated carcinoma nuclear grade I (Gleason pattern 2 or 3).

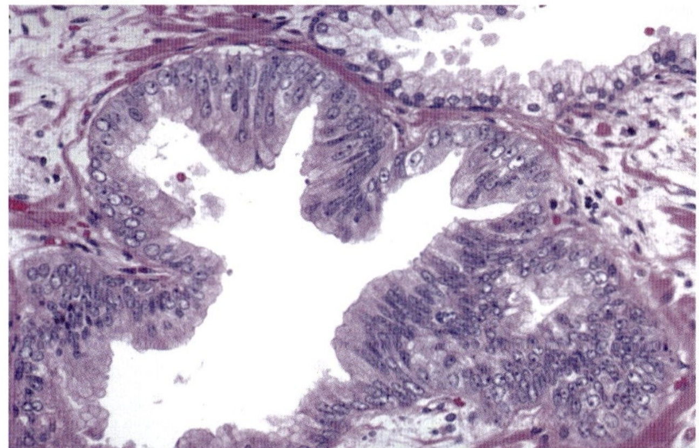

**FIGURE 6–2.** Prostatic intraepithelial neoplasia. The large gland is lined in part by piled-up malignant epithelial cells and partly by a layer of normal secretory cells.

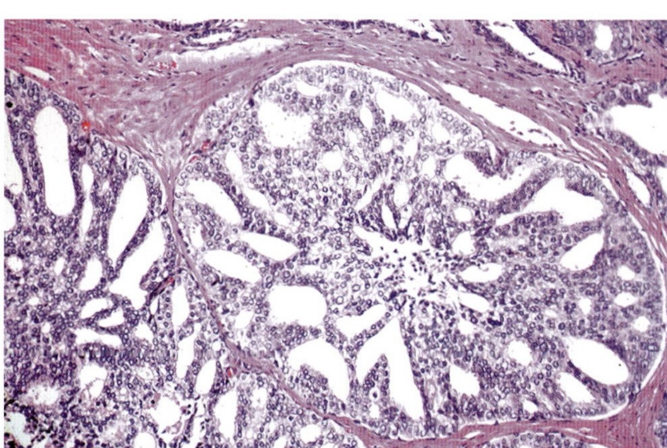

**FIGURE 6–5.** Cribriform carcinoma, moderately differentiated nuclear grade II (Gleason pattern 3).

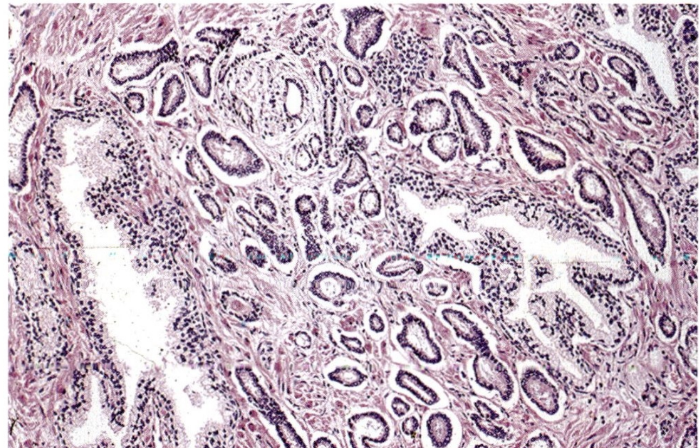

**FIGURE 6–3.** Small acinar well-differentiated nuclear grade I carcinoma, side by side with benign hyperplastic glands (Gleason pattern 2).

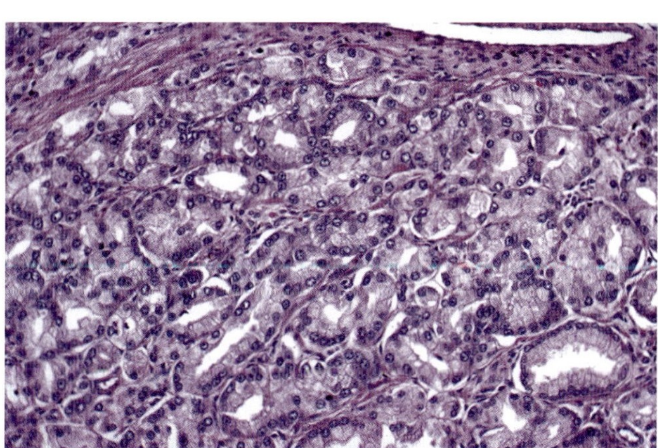

**FIGURE 6–6.** Fused gland carcinoma of the prostate, moderately differentiated nuclear grade II (Gleason pattern 4).

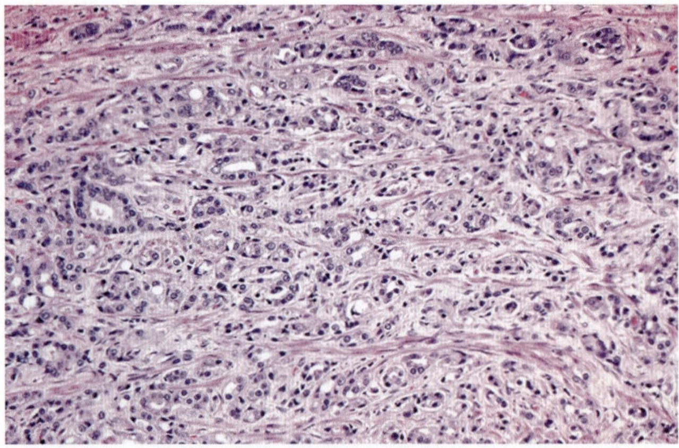

**FIGURE 6–7.** Poorly differentiated carcinoma of the prostate with occasional gland formation nuclear grades II and III (Gleason pattern 5).

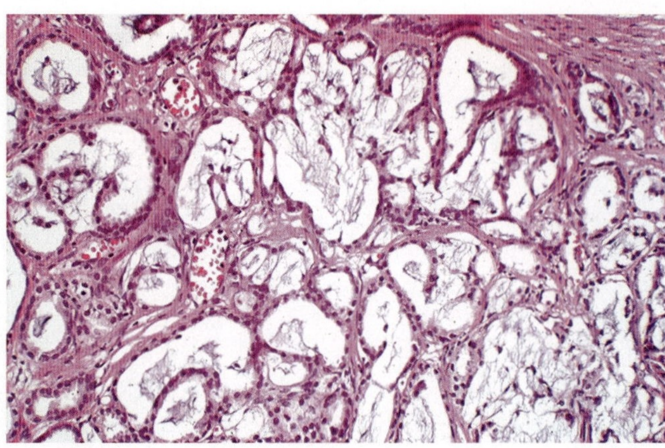

**FIGURE 6–10.** Mucinous carcinoma nuclear grade II, no Gleason grade.

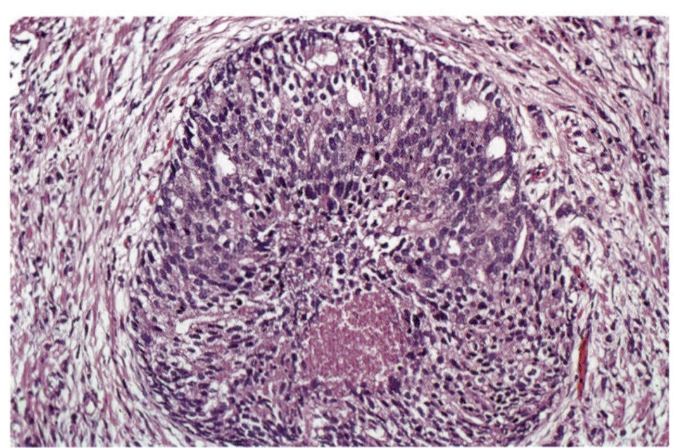

**FIGURE 6–8.** Undifferentiated nuclear grade II carcinoma showing solid sheets of tumor cells with necrosis (Gleason pattern 5).

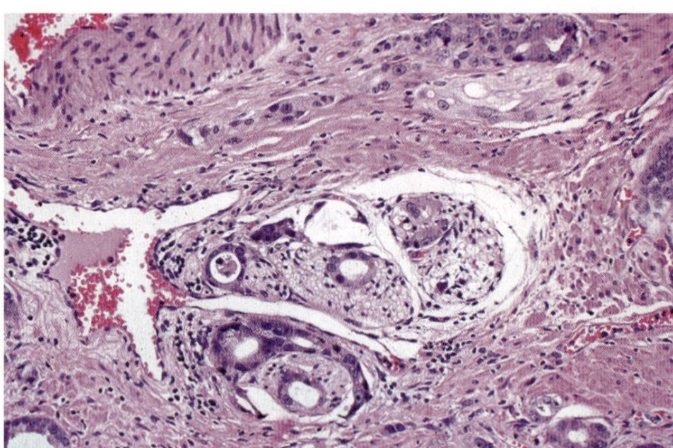

**FIGURE 6–11.** Prostate carcinoma showing perineural invasion.

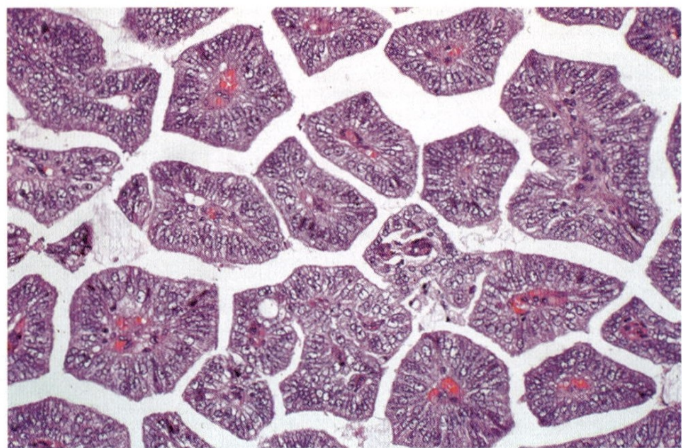

**FIGURE 6–9.** Papillary carcinoma nuclear grade II (endometroid type), no Gleason grade.

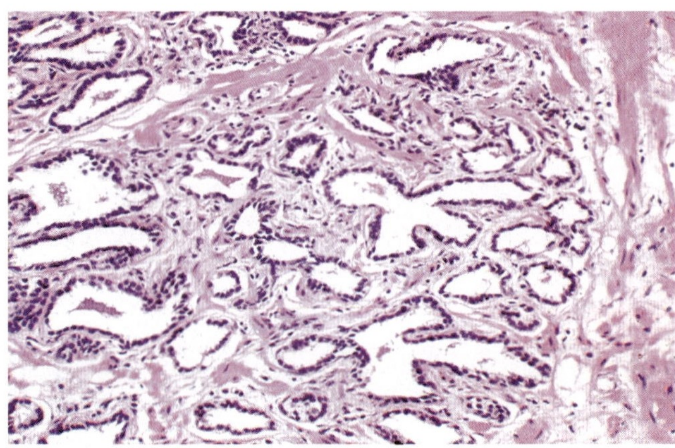

**FIGURE 6–12.** Prostatic atrophy showing lobules of small glands with a single layer of epithelial cells with little cytoplasm and small dark-staining nuclei. The lesion is often misdiagnosed as carcinoma.

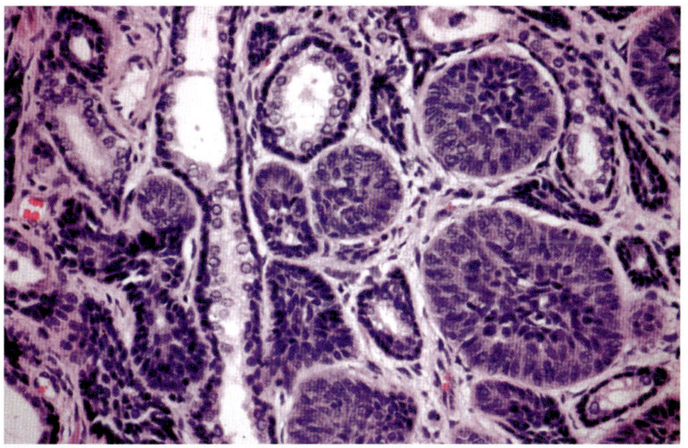

**FIGURE 6–13.** Basal cell hyperplasia. Many of the acini are filled with elongated basal cells occasionally differentiating into secretory cells. This appearance is often misdiagnosed as carcinoma of the prostate.

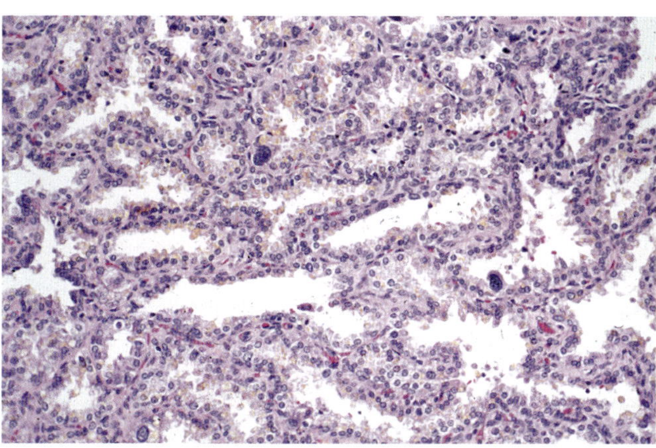

**FIGURE 6–14.** Seminal vesicle showing involutional changes. Tubular structures with dark-staining luminal cells. This change in the seminal vesicle is often misdiagnosed as carcinoma of the prostate.

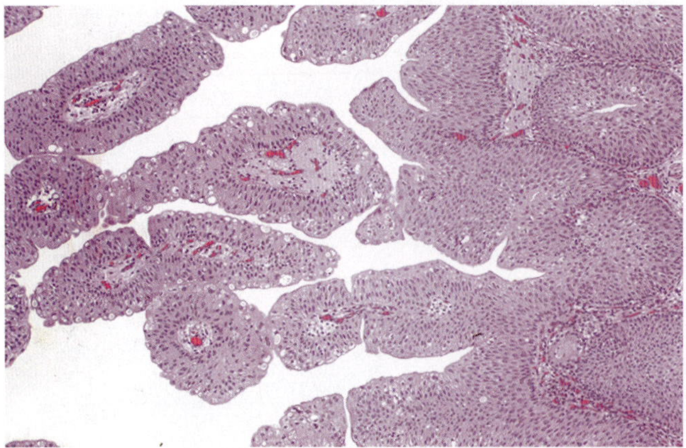

**FIGURE 6–16.** Transitional (urothelial) cell papilloma. The tumor has a delicate fibrovascular-stroma covered by transitional epithelium indistinguishable from that of normal bladder.

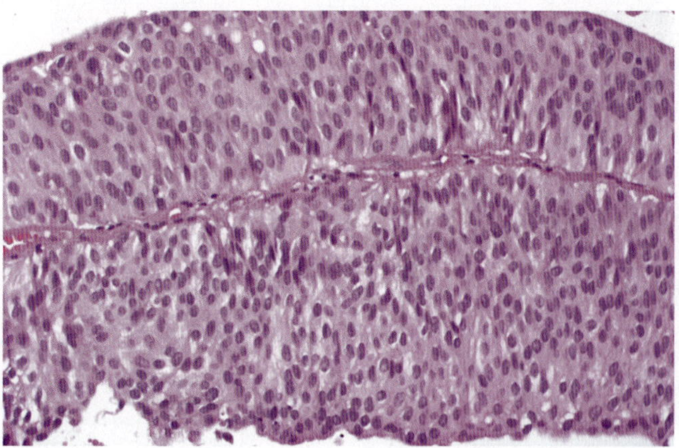

**FIGURE 6–19.** Papillary transitional cell carcinoma grade I. The epithelium has an overall orderly appearance, but with easily recognizable variations of nuclear polarity, size, shape, and chromatin. Mitoses are infrequent, but may occur at any level of the epithelium, usually the basal third.

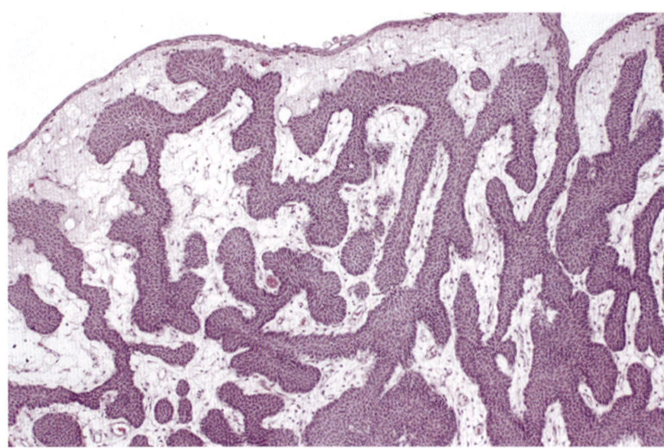

**FIGURE 6–17.** Inverted papilloma. The tumor has the characteristic of papilloma but with an endophytic rather than exophytic growth pattern.

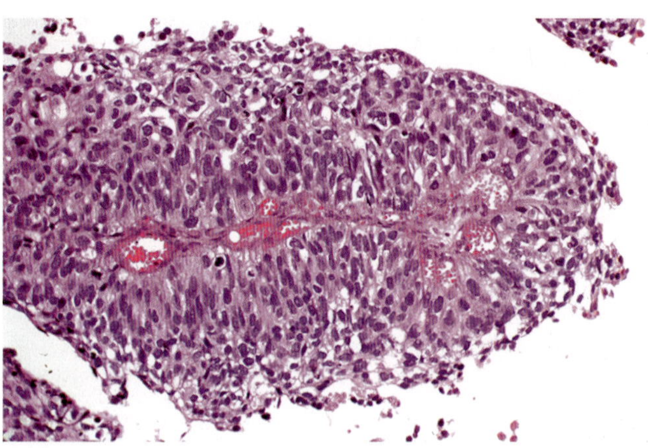

**FIGURE 6–20.** Papillary transitional cell carcinoma grade II. The tumor is distinguishable from grade I by a predominantly disordered architectural pattern, but with retention of some elements of organization, e.g., polarity and nuclear uniformity.

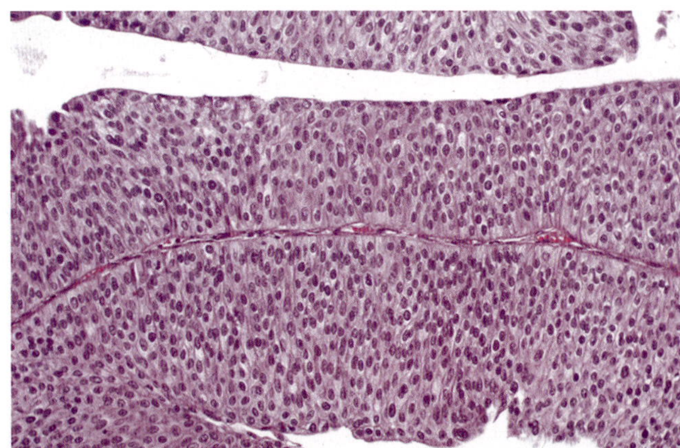

**FIGURE 6–18.** Papillary transitional (urothelial) cell neoplasm of low malignant potential. This tumor resembles the typical papilloma but shows increased cellular proliferation exceeding six layers in thickness.

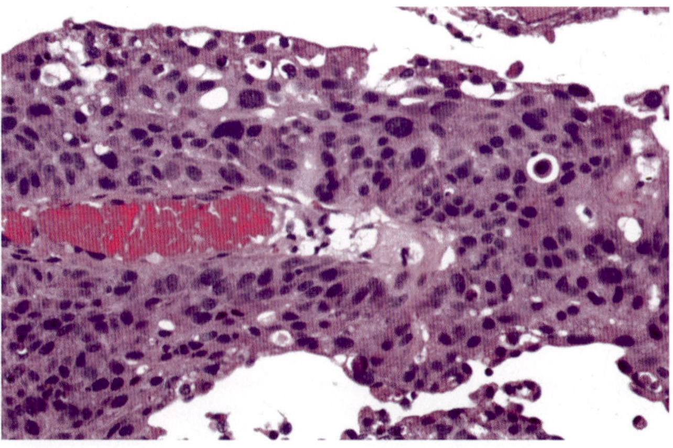

**FIGURE 6–21.** Papillary transitional cell carcinoma grade III. The tumor presents an overall impression of complete disorder or chaos with absence of polarity and, commonly, loss of superficial cells, marked variations of all nuclear parameters and, usually, numerous irregularly distributed mitoses.

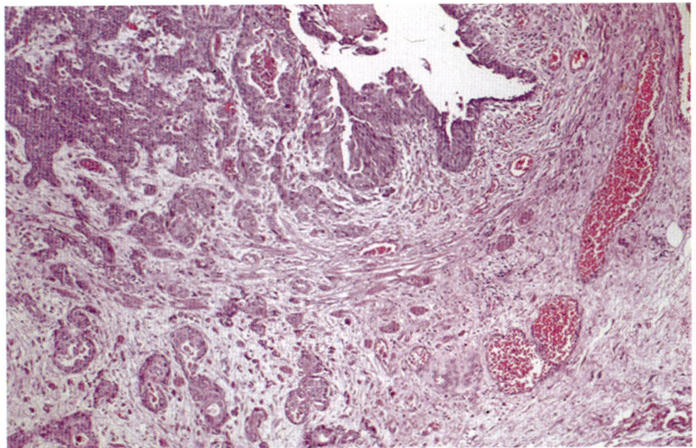

**FIGURE 6–22.** Transitional cell carcinoma infiltrating lamina propria.

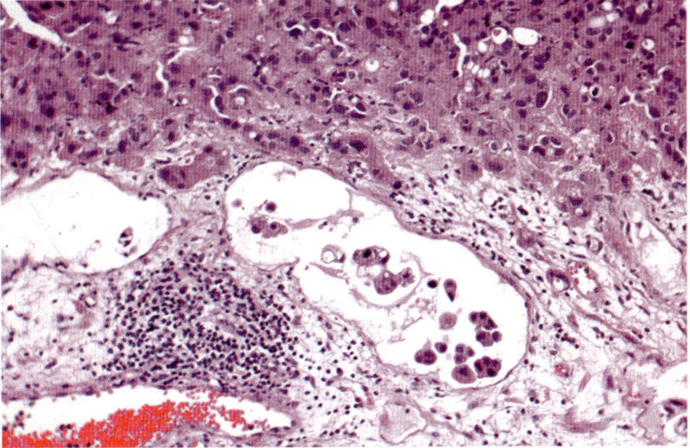

**FIGURE 6–25.** Transitional cell carcinoma with lymphatic invasion.

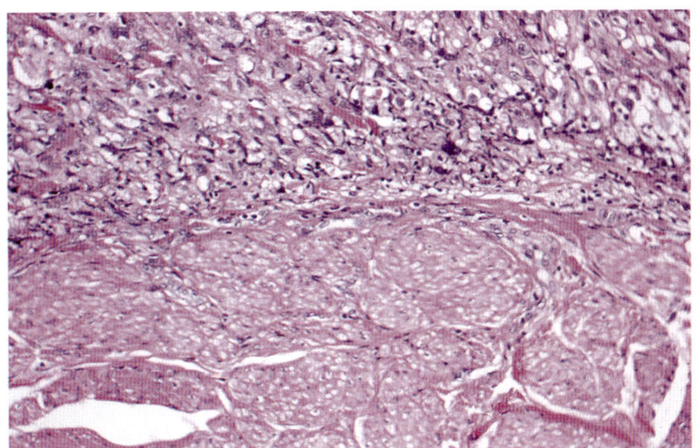

**FIGURE 6–23.** Transitional cell carcinoma infiltrating muscular propria in a broad front manner.

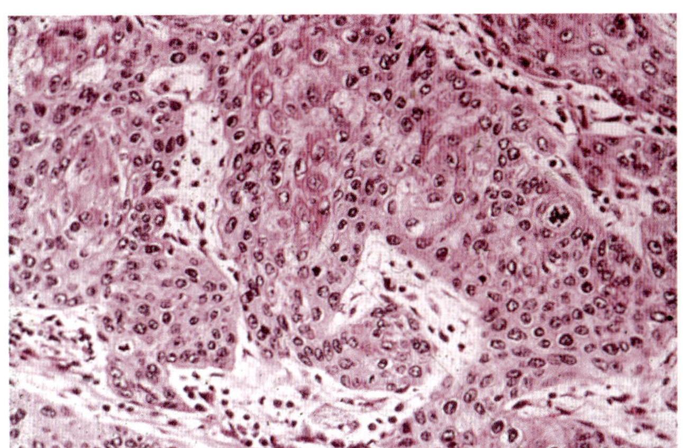

**FIGURE 6–26.** Squamous cell carcinoma. This tumor forms keratin. It is typically sessile and nodular and may be ulcerated.

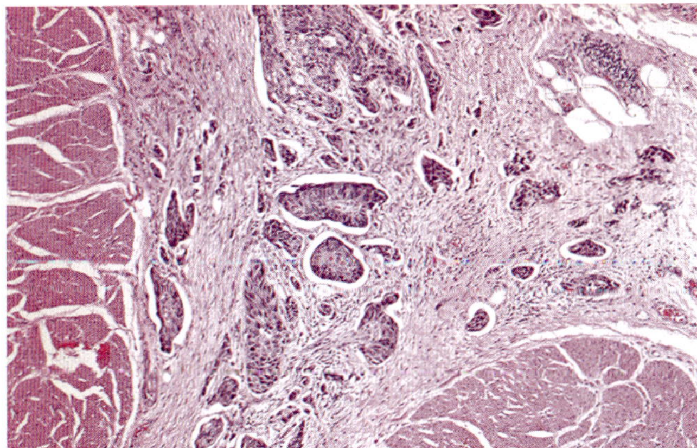

**FIGURE 6–24.** Transitional cell carcinoma infiltrating muscular propria in a tentacular manner.

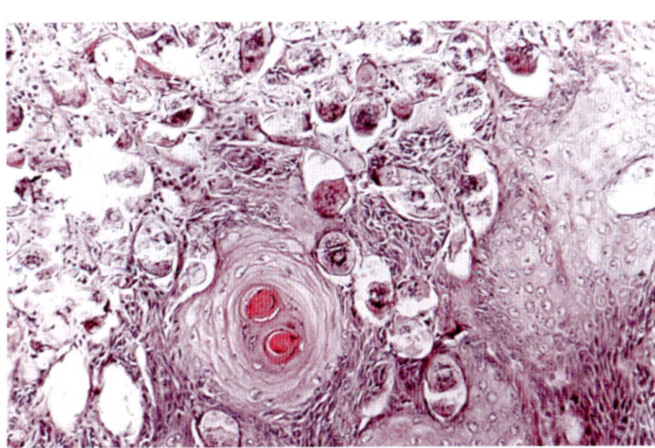

**FIGURE 6–27.** Squamous cell carcinoma with schistosomiasis.

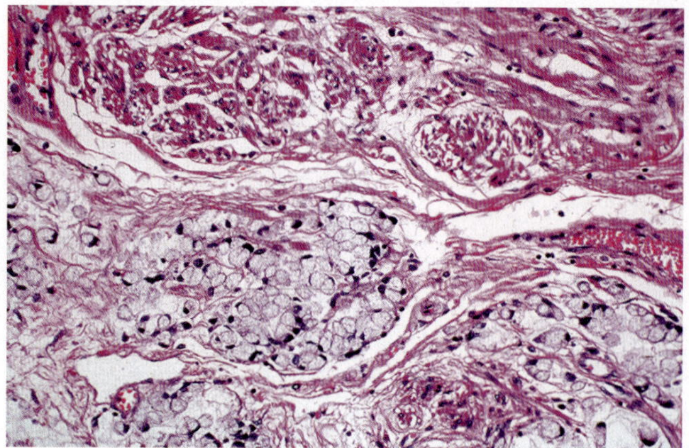

**FIGURE 6–28.** Adenocarcinoma of the bladder. The tumor consists of signet ring cells.

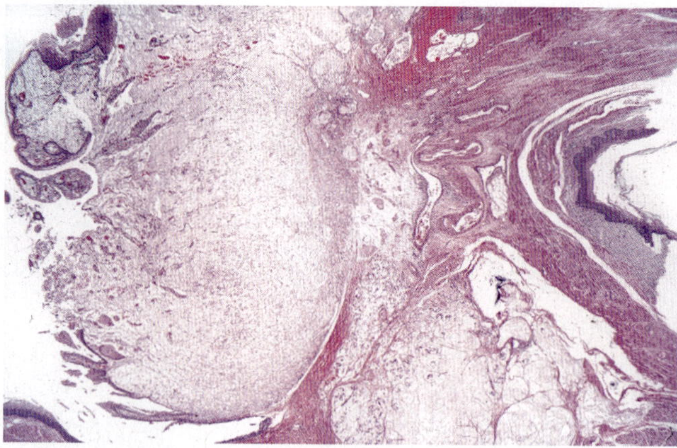

**FIGURE 6–29.** Urachal adenocarcinoma. This tumor is intramural. It is located in the dome or the adjacent anterior wall.

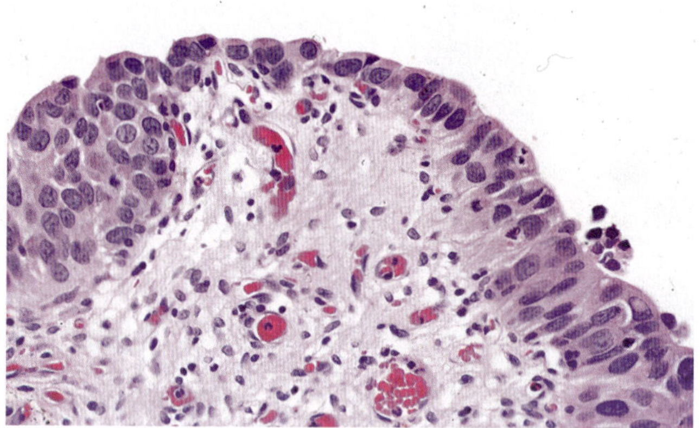

**FIGURE 6–30.** Carcinoma in situ. In this flat lesion the surface epithelium is replaced by malignant cells involving the entire thickness of the epithelial layer. In other words, the malignant cells may be at the base or the surface, and they may be pagetoid or involve Brunn's nests.

# Kidney

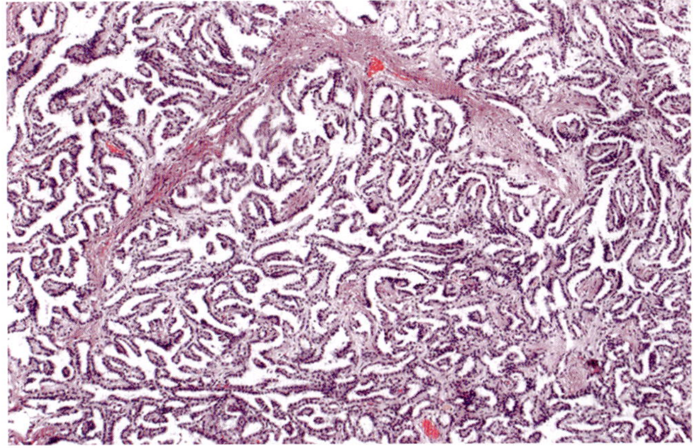

**FIGURE 6–32.** Papillary tubulopapillary adenoma. The tumor is composed of small cells with little cytoplasm with small, uniform, dark-staining nuclei and forming tubulopapillary structure.

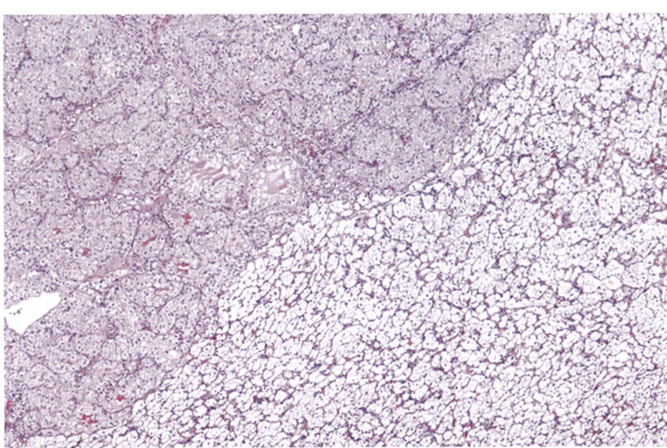

**FIGURE 6–35.** Renal cell carcinoma. Clear cell and granular cell type.

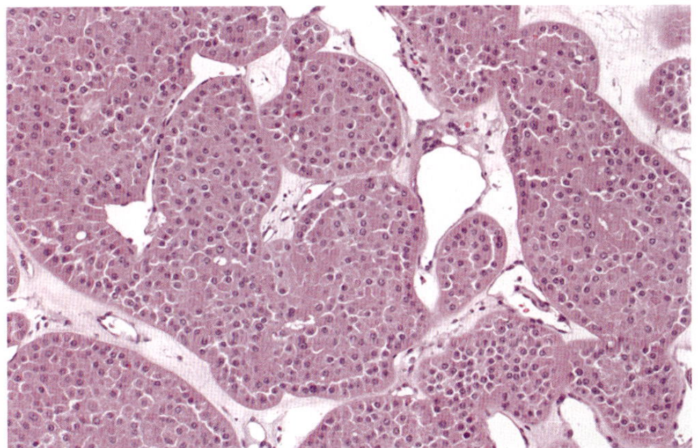

**FIGURE 6–33.** Oncocytoma. The tumor is composed of cells with intensely granular eosinophilic cytoplasm forming solid sheets.

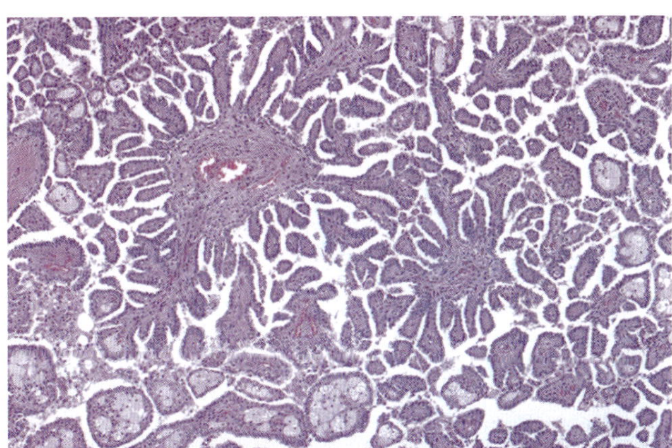

**FIGURE 6–36.** Papillary renal cell carcinoma. The tumor consists of rows of cuboidal or low columnar cells forming papillary structures.

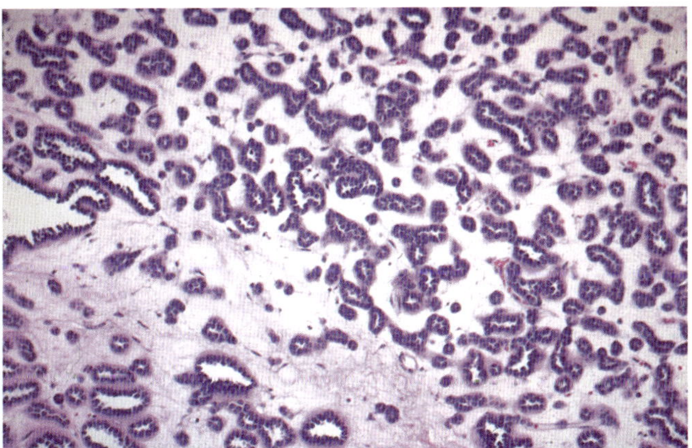

**FIGURE 6–34.** Metanephric adenoma. This tumor is composed of small cells with very little pink cytoplasm forming small tubules in an acellular stroma.

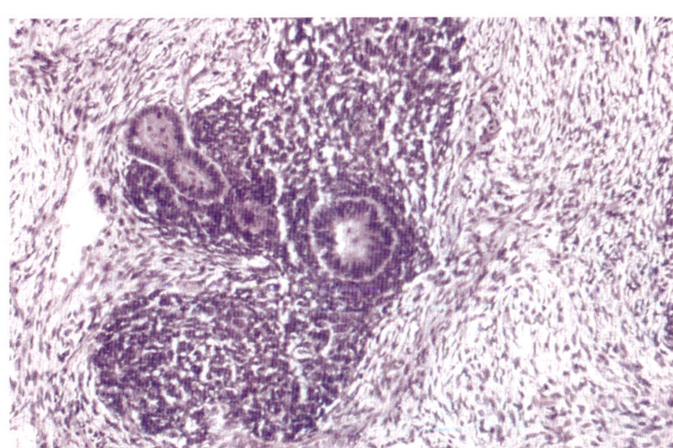

**FIGURE 6–37.** Wilms' tumor (nephroblastoma). The tumor consists of three elements: Blastemal, mesenchymal, and primitive tubular elements.

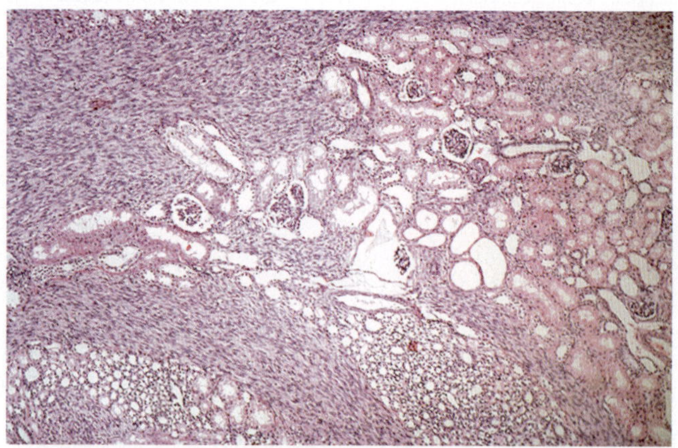

**FIGURE 6–38.** Mesoblastic nephroma. This tumor consists of fascicles of spindle-shaped cells intermingled with groups of nephrons.

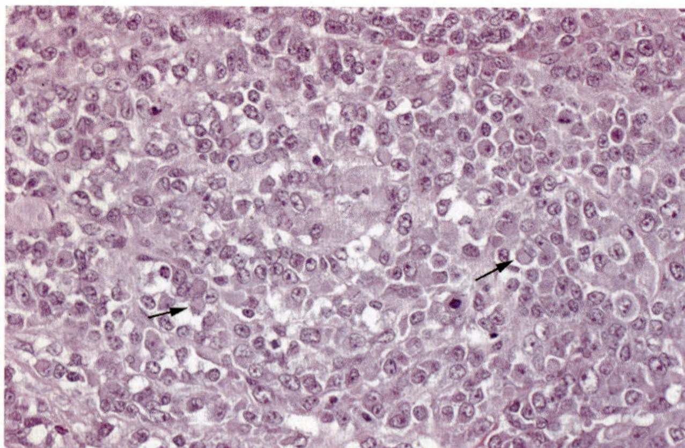

**FIGURE 6–40.** Rhabdoid tumor. The tumor has a monomorphic population of noncohesive cells that have large vesicular nuclei, prominent nucleoli, and scattered cytoplasmic inclusions.

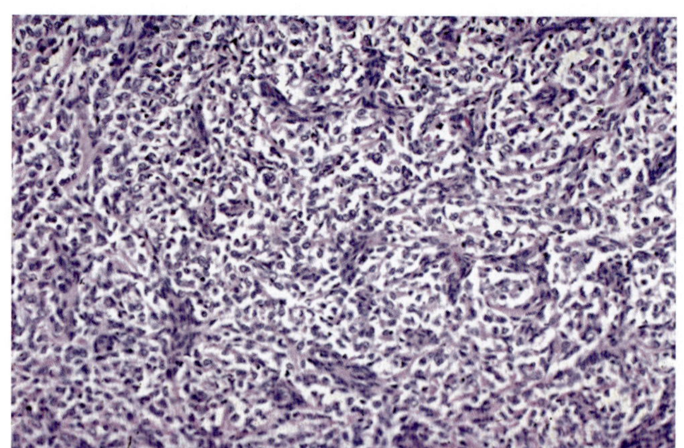

**FIGURE 6–39.** Clear cell sarcoma. The tumor presents cords of undifferentiated cells with vacuolated cytoplasm within a network of vascular channels.

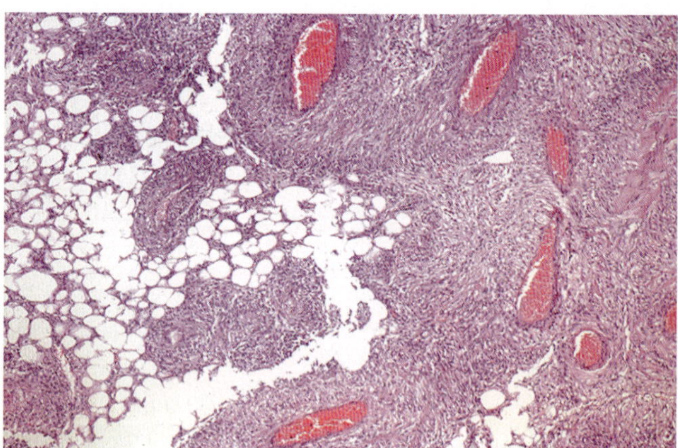

**FIGURE 6–41.** Angiomyolipoma. This tumor is composed of three elements: adipose tissue, thick-walled blood vessels, and smooth muscle cells.

# Testis

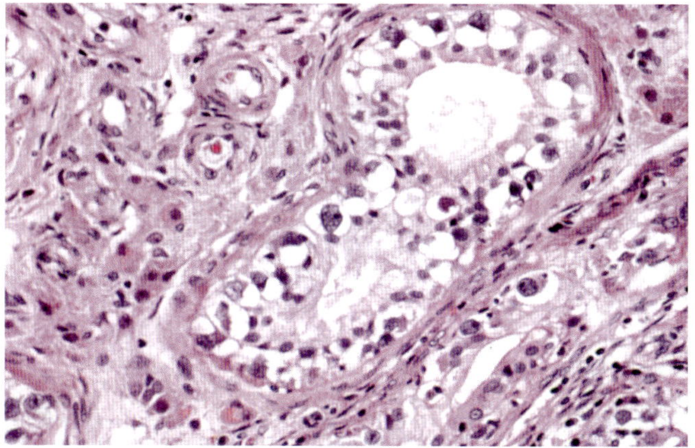

**FIGURE 6–43.** Intratubular malignant germ cells (carcinoma in situ). The germ cells contain abundant vacuolated cytoplasm and large, irregular nuclei located within the seminiferous tubules.

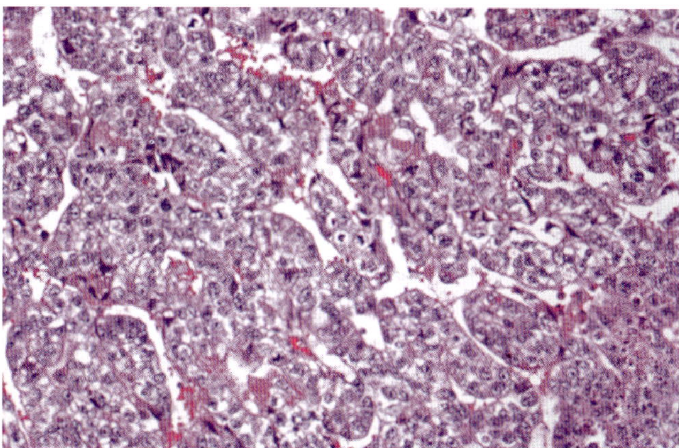

**FIGURE 6–46.** Embryonal carcinoma. Tumor composed of undifferentiated epithelial cells with abundant clear to granular cytoplasm.

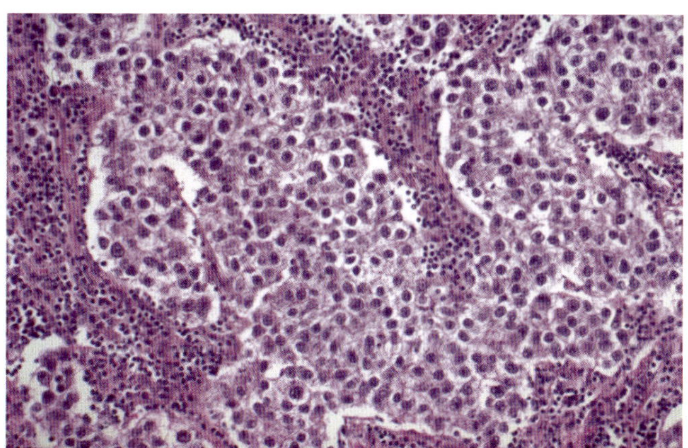

**FIGURE 6–44.** Seminoma. The tumor consists of fairly uniform cells with clear or dense eosinophilic cytoplasm, a large regular nucleus.

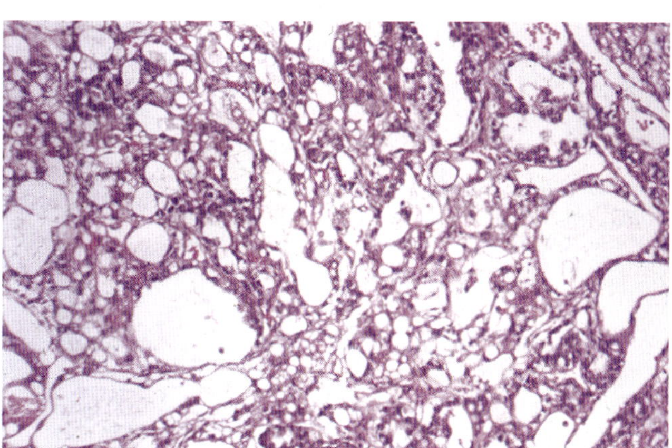

**FIGURE 6–47.** Yolk sac tumor is characterized by a loose vacuolated network of small cells forming anastomosing tubuloacinar structures.

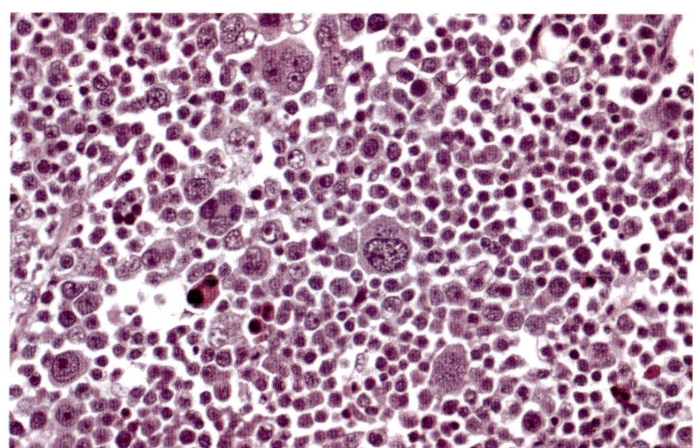

**FIGURE 6–45.** Spermatocytic seminoma. The tumor is composed of germ cells that vary in size from lymphocyte-like to giant cells with the bulk of the tumor composed of cells of intermediate size.

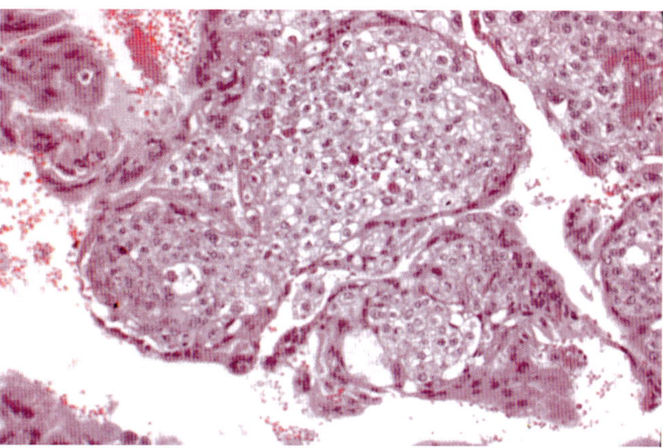

**FIGURE 6–48.** Choriocarcinoma is composed entirely of syncytiotrophoblastic cells and cytotrophoblastic cells.

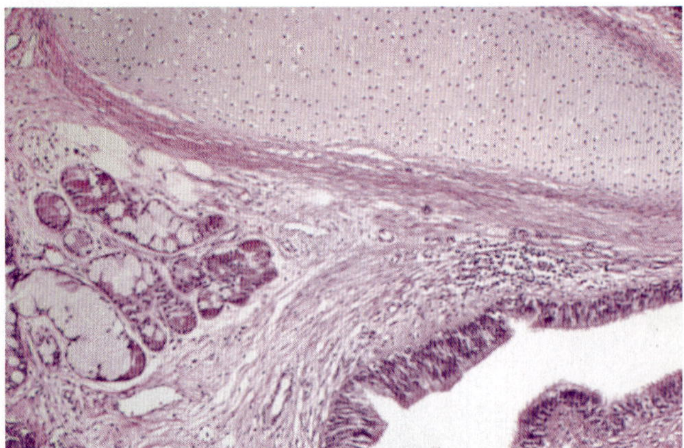

**FIGURE 6–49.** Mature teratoma. This tumor is composed of mucous glands, cartilage, and a tubular structure.

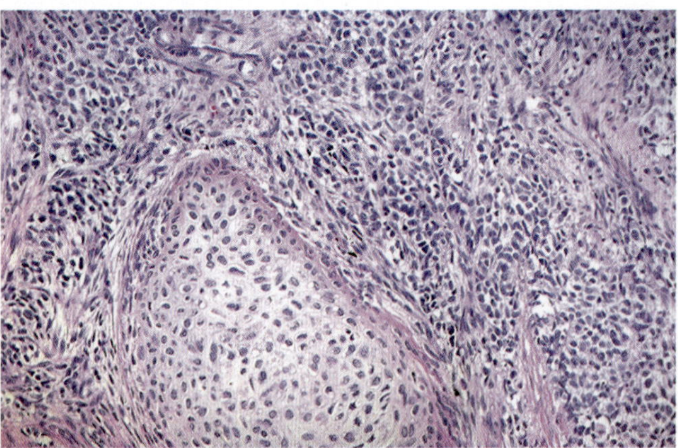

**FIGURE 6–51.** Teratoma with malignant areas. This tumor consists of tubular structures and rhabdomyosarcomatous elements.

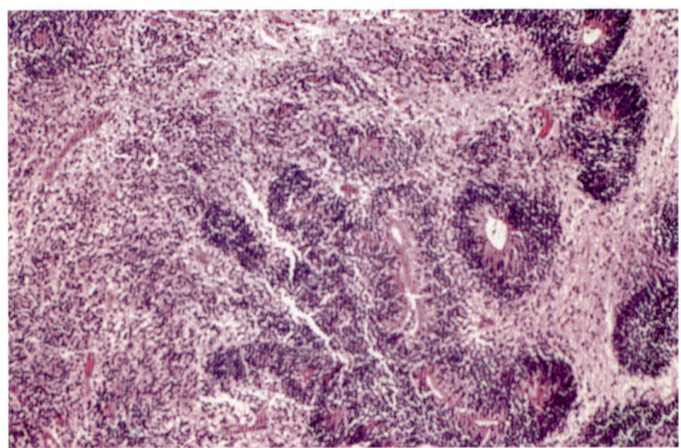

**FIGURE 6–50.** Immature teratoma consists of primitive embryonic neuroepithelial elements.

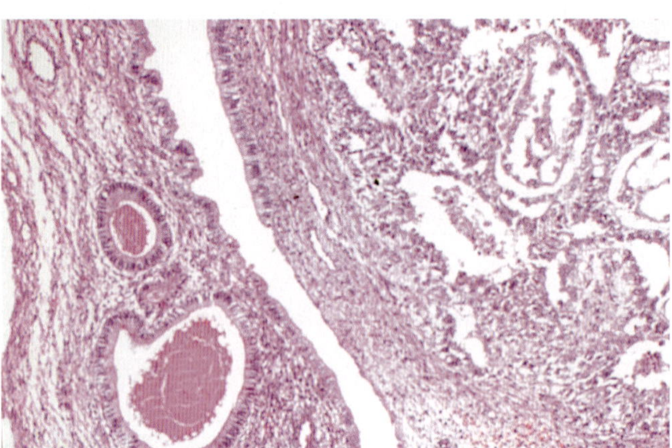

**FIGURE 6–52.** Germ cell tumor of more than one histologic type. Teratoma on the right and embryonal carcinoma on the left.

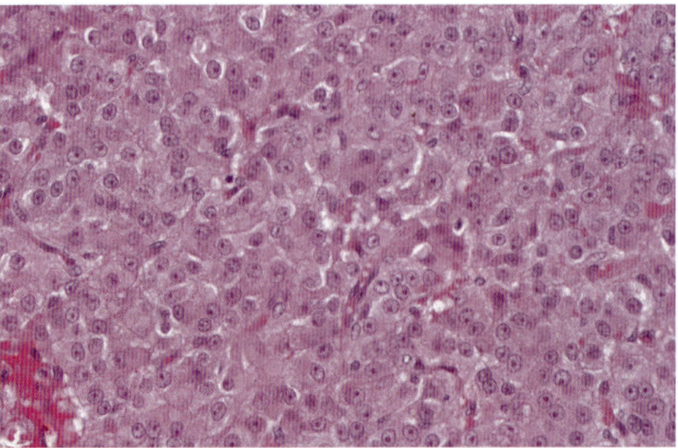

**FIGURE 6–53.** Leydig cell tumor. This tumor consists of uniform cells with eosinophilic cytoplasm and small uniform nuclei.

is forming. We initially coded some oncocytomas as "atypical" before the full spectrum was appreciated. In these, the cells were much larger and often had prominent nucleoli, but they are also benign. Lack of intercellular cohesion is the most helpful feature in distinguishing these tumors from carcinomas with granular cytoplasm. Bizarre clones of cells are common. Tumors may expand into perinephric fat or may herniate into vascular spaces without affecting the prognosis. We have found foci of renal cell carcinoma (RCC) in several cases, but our material is highly selective. For purposes of patient care, a diagnosis of oncocytoma on a needle biopsy can be managed as such, although it can never be entirely devoid of risk.

## Metanephric Adenoma

Pathologically, these sharply circumscribed tumors are sometimes lobulated or bosselated, appearing tan, gray, or yellow. Calcification is very common. The usual microscopic appearance is that of multiple, very small acini, which are formed by very small cells within an acellular stroma (either dense collagen or edematous fluid). It may be papillary or glomeruloid in areas, but all the cells are small. Signs of regression are frequently present, and this is manifested as areas of scarring with calcification or bone. These tumors are benign, but the main concern for the pathologist is to exclude an epithelial Wilms' tumor. In the latter, the tumor cells will be mitotically active and much larger than those of the adenoma. These tumors range from 0.3 to 15.0 cm with a mean size of 5.5 cm. They are seen chiefly in adult females with a mean age of 41 years (range, 5 to 83). Twenty of 50 were found incidentally, 11 had pain, 5 had hematuria, and 5 had a palpable mass. In 6 patients, the tumor was discovered during an evaluation for polycythemia. We designated them as metanephric adenomas to avoid confusion with common cortical adenomas and because they are identical to the epithelial elements of sclerosing nephrogenic nests and to more mature areas of some epithelial Wilms' tumors. They have no malignant potential.

## Renal Cell Carcinomas

### Clear Cell or Granular Cell Types

Grossly, the average RCC is about 7 cm in diameter. There is often bulging of the renal surface, but in the early stages the surface may be smooth or there may actually be a depression or dimple effect from cortical ischemia overlying a deep-seated tumor. The renal capsule is markedly congested with dilated veins. The cut surfaces of the tumor have a variegated appearance, depending on the amount of lipid in the tumor and the extent of hemorrhage and necrosis.

Microscopically, most tumors have a rich vascular supply, and the small vessels compartmentalize the tumor cells into aggregates. Such aggregates may be tubular, trabecular, or alveolar in configuration. When a lumen is formed by the cells, it may be small or large to the point of forming a cyst of variable size. This pattern has been described as an endocrine vascular pattern; in a three-dimensional view one can imagine that most of the cells are in continuity with a vessel. In some cases, a single layer of cells line the vessel wall to produce a papillary pattern. The tumor cells may have clear or eosinophilic cytoplasm. In about half the tumors, it is one or the other; in the rest, both types are present. In higher grade tumors, the quantity of cytoplasm increases, as does the size and variability of the nucleus. In the most anaplastic and spindle cell (sarcomatoid) carcinomas, the characteristic vascularity is lost. The latter is reflected in the gross pathology by a more firm and relatively less colorful neoplasm. These are much more lethal than the clear and granular cell types.

### Chromophobe Cell Type

The chromophobe cell type of RCC consists of two types of cell: large, pale-staining cells with a ballooned appearance (the chromophobe cells) and smaller eosinophilic cells that usually have a perinuclear clear zone. Some tumors may consist largely of one or the other, but most contain both types. The most repetitive pattern shows the pale cells arranged along the vessels. These lesions have distinct cell borders and tight intercellular cohesion. They are positive with Hales colloidal iron stain and with epithelial membrane antigens (EMA) and keratin (A1/A3). We previously classified this type as a variety of granular cell RCC, but it merits segregation from other RCCs because it seems to be less aggressive. Most of these tumors are grade II and, compared to the more common clear cell–granular cell carcinomas, they metastasize less frequently. However, a few have been aggressive. Most have been described on gross examination as beige, tan, or brown, and they often show no necrosis. By light microscopy this lesion differs from oncocytoma chiefly by the presence of tight intercellular cohesion. In uncrowded areas, oncocytomas will show a lack of such cohesion, i.e., the cells may be crowded together but they are not stuck together. Ultrastructurally, the chromophobe tumors have numerous cytoplasmic vesicles.

### Spindle Cell or Sarcomatoid Types

Wide sampling is the best way to distinguish these types from sarcomas because the majority will show focal areas of differentiated RCC. Immunostains for keratins and EMA most often seem to highlight overlooked foci of the latter. A positive vimentin immunostain can be expected, and one should recall that some angiomyolipomas contain little or no fat, so an HMB-45 or the smooth muscle immunostains may be indicated. In addition to the clear cell–granular cell tumors, Bellini duct tumors and less commonly the chromophobic cell lesion may demonstrate spindle cell morphology. Spindling is rarely a feature of papillary RCC.

### Cystic Tumors

These tumors have a multiloculated gross morphology and, microscopically, extensive evidence of regression: hyalinized scar tissue, new or old hemorrhage, calcification, or ossification. Variable amounts of viable tumor will be found—almost always a clear cell lesion—lining some of the cysts or within the scarred septae. This lesion is frequently misdiagnosed as a multilocular cyst (or cystic nephroma). The latter has eosinophilic cells, flattened or hobnail, lining the cysts and a fibroblastic (ovarian-like) stroma. The cystic nephroma is thus a biphasic neoplasm. Some solid RCC will undergo hemorrhage and necrosis with central resorption, leaving a solitary or unilocular cyst. Such cysts are lined with fibrotic or granular tissue, with a band of viable tumor beneath this organized exudate.

### Papillary Tumors

Cytologically these tumors are similar to the common type of RCC, but they are arranged as a single cell layer over papillary fronds. Most are eosinophilic cell lesions, but a few consist of clear cells. Most are of low nuclear grade, but some are not and this likely determines their aggressiveness. Foamy macrophages often distend the papillary fronds. Some of these tumors will have a mixed tubular-papillary morphology, and one frequently sees multiple smaller lesions in the adjacent renal cortex.

## Collecting Duct Carcinoma

Currently a wide variety of apparently different morphologies are being classified as such.[114] The lesion that we have been coding as CDC shows a much more restricted morphology.[130] The tumor cells may be clear or granular, which is similar to RCC except that cell borders are indistinct. Most show moderate to severe nuclear anaplasia. They show a tubular or duct-like structure, usually associated with a papillary element. Unlike RCC, there usually is some stroma between the tubules, and in both the tubules and the papillations, the cells are stratified. The papillary element frequently projects into the renal pelvis. These tumors react with broad-spectrum cytokeratins and peanut lectin, but we do not believe this distinguishes them from RCC. As a group, they are more aggressive than RCC, and a much

larger proportion of them present initially with positive nodes. In most cases, the tumor is located largely in the medulla, but extensive disease may obscure this feature. The collecting ducts and tubules extend to the capsule of the kidney normally, and this distribution seems to explain the few cases that appear to be entirely cortical.

## Renal Medullary Carcinoma

This type of adenocarcinoma of the kidney is seen almost exclusively in patients with sickle cell trait. Because it produces a dominant tumor mass in the renal medulla, we have designated it as renal medullary carcinoma in order to avoid confusion with collecting duct carcinomas, which also occupy chiefly the renal medulla. The histology is such that one can usually anticipate when a search will reveal sickled erythrocytes. The most common microscopic picture is that of a reticular growth pattern (reminiscent of the reticular yolk sac testicular tumor) usually associated with a more compact, adenocystic element. Many will also have poorly differentiated areas composed of cells with a squamous or rhabdoid appearance. Many microscopic fields of tumor are admixed with neutrophils, and the tumors exhibit a desmoplastic stromal reaction that forms a significant bulk of the mass. These features, together with the frequent satellite nodules in the cortex and adjacent pelvic soft tissue, produce a picture unlike that of any other renal neoplasm. Most of the 33 cases we reported had metastasized (chiefly nodes, liver, and lungs) when initially diagnosed, and none were confined to the kidney. The mean survival after nephrectomy was only 13 weeks. Although a diagnosis of sickle cell disorder was not clinically confirmed in all cases, the vast majority had sickle cell trait. They ranged in age from 11 to 39 years with a mean of 22 years. Males predominated by 3:1 under age 25; beyond that the male-female ratio was 1:1. Race was known in 25 of the 33 cases, and they were African-American. A 34th patient was a 31-year-old Caucasian woman without sickling, so the tumor is not entirely specific for sickle cell disorders.

## Nephroblastic Lesions

### Nephroblastoma (Wilms' Tumor)

Grossly, these tumors are pale gray or tan, are not encapsulated, and typically show a lobulated, encephaloid appearance. Varying amounts of hemorrhage, necrosis and cyst formation may be present. The histologic appearance is usually very distinctive, because they recapitulate to a remarkable degree the developing fetal kidney. Thus, the classical triphasic Wilms' tumor will be composed of variable quantities of the small, undifferentiated blastemal cells occurring usually in aggregates, epithelial cells with elongated nuclei arranged in ribbons, tubules, and rosettes. The presence of cellular anaplasia identifies the unfavorable histologic finding: nuclei that are markedly enlarged and dark and multipolar mitoses. The National Wilms' Tumor Study Group has recently redefined focal and diffuse anaplasia.[136]

### Focal Anaplasia

Anaplastic nuclear changes are confined to one or more clearly defined loci within the primary tumor, without evidence of anaplasia or prominent nuclear atypia in extratumoral or extrarenal sites. A tumor with more than one anaplastic focus is acceptable when each is small enough to be contained on a single microscopic section, provided that the other criteria for focal anaplasia are met.

### Diffuse Anaplasia

Anaplastic changes are present but do not meet the revised criteria for focal anaplasia for one or more of the following reasons:

1. Anaplastic changes in the primary tumor are less confined than required by the definition of focal anaplasia.
2. Tumor cells with anaplastic nuclear changes are present in intrarenal or extrarenal vessels, renal sinus, extracapsular invasive sites, or metastatic deposits.
3. Anaplasia is focal, but nuclear atypia approaching the criteria for anaplasia is present elsewhere in the tumor.
4. Anaplasia is present in a biopsy or other incomplete tumor sample.
5. Nondemarcated anaplastic nuclear changes extend to the edge of more than one section.

The report does not document that the involved sections were from the same tumor locus. If multicentric, each tumor should be similarly sampled.

### Mesoblastic Nephroma

The classic type is characterized by interlacing fascicles of spindle cells resembling fibroblasts or myofibroblasts interspersed with scanty collagen. The cells are fairly uniform with little or no pleomorphism. Hemorrhages, necrosis, and cysts are common. The characteristic distinguishing feature is the peculiar growth pattern in which the spindle cell bundles interdigitate with groups of nephrons. The latter often have an embryonic appearance and papillary hyperplasia. The tumor margins are irregular, with radiating bands of spindle cells often extending into the perirenal or hilar region. Nodules of hyaline cartilage are frequent.

The cellular or atypical variant is more common than the classic type described here and differs from it chiefly in the fact that it exhibits increased cellular density and a loss of fascicular morphology. The cellular type usually consists of plump cells with large vesicular nuclei and moderate amounts of cytoplasm. Some nuclear pleomorphism may also be present. The cellular type tends to be more sharply circumscribed than the classic type with little or no interdigitation with parenchymal elements. However, it is not uncommon to see both classic and cellular types within the same tumor. In older infants, the tumors tend to be somewhat more aggressive, but several neonates have also had recurrences. Material in the National Wilms' Tumor Study Pathology Center indicates that the proportion of cellular and classical patterns is similar in the recurrent and nonrecurrent cases.

### Cystic Nephroma

Previously known as the multilocular cyst and then as benign multilocular cystic nephroma, this tumor now is properly termed cystic nephroma. This term is appropriate partly because the word multilocular is often used descriptively for unrelated lesions such as the multicystic (dysplastic) kidney, for cystic RCCs, and for aggregates of simple cysts. This expansile, encapsulated tumor has a fibroblastic stroma and locules that are lined by eosinophilic cells having either a teardrop or flattened appearance. The cellularity of the stroma is such that the tumors are sometimes mistaken for ovarian or müllerian tissue. In infants, these lesions sometimes include foci of Wilms' tumor within the stroma, and this is designated cystic, partially differentiated nephroblastoma. If such foci are large enough to show nodules in the gross specimen, the diagnosis is cystic nephroblastoma. Except for the latter, these tumors have all proved to lack aggressive behavior, but in a few of the adult patients the ovarian-like stroma shows features of sarcoma and metastasizes (to nodes, liver, or lungs usually). The diagnosis is based upon the fact that the stroma shows anaplasia, mitosis, or necrosis and the stromal overgrowth compresses the locules to slit-like spaces and invades into the adjacent renal parenchyma.

### Clear Cell Sarcoma

The classic pattern is the diagnostic lesion, present at least focally in most tumors. The cells are small, with vacuoles in the cytoplasm, and there are no nucleoli. These are the cord cells and they are compartmentalized by narrow vascular channels and their supporting spindle cells (the septal cells). The many variants of this tumor result from spindling of either of the cell types, from cystic degeneration, or from cohesive alterations that produce epithelial-like aggregates of cells.

### Rhabdoid Tumor

In this tumor the individual cells are noncohesive, with large vesicular nuclei and prominent nucleoli. Some cells have pale-staining cytoplasmic inclusions, but these are often few and require some searching. This lesion also has its variants. Stromal changes may assume an osteoid or chondroid-like appearance, and it (the stroma) may induce cell aggregations that impart an epithelial-like structure.

### Angiomyolipoma

These tumors are multifocal and bilateral in patients who have tuberous sclerosis. In this group, the sexes are about equally affected, and the renal tumors, often associated with bilateral renal cysts, generally make their presence known in the first two to three decades of life. However, most of the AMLs that come to the attention of the surgeon are in older patients with no evidence of tuberous sclerosis. Age ranges from 20 to 70 years, the female-male ratio is nearly 4:1, and the tumors are usually solitary and unilateral. Symptoms may be related to mass but frequently are due to rapid or slow bleeding into the tumor and adjacent tissue. Grossly, these tumors vary from minute to large in size, filling much of one side of the abdomen. Average size is around 9 cm. When discovered, they frequently have already extended into the perinephric tissue. Large blood clots with a renal tumor suggest this diagnosis. The color varies from yellow to gray, corresponding to the fat and muscle elements, respectively. There is no tumor capsule. Microscopically, the tumor is composed of vessels, smooth muscle, and fat in varying proportions. Muscle or fat may predominate. The vessels are tortuous and usually occur in aggregates. The muscle occurs in sheets or as collars around the vessels. Nuclear pleomorphism is usually present, and mitoses are usually absent. HMB-45 immunostains are invariably positive.

## TESTICULAR TUMORS

## Staging

TNM classification of testicular tumors has recently been revised (Fig. 6–54).

Primary tumor is represented as pT.

pTX    Primary tumor cannot be assessed (if no radical orchiectomy has been performed, TX is used)

pT0    No evidence of primary tumor (e.g., histologic scar in testis)

pTis    Intratubular germ cell neoplasia (carcinoma in situ)

pT1    Tumor limited to testis and epididymis without vascular/lymphatic invasion; tumor may invade tunica albuginea but not tunica vaginalis

pT2    Tumor limited to testis and epididymis with vascular/lymphatic invasion; tumor may extend through tunica albuginea with involvement of tunica vaginalis

pT3    Tumor invades spermatic cord with or without vascular/lymphatic invasion

pT4    Tumor invades scrotum with or without vascular/lymphatic invasion

Regional lymph nodes are designated as pN.

pNX    Regional lymph nodes cannot be assessed

pN0    No regional lymph node metastasis

pN1    Metastasis with a lymph node mass 2 cm or less in greatest dimension and five or fewer positive nodes, none more than 2 cm in greatest dimension

pN2    Metastasis with a lymph node mass more than 2 cm but not more than 5 cm in greatest dimension; or more than five nodes positive, none more than 5 cm; or evidence of extranodal extension of tumor

pN3    Metastasis with a lymph node mass more than 5 cm in greatest dimension

## Tumors of Germ Cell Origin

Testicular germ cell tumors begin as intratubular malignant germ cells and progress into one or more of the basic histologic types. Germ cell tumors constitute 94% of testicular tumors. They are divided into tumors of a single histologic type (38%) and those of more than one histologic type (62%).

### Tumors of One Histologic Type

1. *Seminoma.* About 60% of these tumors occur in men (typically age 30 to 50), mostly in pure form; none are found in infants. In seminoma, placental alkaline phosphatase may be elevated and demonstrated in the cells, but in pure seminoma (i.e., when the tumor consists entirely of seminoma), alpha-fetoprotein (AFP) is negative.

Seminomas consist of fairly uniform cells typically with clear cytoplasm and well-defined cell borders resembling primitive germ cells. The cytoplasm has much glycogen. The nucleus is large and vesicular with one or two nucleoli.

The tumor cells occur in lobules supported by fibrovascular stroma, in which almost invariably some lymphoid infiltration and granulomatous reaction are

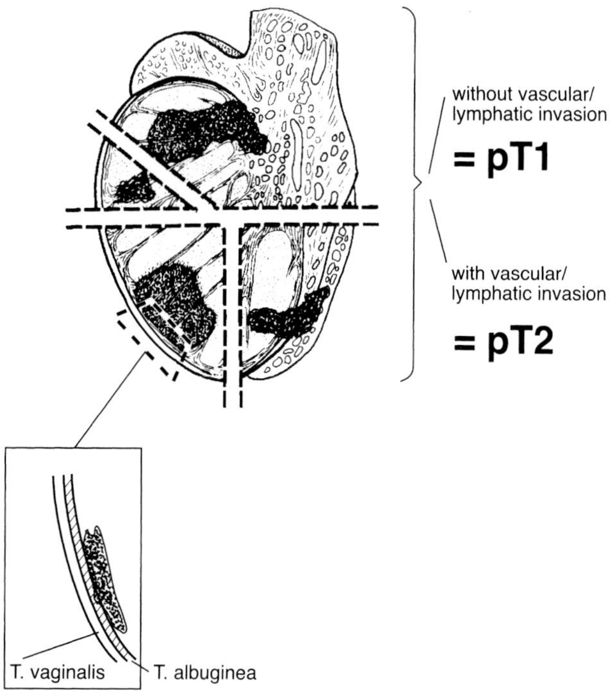



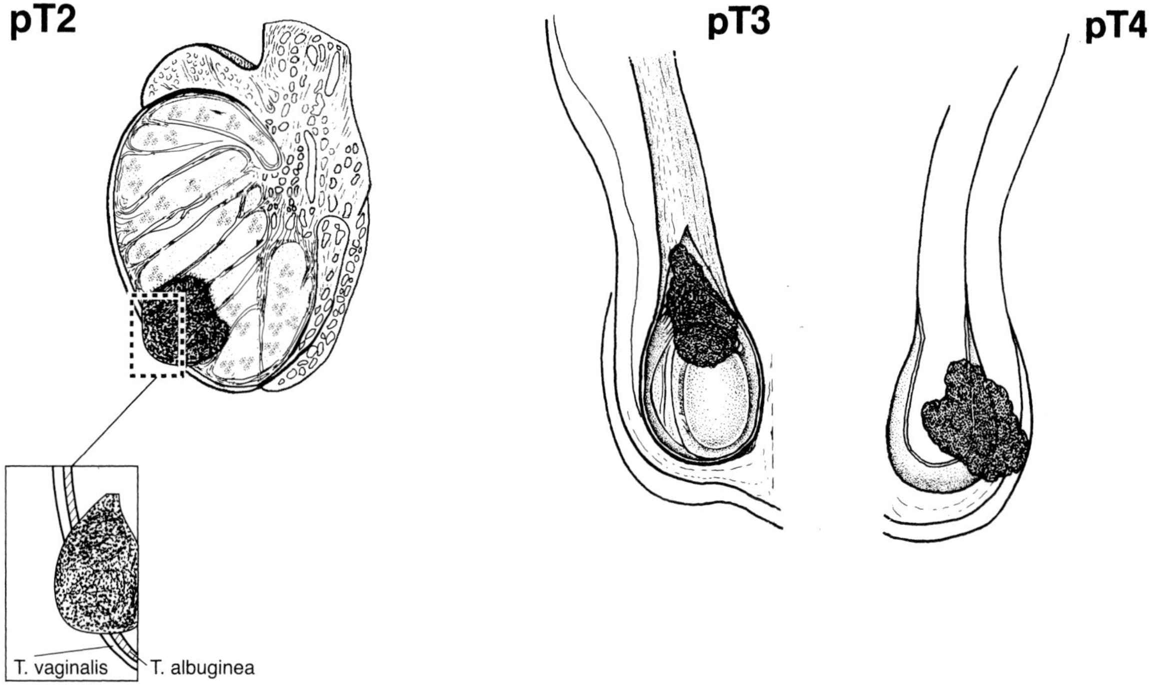



**Figure 6–54**

seen, indicating immunologic response. The tumor is very radiosensitive.

2. *Spermatocytic seminoma.* Usually seen in older men, this type accounts for 2% to 4% of germ cell tumors. The tumor seems to recapitulate spermatogenesis. Three cell types are seen—large cells, intermediate cells, and very small cells—resembling spermatids with no lymphocytic or granulomatous reaction. The nuclei have filamentous chromatin distribution. A rare spermatocytic seminoma is associated with an undifferentiated sarcoma, which may metastasize.

3. *Embryonal carcinoma* (ECa). In pure form, this tumor constitutes only 3% of germ cell tumors, but it is present in 47% of all testicular tumors. It is not seen in infants or children. The tumor consists of primitive epithelial cells forming carcinoma that is usually glan-

dular but may be papillary, tubular, or solid. There is much confusion about AFP and embryonal carcinoma. Our group could demonstrate AFP in only 13% of ECa cells. The reported elevation of AFP in ECa is almost invariably due to yolk sac tumor elements that are often present in these tumors, but overlooked. We have not found hCG in any ECa cells.

4. *Yolk sac tumor* (endodermal sinus tumor, infantile embryonal carcinoma). This tumor accounts for 60% of testis tumors in children. In its pure form the incidence in adults is 2.4%, but it is present in 41% of all germ cell tumors. The tumor consists of anastomosing tubuloacinar structures lined with epithelium that varies from thin to highly cuboidal. Some may have papillary structures—Schiller-Duval bodies. AFP is almost invariably elevated and demonstrable in the cells, but rarely, AFP may be negative in serum and in the tumor cells.

5. *Choriocarcinoma.* This rare (18 in 6000) primary tumor is usually asymptomatic and may be missed. The metastases usually cause symptoms. Levels of hCG are very high, and AFP is negative. The tumor consists of two cell types: syncytiotrophoblasts and cytotrophoblasts.

6. *Teratoma.* In infants and children, teratoma constitutes about 40% of testicular tumors. In adults, in its pure form the incidence is 3%, but it is present in 47% of all germ cell tumors. Teratoma is a complex tumor showing disorderly arrangement of fetal and adult tissues and structures representing three germ layers: endoderm, mesoderm, and ectoderm. We subclassify teratomas into mature teratoma, immature teratoma, and teratoma with malignant areas (sarcoma, adenocarcinoma, squamous cell carcinoma). AFP can be demonstrated in mucous glands of mature and immature teratomas. Although in infants testicular teratomas seem to be benign, in adults they can invade vascular spaces and metastasize. It should be emphasized that irrespective of the benign histologic appearance, every element in a teratoma—mature or immature—as well as the sarcomas that may be found, can metastasize. Identification of the unusual elements, i.e., sarcomas of various types, is very important because they may (and often do) metastasize. They do not respond to the standard treatment for nonseminomatous germ cell tumors. It should be noted that the WHO classification of teratoma is not the same as the British classification of teratoma, which includes all nonseminiferous tumors. Dermoid cyst is the most common teratoma in the ovary but is rare in the testes. It consists of a cyst lined with keratinizing, stratified, squamous epithelium and skin appendages (hair, sebaceous glands, teeth, and the like). There may be some other tissues also, but the main tumor is the cyst. Epidermal (epidermoid) cyst is also lined with keratinizing, stratified, squamous epithelium; there are no skin appendages.

Either one may rupture, with resultant foreign body granulomatous reaction.

7. *Polyembryoma* refers to very rare tumors that have some peculiar structures—embryoid bodies that resemble 15-day-old embryos. Embryoid bodies are not infrequent in association with ECa.

## Tumors of More Than One Histologic Type

From the practical point of view, seminoma, embryonal carcinoma, yolk sac tumor, teratoma, and choriocarcinoma are the main tumors that are seen in general practice. Next in frequency are seminoma and syncytiotrophoblasts. In a recent study of over 1000 testicular tumors evaluated by the WHO classification, we found that only 38% had a single cell type, and 62% had more than one histologic type. The frequency of the types was as follows:

| | |
|---|---|
| Pure seminoma (S) | 26.9% |
| Spermatocytic seminoma (SS) | 2.4% |
| Embryonal carcinoma (ECa) | 3.1% |
| Yolk sac tumor (YST) | 2.4% |
| Teratoma (T) | 2.7% |
| Choriocarcinoma | 0.004% |
| Syncytiotrophoblast (SCT) | 42% |
| Intratubular malignant germ cells (ITMGC) | 0.6% |
| ECa + YST + T + SCT | 14.3% |
| Seminoma + SCT | 8.1% |
| ECa + YST + T + S + SCT | 7.4% |
| ECa + YST + teratoma | 4.7% |
| YST + teratoma | 2.5% |
| ECA + T | 1.4% |
| Other combinations | 24.0% |

We found that yolk sac tumor elements were present in 41% of tumors, embryonal carcinoma in 47%, teratoma in 47%, and syncytiotrophoblasts in 42%. As far as markers are concerned, AFP was demonstrable in 92% of yolk sac tumors, 19% of teratomas (in mucous glands), and 13% of embryonal carcinomas; all but 2 of 24 pure ECas were negative for AFP; chorionic gonadotropin was demonstrable in 94% of syncytiotrophoblasts; and in testicular tumors, hCG was demonstrable only in syncytiotrophoblasts and in no other cells. This finding suggests that two markers (AFP and hCG) can reliably monitor yolk sac tumors and choriocarcinoma, respectively. However, no reliable markers are present for seminoma, spermatocytic seminoma, or ECa.

Mature and immature teratomas can actually invade vascular channels and metastasize; in over 95% of cases, the histology of metastases is identical to that of the primary tumor.

Syncytiotrophoblasts frequently are seen in association with seminoma. This group has caused much confusion in that reports in the literature have found pure seminoma with elevated hCG levels. All such seminomas that we have seen have had syncytiotrophoblasts, which were the only cells that reacted positively with hCG stain. The same applies to ECa with elevated hCG. In seminomas with elevated AFP, yolk sac tumor elements may explain the source of AFP. The source of hCG in testicular tumors is syncytiotrophoblasts. The main source of AFP is yolk sac tumor.

In infants and children, yolk sac tumor is the most common germ cell tumor of testes, followed by teratoma.

## Prognostic Factors

Testicular tumors spread through the lymphatics and blood vessels. Deaths in testicular tumors are entirely secondary to metastases. The mortality rate from testicular tumors has dropped dramatically because of chemotherapy. In a number of patients with metastatic tumors, it has been found that metastasis failed to respond to chemotherapy or radiation therapy. Some of these metastases consist of cystic teratoma and others of nongerminal malignant tumors (e.g., rhabdomyosarcoma, Wilms' tumor, undifferentiated sarcoma). It has been postulated that chemotherapy or radiation therapy converts embryonal carcinoma to teratoma or sarcoma. We have reported the same phenomena in untreated patients, i.e., mature teratoma, sometimes in pure form, and nongerminal tumors in the metastases before the patient had received any treatment. Because we have demonstrated these elements in vascular spaces in the testes and have seen them in the metastases before any treatment was given, we hypothesize that chemotherapy and radiation destroyed the seminoma, embryonal carcinoma, choriocarcinoma, and yolk sac elements in the metastases, permitting the resistant teratoma and nongerminal tumors to propagate. The significance of these observations is that germ cell tumors of testes should be examined thoroughly and these elements looked for and reported. To understand the pathology of germ cell tumors of the testes, it is important to remember the potentialities of germ cells. Normally, the fertilized germ cell divides into a number of cell lines to produce germ cells and embryonic (somatic) or extraembryonic elements, eventually producing the placenta on the one hand and the embryo on the other. Germ cell tumors recapitulate the same potentialities.

## Intratubular Malignant Germ Cells: Carcinoma in Situ

Examination of nontumorous portions of a tumor-bearing testis often shows large cells with hyperchromatic irregularly shaped nuclei surrounded by clear cytoplasm. Such cells may be seen in association with any tumor cell type. Less frequently in patients with seminoma, ECa, or yolk sac tumor, cells resembling the main tumor may be found in the surrounding seminiferous tubules.

Skakkebaek has written extensively about the undifferentiated cells, which he has designated as carcinoma in situ.[168] He has reported them in 1% of biopsies of infertile men, 5% of contralateral testes of patients with testicular tumors, and in a number of patients with undescended testes. Of note, Bunge and Bradbury were the first to report these cells in an infertile man who developed seminoma 3 years later.[149] They called them early seminoma cells.

## Extratesticular Germ Cell Tumors

Occasionally, a tumor in the retroperitoneum or mediastinum on biopsy turns out to be a germ cell tumor. In a number of such cases, examination of the testis shows a scar with or without a small area of seminoma or teratoma at the edge. The adjacent seminiferous tubules many times will show malignant intratubular germ cells. Such areas likely represent burned-out testicular tumor.

## Tumors of Specialized Gonadal Stroma

### Differentiated Forms

#### Leydig Cell Tumors

Leydig cell tumors constitute about 3% of testicular tumors. They are associated with the following characteristics:

- They occur at any age, but more often in older patients.
- All children show macrogenitosomia.
- About 40% of adults with these tumors have gynecomastia.
- Tumors produce androgens, estrogens, progesterone, and corticosteroids.

The most common appearance is that of medium-sized cells with distinct cell borders, eosinophilic cytoplasm, and a round or oval vesicular and rarely grooved nucleus frequently containing a prominent nucleolus.

Reinke crystal is helpful in the identification of Leydig cell tumors but is detectable in only about 40% of cases. Lipofuscin pigment is often present. The cells occur in sheets, columns, cords, and trabeculae. One of the distinguishing features of Leydig cell tumors is the delicate endocrine type of vascularity, best observed when the tumor occurs in sheets.

About 10% of Leydig cell tumors are malignant. The criteria for the diagnosis of malignancy are anaplasia of the cells, individual cell necrosis, larger areas of tumor necrosis, extension to the tunica or epididymis, increased mitotic activity, and vascular invasion.

However, rarely the tumor shows none of these features but does metastasize. In such cases, the metastases are usually delayed 5 or more years.

Leydig cell tumors have to be distinguished from nodular aggregates of Leydig cells found in the testes of persons with atrophy, cryptorchidism, the Klinefelter syndrome, and Klinefelter-like syndrome. In such cases, the testes are small and the seminiferous tubules are small and often sclerotic. Hyperplasia differs from neoplasia in that the tubules are entrapped in the former but not in the latter, although a few entrapped tubules may be seen in the periphery of a tumor.

Leydig cell tumors and hyperplasia can be distinguished from similar changes in the androgen insensitivity and the adrenogenital syndromes by the absence of clinical symptoms or laboratory evidence of those syndromes.

### Sertoli Cell Tumors

Sertoli cell tumors constitute about 3% of testicular tumors; they occur in all ages but mostly in infants and children. In adults, 40% show gynecomastia. In a few instances, estrogen and pregnanediol levels are elevated. They are usually benign, but 10% are malignant.

The tumor cells range in shape from oval to columnar. They have a small or medium-sized, round or oval vesicular nucleus containing a fine chromatin network and a solitary, small basophilic nucleolus. The cytoplasm may be scanty or abundant, with a single large or multiple small lipid vacuoles. The cells form tubules with a more or less distinct lumen, which may contain basement membrane–like material, or the tubules appear solid as in the prepubertal testis. The tumor may occur in sheets with only occasional tubule formation. The stroma can be scanty or composed of abundant, sometimes hyalinized, fibrous tissue.

Sertoli cell tumors must be distinguished from the small nodules of coiled tubules lined by immature Sertoli cells found in over 20% of cryptorchid testes and occasionally in descended testes. Such nodules are sometimes mislabeled Sertoli cell or tubular adenoma, but represent residual nodules of immature tubules. Occasionally, scattered spermatogonia are found within the tubules of the Sertoli cell nodules.

### *Variant*

In large cell calcifying Sertoli cell tumor the cells are large with cuboidal, hexagonal, columnar, or spindle shapes. The cytoplasm is abundant, finely granular, and eosinophilic, but may be amphophilic and slightly vacuolated and contain abundant lipid in fine droplets or large vacuoles. The nuclei are round, oval, or elongated with one or two small nucleoli. Mitoses are generally absent or rare. The neoplastic cells often form tubules or cords, clusters, trabeculae, or solid sheets. The stroma may be loose, myxoid, or densely collagenous with varying degrees of calcification. Calcification appears as large, wavy, laminated nodules or massive deposits; sometimes it is sparse. In the absence of prominent tubule formation and minimal calcification, the tumor may simulate a Leydig cell tumor, especially in a child with precocious puberty.

The large cell calcifying Sertoli cell tumor is most common in children and is often associated with hyperplasia and neoplasia of other endocrine organs, including testicular Leydig cell tumors, bilateral primary adrenocortical hyperplasia and pituitary adenomas, spotty mucocutaneous pigmentation, and cardiac myxomas. Clinical associations have included sexual precocity, acromegaly, pituitary gigantism, hypercortisolemia, Peutz-Jeghers syndrome, and sudden death.

### Granulosa Cell Tumors

Two types are recognized: adult and juvenile. Both display the same histologic patterns as their ovarian counterparts.

**Adult Type Granulosa Cell Tumor.** The nuclei are vesicular and grooved, but they may be large, round, and hyperchromatic. The cells are small, round, or hexagonal; the cytoplasm is generally scant. The tumor may have a diffuse or microfollicular pattern with Call-Exner bodies. About half of the patients have gynecomastia.

**Juvenile Type Granulosa Cell Tumor.** The cells are polyhedral or round and contain abundant pale to eosinophilic cytoplasm. The nuclei are round or oval and hyperchromatic with occasional nucleoli. There may be many mitoses. Histologically, the tumor is usually cystic but may be follicular or have solid areas. The follicles are usually large and round. The tumor is almost always encountered before the age of 2 years. It is the most common testicular tumor of the newborn. A few have been reported in cryptorchid testes with intersex disorders.

### *Mixtures*

1. Leydig cell and Sertoli cell tumors
2. Others (granulosa, theca cell tumors of testes)

To explain the range of histology of these tumors, many years ago one of us (F.K.M.) postulated that these tumors had a common origin—the specialized stroma of the primitive gonad—which in the male normally develops into Leydig and Sertoli cells and in the female develops into theca-granulosa cells. Either cell may occur in either organ. The tumors recapitulate the same potentialities.

## Tumors with Germ Cell and Gonadal Stromal Elements

Gonadoblastoma is composed of two principal cell types: large germ cells similar to those of seminoma and small cells resembling immature Sertoli and granulosa cells; elements resembling Leydig and lutein cells may also be present.

The two cells (germ cell and sex cord/gonadal stromal elements) are usually in irregular or rounded discrete nests presenting one or more of three patterns. Most often the sex cord cells surround rounded hyaline nodules of basement membrane substance, which merges with the surrounding basement membrane. The second pattern consists of nests composed of large germ cells surrounded by many smaller Sertoli cells. In the third growth pattern, the Sertoli cells form a ring of single cells at the periphery of a central nest of germ cells. Focal calcification may begin in hyaline bodies, sometimes forming large, wavy, laminated masses separated by dense fibrous tissue. Large polyhedral cells resembling Leydig cells but without Reinke crystals may be present after puberty. Sometimes the germ cells of a gonadoblastoma transgress the margins of the nests and grow as a seminoma or embryonal carcinoma with only small foci of gonadoblastoma within them or at their margins. The type of germ cell tumor should be specified.

Gonadoblastomas arise almost exclusively in patients with rudimentary or streak gonads, most of whom are phenotypic females and almost all of whom are X chromatin negative and have a Y chromosome.

Rarely, the tumor may occur in testes of normal males.

## Metastatic Tumors of the Testicle

These tumors are most often seen in older patients, but are rarely of clinical importance. The primary site is typically the prostate, lung, pancreas, or gastrointestinal tract.

## Lymphomas

Lymphomas may occur at any age, but most frequently are seen in older patients. In 25%, the opposite testis is involved. The tumor cells infiltrate the stroma heavily.

# REFERENCES

## Tumors of the Prostate


1. Abrahamsson PA, Wadstrom LB, Alumets J: Peptide-hormone and serotonin-immunoreactive tumour cells in carcinoma of the prostate. Pathol Res Pract 182:298–307, 1987.
2. Allsbrook WC, Simms WW: Histochemistry of the prostate. Human Pathol 23:297–305, 1992.
3. Armas OA, Aprikinn AG, Melamed J: Clinical and pathobiological effects of neoadjuvant total androgen ablation therapy on clinically localized prostatic adenocarcinoma. Am J Surg Pathol 18:979–991, 1994.
4. Azzopardi JG, Evans DJ: Argentaffin cells in prostate carcinoma: Differentiation from lipofuscin and melanin in prostatic epithelium. J Pathol 4:247–251, 1971.
5. Bostwick DG: High grade prostatic intraepithelial neoplasia (PIN): The most likely precursor of prostate cancer. Cancer 75:1823–1836, 1995.
6. Bostwick DG, Srigley J, Grignon D: Atypical adenomatous hyperplasia of prostate. Human Pathol 24:819–832, 1993.
7. Brawn PN: Histologic grading study of prostatic adenocarcinoma: Development of a new system and comparison with other methods. Cancer 49:525–532, 1982.
8. Byar DP, Mostofi FK (VA Cooperative Urological Research Group): Carcinoma of the prostate: Prognostic evaluation of certain pathologic features in 208 radical prostatectomies. Cancer 30:5–13, 1972.
9. Choe BK: Immunological approaches to human prostatic epithelial cells. Prostate 1:383–398, 1980.
10. Christensson A, Lilja H: Complex formation between protein C inhibitor and prostate-specific antigen in vitro and in human semen. Eur J Biochem 220:45–53, 1994.
11. Cohen RS, Glezerson G, Haffe JEE: Neuroendocrine cells: A new prognostic parameter in prostatic cancer. Br J Urol 68:258–262, 1991.
12. Correa RJ Jr: Latent carcinoma of the prostate. Why the controversy? J Urol 111:644–646, 1974.
13. Daniels GF Jr, McNeal JE, Stamey TA: Predictive value of contralateral biopsies in unilaterally palpable prostate cancer. J Urol 147:870–874, 1992.
14. DeBruyne FMJ, Collins VP, van Dekken H, et al: Cytogenetics of prostate cancer. Scand J Urol Nephrol Suppl 162:65–71, 1994.
15. Dhom G: Classification and grading of prostatic carcinoma: Recent results. Cancer Res 60:14–26, 1977.
16. di Sant'Agnese PA: Neuroendocrine differentiation in prostatic carcinoma. Cancer 75:1850–1859, 1995.
17. Diamond DA, Berry SJ, Embricht C, et al: Computerized image analysis of nuclear shape as a prognostic factor for prostatic cancer. Prostate 3:321–332, 1982.
18. Drago JR: Introductory remarks and workshop summary. Urology 34:2–3, 1987.
19. Epstein JI, Pizov G, Walsh PC: Correlation of pathologic findings with progression following radical prostatectomy. Cancer 71:3582–3593, 1993.
20. Epstein JI, Paull G, Eggleston JC, et al: Prognosis of untreated stage AI prostate carcinoma: A study of 94 cases with extended follow-up. J Urol 136:837–839, 1986.
21. Epstein JI, Grignon DJ, Humphrey PA, et al: Interobserver reproducibility in the diagnosis of prostatic intraepithelial neoplasia. Am J Surg Pathol 19(8):873–886, 1995.
22. Franks LM: Estrogen-treated prostatic cancer. Cancer 13:490–491, 1960.
23. Furusato M, Mostofi FK: Intraprostatic lymphatics in man, light and ultra-structural observations. Prostate 1:15–23, 1980.
24. Gaeta JF, Asirwatham JE, Miller G, Murphy GP: Histologic grading of primary prostatic cancer: A new approach to an old problem. J Urol 123:689–693, 1980.
25. Gleason DF: Classification of prostatic carcinoma. Cancer Chemother Rep 50:125–128, 1966.
26. Grayhack JF, Assimos DC: Prognostic significance of tumor grade and stage in patients with carcinoma of the prostate. Prostate 4:13–31, 1983.
27. Helpap B, Koch V: Histological and immunohistochemical find-

ings of prostatic carcinoma after external or interstitial radiotherapy. J Cancer Res Clin Oncol 117:608–614, 1991.

28. Kastendieck H, Altenahr E: Cyto- and histomorphogenesis of the prostate carcinoma. A comparative light and electron microscopic study. Virchow's Arch (Pathol Anat) 370:207–224, 1976.

29. Kastendieck H, Helpap B: Prostatic dysplasia–Atypical hyperplasia. Terminology, histopathology, pathobiology and significance. Urology Suppl 34:28–42, 1989.

30. Kastendieck H, Altenahr E, Husselman H, Bressel M: Carcinoma and dysplastic lesions of the prostate. A histomorphological analysis of 50 prostatectomies by step section technique. Z Krebsforsch 88:33–54, 1976.

31. Kastendieck H, Altenahr E, Husselmann H: Carcinoma and dysplastic lesions of the prostate. Z Krebsforsch 88:33–54, 1976.

32. Kastendieck H, Helpap B: Prostatic dysplasia—Atypical hyperplasia. Terminology, histopathology, pathobiology and significance. Urology Suppl 34:28–42, 1989.

33. Kastendieck H: Correlations between atypical primary hyperplasia and carcinoma of the prostate. Pathol Res Pract 169:366–387, 1980.

34. Kovi J, Mostofi FK, Heshmat MY: Large acinar atypical hyperplasia and carcinoma of the prostate. Cancer 61:555–561, 1988.

35. Lange PH: Tumor markers in prostate cancer. Amsterdam Excerpta Med 1986.

36. Lee CL, Wang MC, Killian CS: Solid-phase immunofluorescent and immunoabsorbent assays of serum prostatic acid phosphatase. Prostate 1:427–439, 1980.

37. Lilja H: Improved separation between normals, benign prostatic hyperplasia (BPH) and carcinoma of the prostate (CAP) by measuring free (F), complexed (C) and total (T) concentrations of prostate-specific antigen (PSA). J Urol 151:400A, 1994.

38. McNeal JE: Cancer volume and site of origin of adenocarcinoma in the prostate. Relationship to local and distant spread. Human Pathol 23:258–266, 1992.

39. McNeal JE: Significance of duct acinar dysplasia in prostatic carcinoma. Prostate 13:91–102, 1988.

40. McNeal JE, Bostwick DG: Intraductal dysplasia: A premalignant lesion of the prostate. Human Pathol 17:64–71, 1986.

41. McNeal JE, Villers AA, Redwine EA, et al: Histologic differentiation, cancer volume and pelvic lymph node metastasis in adenocarcinoma of the prostate. Cancer 66:1225–1233, 1990.

42. Melicow MM, Tannenbaum M: Endometrioid carcinoma of uterus masculinus (prostatic utricle): Report of 6 cases. J Urol 106:892–902, 1971.

43. Moore GH, Lawshe B, Murphy J: Diagnosis of adenocarcinoma in transurethral resections of the prostate gland. Am J Surg Pathol 10:165–169, 1986.

44. Mostofi FK, Price EB Jr: Tumors of the Male Genital System (Fascicle 8), Atlas of Tumor Pathology, 2nd Series. Washington, DC, Armed Forces Institute of Pathology, 1973, pp 236–338.

45. Mostofi FK: Can pathology predict response? Role of classic methods and modern techniques. In Smith PH, Pavone-Macaluso M: EORTC Genitourinary Group Monograph 10—Urologic Oncology: Reconstructive Surgery Organ Conservation and Restoration of Function. New York, Wiley-Liss, 1991, pp 237–248.

46. Mostofi FK: Precancerous lesions of the prostate. In Carter RL (ed): Precancerous States. London, Oxford University Press, 1984, pp 303–316.

47. Mostofi FK, Sesterbenn IA, Davis CJ, Jr.: A pathologist's view of prostatic carcinoma. Cancer 71:906–932, 1993.

48. Mostofi FK: Problems in grading carcinoma of the prostate. Semin Oncol 3:161–169, 1976.

49. Mostofi FK, Davis CJ, Sesterhenn IA, Sobin LH: Histological Typing of Prostate Tumours. In World Health Organization International Classification of Tumours. Heidelberg, Springer Verlag, 2001.

50. Murphy GP, Whitmore WF, Jr.: A report of workshops on the current status of the histological grading of prostate cancer. Cancer 44:1490–1494, 1979.

51. Murphy WM, Dean PJ, Brasfield JA: Incidental carcinoma of prostate. How much sampling is adequate? Am J Surg Pathol 10:170–174, 1986.

52. Murphy WM, Soloway MS, Barrows GH: Pathologic changes associated with androgen deprivation therapy for prostate cancer. Cancer 68:821–828, 1991.

53. Schroeder FH, Hop WC, Blom JH: Grading of prostatic carcinoma. Multivariant analysis of prognostic parameters. Prostate 7:13–20, 1985.

54. Schroeder FH: The TNM classification of prostate cancer. Prostate (suppl 4):129–139, 1992.

55. Sesterhenn IA: Immunopathology of prostate and bladder tumors. In Russo J (ed): Immunocytochemistry in Tumor Diagnosis. Boston, Martinus Nijhoff, 1985, pp 337–350.

56. Sherwood ER, Theyer G, Steiner G: Differential expression of specific cytokeratin polypeptides in the basal and luminal epithelia of the human prostate. Prostate 18:303–314, 1991.

57. Sobin LH, Wjermstad BM, Sesterbenn IA: Prostatic acid phosphatase activity in carcinoid tumors. Cancer 58:136–138, 1986.

58. Sobin LH: TNM Classification of Malignant Tumours, 5th ed. New York, Wiley-Liss, Inc, 1997.

59. Stamey TA, Freiha FS, McNeal JE, et al: Localized prostate cancer: Relationship of tumor volume to clinical significance for treatment of prostate cancer. Cancer (suppl) 71:933–938, 1993.

60. Tetu B, Srigley JR, Boirin JC: Effect of combination endocrine therapy (LHRH agonist and flutamide) on normal prostate and prostatic adenocarcinoma. A histopathologic and immunohistochemical study. Am J Surg Pathol 15:111–120, 1991.

61. Visakorpi T, Hyytinen E, Koivisto P: In vivo amplification of the androgen receptor gene and progression of human prostate cancer. Nature Genet 9:401–406, 1995.

62. Visakorpi T, Hyytinen L, Kallioniemi A: Sensitive detection of chromosome copy number aberrations in prostate cancer by fluorescence in situ hybridization. Am J Pathol 145:624–630, 1994.

63. Wang MC, Papsidero LD, Kuriyama M: Prostate antigen: A new potential marker for prostatic cancer. Prostate 2:89–96, 1981.

64. Watt KWK, Lee PJ, M'Timkulu T: Human prostatic specific antigen: Structural and functional similarity with serine proteases. Proc Natl Acad Sci 83:3166–3170, 1986.

65. Wolman SR, Macoska JA, Micale MA: An approach to definition of genetic alterations in prostate cancer. Diagn Mol Pathol 1:192–199, 1992.

66. Yam LT, Janekila AJ, Lam WK: Immunohistochemistry of prostatic acid phosphatase. Prostate 2:97–107, 1981.


# Tumors of the Bladder


67. Amin MB, Ro JY, Lee KM: Lymphoepithelioma-like carcinoma of the urinary bladder. Am J Surg Pathol 18:466–473, 1994.

68. Amin MB, Ro JY, el-Sharkamy T: Micropapillary variant of transitional cell carcinoma of the urinary bladder. Histologic pattern resembling ovarian papillary serous carcinoma. Am J Surg Pathol 18:1224–1232, 1994.

69. Bannach B: Sarcomatoid transitional cell carcinoma vs. pseudosarcomatous stromal reaction in bladder carcinoma: An immunohistochemistry study. J Urol Pathol 1:105–119, 1993.

70. Blomjous CEM, Vos W, De Voogt HJ: Small cell carcinoma of the urinary bladder: A clinicopathologic, morphometric, immunohistochemical, and ultra structural study of 18 cases. Cancer 64:1347–1357, 1989.

71. Campo E, Algaba F, Palacin A: Placental proteins in high-grade urothelial neoplasm: An immunohistochemical study of human chorionic gonadotropin, human placental lactogen, and pregnancy-specific beta-1 glycoprotein. Cancer 63:2497–2504, 1989.

72. Dinney CPN, Ro JY, Babaian RJ: Lymphoepithelioma of the bladder: A clinicopathological study of 3 cases. J Urol 149:840–842, 1993.

73. Drew PA, Murphy WM, Civantos F: The histogenesis of clear cell adenocarcinoma of the lower urinary tract: Case series and review of the literature. Human Pathol 27:248–252, 1996.

74. Drew PA, Furman J, Civantos F: The nested variant of transitional cell carcinoma: An aggressive neoplasm with innocuous histology. Mod Pathol 9:989–994, 1996.

75. Eble JN, Young RH: Carcinoma of the urinary bladder: A review of its diverse morphology. Semin Diagn Pathol 14:98–108, 1997.

76. Elem B, Alam SZ: Total intestinal metaplasia with focal adenocarcinoma in a schistosoma-infested defunctioned urinary bladder. Br J Urol 56:331–343, 1984.

77. Epstein JI, Amin MB, Reuter VR, Mostofi FK: The World Health Organization/International Society of Urological Pathology

Consensus Classification of Urothelial (Transitional Cell) Neoplasms of the Urinary Bladder. Am J Surg Pathol 22(12):1435–1448, 1998.

78. Grignon DJ: Neoplasms of the urinary bladder. In Bostwick DG, Eble JN (eds): Urologic Surgical Pathology. St. Louis, Mosby–Year Book, 1997.

79. Grignon DJ, Ro JY, Ayala AG: Primary adenocarcinoma of the urinary bladder: A clinicopathologic analysis of 72 cases. Cancer 67:2165–2172, 1991.

80. Jacobsen A-B, Nesland JM, Fossa SD: Human chorionic gonadotropin, neuron specific enolase and deoxyribonucleic acid flow cytometry in patients with high grade bladder carcinoma. J Urol 143:706–709, 1990.

81. Jones EC, Young RH: Myxoid and sclerosing sarcomatoid transitional cell carcinoma of the urinary bladder. A clinicopathological and immunohistochemical study of 25 cases. Mod Pathol 10:908–916, 1997.

82. Kotliar SN: Transitional cell carcinoma exhibiting clear cell features: A differential diagnosis for clear cell adenocarcinoma of the urinary tract. Arch Pathol Lab Med 119:79–81, 1989.

83. Martin JE, Jenkins BJ, Zuk RJ: Clinical importance of squamous metaplasia in invasive transitional cell carcinoma of the bladder. J Clin Pathol 42:250–253, 1989.

84. Martin JE, Jenkins BJ, Zuk RJ: Human chorionic gonadotropin expression and histological findings a predictor of response to radiotherapy in carcinoma of the bladder. Virchows Arch [A] 414:273–277, 1989.

85. Mostofi FK: Mucous adenocarcinoma of the urinary bladder. Cancer 8:741–758, 1995.

86. Mostofi FK, Davis CJ, Sesterhenn IA, Sobin LH: Histological typing of urinary bladder tumours, 2nd ed. In World Health Organization International Histological Classification of Tumours. Heidelberg, Springer Verlag, 1999.

87. Mostofi FK: Dysplasia versus atypia versus carcinoma in situ of bladder. In McCullough DL (ed): Difficult Diagnoses in Urology. New York, Churchill Livingstone, 1988, pp 165–172.

88. Mostofi FK, Sesterhenn IA: Lymphocytic Infiltration in Relationship to Urologic Tumors, Monograph 349. Bethesda, MD, National Cancer Institute, 1978.

89. Murphy WM, Deana DG: The nested variant of transitional cell carcinoma: A neoplasm resembling proliferation of Brunn's nests. Mod Pathol 5:240–243, 1992.

90. Nakanishi K, Kawai T, Suzuki M: Prognostic factors in urachal adenocarcinoma; a study in 41 specimens of DNA status, proliferating cell-nuclear antigen immunostaining, and argyrophilic nucleolar-organizer region counts. Human Pathol 27:240–247, 1996.

91. Ordóñez NG: Oat cell carcinoma of the urinary tract: An immuno-histochemical and electron microscopic study. Cancer 58:2519–2530, 1985.

92. Paik SS, Park MH: The nested variant of transitional cell carcinoma of the urinary bladder. Br J Urol 78:793–794, 1996.

93. Paz A, Rath-Wolfson L, Lask D: The clinical and histological features of transitional cell carcinoma of the bladder with microcysts: Analysis of 12 cases. Br J Urol 79:722–725, 1997.

94. Perret L, Chaubert P, Wessler D: Primary heterologous carcinosarcoma (metaplastic carcinoma) of the urinary bladder: A clinicopathologic, immunohistochemical, and ultra structural analysis of eight cases and a review of literature. Cancer 82:1535–1549, 1998.

95. Podesta AH, Lawrence DT: Small cell carcinoma of the bladder: report of five cases with immunohistochemistry and review of literature with evaluation of prognosis according to stage. Cancer 65:710–714, 1989.

96. Reyes CV, Soneru I: Small cell carcinoma of the urinary bladder with hypercalcemia. Cancer 56:2530–2533, 1985.

97. Sheldon CA, Clayman RV, Gonzalez R: Malignant urachal lesions. J Urol 131:1–8, 1984.

98. Talbert ML, Young RH: Carcinomas of the urinary bladder with deceptively benign-appearing foci. A report of three cases. Am J Surg Pathol 13:374–381, 1989.

99. Thomas DG, Ward AM, Williams JL: A study of 52 cases of adenocarcinoma of the bladder. Br J Urol 43:4–15, 1971.

100. Young RH, Wick MR: Transitional cell carcinoma of the bladder with pseudo-sarcomatous stroma. Am J Clin Pathol 90:216–219, 1988.

101. Young RH, Scully RE: Clear cell adenocarcinoma of the bladder and urethra. Am J Surg Pathol 9:816–826, 1985.

102. Young RH, Zukerberg LR: Microcystic transitional cell carcinoma of the urinary bladder. A report of four cases. Am J Clin Pathol 96:635–639, 1991.

103. Young RH, Oliva E: Transitional cell carcinomas of the urinary bladder that may be underdiagnosed: A report of four cases exemplifying the homology between neoplastic and non-neoplastic transitional cell lesions. Am J Surg Pathol 20:1448–1454, 1996.

104. Young RH, Eble JN: Unusual forms of carcinoma of the urinary bladder. Human Pathol 22:948–965, 1991.

105. Young RH, Parkburst EC: Mucinous adenocarcinoma of bladder. Case associated with extensive intestinal metaplasia of urothelium in patient with nonfunctioning bladder for twelve years. Urology 24:192–195, 1984.

106. Young RH: Lymphoepithelioma-like carcinoma of the urinary bladder. J Urol Pathol 1:63–67, 1993.

107. Young RH: Sarcomatoid carcinoma of the urinary bladder: A clinicopathologic analysis of 12 cases and review of the literature. Am J Clin Pathol 90:653–661, 1998.

108. Zukerberg LR, Harris NL, Young RH: Carcinomas of the urinary bladder simulating malignant lymphoma: A report of five cases. Am J Surg Pathol 15:569–576, 1991.

## Tumors of the Kidney

109. Amin MB, Crotty TB, Tickoo SK, Farrow GM: Renal oncocytoma: A reappraisal of morphologic features with clinicopathologic findings in 80 cases. Am J Surg Pathol 21:1–12, 1997.

110. Bell ET: Renal Disease, 2nd ed. Philadelphia, Lea & Febiger, 1950, p 431.

111. Davis CJ, Barton JH, Sesterhenn IA, Mostofi FK: Metanephric adenoma. Clinicopathological study of 50 patients. Am J Surg Pathol 19:1101–1114, 1995.

112. Davis CJ, Sesterhenn IA, Mostofi FK, Ho CK: Renal oncocytoma: Clinicopathological study of 166 patients. J Urogenital Pathol 1:41–52, 1991.

113. Jones EC, Pins M, Dickerson GR, Young RH: Metanephric adenoma of the kidney. A clinicopathological, immunohistochemical, flow cytometric, cytogenetic, and electron microscopic study of seven cases. Am J Surg Pathol 19:615–626, 1995.

114. Murphy WM, Beckwith JB, Farrow GM: Tumors of the kidney, bladder, and related structures. Atlas of Tumor Pathology, Third Series, Fascicle II, Washington, D.C., Armed Forces Institute of Pathology, 1994, pp 132–135.

115. Aizawa S, Chigusa M, Ohno Y: Chromophobe cell renal carcinoma with sarcomatoid component. J Urol Pathol 6:51–59, 1997.

116. Amin MB, Corless CL, Renshaw AA, et al: Papillary (chromophil) renal cell carcinoma: Histomorphologic characteristics and evaluation of conventional pathologic parameters in 62 cases. Am J Surg Pathol 21:621–635, 1997.

117. Baer SC, Ro JY, Ordoney NG, et al: Sarcomatoid collecting duct carcinoma. A clinicopathologic and immunohistochemical study of five cases. Human Pathol 24:1017–1022, 1993.

118. Cochand-Priollet B, Molinie V, Bougaran J: Renal chromophobe cell carcinoma and oncocytoma. A comparative morphologic, histochemical, and immunohistochemical study of 124 cases. Arch Pathol Lab Med 121:1081–1086, 1997.

119. DeLong WH, Sakr W, Grignon DJ: Chromophobe renal cell carcinoma: A comparative histochemical and immunohistochemical study. J Urol Pathol 4:1–8, 1996.

120. Eble JN: Neoplasms of the kidney. In Bostwick DG, Eble JN (eds): Urologic Surgical Pathology. St. Louis, Mosby–Year Book, 1997, pp 83–106.

121. Hartman DS, Davis CJ, Johns T, Goldman SM: Cystic renal cell carcinoma. Urology 28:145–153, 1986.

122. Renshaw AA, Henske EP, Loughlin KR, et al: Aggressive variants of chromophobe renal cell carcinoma. Cancer 78:1756–1761, 1996.

123. Mostofi FK, Davis CJ, Sesterhenn IA, Sobin LH: Histological Typing of Kidney Tumours. In World Health Organization International Histological Classification of Tumours. Heidelberg, Springer Verlag, 1998.

Thoenes W, Storkel ST, Rumpelt H-J: Human chromophobe cell renal carcinoma. Virchows Arch [Cell Pathol] 48:207–217, 1985.

124. Thoenes W, Storkel ST, Rumpelt H-J, et al: Chromophobe cell renal carcinoma and its variants—A report on 32 cases. J Pathol 155:277–287, 1988.

125. Tomera KM, Farrow GM, Lieber MM: Sarcomatoid renal carcinoma. J Urol 130:657–659, 1983.

126. Weiss LM, Gelb AB, Medeiros LJ: Adult renal epithelial neoplasms. Am J Clin Pathol 103:624–635, 1995.

127. Cromie WJ, Davis CJ, DeTure FA: Atypical carcinoma of kidney: Possibly originating from collecting duct epithelium. Urology 13:315–317, 1979.

128. Dimopoulos MA, Logothetis CJ, Markowitz A, et al: Collecting duct carcinoma of the kidney. Br J Urol 71:388–391, 1993.

129. Fleming S, Lewi HJE: Collecting duct carcinoma of the kidney. Histopathology 10:1131–1141, 1986.

130. Kennedy SM, Merino MJ, Linehan WM, et al: Collecting duct carcinoma of the kidney. Human Pathol 21:449–456, 1990.

131. Rumpelt HJ, Storkel S, Moll R, et al: Bellini duct carcinoma: Further evidence for this rare variant of renal cell carcinoma. Histopathology 18:115–122, 1991.

132. Avery RA, Harris JE, Davis CJ: Renal medullary carcinoma: Clinical and therapeutic aspects of a newly described tumor. Cancer 78:128–132, 1996.

133. Davidson AJ, Choyke PL, Hartman DS, Davis CJ: Renal medullary carcinoma associated with sickle cell trait: Radiologic findings. Radiology 195:83–85, 1995.

134. Davis CJ, Mostofi FK, Sesterhenn IA: Renal medullary carcinoma. The seventh sickle cell nephropathy. Am J Surg Pathol 19:1–11, 1995.

135. Rodriguez-Jurado R, Gonzalez-Crussi F: Renal medullary carcinoma: Immunohistochemical and ultrastructural observations. J Urol Pathol 4:191–203, 1996.

136. Faria P, Beckwith B, Mishra K, et al: Focal versus diffuse anaplasia in Wilms' tumor—New definitions with prognostic significance—A report from the National Wilms' Tumor Study Group. Am J Surg Pathol 20:909–920, 1996.

137. Joshi VV, Beckwith JB: Multilocular cyst of the kidney (cystic nephroma) and cystic, partially differentiated nephroblastoma: terminology and criteria for diagnosis. Cancer 64:466–479, 1989.

138. Madewell JE, Goldman SM, Davis CJ, et al: Multilocular cystic nephroma: A radiographic-pathologic correlation of 58 patients. Radiology 146:309–321, 1983.

139. Pettinato G, Manivel JC, Wick MR, Dehner LP: Classical and cellular (atypical) congenital mesoblastic nephroma. A clinicopathologic, ultrastructural, immunohistochemical, and flow cytometric study. Human Pathol 20:682–690, 1989.

140. Eble JN, Amin MB, Young RH: Epithelioid angiomyolipoma of the kidney. Am J Surg Pathol 21:1123–1130, 1997.

141. Ferry JA, Malt RA, Young RH: Renal angiomyolipoma with sarcomatous transformation and pulmonary metastases. Am J Surg Pathol 15:1083–1088, 1991.

142. Kragel PJ, Tokes C: Infiltrating recurrent renal angiomyolipoma with fatal outcome. J Urol 133:90–91, 1985.

143. Pea M, Bonetti F, Zamboni G: Melanocyte-marker HMB is regularly expressed in angiomyolipoma of the kidney. Pathology 23:185, 1991.

144. Steiner MS, Goldman SM, Fishman EK, Marshall FF: The natural history of renal angiomyolipoma. J Urol 150:1782–1786, 1993.

145. Beckwith JB: Wilms' tumor and other renal tumors of childhood. Human Pathol 14:481–492, 1983.

146. Marsden HB, Lawler W: Bone metastasizing renal tumors of childhood. Virchows Arch (Pathol Anat) 387:341–351, 1980.

147. Weeks DA, Beckwith JB, Mierau GW, Luckey DW: Rhabdoid tumor of kidney: A report of 111 cases from the National Wilms' Tumor Study Pathology Center. Am J Surg Pathol 13:439–458, 1989.

## Testicular Tumors

148. Azzopardi JD, Mostofi FK, Theiss EA: Lesions of testis observed in certain patients with widespread choriocarcinoma and related tumors. Am J Pathol 38:207–225, 1961.

149. Bunge RG, Bradbury JT: An early human seminoma. JAMA 193:960–962, 1961.

150. Burke AP, Mostofi FK: Intratubular malignant germ cells in testicular biopsies: Clinical course and identification by staining for placental alkaline phosphatase. Mod Pathol 1:475–479, 1988.

151. Burke AP, Mostofi FK: Spermatocytic seminoma: A clinicopathologic study of 79 cases. J Urol Pathol 1:21–32, 1993.

152. Freedman LS, Parkinson MC, Jones WG, et al: Histopathology in the prediction of relapse of patients with stage I testicular teratoma treated by orchidectomy alone. Lancet 2:294–298, 1987.

153. Fung CY, Kalish LA, Brodsky GL, et al: Stage I nonseminomatous germ cell testicular tumor: Prediction of metastatic potential by primary histopathology. J Clin Oncol 6:1467–1473, 1988.

154. Gondos B, Berthelsen JG, Skakkebaek NE: Intratubular germ cell neoplasia (carcinoma in situ): A preinvasive lesion of the testis. Am Clin Lab Sci 13:185–192, 1983.

155. Hermanek P, Hutter RVP, Sobin LH, et al (eds): International Union Against Cancer. TNM Atlas, 4th ed. New York, Springer Verlag, 1997.

156. Jacobsen GK, Henriksen OB, der Maase HV: Carcinoma in situ of testicular tissue adjacent to malignant germ cell tumors. A study of 105 cases. Cancer 47:2660–2662, 1981.

157. Lawrence WD, Young RH, Scully RE: Juvenile granulosa cell tumor of the infantile testis: A report of 14 cases. Am J Surg Pathol 9:87–94, 1985.

158. Mostofi FK, Price ER Jr: Tumors of the male genital system. In Atlas of Tumor Pathology, 2nd series, fascicle 8. Washington, DC, Armed Forces Institute of Pathology, 1973.

159. Mostofi FK: Histological changes ostensibly produced by therapy in the metastases of germ cell tumors of testes. Progr Clin Biol Res 203:57–60, 1985.

160. Mostofi FK, Sesterhenn IA, Sobin LH: Histological typing of testis tumors. In World Health Organization: International Histological Classification of Tumors, 2nd ed. New York, Springer Verlag, 1998.

161. Mostofi FK, Sesterhenn IA, Davis CJ Jr: Immunopathology of germ cell tumors of the testis: Semin Diagn Pathol 4:320–341, 1987.

162. Mostofi FK: Pathology of germ cell tumors of testis. A progress report. Cancer 45:1735–1754, 1980.

163. Moul JW, McCarthy WF, Fernandez EB, Sesterhenn IA: Percentage of embryonal carcinoma and of vascular invasion predicts pathological stage in clinical stage I nonseminomatous testicular cancer. Cancer Res 54:362–364, 1994.

164. Percarpio B, Clements JC, McLeod DG, et al: Anaplastic seminoma: An analysis of 77 patients. Cancer 43:2510–2513, 1979.

165. Proppe KH, Scully RE: Large-cell calcifying Sertoli cell tumor of the testis. Am J Clin Pathol 74:607–619, 1980.

166. Scully RE: Gonadoblastoma: A review of 74 cases. Cancer 25:1340–1356, 1970.

167. Sesterhenn IA, Weiss RB, Mostofi FK, et al: Prognosis and other clinical correlates of pathologic review in stage I and II testicular carcinoma: A report from the Testicular Cancer Intergroup Study. J Clin Oncol 10:69–78, 1992.

168. Skakkebaek NE: Carcinoma in situ of the testis: Frequency and relationship to invasive germ cell tumors in infertile men. Histopathology 2:157, 1978.

169. Sobin LH, Wittekind CH (eds): TNM Classification of Malignant Tumors, 5th ed. New York, Wiley, 1997.

170. Talerman A: Endodermal sinus (yolk sac) tumor elements in testicular germ-cell tumors in adults: Comparison of prospective and retrospective studies. Cancer 46:1213–1217, 1980.

171. Talerman A: Germ cell tumors. In Talerman A, Roth LM (eds): Pathology of the Testis and Its Adnexa. New York, Churchill Livingstone. 1986, pp 28–65.

172. Thackray AC, Crane WAJ: Seminoma. In Pugh RCB (ed): Pathology of the Testis. Oxford, Blackwell Scientific Publications, 1976, pp 164–198.

173. Ulbright TM, Loehrer PJ, Roth LM, et al: The development of nongerm cell malignancies within germ cell tumors. A clinicopathologic study of 11 cases. Cancer 54:1824–1833, 1984.

174. Wishnow KI, Johnson DE, Swanson DA, et al: Identifying patients with low-risk clinical stage I non-seminomatous testicular tumors who should be treated by surveillance. Urology 34:339–343, 1989.

175. Young RH, Scully RE: Testicular and paratesticular tumors and tumor-like lesions of ovarian common epithelial and müllerian types. Am J Clin Pathol 86:146–152, 1986.

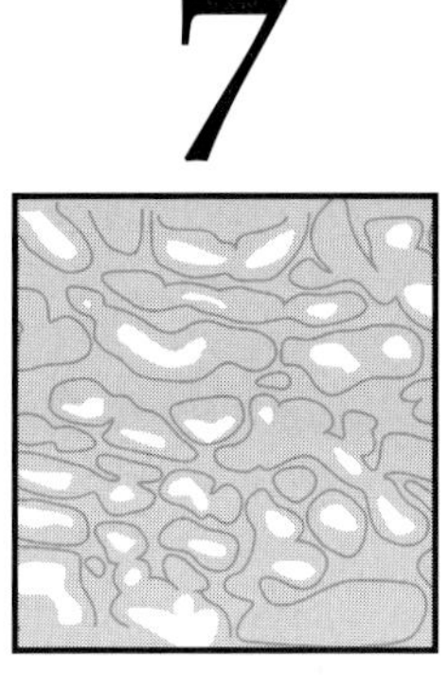

# 7

# Renal and Adrenal Carcinoma: Genetics, Staging, and Surgical Management

*John Naitoh*

*Diane Carter*

*Arie Belldegrun*

## RENAL CANCER

It has been estimated that approximately 30,800 new cases of kidney cancer (both renal cell carcinoma and transitional cell carcinoma) will be diagnosed in the year 2001, and that 12,100 patients will die from this disease.[1] The cause of renal cell carcinoma in the majority of patients is unknown, although familial forms of the cancer are well described.[15] Renal cell carcinoma is rare in children, with the peak incidence occurring in patients who are over the age of 60. Men develop the tumor twice as often as women. Some cases of renal cell carcinoma appear to be hereditary, such as in families who have von Hippel–Lindau disease.[2, 15] Additionally, patients who have tuberous sclerosis, acquired cystic diseases of the kidney, and autosomal dominant polycystic kidney disease also have an increased risk of renal cell carcinoma. Studies of these familial cancer cases have permitted the identification of many genetic lesions that are associated with the initiation and promotion of this cancer: specifically, changes in the von Hippel–Lindau gene have been implicated in the pathogenesis of renal cell carcinoma.[15] Although the description of the genetic alterations in these tumors has yet to translate into advances for the treatment of these cancers, we can hope that future treatments will be developed eventually that will be based on the replacement of these dysfunctional genes.

Because of the kidney's well-protected position deep in the retroperitoneum, most kidney tumors remain asymptomatic until they become large or have metastasized. Prior to the advent of computed tomographic (CT) scanning or ultrasound, most renal cell carcinomas were found only when they became large enough to cause flank pain, a palpable mass, or gross hematuria. Symptoms such as chronic cough, bone pains, and weight loss were also common symptoms in those renal cell cancer patients who already had widespread disease at the time of diagnosis.

Unfortunately, beyond checking the urinalysis for blood, there is no simple, cost-effective, and reliable way to screen asymptomatic patients for renal cell carcinoma so that tumors can be detected while they are still small and confined to the kidney. However, because of the widespread availability of noninvasive imaging tests such as renal ultrasound and CT scan, many renal cell carcinomas are now being found incidentally in patients who are undergoing radiologic evaluation for unrelated reasons. These incidentally found tumors tend to be smaller and thus have a higher probability of being cured following surgical resection.

The improvements in radiologic imaging have also facilitated the diagnostic evaluation of renal masses. In the majority of patients, the diagnosis of renal cell carcinoma can be made with a high degree of certainty prior to surgical exploration. On occasion, a patient may present with a complex renal cyst or a mass that is less than 2 cm in diameter; these smaller, indeterminate lesions present a more significant diagnostic challenge. Once the diagnosis of renal cell carcinoma has been made, chest x-ray, bone scan, magnetic resonance imaging (MRI), and vena cavagram can be selectively used to stage the lesion. Although renal cell cancer can spread to any part of the body, the lungs, bones, liver, lymph nodes, adrenal glands, and brain are the most common sites of metastasis.

The treatment of localized tumors involves the surgical resection of the tumor (including resection of adjacent organs such as the colon or spleen when they are involved with tumors), and widely metastatic cancers are usually treated with a combination of surgery and immunologic treatments. Immunotherapy using interleukin 2 regimens have been 15% to 20% effective, and newer techniques that use adoptive cell therapy (in which patients are treated with antitumor lymphocytes that are harvested directly from the patient's tumor) are reported to have response rates of 35%.[3, 4]

In contrast to renal cell carcinoma, little is known about the genetics of transitional cell carcinoma. There appears to be no familial form of this tumor.[5] However, unlike the case for kidney cancer, the risk factors for the occurrence of transitional cell cancer have been well defined. A prior history of cigarette smoking, phenacetin abuse, and industrial solvent or dye exposure have all been implicated in the pathogenesis of transitional cell cancer. Transitional cell carcinoma can occur anywhere along the urinary tract, because the tumor originates from the cells of the urothelium, which lines the entire collecting system from the kidney to the bladder and urethra. Approximately 5% of all transitional cell carcinomas occur in the kidney.[6] When a TCC of the kidney is diagnosed via endoscopy, cytology, or biopsy, a metastatic survey as well as a complete survey of the remainder of the urothelium is required to rule out the existence of other tumor foci elsewhere in the urinary tract. The standard treatment for TCC of the kidney involves nephroureterectomy, although endoscopic resection can be used successfully in specific circumstances.[7] For patients with more advanced disease, combinations of surgery and chemotherapy can be very effective.

## ADRENAL CANCER

In comparison to kidney tumors, tumors of the adrenal gland are relatively rare, with malignant tumors of the adrenal gland even more uncommon. However, although they are rare, they tend to have a poor prognosis, given that they usually do not cause specific symptoms and given that they are rapidly growing and can be quite large at presentation. Because the normal function of the adrenal gland involves the synthesis of catecholamines and steroid hormones, some

tumors of the adrenal gland secrete excess amounts of these compounds, causing symptoms. The suspicion of an adrenal tumor must be raised for any patient who has severe, uncontrollable hypertension (suggesting the presence of a pheochromocytoma or aldosteronoma), signs of virilization or feminization (suggesting the presence of an adrenocorticocarcinoma), or unexplained Cushing's syndrome. Diagnostic evaluation involves the use of an ultrasound or CT scan to determine the presence or absence of a mass lesion in the adrenal gland, with MRI, nuclear function scans, and metabolic studies also used when indicated by the clinical situation. Once the diagnosis and staging evaluation are completed, the treatment of these tumors involves the correction of any metabolic abnormalities and the surgical resection of the tumor.

With the advent of ultrasound and CT scanning, many adrenal tumors are also being diagnosed incidentally.[8] Although the widespread use of these imaging modalities has enabled the detection of smaller adrenal lesions that are more amenable to surgical resection, many of these tumors are so small that the malignant nature of these lesions is uncertain. In general, all hormone-producing tumors should be removed, and nonfunctioning tumors that are less than 5 cm in diameter can be observed as long as there is no sign of growth over time.

**Figure 7–1:** Adrenal hormone biosynthesis from the cortex and medulla. The adrenal gland is divided into the outer cortex and inner medulla. The cortex is derived from the mesoderm and is involved in steroid hormone biosynthesis (aldosterone from the zona glomerulosa, cortisol from the zona fasciculata, and sex hormones from the zona reticularis). Approximately 80% of adrenocorticocarcinomas are functional; those types produce excess steroid hormone and cause symptoms secondary to the endocrinologic abnormality.[9] The adrenal medulla is derived from the neuroectoderm and is involved in catecholamine production as part of the sympathetic chain. Pheochromocytomas can originate from anywhere along the sympathetic chain, and can cause symptoms secondary to excess catecholamine production. In general, an elevated norepinephrine level suggests that the pheochromocytoma is extra-adrenal, because the methylating enzyme that converts norepinephrine to epinephrine is found only in the adrenal medulla.[8] (From Vaughan ED, Blumenfeld JD: The adrenals. In Walsh PC, Retik AB, Stamey TA, Vaughan ED [eds]: Campbell's Urology, 6th ed. Philadelphia, WB Saunders, 1992, Figs. 64–6, 64–8, 64–9, 64–16.)

**Figure 7–2:** The anatomic relationships of the adrenal gland to the structures of the retroperitoneum and its blood supply. The adrenal glands are paired organs that lie on the superior, anteromedial aspect of each kidney. They are loosely adherent to the upper pole of the kidney, and are enveloped by Gerota's fascia, which

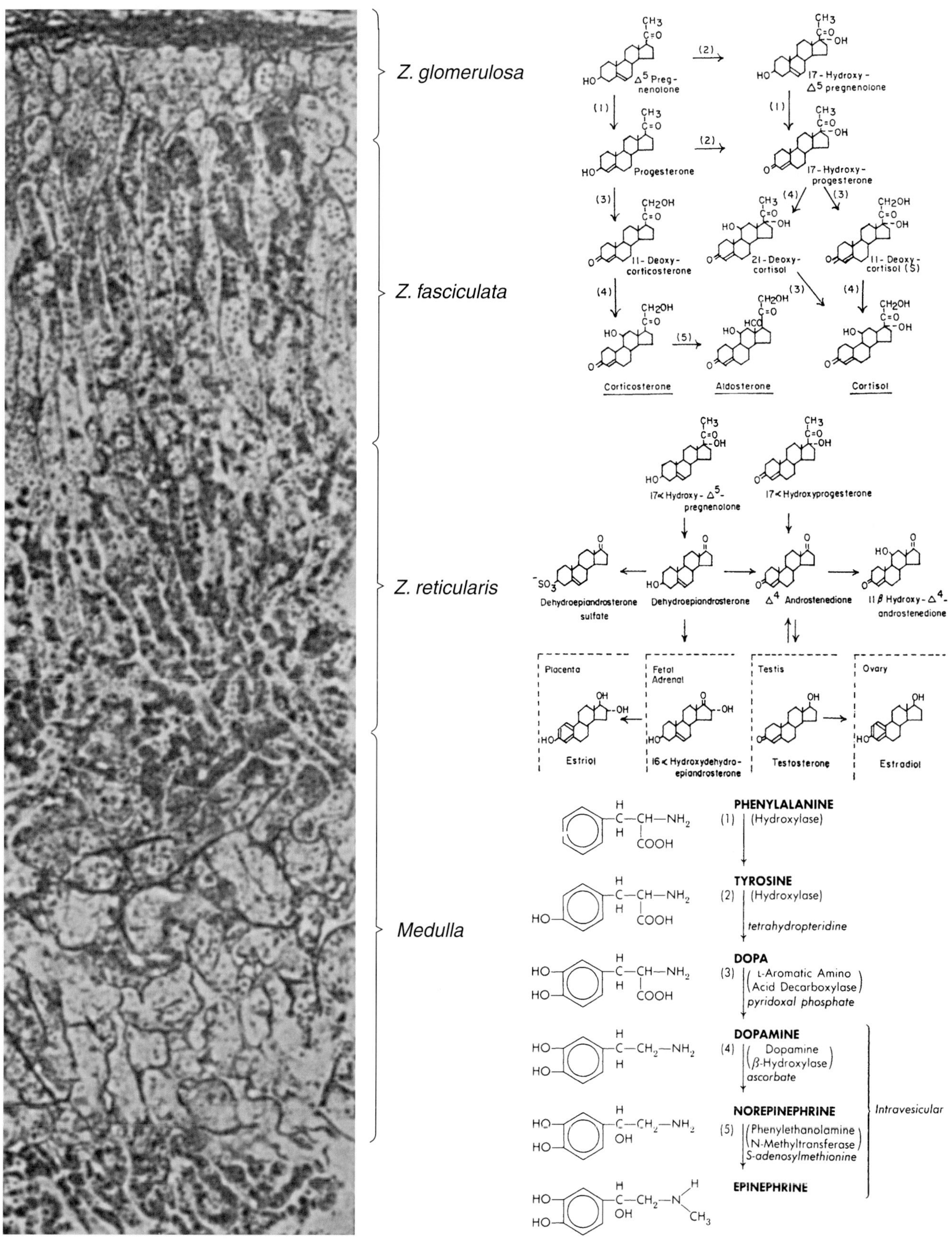


Figure 7–1

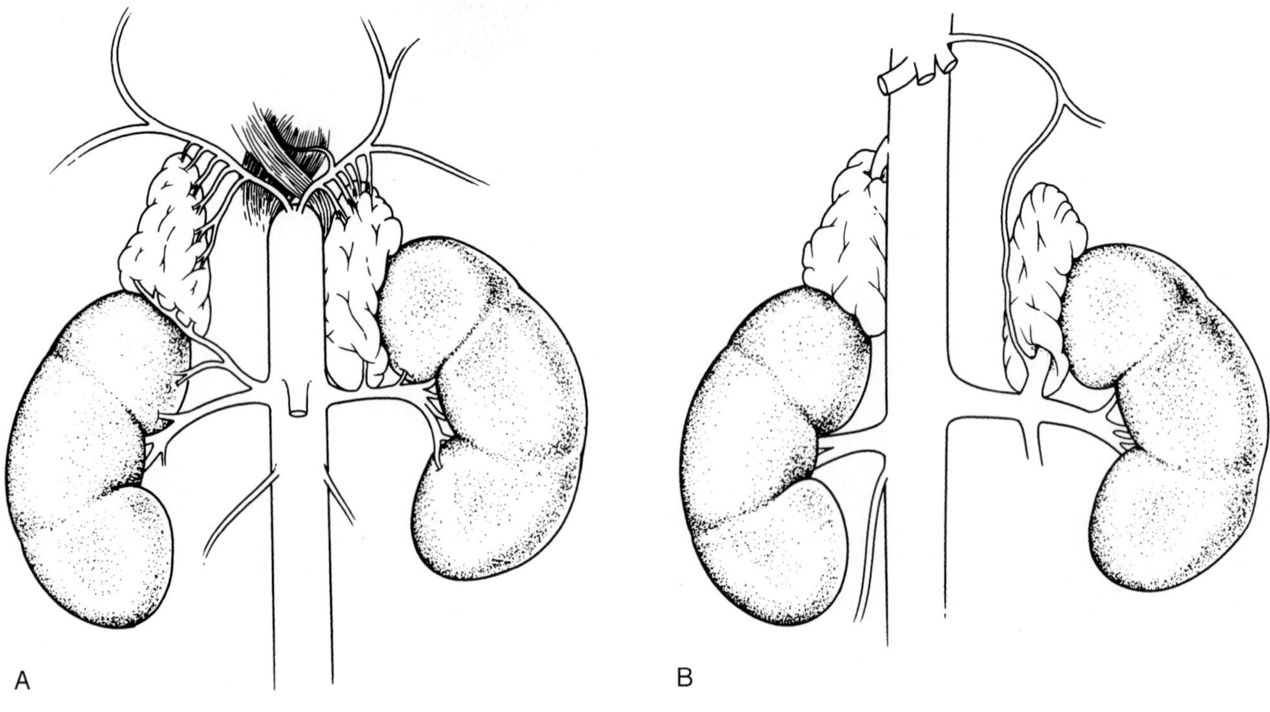

**Figure 7–2**

also surrounds the kidney. The arterial supply to each adrenal gland (*A*) is derived from multiple and highly variable branches of the phrenic artery, the renal artery, and the aorta. *B,* In contrast, each adrenal gland is drained by a single central vein: the left adrenal gland is connected to the left renal vein, and the right renal vein is connected directly to the inferior vena cava. (From Vaughan ED Jr, Carey RM: Adrenal Disorders. New York, Thieme Medical Publishers, 1989, Figs. 9–1, 9–2.)

**Figure 7–3:** The normal appearance of the adrenal glands as seen on CT scan. The right adrenal gland is pyramidal in shape, but the left is more flattened and elongated. The anteromedial aspect of the right adrenal gland extends behind the vena cava, while the left adrenal gland extends below the spleen to the crus of the diaphragm.[8] (From Belldegrun A, Richie JP: Tumors of the adrenal gland. In Graham SD [ed]: Urologic Oncology. New York, Raven Press, 1986, p 248, Fig. 1.)

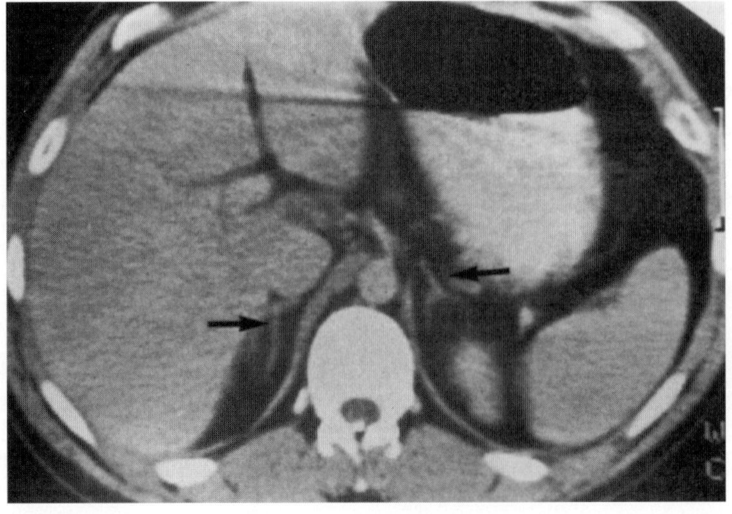

**Figure 7–3**

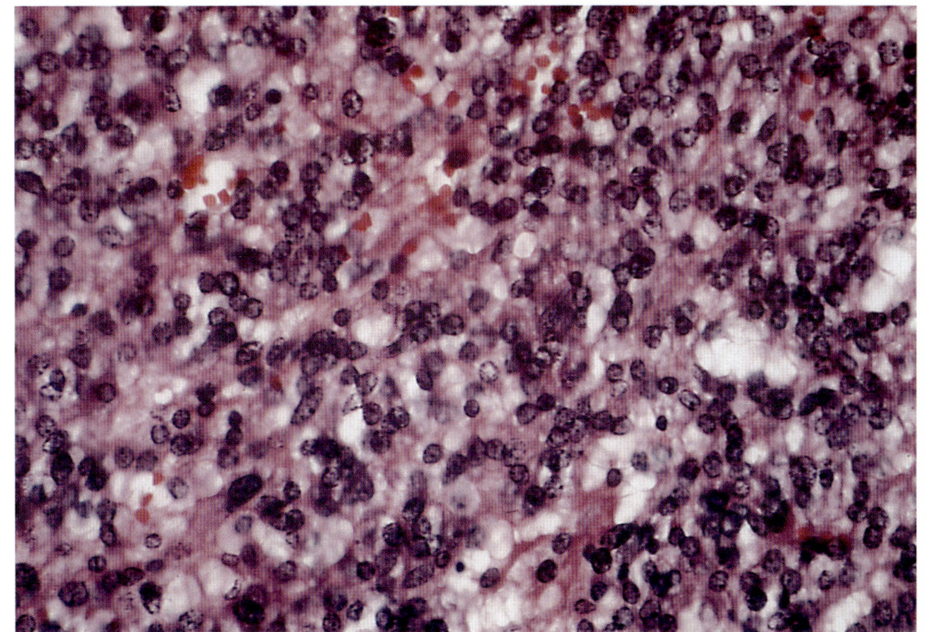

FIGURE 7–12

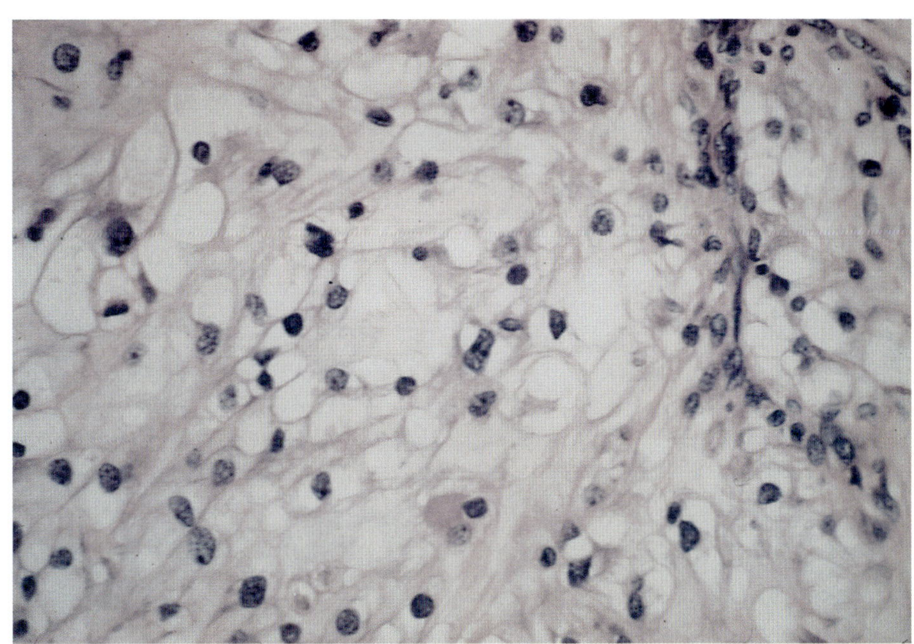

FIGURE 7–15

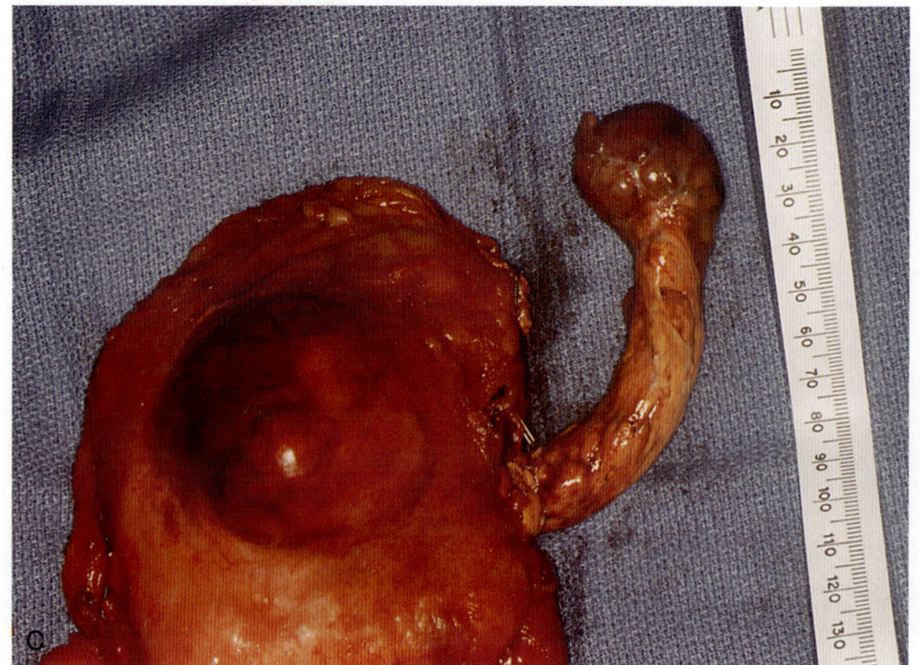

FIGURE 7–21C

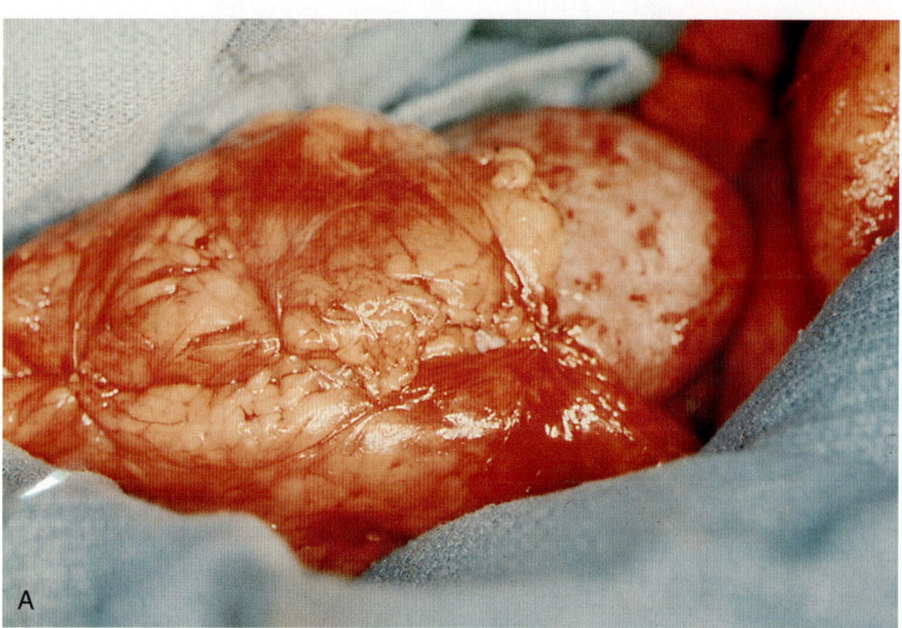

FIGURE 7–23A

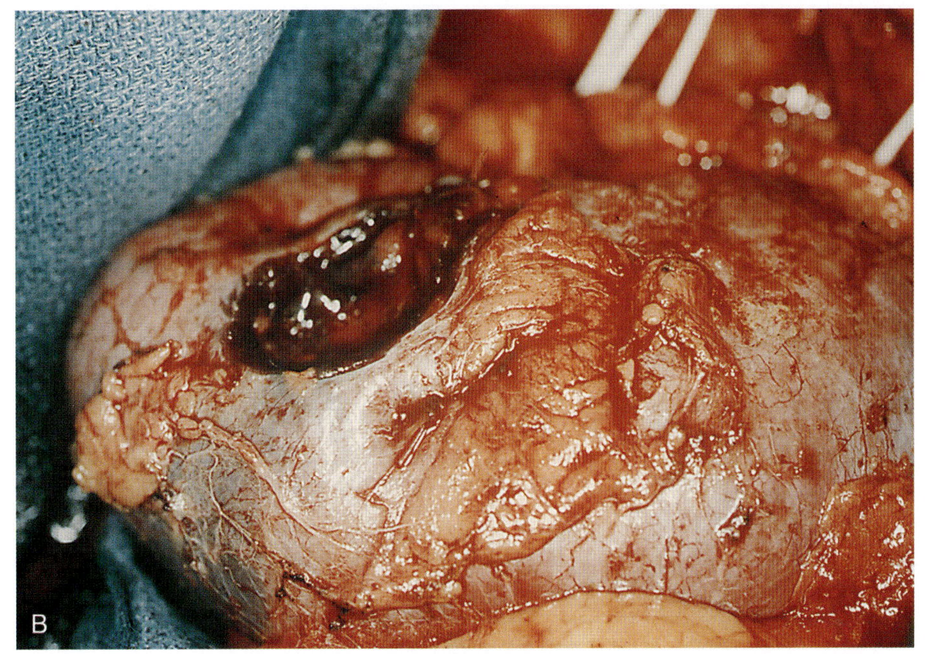

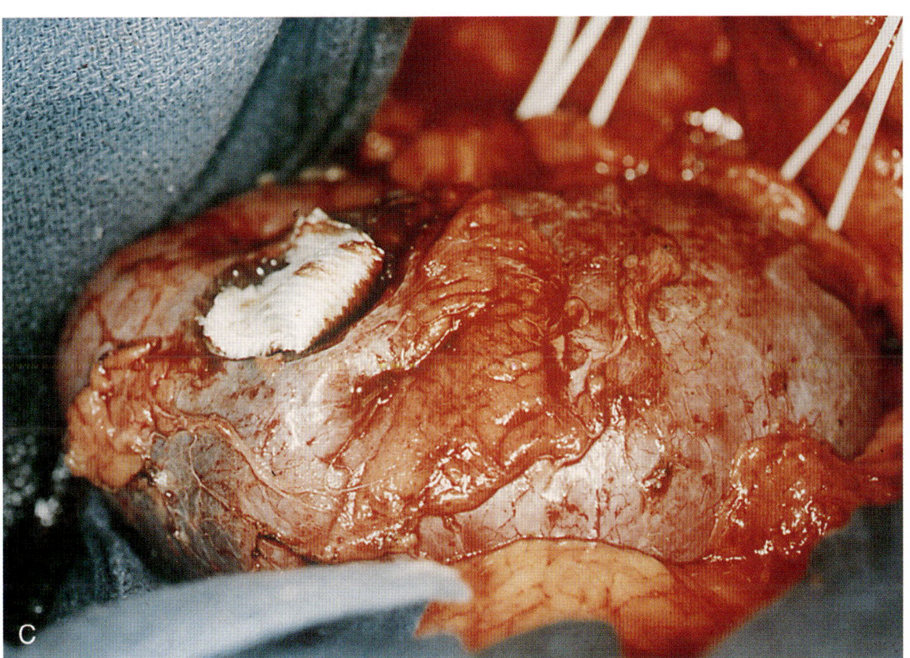

FIGURE 7–23 B & C

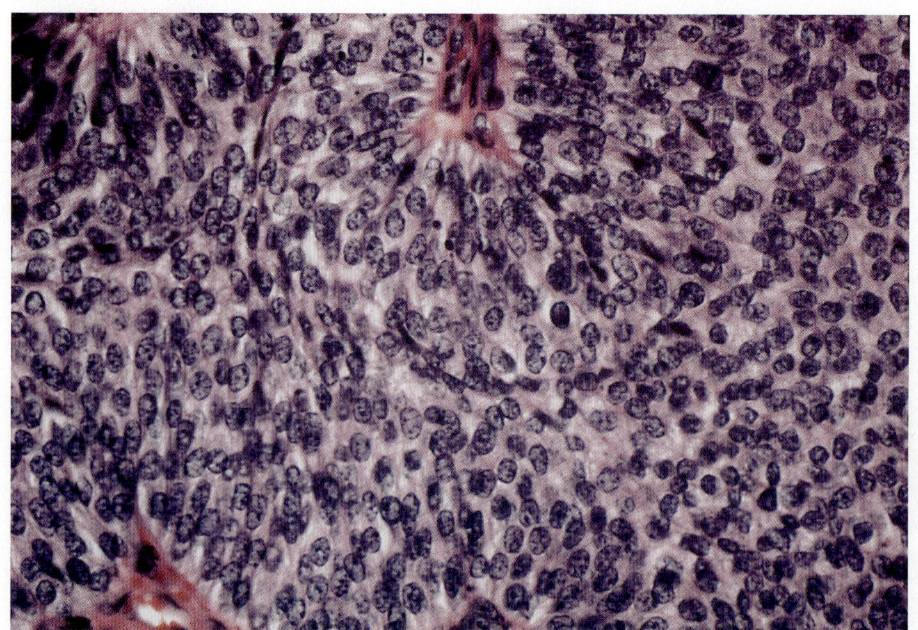

**FIGURE 7–27**

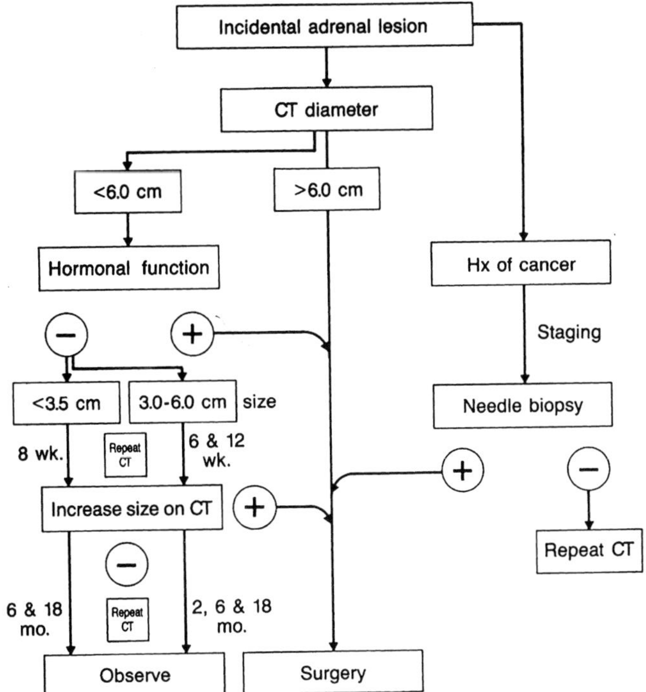


**Figure 7–4**

**Figure 7–4:** The diagnostic evaluation of the incidental adrenal mass. The initial work-up involves the determination of the functional status of the tumor, the nature of the lesion (cystic versus solid), and the maximum diameter of the lesion. Serum and urinary catecholamine levels (metanephrine, vanillymandelic acid, norepinephrine, and epinephrine levels) are determined to diagnose the presence of a pheochromocytoma. Morning cortisol levels can be used to detect Cushing's disease. Serum aldosterone levels and potassium levels can be obtained to detect an aldosterone-producing tumor, and sex steroid levels (estrogen, testosterone) can be used to detect a sex steroid–producing adrenocorticocarcinoma. Once the functional status of the tumor is established, treatment decisions are based on the size and nature of the adrenal mass. Cystic lesions can be aspirated, and an abnormal cytologic finding or hemorrhagic aspirate is an indication for adrenalectomy.[8] If the patient has a prior history of malignancy (especially of breast cancer, melanoma, or kidney cancer), needle biopsy of the mass can then be considered to rule out an adrenal metastasis. All hormonally active tumors should be removed surgically as long as the patient can tolerate the stresses of the procedure. Finally, all nonfunctional tumors larger than 5 cm in diameter should be removed, given the higher risk that they are malignant. In contrast, smaller lesions can be followed serially with CT scans, and growth of the mass over time is also an indication that the lesion should be removed.

**Table 7–1:** Hereditary syndromes that involve pheochromocytoma are listed. Familial pheochromocytoma has been associated with multiple endocrine neoplasia (MEN) type 2, as well as neurofibromatosis, and von Hippel–Lindau (VHL) disease.

**Figure 7–5:** The diagnostic evaluation of a pheochromocytoma. Pheochromocytomas follow the 10% rule: approximately 10% are malignant, 10% are extra-adrenal, 10% are bilateral, and 10% occur in children. Although the classic symptoms of a pheochromocytoma are paroxysms of tachycardia, diaphoresis, headache, and severe hypertension, such symptoms are found in

## TABLE 7–1

### HEREDITARY PHEOCHROMOCYTOMA SYNDROMES

| SYNDROME | SIGNS | GENE DEFECT |
|---|---|---|
| Multiple endocrine neoplasia 2A | Medullary carcinoma of the thyroid, pheochromocytoma, hyperparathyroidism | Loss of RET proto-oncogene at chromosome 10q11 |
| Neurofibromatosis | Café au lait spots, skin nodules, optic gliomas, acoustic neuromas, pheochromocytoma | Loss of NF1 tumor suppressor gene at chromosome 17q11 |
| von Hippel-Lindau | Cerebellar hemangioblastomas, retinal angiomas, cysts of the pancreas, kidney and epididymis, renal cell carcinoma, pheochromocytoma | Autosomal dominant transmission

Loss of VHL gene at chromosome 3p26 |

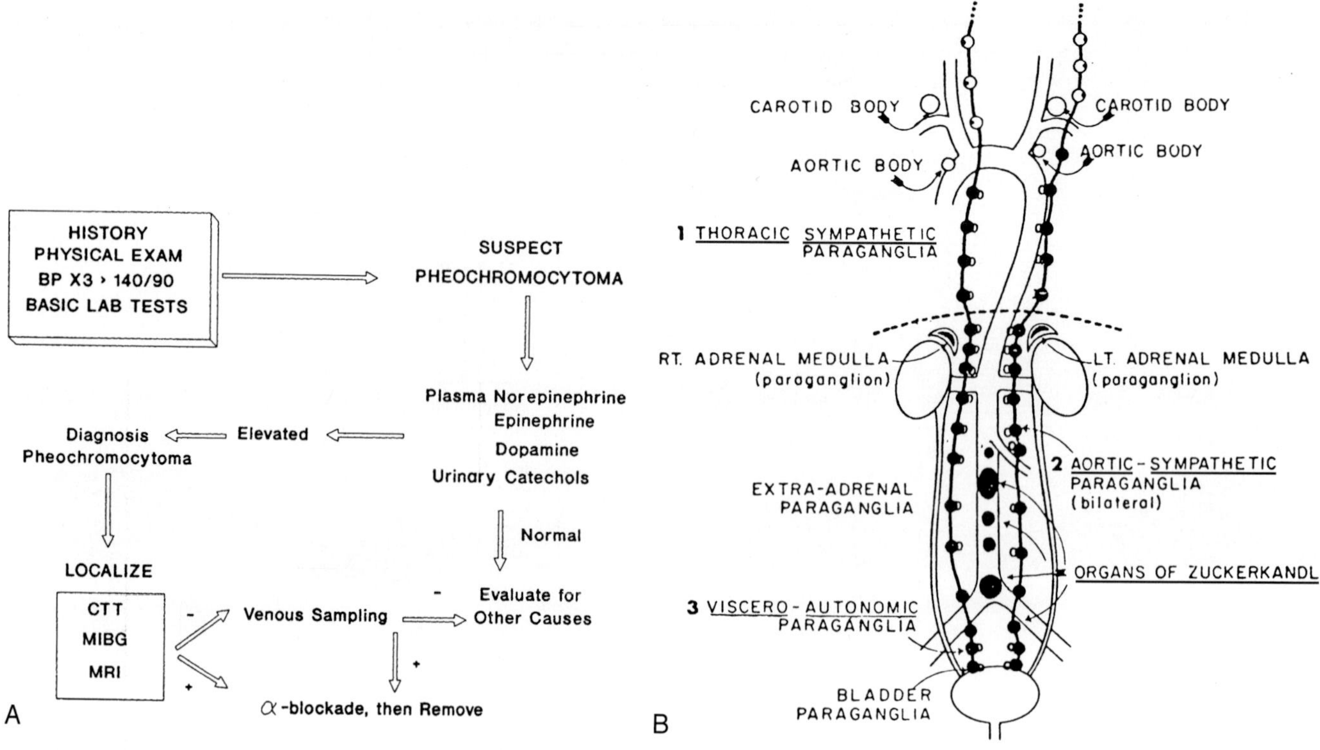


**Figure 7–5**

only about 50% of these patients **(Table 7–2)**.[10] The rest of the patients present with hypertension that is difficult to control or the sequelae of prolonged catecholamine stimulation, such as cardiomyopathy or stroke. The diagnosis is made based on the measurement of plasma norepinephrine and epinephrine levels, as well as measurement of urinary catecholamines and the metabolites metanephrine and vanillylmandelic acid (*A*). Subsequent radiologic tests and nuclear scans are then done to localize the tumor, because a pheochromocytoma can occur anywhere along the sympathetic chain (*B*). (*A* from Vaughan ED, Blumenfeld JD: The Adrenals. In Walsh PC, Retik AB, Stamey TA, Vaughan ED [eds]: Campbell's Urology, 6th ed. Philadelphia, WB Saunders, 1992, p 2394, Fig. 64–40.)

**Figure 7–6:** Gross (*A*) and histologic (*B*) appearance of pheochromocytoma. No histologic feature discriminates a malignant pheochromocytoma from its benign counterpart. The diagnosis of malignancy is made only from the presence of metastatic lesions into the lymphatics. Histologic evaluation of a pheochromocytoma reveals a vague nesting pattern with marked nuclear and cellular pleomorphism. Immunohistochemical staining is strongly positive for chromogranin (*B*).

**Figure 7–7:** Radiologic localization of a pheochromocytoma using metaiodobenzylguanidine (MIBG) scanning. Historically, the preoperative localization of a pheochromocytoma has been difficult, because they can originate either from the adrenal gland or from anywhere else along the sympathetic chain. Classically, 90% of pheochromocytomas originate in the adrenal gland, with adrenal pheochromocytomas producing excess epinephrine. In contrast, extra-adrenal pheochromocytomas produce excess norepinephrine owing to a lack of the methylation enzyme in extra-adrenal sites that converts norepinephrine to epinephrine. However, most tumors were not accurately localized

## TABLE 7–2

### SYMPTOMS ASSOCIATED WITH PHEOCHROMOCYTOMA

| SYMPTOM | PATIENTS WITH PAROXYSMAL HYPERTENSION (%) | PATIENTS WITH PERSISTENT HYPERTENSION (%) |
|---|---|---|
| Severe headache | 92 | 72 |
| Excessive sweating | 65 | 69 |
| Palpitations | 73 | 51 |
| Anxiety/nervousness | 60 | 28 |
| Tremulousness | 51 | 26 |
| Chest/abdominal pain | 48 | 28 |
| Nausea/vomiting | 43 | 26 |
| Weakness/fatigue | 38 | 15 |
| Weight loss | 14 | 15 |
| Warmth/heat intolerance | 13 | 15 |

Adapted from Vaughan ED, Blumenfeld JD: The adrenals. In Walsh PC, Retik AB, Stamey TA, Vaughan ED (eds): Campbell's Urology, 6th ed. Philadelphia, WB Saunders, 1992, p 2389, Table 64–12.

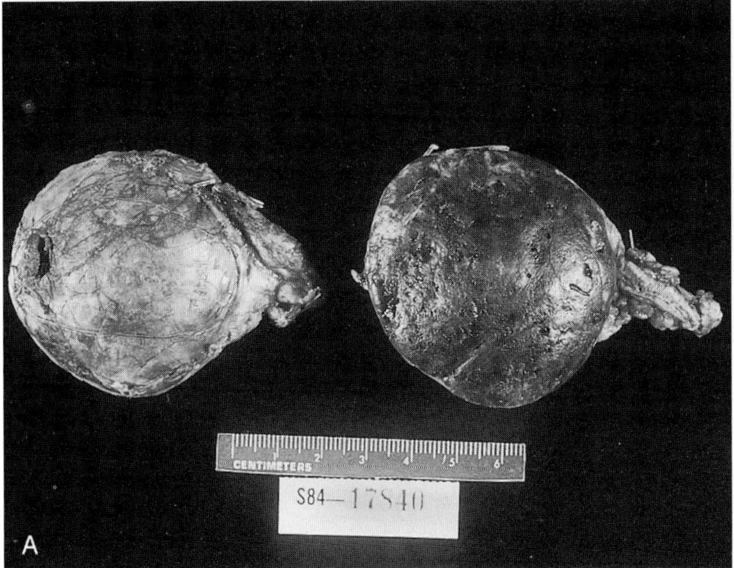

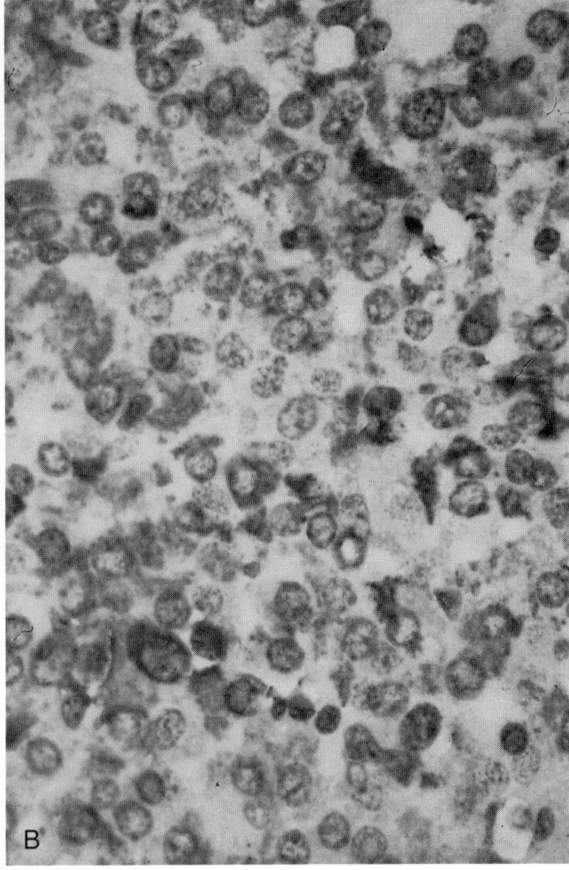

**Figure 7-6**

until the time of abdominal exploration, when manipulation of the tumor and the consequent, rapid changes in blood pressure and heart rate allow identification of the tumor. Currently, with the advent of MIBG scanning and magnetic resonance imaging (MRI) the majority of pheochromocytomas can be localized prior to surgical exploration.[11] In the early MIBG image (*left*), abnormally increased uptake can be seen in the adrenal gland (A), with some normal uptake in the liver (L). In the delayed MIBG image (*right*), some normal uptake can also be seen in the kidney (K) just beneath the adrenal (A).

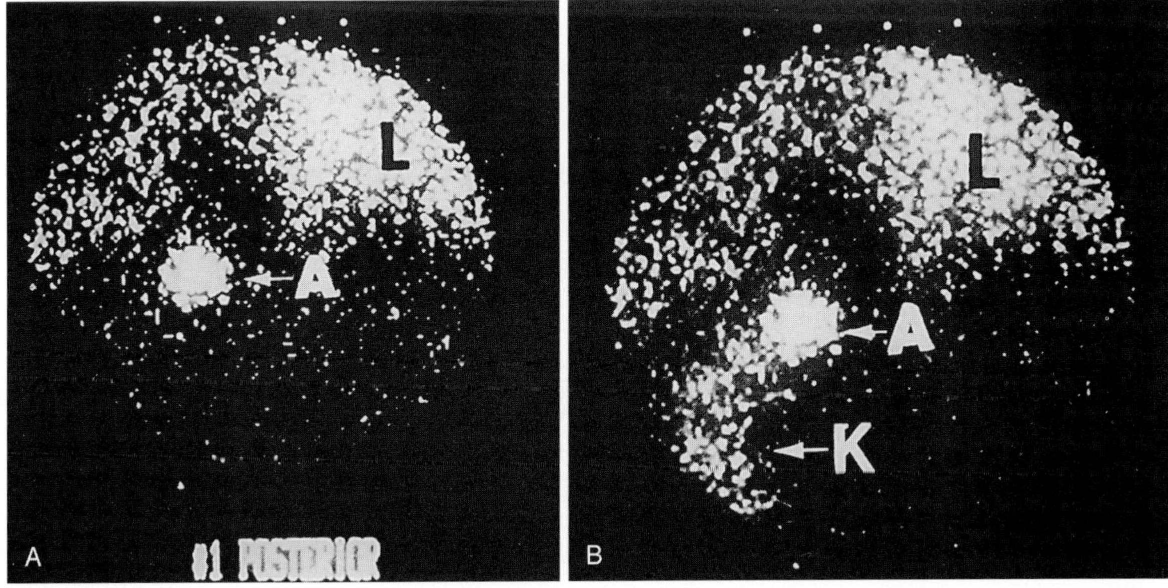


**Figure 7-7**

**Figure 7–8:** Radiologic appearance of a pheochromocytoma on a $T_1$-weighted (*A*) and $T_2$-weighted (*B*) MRI. MRI has become the test of choice to localize pheochromocytomas, because pheochromocytomas create a strong, bright signal (*arrow*) on the $T_2$-weighted image (*B*). In contrast, the tumor appears dark on the $T_1$-weighted image. This "light bulb" sign on MRI is, in fact, diagnostic for pheochromocytoma.[12]

**Figure 7–9:** Surgical treatment of pheochromocytomas: the chevron incision (*A, B*) and the thoracoabdominal incision (*C*). Once the diagnosis of pheochromocytoma is made, blood pressure must be normalized prior to any attempt at surgical extirpation of the tumor. The hypertension secondary to pheochromocytoma is best controlled by first using a selective alpha-adrenergic blocker such as phenoxybenzamine: other alpha blockers such as prazosin may not be as effective, because phenoxybenzamine binds irreversibly to the alpha receptor and can decrease the blood pressure swings that can occur as the tumor is mobilized. Once alpha blockade is achieved, beta-adrenergic blockers such as propanolol can then be added to decrease the risk of

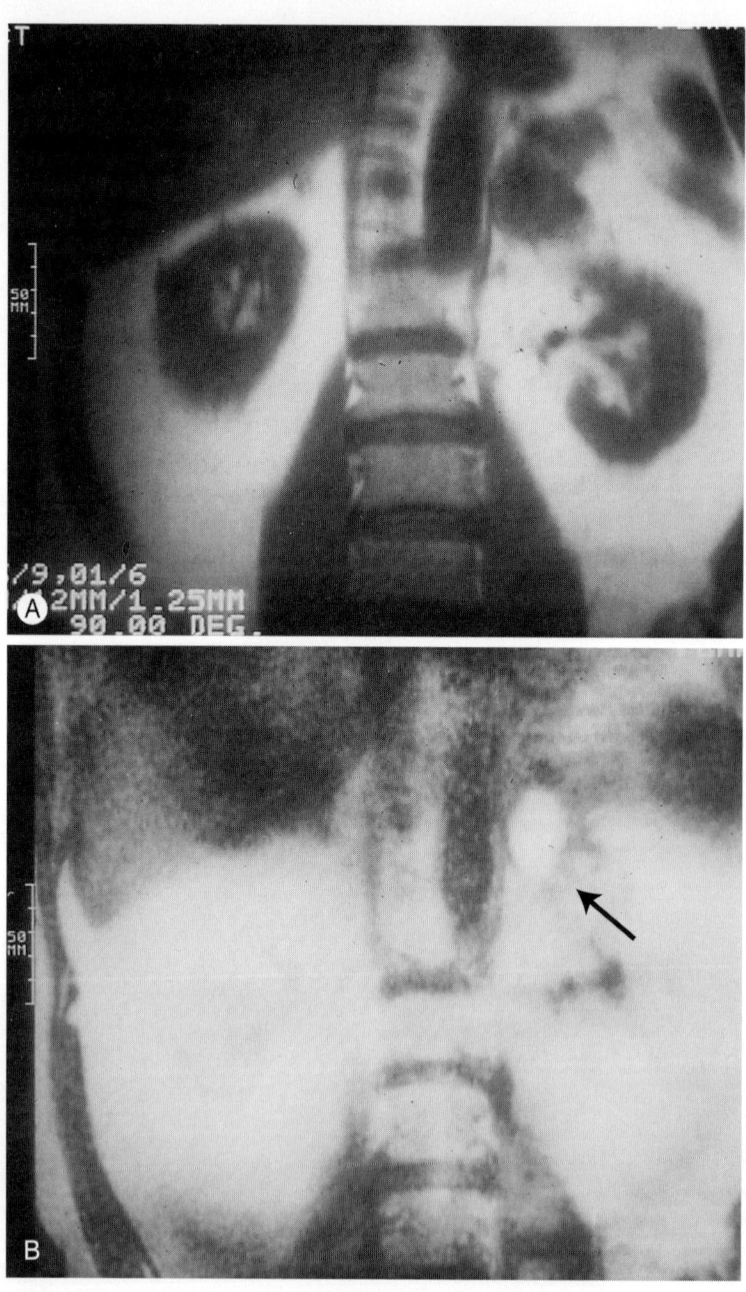


**Figure 7–8**

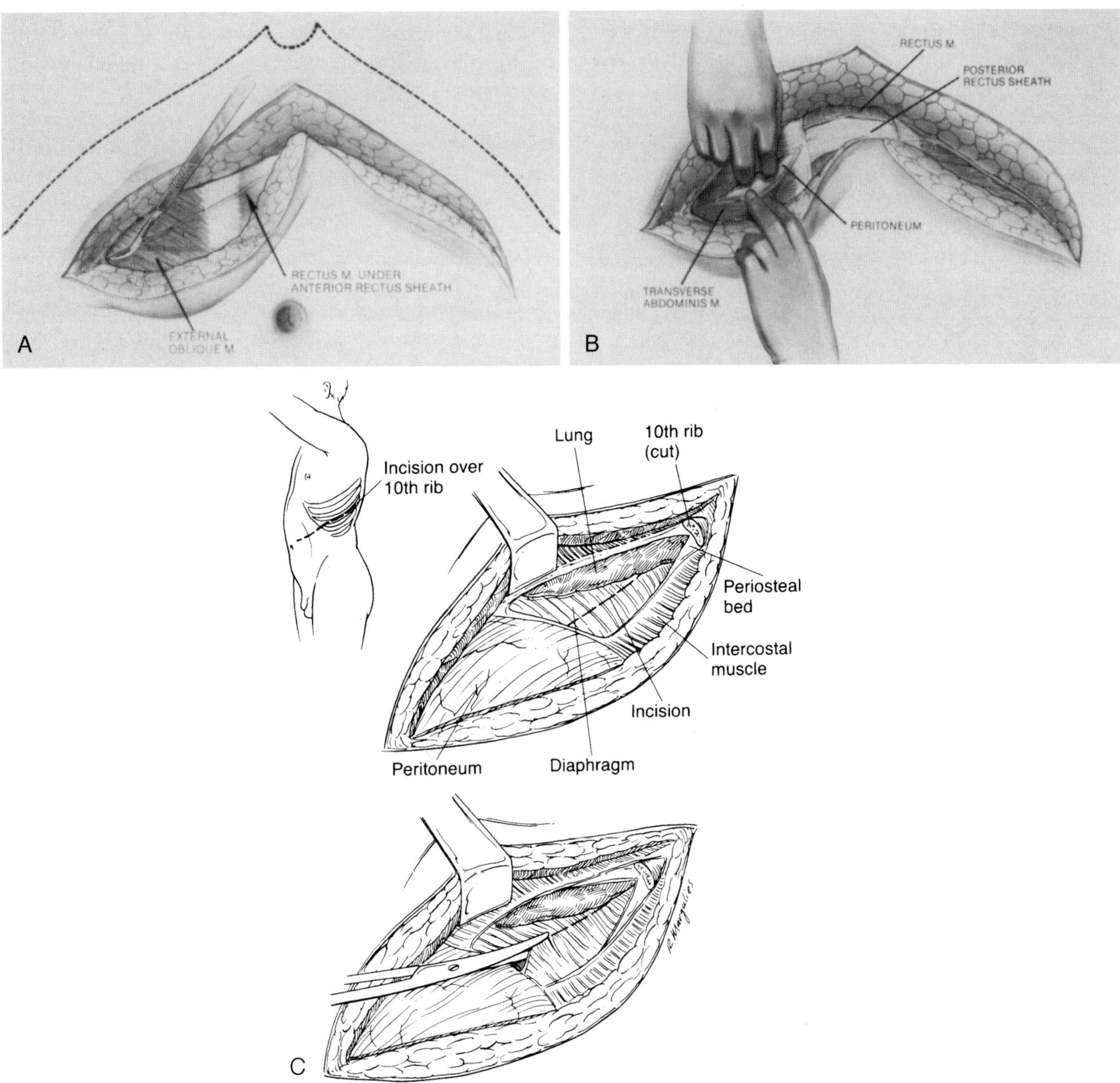



**Figure 7–9**

arrhythmia and further improve blood pressure control. Unopposed beta blockade should be avoided because of the risk of precipitating a hypertensive crisis due to unopposed alpha-adrenergic stimulation. Prior to surgery, intravascular volume must also be restored because these patients are usually vasoconstricted owing to the catecholamine stimulation. Once the pheochromocytoma is removed, vasodilation and hypotension may result if the intravascular volume is not adequate in the preoperative setting. The surgical treatment of pheochromocytoma historically involved the use of transabdominal (*A*) or thoracoabdominal (*B*) approaches, which permit abdominal exploration and the identification of additional, unsuspected lesions. However, given the improved ability to localize the tumor prior to surgery, abdominal exploration is no longer mandatory for pheochromocytoma. Thus, while transabdominal approaches are still preferable for larger lesions, laparoscopic approaches are suitable for smaller adrenal lesions (<5 cm in size).[13, 14] (From Vaughan ED, Blumenfeld JD: The adrenals. In Walsh PC, Retik AB, Stamey TA, Vaughan ED [eds]: Philadelphia, WB Saunders, 1992, pp 2303–2304, Figs. 64–51, 64–52.)

**Figure 7–10:** Trocar placement (*A*) and the intraoperative technique (*B*) of laparoscopic adrenalectomy. Given the deep position of the adrenal gland, large incisions are often needed to obtain access to the gland. Thus, even though the adrenal mass is small (less than 6 cm), a small tumor is removed through an incision that is many times the size of the involved organ. Laparoscopic techniques provide access to the adrenal gland while avoiding the trauma of a large abdominal incision. An umbilical port is first placed, after which four additional ports are placed along the costal margin (*A*). To gain access to the adrenal gland, the colon is mobilized medially along the white line of Toldt. Gerota's fascia is then opened, with dissection along the medial aspect of the kidney, resulting in identification of the adrenal vein. *B*, Dissection along the vein allows identification of the adrenal gland among all the perirenal adipose tissue. Clips are then used to control the remaining blood supply to the adrenal gland from the medial and superior surface of the gland. *C*, The entire gland is then removed through one of the laparoscopic trocar ports. (*B* and *C* from Heniford BT, Arca MJ, Walsh RM, Grill IS: Laparoscopic adrenalectomy for cancer. Semin Surg Oncol 16:298, 1999.)

**Figure 7–11:** CT scan appearance of adrenocorticocarcinoma. Because of their clinically silent course, most adrenal carcinomas are not detected until they become quite large and locally advanced. Once they

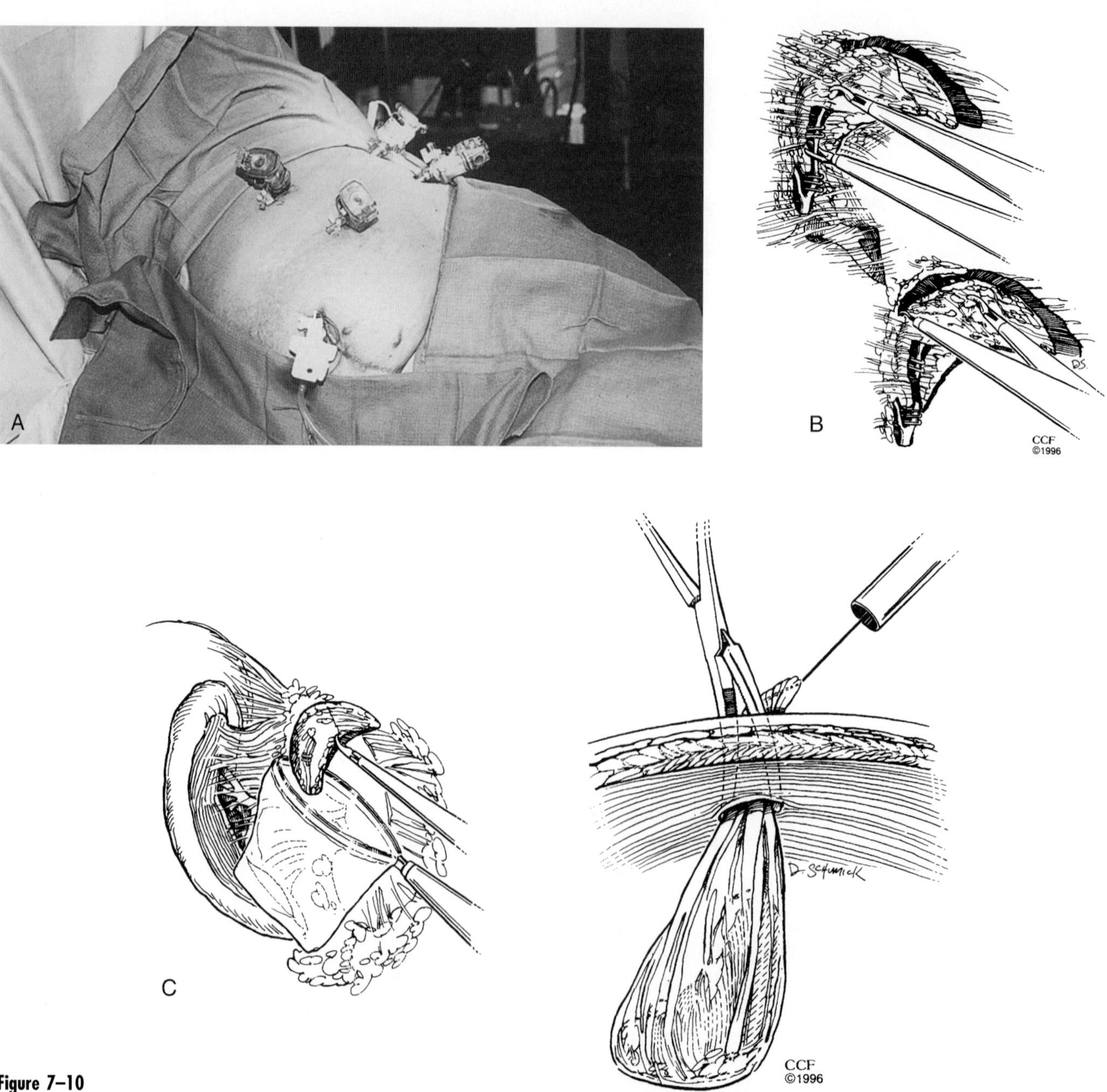

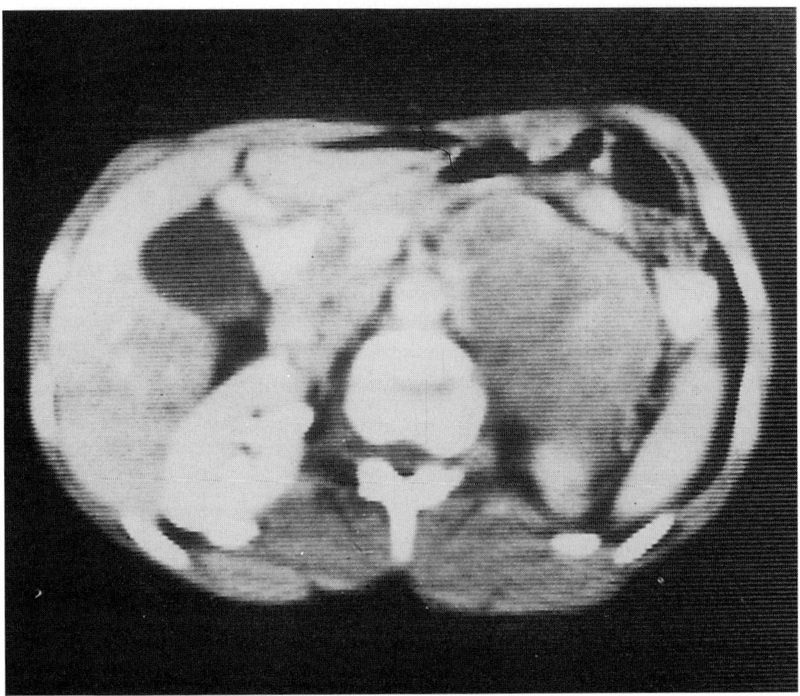

**Figure 7–11**

become large, symptoms can occur as a result of the steroid hormones that they produce, or they can cause pain secondary to hemorrhage and necrosis within the mass. Tumors of the adrenal cortex are derived from cells of the zona glomerulosa, reticularis, and fasciculata, with 80% of such tumors therefore secreting hormones such as cortisol, aldosterone, or the sex steroids.[8] The most common hormonal abnormalities involve excess 17-hydroxycorticoid, excess 17-ketosteroid, and excess dihydroepiandrosterone production. Additionally, steroid production tends to be resistant even to high-dose dexamethasone suppression because of the autonomous hormone production of the tumor. Besides Cushing's syndrome and hypertension secondary to hyperaldosteronism, males with adrenal cancer can also present with gynecomastia, and women can present with hirsutism. Because of their large size, an adrenal cancer can be difficult to differentiate from an upper pole renal cell carcinoma, given that both types of tumor tend to be large, locally invasive, and heterogeneous in appearance, and they enhance with the administration of intravenous contrast material. However, making the correct preoperative diagnosis is irrelevant to a point, because surgical excision of the mass is the treatment of choice for either type of malignancy.

**Table 7–3:** The surgical treatment of adrenal tumors.

The treatment of adrenocorticocarcinoma is largely surgical, involving the removal of the tumor and surrounding involved tissue (Table 7–3). Given the large size and locally invasive nature of these cancers, wide surgical exposure is mandatory, using a transabdominal incision. On occasion, bowel resection, splenec-

tomy, nephrectomy, and partial pancreatectomy may be needed to render the patient free of tumor. Smaller tumors can be resected using a lumbotomy approach or a laparoscopic technique, although such minimally invasive approaches are probably best reserved for patients who have benign adrenal lesions and no masses that are suspected of being cancerous. For patients with metastatic cancer, the results of chemotherapy and radiotherapy have been poor, with only mitotane and aminoglutethimide showing biologic activity against the cancer.

## TABLE 7–3

### SURGICAL OPTIONS FOR ADRENAL TUMORS

| TUMOR TYPE | SURGICAL APPROACH |
| --- | --- |
| Benign, functional adenoma | Posterior dorsal lumbotomy<br>Laparoscopic<br>Eleventh rib flank approach<br>Transthoracic |
| Adrenal carcinoma | Thoracoabdominal<br>Bilateral transabdominal chevron<br>Anterior subcostal<br>Eleventh rib flank approach |
| Pheochromocytoma | Thoracoabdominal<br>Bilateral transabdominal chevron<br>Eleventh rib flank approach<br>Laparoscopic (smaller lesions) |

**Figure 7–12:** See Color Section. Histologic appearance of adrenocorticocarcinoma. High-power (400×) magnification shows moderate nuclear pleomorphism and hyperchromasia, which are characteristic for carcinoma.

**Figure 7–13:** Evaluation of the incidental renal mass. The initial work-up primarily involves the determination of whether the renal mass is cystic or solid. Purely simple cysts are benign and need no further evaluation. In contrast, more complex cystic lesions need evaluation. Although such cysts can be aspirated, the reliability of cyst aspiration to predict the presence or absence of malignancy is poor. Most complex cysts should be considered malignant until proved otherwise. In general, all solid masses of the kidney (especially those that enhance with the administration of intravenous contrast material) should also be considered malignant. The treatment of these lesions involves either radical or partial nephrectomy, depending on the size and location of the tumor. However, for very small lesions, for which ultrasound or CT scanning is unable to determine the solid or cystic nature, serial observation can be used. Surgical removal of the lesion is then performed if the mass grows in size over time. Additionally, if the patient has a prior history of malignancy (especially of breast cancer, melanoma, or kidney cancer), needle biopsy of the mass can also be considered to rule out a metastasis to the kidney. For patients in whom there is a history of lymphoma, or with multiple intraparenchymal nodules, diffuse replacement of the kidney with tumor, or significant adenopathy, the diagnosis of renal lymphoma should also be considered with percutaneous biopsy appropriate in that circumstance as well.[15] For patients with metastatic cancer or lymphoma of the kidney, systemic chemotherapy might be a more appropriate treatment option than nephrectomy.

**Figure 7–14:** Genetics of renal cell carcinoma, showing the familial occurrence of renal cell carcinoma in multiple von Hippel–Lindau kindreds (*A*) and the location of the von Hippel–Lindau (VHL) gene on chromosome 11p25 (*B*). Because of the existence of familial renal cell carcinoma, as well as hereditary cancers that occur in syndromes such as the von Hippel–Lindau syndrome, some of the genes that are involved in the initiation and promotion of renal cell carcinoma have been identified. The *VHL* gene is transmitted in an autosomally dominant manner but has incomplete penetrance. Patients who carry the *VHL* gene tend to suffer from multifocal, bilateral renal cell carcinomas that strike at an early age. Besides the VHL syndrome, patients who have tuberous sclerosis, acquired cystic diseases of the kidney, or autosomal dominant polycystic kidney disease also have an increased risk for renal cell carcinoma. Through intense study of these kindreds that have familial renal cell carcinoma, the *VHL* gene was recently identified and was found to be located at chromosome 3p25.[16] It has been hypothesized that the VHL protein functions as a cell-cycle regulator, able to control cellular proliferation by restricting gene transcription, translation, or repair. Unfortunately, only 45% to 60% of all patients with sporadic renal call cancer have a detectable mutation in the VHL gene, with other genetic lesions in the Pax2 oncogene, or in the G250 gene also probably related to the initiation or promotion of kidney cancer.[17, 18] (From Linehan WM, et al: Genetic basis of renal cell cancer. In Devita VT, Hellman S, Rosenberg SA [eds]: Important Advances in Oncology. Philadelphia, JB Lippincott, 1993, pp 47–70.)

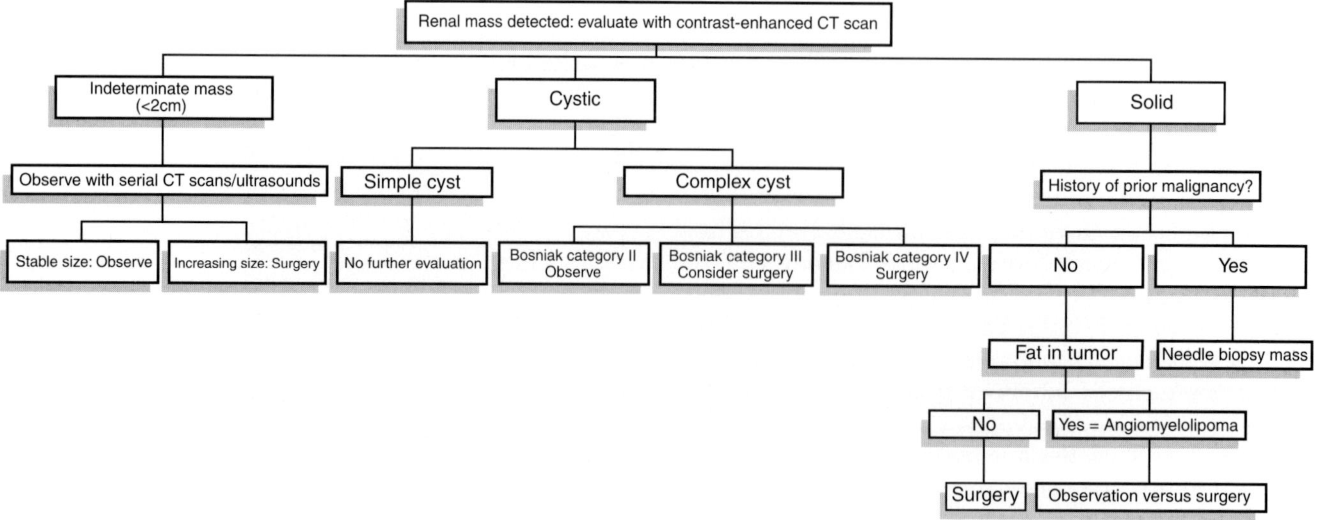



**Figure 7–13**

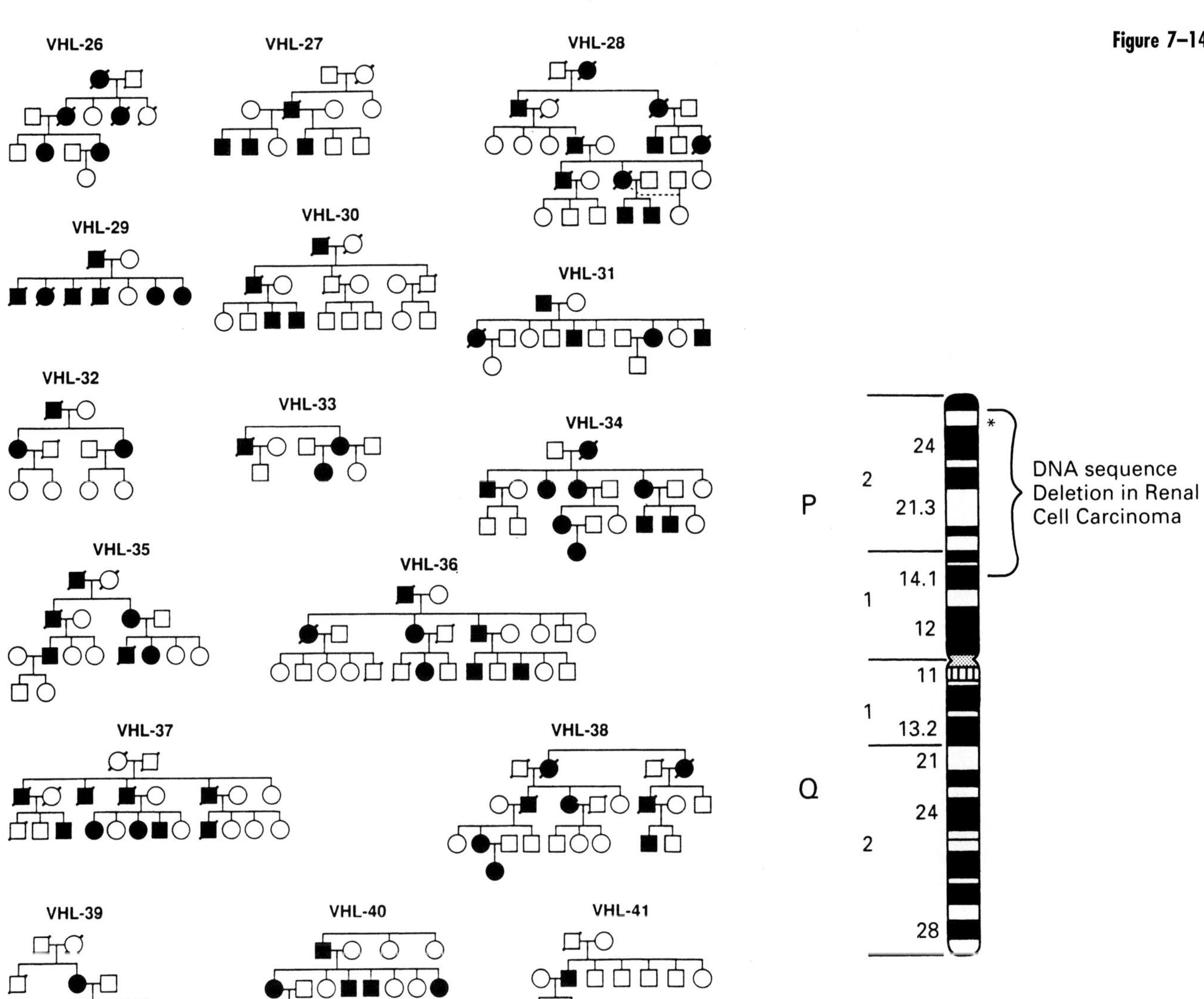



**Figure 7–15:** See Color Section. Histology of renal cell carcinoma. High-power magnification shows clear cell carcinoma exhibiting an alveolar pattern. Cells are in compact nests with clear cytoplasm and enlarged, irregular nuclei. Nucleoli are prominent.

**Table 7–4:** Signs and symptoms of renal cell carcinoma. Renal cell carcinoma presents with a wide variety of symptoms and signs. Because of the kidney's well-protected position deep in the retroperitoneum, the classic findings of flank pain, hematuria, and a palpable mass usually do not occur together until the tumor becomes large and advanced. However, at least one or two of these signs will usually occur in patients with renal cell carcinoma, and the problem will then initiate a diagnostic search for the cause of the symptoms. Hypercalcemia, polycythemia, elevated liver function tests (Stauffer's syndrome), and an elevated erythrocyte sedimentation rate are some of the other findings that can be associated with renal cell carci-

noma. The diagnosis of renal cell cancer can be made by intravenous pyelography (IVP) or on renal ultrasound, although a CT scan is usually required to confirm the diagnosis.

## TABLE 7–4

### SYMPTOMS OF RENAL CELL CARCINOMA

| SYMPTOM | FREQUENCY (%) |
| --- | --- |
| Classic triad of hematuria, flank pain, and abdominal mass | 10% |
| Pain | 41% |
| Hematuria | 38% |
| Mass | 24% |
| Weight loss | 36% |
| Fever | 18% |
| Hypertension | 22% |
| Hypercalcemia | 6% |

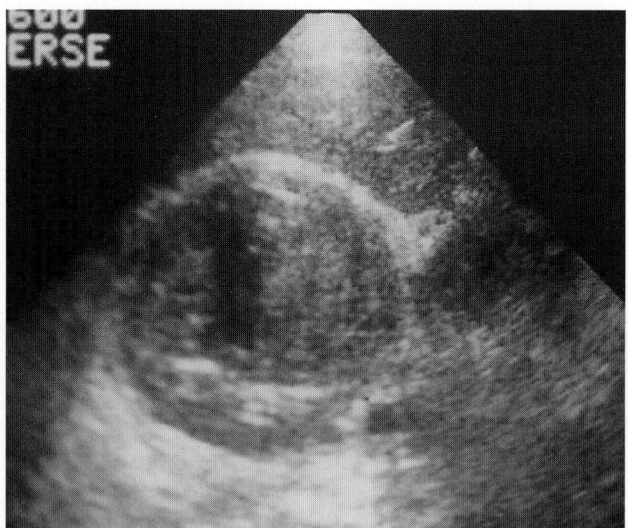

**Figure 7–16**

**Figure 7–16:** Diagnosis of renal cell carcinoma, showing a renal mass on ultrasound. With the widespread use of ultrasound to evaluate a multitude of patient symptoms, the number of renal masses that are found incidentally is increasing. Renal ultrasound is safe, rapid, and noninvasive: furthermore, there is no risk secondary to radiation exposure or iodine dye allergy. Ultrasound can provide accurate information about the size and character of a mass (cystic versus solid), and can detect the presence of obstruction. However, because of the limitations of ultrasound, most patients will need radiologic evaluation with CT scanning or MRI if a solid mass or complex cyst is found on ultrasound.

**Figure 7–17:** Diagnosis and clinical staging of renal cell carcinoma, showing a renal mass on contrast-enhanced CT scanning. The contrast-enhanced CT scan permits (1) confirmation of the solid, heterogeneous, contrast-enhancing nature of the mass and allows for (2) evaluation of the liver, adrenal glands, contralateral kidney, and lymphatics for signs of metastasis. The appearance of renal cell carcinoma on CT scan can be considered diagnostic for the disease. Local extension of the tumor and renal vein/vena caval involvement can also be inferred from the CT scan.

The staging system for renal cell carcinoma is discussed in Chapter 6. Prior to treatment of the renal lesion, a chest x-ray with oblique films (or a chest CT scan) is required to complete the metastatic survey; bone scans, head CT scans, renal angiograms, abdominal MRIs, vena cavagrams, and transesophageal cardiac ultrasound scans can also be obtained as clinically indicated. Tumor stage is based on the size of the primary tumor, extent of local disease, and the presence or absence of metastasis to the lymphatics, lung, liver, bone, or brain.

**Figure 7–18:** Bosniak classification of renal cysts. The classic Bosniak system was used to categorize cystic lesions as seen on CT scanning, but the classification system can also be used to categorize lesions that are seen on renal ultrasound.[19] A category I cyst is a simple, benign cyst that is anechoic on ultrasound with a sharply defined, smooth, thin wall. Category II cysts

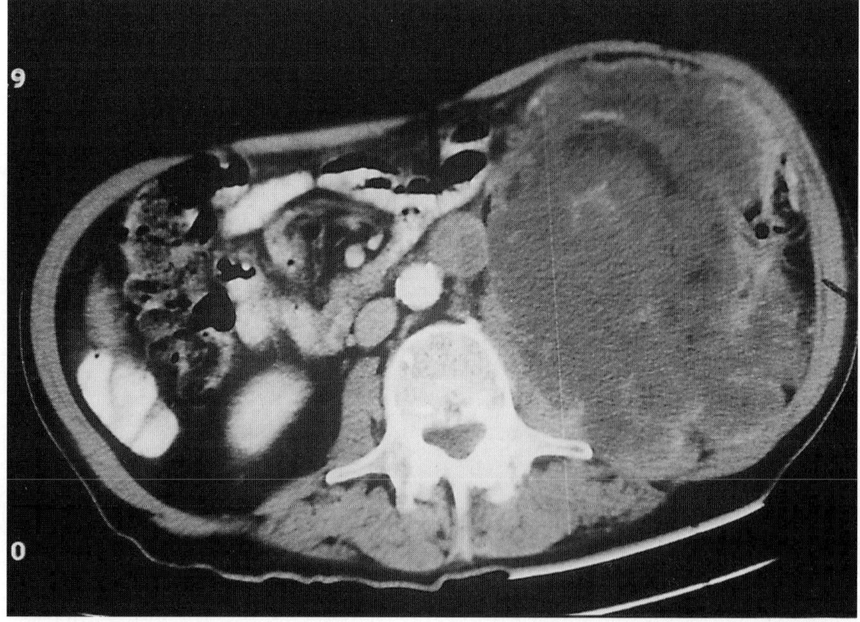

**Figure 7–17**

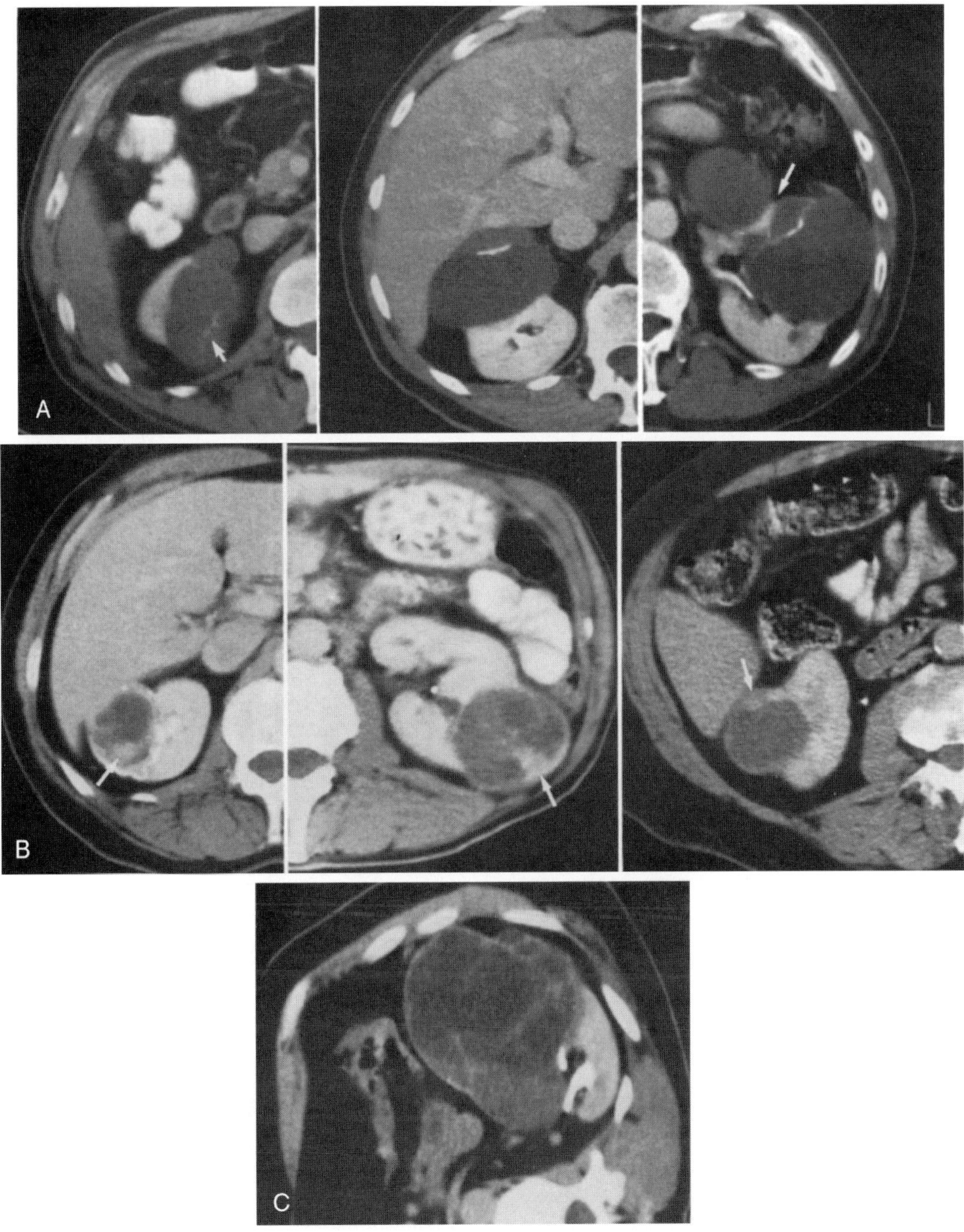

**Figure 7–18**

are only minimally complex, with thin septae, anechoic contents, and small amounts of calcification in the wall (*A*). These cysts can also be considered benign. In contrast, the risk of malignancy is increased with category III or IV lesions (*B* and *C*). Features that put a mass into these categories include the presence of a thickened and irregular cyst wall, thickened septae, nodularity within the cyst, large or non–border-forming calcifications, or contrast enhancement seen on CT scanning. Category IV lesions have at least three of these features and have a 95% probability that they are malignant, and category III lesions have one or two features and have a 50% risk that they are cancerous. In general, category I lesions are treated as benign, and category IV lesions are treated as malignant, with relative degrees of uncertainty existing regarding the best treatment approach for category II and III lesions. (From Bosniak MA: Problems in the radiologic diagnosis of renal parenchymal tumors. Urol Clin North Am 20[2]:218–220, 1993.)

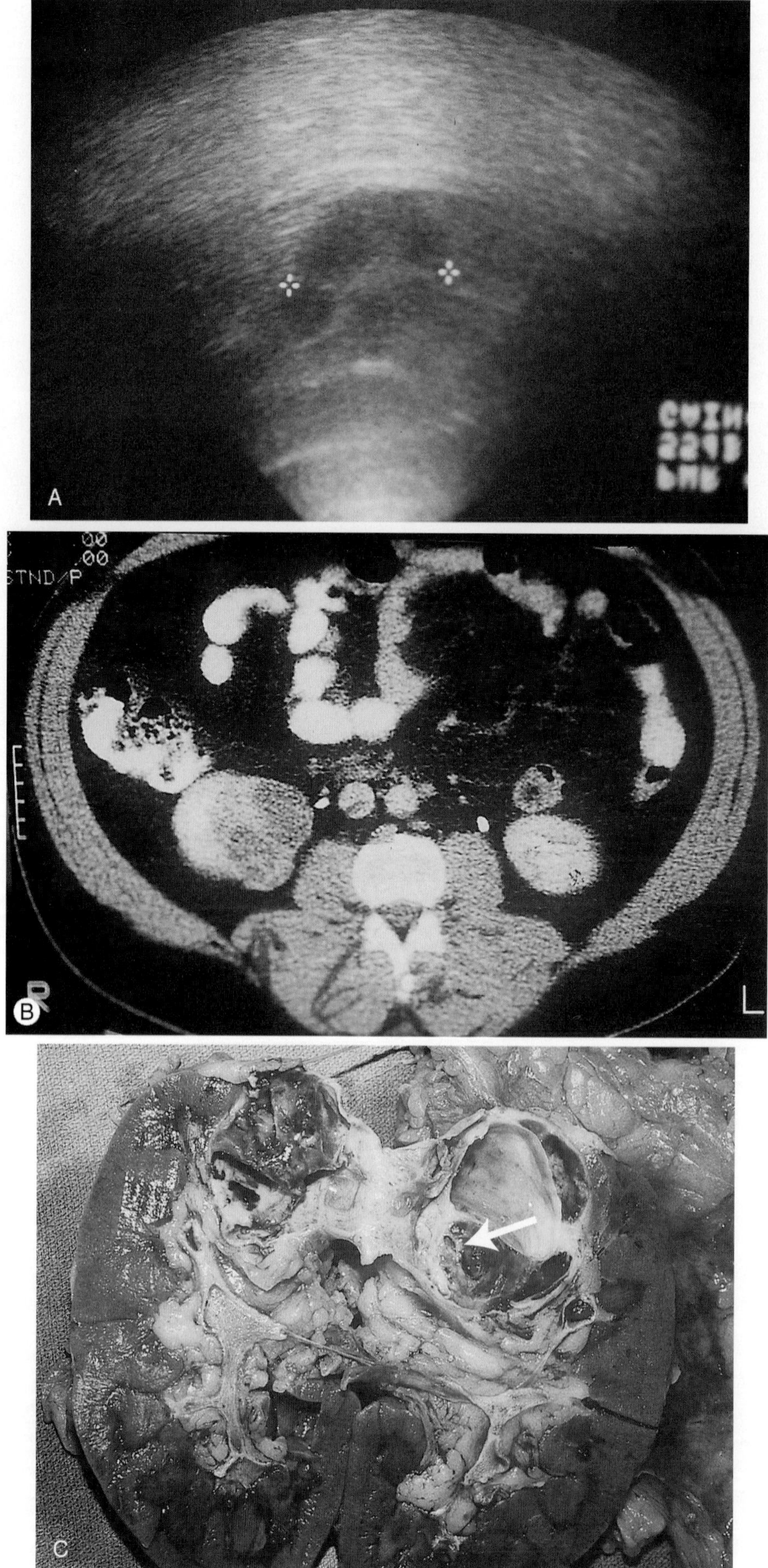

**Figure 7–19**

**Figure 7–19:** Cystic renal cell cancer, as imaged on ultrasound (*A*) and on CT scanning (*B*), with the tumor seen on the cyst wall (*arrow*) in the bisected pathologic specimen (*C*). The presence of thick septations, internal echoes, and a cyst wall that enhances on CT scanning with the administration of intravenous contrast material made this a Bosniak 4 lesion. The presence of a mass on the cyst wall or calcifications in the cyst are also highly suspicious for malignancy. The radiologic findings shown in *A* and *B* were considered pathognomonic for cystic renal cell carcinoma, which was confirmed at the time of radical nephrectomy (*C*).

**Figure 7–20:** Staging on vena caval extension for renal cell carcinoma. Renal cell carcinoma is one of the few cancers that has the propensity for invading vascular structures. However, if the tumor thrombus can be extracted completely from the vena cava, the impact on prognosis appears to be minimal as long as complete resection of the primary tumor is also achievable.[20] The level of vena caval involvement of the tumor is important to determine prior to surgery, because the surgical approach will be largely determined by the degree that the vena cava is involved. Because extraction of the tumor thrombus involves the performance of wide incision in the vena cava, the key to the operation involves proximal and distal control of the cava to minimize intraoperative blood loss. For tumor thrombi that extend either just into the vena cava or at a level below the hepatic veins, control of the vena cava can be obtained through the simple application of vascular clamps above and below the tumor. However, for tumors that extend behind the liver and into the chest, cardiopulmonary bypass, hypothermic cardiac arrest, and exsanguination of the patient may be needed to empty the cava of blood and therefore permit safe extraction of the tumor thrombus. (From Libertino JA, Cyr J, Zinman L: Renal cell carcinoma with extension into the vena cava. In Libertino JA [ed]: Pediatric and Adult Reconstructive Urology. Baltimore, Williams & Wilkins, 1987, p 111, Fig. 11.1.)

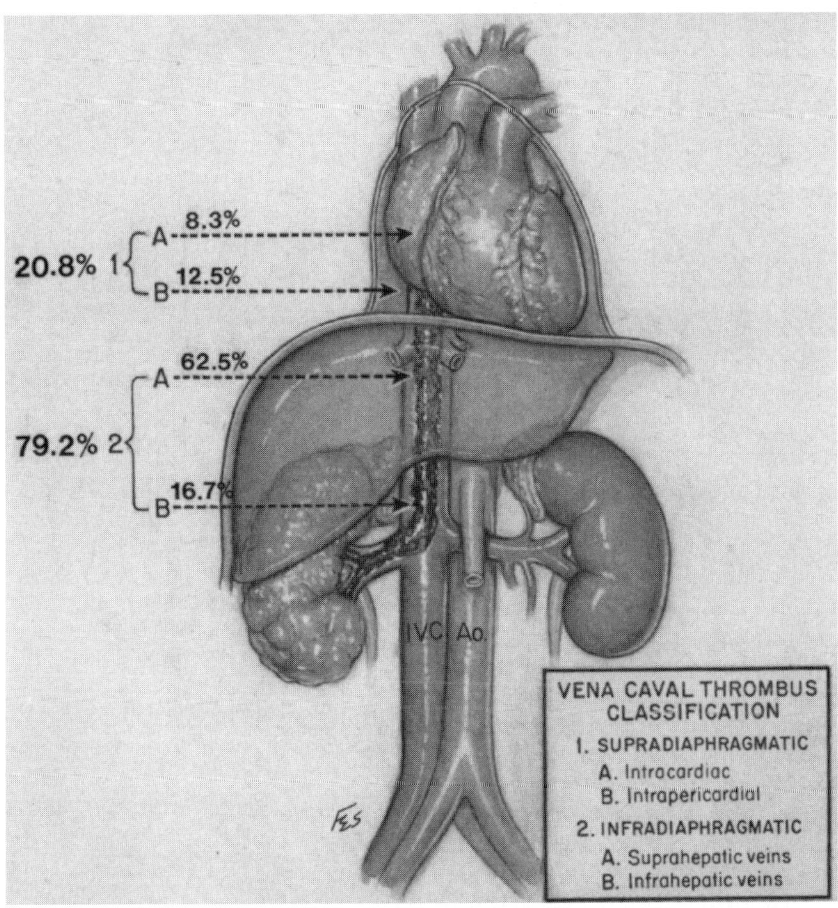


**Figure 7–20**

**Figure 7–21:** Patient with tumor thrombus extending into the right atrium on MRI on a coronal view (*A*), with atriotomy showing tumor growing into the heart (*B*), and the final pathologic specimen showing the tongue of tumor growing out of the renal vein (*C*) [see Color Section]. This patient presented with a relatively small primary tumor but had a caval thrombus extending into the atrium. Although CT scanning can often suggest that a thrombus is present, a vena cavagram, abdominal MRI, or transesophageal echocardiogram are necessary to fully evaluate the extent of the thrombus in the vena cava. *A*, In this patient, tumor can be seen running in the vena cava behind the liver and up into the right atrium (*arrow*) on MRI. Given the extension into the heart, the patient was approached through a midline transabdominal incision that extended into the chest to expose the heart. The patient was subsequently placed on cardiopulmonary bypass and hypothermic cardiac arrest. *B*, Upon opening the atrium, the tip of the tumor could be seen entering the right atrium from the inferior vena cava. After performing a wide cavotomy, the thrombus was fully exposed and extracted intact from the patient. Since there was no other sign of cancer, the patient's long-term prognosis for cure after the surgery is good.

**Figure 7–22:** Treatment of renal cell carcinoma. The treatment of kidney cancer is largely surgical because there is no effective chemotherapy, hormone-based

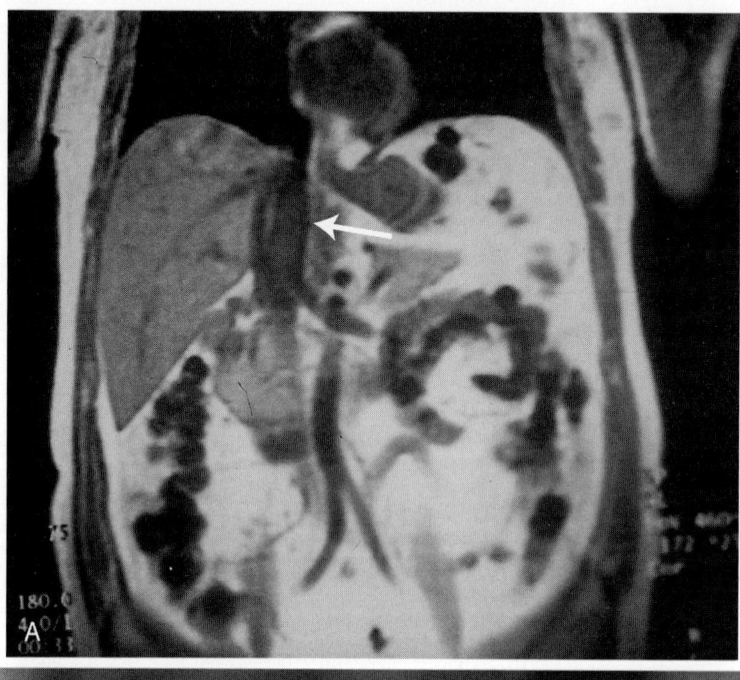

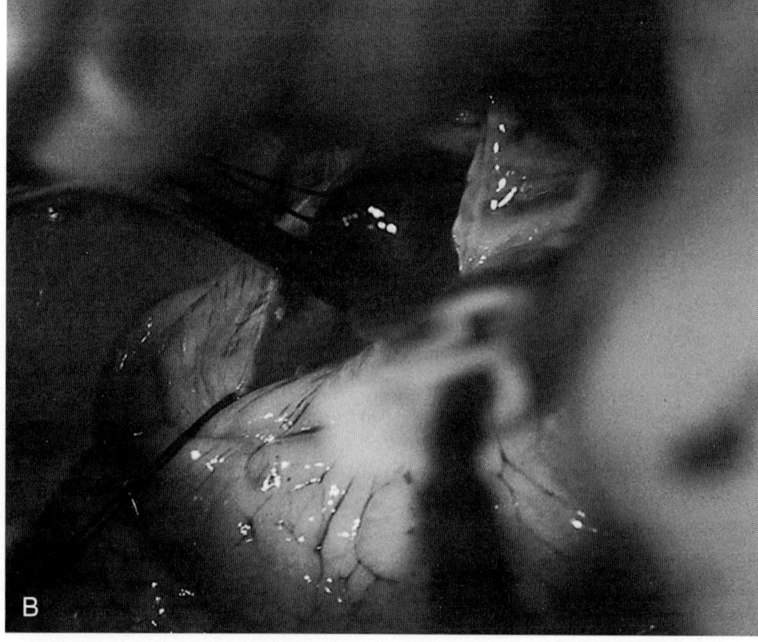

Figure 7–21

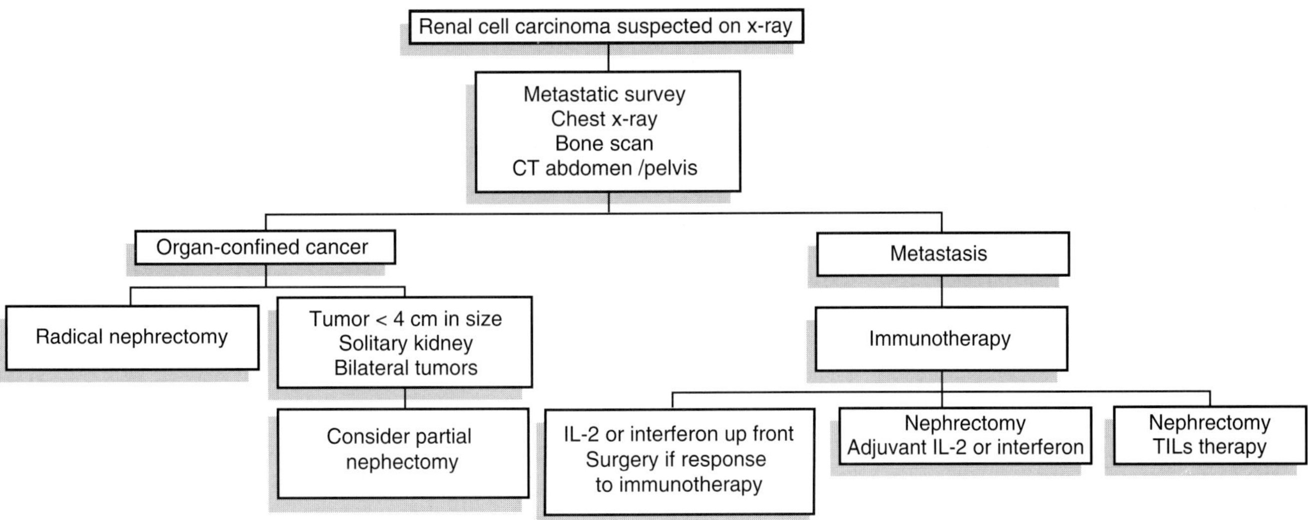


**Figure 7–22**

therapy, or radiotherapy for the patient who has metastatic kidney cancer. The standard treatment for the patient who has a localized, solid mass in the kidney is radical nephrectomy, although for some patients, a partial nephrectomy may also be considered. Surgery offers the best chance at cure, and removal of the tumor may also involve a simultaneous, en bloc resection of the spleen, distal pancreas, liver, bowel, vena cava, or abdominal wall in addition to the radical nephrectomy. For the patient who has metastatic cancer at the time of diagnosis, interleukin 2 and interferon-based immunotherapies offer some hope for cure. The options for the patient with advanced renal cell carcinoma include up-front immunotherapy using systemic interleukin 2 or interferon (reserving nephrectomy for the patients in whom the distant metastasis resolved with IL-2 treatment), nephrectomy followed by adjuvant IL-2 or interferon immunotherapy, or nephrectomy followed by treatment with tumor-infiltrating lymphocytes (TILs). Using these immunologically based treatments for metastatic disease, response rates between 14% and 40% have been reported, with cellular based TILs therapy having the highest rates of cure so far.[21]

**Table 7–5:** Indications for partial nephrectomy for renal cell carcinoma. The absolute indications for partial nephrectomy in cases of renal cell carcinoma involve circumstances in which the patient is at risk for renal failure if radical nephrectomy were to be performed. If there are bilateral renal tumors, tumors in a functionally or anatomically solitary kidney, or if the risk of a contralateral tumor in the future is high (such as in patients who have the von Hippel–Lindau syndrome), a nephron-sparing approach should be considered. However, as more tumors are discovered incidentally, smaller renal lesions are being detected that are amenable to partial nephrectomy, even when the contralateral kidney is normal. Although many renal lesions may be suitable for partial nephrectomy, such surgery should be reserved for patients who have

lesions that are smaller than 3 to 4 cm in diameter, because of the increased risk of multifocality with larger lesions. Currently, disease-free survival of patients does not appear to be compromised when nephron-sparing surgery is applied to lesions that are smaller than 3.5 to 4 cm in diameter.[22] In a recent analysis, patients who underwent partial nephrectomies with T2 lesions (1997 TNM) demonstrated a significant decrease in survival (66%) when compared to patients with T1 lesions (100%, $p < 0.001$).[23] The preoperative evaluation for the patient being considered for partial nephrectomy consists of the standard metastatic evaluation, including a search for satellite lesions in the ipsilateral kidney. For polar lesions and smaller peripherally based tumors, a preoperative renal artery angiogram is not routinely necessary. All other lesions should have a preoperative evaluation of the renal vasculature to determine the feasibility of partial nephrectomy, and to assist in the preservation of the blood supply to the remaining renal parenchyma.

## TABLE 7–5

### INDICATIONS FOR PARTIAL NEPHRECTOMY

| ABSOLUTE INDICATIONS | RELATIVE INDICATIONS |
| --- | --- |
| Tumor in an anatomically or functionally solitary kidney (congenital absence, prior surgery or trauma, chronic obstruction or infection in the contralateral kidney) | Tumor in patient in whom future renal function is at risk (renal artery stenosis, hydronephrosis, recurrent pyelonephritis, calculous disease) |
| Bilateral renal tumors, or tumors in patients with familial RCC syndromes (von Hippel–Lindau) | Incidental renal mass < 4 cm in diameter, when the lesion is positioned so that it is amenable to partial nephrectomy |

**Figure 7–23:** See Color Section. Technique of partial nephrectomy, involving complete exposure of the kidney (A), excision of the tumor with a margin of normal parenchyma (B), and placement of a hemostatic sponge into the parenchymal defect (C). Once the vasculature to the kidney is identified and controlled, the kidney itself is fully exposed by removing Gerota's fascia from the entire kidney (A). Gerota's fascia is left intact only above the tumor, with intraoperative ultrasound very helpful in pinpointing the location of the mass. Subsequently, the renal capsule is incised around the tumor, and blunt dissection is used to remove the tumor along with a margin of normal renal parenchyma (B). Individual bleeding sites are then controlled with suture ligatures, and a hemostatic sponge, perinephric fat, or omentum is placed into the parenchymal defect in order to provide an additional degree of hemostasis (C).

**Figure 7–24:** Metastatic renal cell cancer: metastasis to cheek (A) and to lung (B). Renal cell cancer spreads by hematogenous and lymphatic routes and can metastasize to any location in the body. The more common sites of metastatic spread involve the lung (B), pleura, lymph nodes, liver, adrenal, bone, and brain. As such, patients with renal cell carcinoma can present with a wide variety of symptoms secondary to metastatic disease, including a chronic cough, hemoptysis, weight loss, bone pain, and seizures. Cutaneous metastases are also not uncommon, with some patients diagnosed with renal cell carcinoma due to the results from a skin biopsy. Cutaneous metastases from renal cell carcinoma tend to be raised, rapidly growing, purple lesions (A):

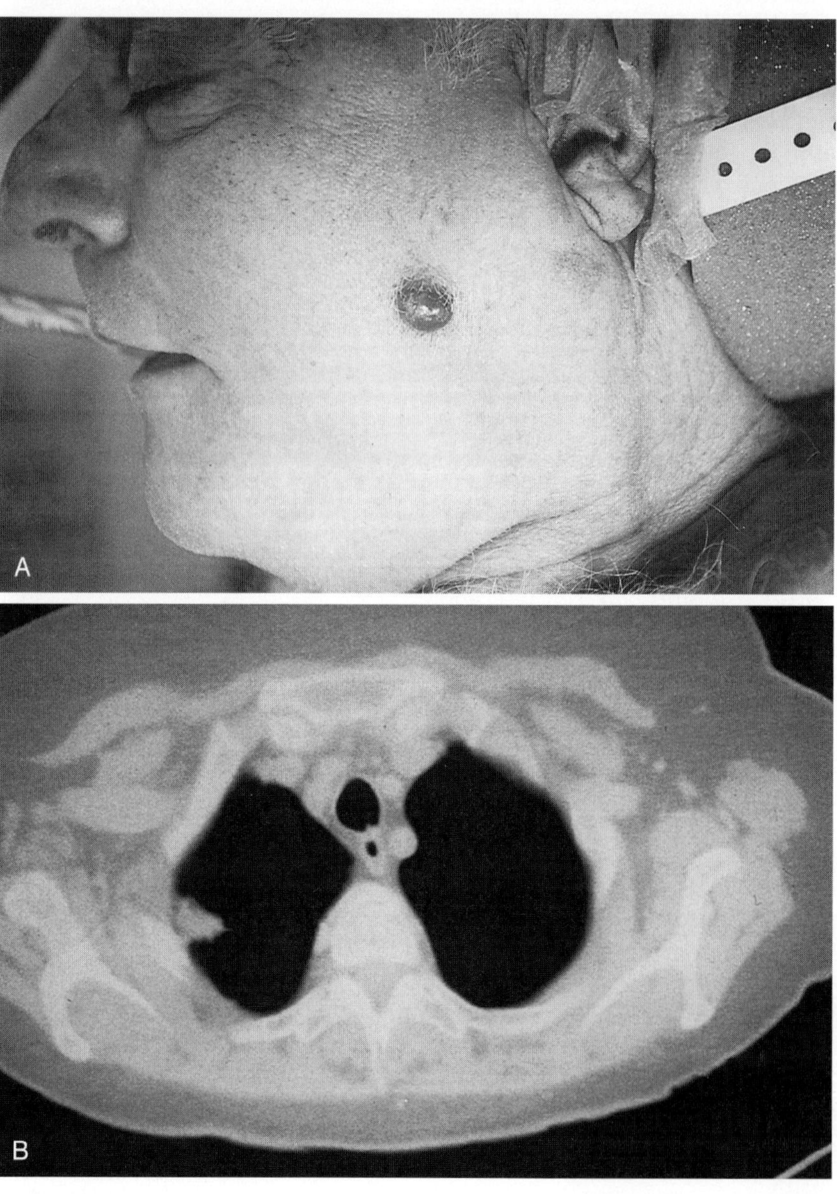


Figure 7–24

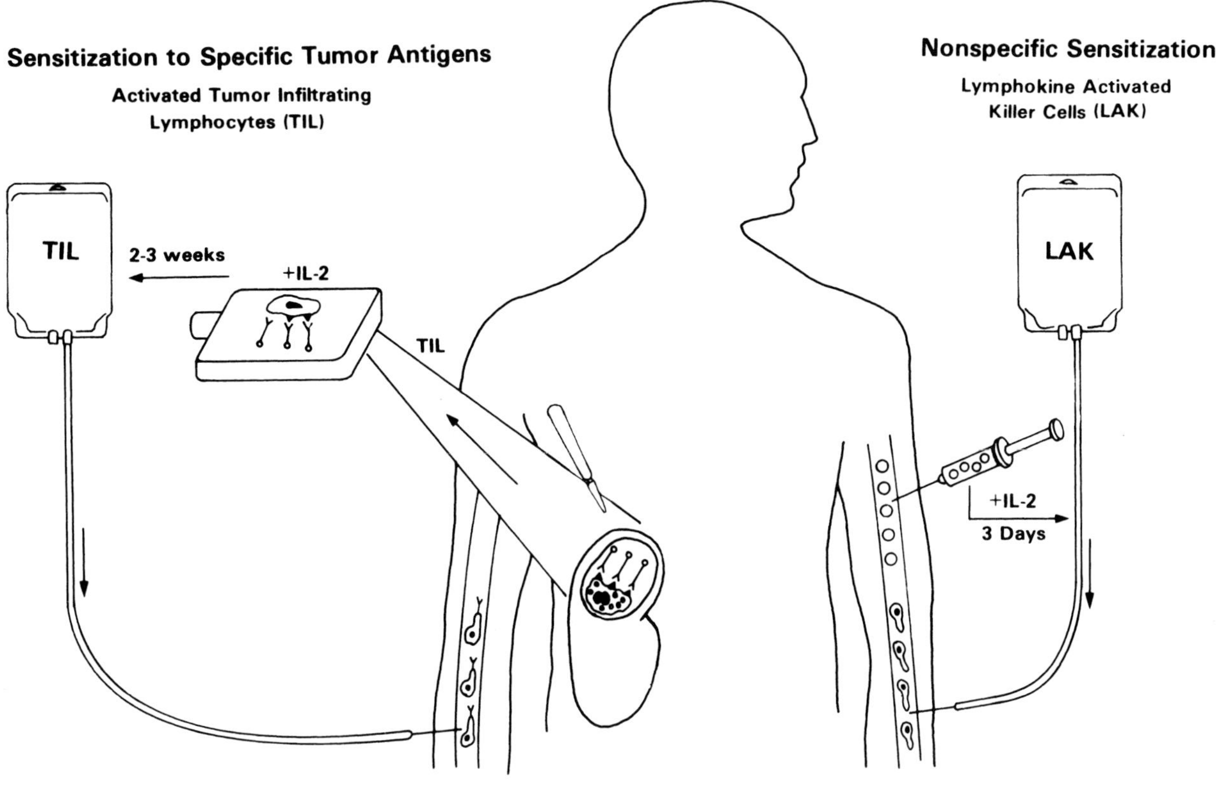


**Figure 7–25**

an excisional biopsy of any such lesion is mandatory so that the correct diagnosis can be made.

**Figure 7–25:** Mechanism for adoptive immunotherapy for renal cell carcinoma. There is no chemotherapy, hormone-based therapy, or radiotherapy that is effective for the treatment of metastatic kidney cancer. However, renal cell carcinoma is one of the few tumors that will respond to immunologic manipulation, in which stimulation of the immune system can result in the regression and even cure of selected patients who have metastatic carcinoma. In this approach, the patient can be given systemic interleukin 2 (IL-2) to stimulate the proliferation of T lymphocytes which then have direct, antitumor activity. Alternately, as depicted in the schematic, tumor-infiltrating lymphocytes (TILs) can be harvested from the primary tumor after radical nephrectomy, cultured, stimulated in the laboratory with cytokines in order to improve their ability to kill cancer cells, and then given back to the patient. In the authors' experience, TIL-based therapy has shown the greatest efficacy in the treatment of metastatic kidney cancer, with response rates of 38% reported.[3, 20] (From Belldegrun A, deKernion JB: Renal tumors. In Walsh PC, Retik AB, Stamey TA, Vaughan ED [eds]: Campbell's Urology, 6th ed. Philadelphia, WB Saunders, 1992, p 1080, Fig. 27–23.)

**Figure 7–26:** Diagnosis of transitional cell carcinoma of the kidney, with tumor apparent on retrograde pyelography (*A*), ureteroscopy (*B*), and CT scan showing filling defect in the renal pelvis (*C*). Transitional cell carcinoma (TCC) originates from the cells of the urothelial lining, and therefore can occur anywhere along the collecting system of the urinary tract. Although only 5% of all transitional cell carcinomas occur in the kidney, between 30% and 70% are associated with either a synchronous or metachronous lesion in the bladder.[5] A prior history of cigarette smoking or phenacetin abuse, or a history of industrial solvent or dye exposure have all been implicated in the pathogenesis of TCC. The most common presenting symptom is hematuria, with irritative voiding symptoms (dysuria, frequency, urgency) also occurring if the patient has an associated tumor in the bladder. Transitional cell carcinoma is usually diagnosed initially via intravenous pyelography, with retrograde pyelography, renal pelvic wash cytology, brush cytology, or retrograde ureterorenoscopy with biopsies used to confirm the diagnosis. When a TCC of the kidney is diagnosed via x-ray evaluation, endoscopy, cytology, or biopsy, a metastatic survey as well as a complete survey of the remainder of the urothelium is required to rule out the existence of other tumor foci elsewhere in the urinary tract.

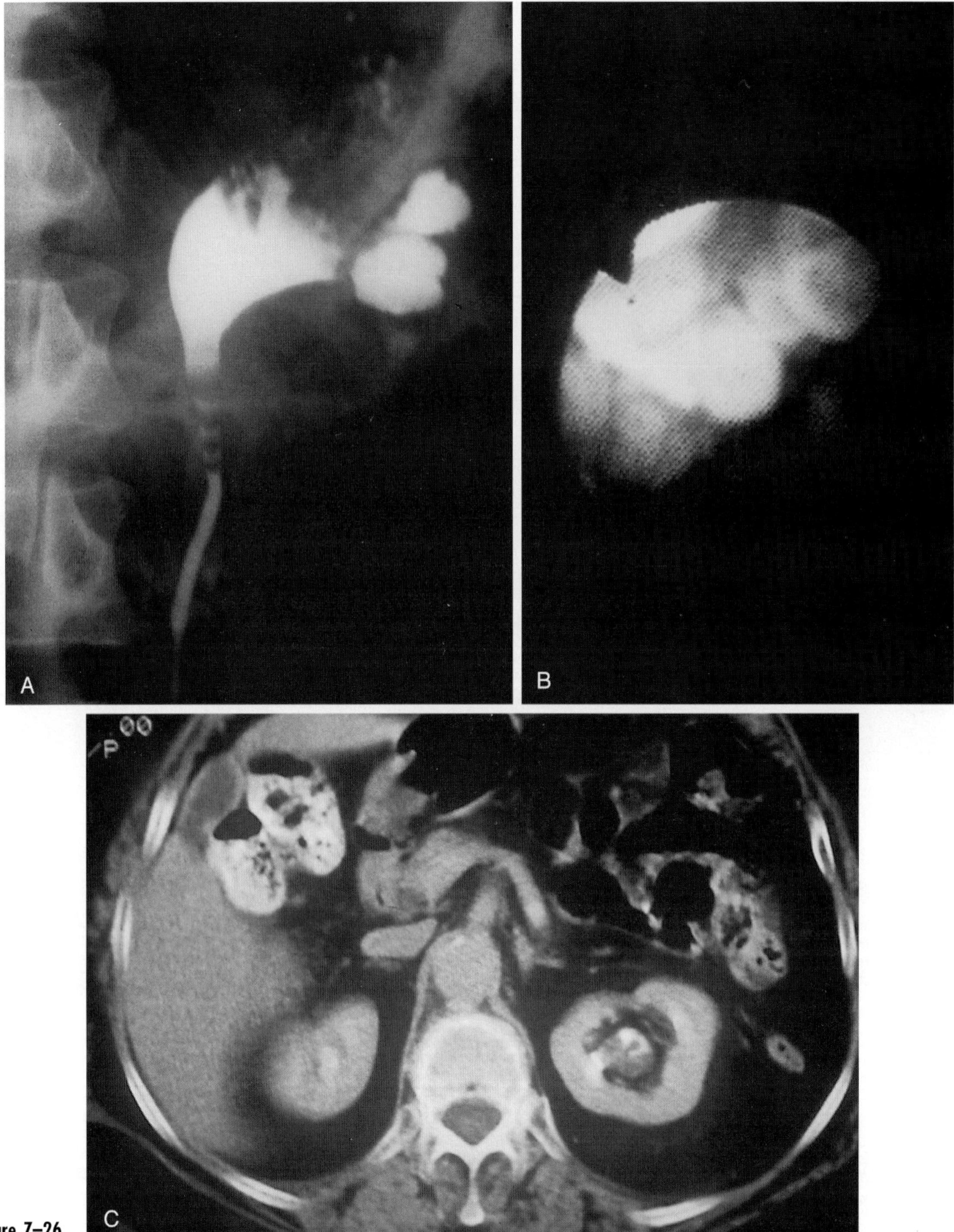

Figure 7–26

Figure 7–27: See Color Section. Histology of TCC of the kidney. High-powered magnification of a renal pelvic tumor shows papillary fronds with central vascular cores. The tumor cells have round to oval shapes and relatively uniform nuclei.

Figure 7–28: Treatment of transitional cell carcinoma of the kidney (A) using percutaneous techniques to visualize and resect the tumor (B), and adjuvant bacillus Calmette-Guérin (BCG) therapy. Three months following endourologic treatment and adjuvant BCG therapy, no evidence of cancer is seen on antegrade nephrostogram.

The standard treatment of upper tract TCC is nephroureterectomy. When TCC involves the kidney, the entire ipsilateral ureter down to the level of the bladder must be removed because of the 30% risk of recurrence if the ureteral stump is left behind, and because of the inherent difficulty that exists in serially monitoring a distal ureteral stump for cancer recurrence.[22] However, in some cases, nephroureterectomy may not be the best option: for the patient with an anatomically or functionally solitary kidney, or for the patient who has low-grade, low-stage TCC of the kidney, renal preservation approaches can also be consid-

164

ered.[6] By using either endoscopic, retrograde intrarenal surgery, or endoscopic, percutaneous approaches to resect and ablate the tumor (in *B,* the fronds of tumor are seen in the endoscopic view), the tumor can be destroyed while leaving a functional renal unit. The addition of BCG into the renal collecting system can also be used as an adjuvant to further decrease the risk of cancer recurrence. Although it was successful in this patient who had a superficial grade II TCC in a solitary kidney (and is now 3 years out from treatment and still without signs of recurrence), this approach should be used with caution and only in patients who have low-grade, low-stage tumors.

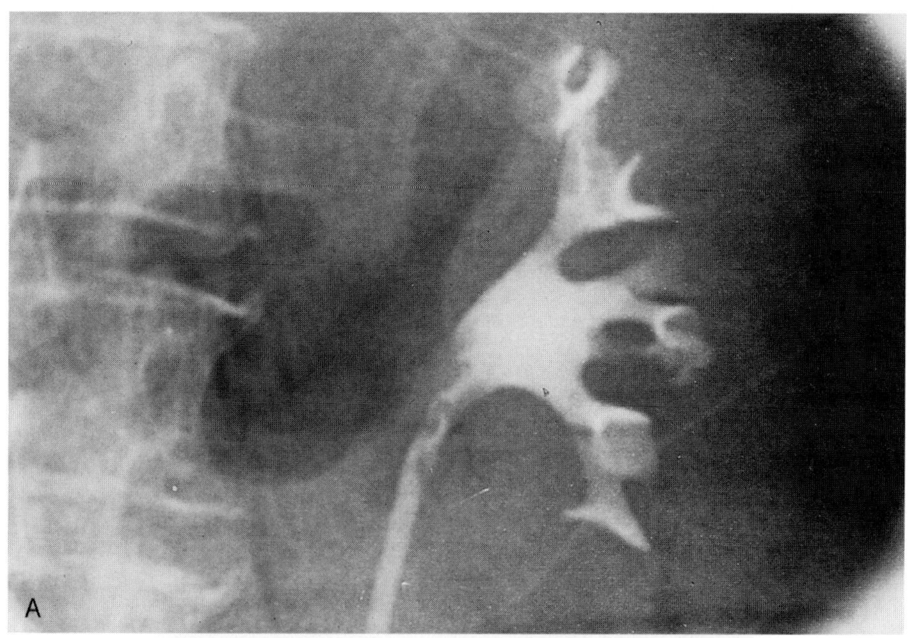

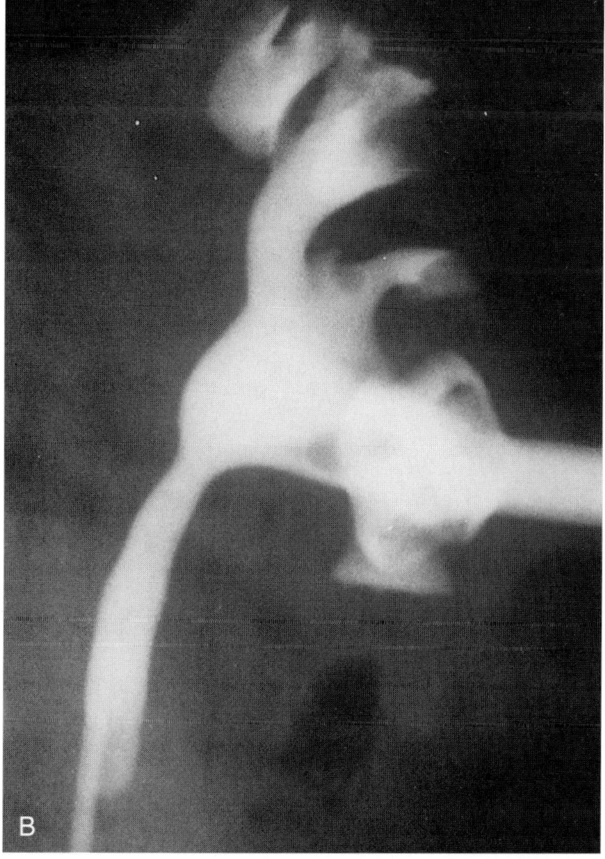

**Figure 7–28**

## REFERENCES

1. Greenlee RT, Hill-Harmon M, Murray T, Thun M: Cancer statistics. CA Cancer J Clin 51(1):15–36, 2001.
2. deKernion JB, Belldegrun A: Renal tumors. In Walsh PC, Retik AB, Stamey TA, Vaughan ED (eds): Campbell's Urology, 7th ed. Philadelphia, WB Saunders, 1997, pp 2283–2326.
3. Gitlitz BJ, Belldegrun A, Figlin RA: Immunotherapy and gene therapy. Semin Urol Oncol 14:237–243, 1996.
4. Figlin RA, Pierce WC, Kaboo R, et al: Treatment of metastatic renal cell carcinoma with nephrectomy, IL-2, and autologous primed or CD8(+) selected tumor infiltrating lymphocytes from primary tumor. J Urol 158:740–745, 1997.
5. Naitoh J, Walzak MP: Hereditary aspects of urologic cancer. Surg Oncol Clin North Am 3:609–640, 1994.
6. Catalona WJ: Urothelial tumors of the urinary tract. In Walsh PC, Retik AB, Stamey TA, Vaughan ED (eds): Campbell's Urology, 7th Ed. Philadelphia, WB Saunders, 1997, pp 2283–2326.
7. Jarrett TW, Seetse PM, Weiss GH, Smith AD: Percutaneous management of transitional cell carcinoma of the renal collecting system: 9 year experience. J Urol 154:1629–1635, 1995.
8. Belldegrun A, Hussain S, Seltzer SC, et al: Incidentally discovered mass of the adrenal gland. Surg Gynecol Obstet 163:203–208, 1986.
9. Belldegrun A, Richie JP: Tumors of the adrenal gland. In Graham SD (ed): Urologic Oncology, New York, Raven Press, 1986, pp 243–266.
10. Vaughan ED, Blumenfeld JD: The adrenals. In Walsh PC, Retik AB, Stamey TA, Vaughan ED (eds): Campbell's Urology, 7th Ed. Philadelphia, WB Saunders, 1997, pp 2915–2957.
11. Shapiro B, Copp JE, Sisson JC, et al: Iodine 131 metaiodobenzylguanidine for the locating of suspected pheochromocytoma: Experience in 400 cases. J Nucl Med 26:576–578, 1985.
12. Whalen RK, Althausen AF, Daniels GH: Extra-adrenal pheochromocytoma. J Urol 147:1–10, 1992.
13. Winfield HN, Hamilton BD, Bravo EL: Technique of laparoscopic adrenalectomy. Urol Clin North Am 24:459–465, 1996.
14. Heniford BT, Arca MJ, Walsh RM, Gill IS: Laparascopic adrenalectomy for cancer. Semin Surg Oncol 16:293–306, 1999.
15. Heiken JP, Gold RP, Schnur MJ, et al: Computed tomography of renal lymphoma with ultrasound correlation. J Comput Assist Tomogr 7:245–250, 1983.
16. Linehan WM, Lerman MI, Zbar B: Identification of the von Hippel Lindau gene. JAMA 273:564–570, 1995.
17. Gnarra JR, Dressler GR: Expression of pax-2 in human renal cell carcinoma and growth inhibition by antisense oligonucleotides. Cancer Res 55:4092–4095, 1995.
18. Oosterwijk E, Bander NH, Divgi CR: Antibody localization in human renal cell carcinoma: A phase I study of the monoclonal antibody G250. J Clin Oncol 11:738–745, 1993.
19. Bosniak MA: Problems in the radiologic diagnosis of renal parenchymal tumors. Urol Clin North Am 20:217–230, 1993.
20. Libertino JA, Cyr J, Zinman L: Renal cell carcinoma with extension into the vena cava. In Libertino JA (ed): Pediatric and Adult Reconstructive Urologic Surgery. Baltimore, Williams & Wilkins, 1987, pp 109–118.
21. Franklin JR, Figlin R, Rauch J, et al: Cytoreductive surgery in the management of metastatic renal cell carcinoma: The UCLA experience. Semin Urol Oncol 14:237–243, 1996.
22. Novick AC: Indications and results of partial nephrectomy for renal cell carcinoma. AUA Update Series 28:222–227, 1996.
23. Belldegrun A, Tsui K-H, deKernion JB, Smith RB: Efficacy of nephron-sparing surgery for renal cell carcinoma: Analysis based on the new 1997 tumor-node metastasis staging system. J Clin Oncol 17(9):2868–2875, 1999.
24. Naitoh J, Smith RB: Complications of renal surgery. In Taneja SS, Smith RB, Ehrlich R (eds): Complications of Urologic Surgery. Philadelphia, WB Saunders, 2001.

# 8

# Systemic Therapy of Renal Cell Carcinoma

*Ronald Bukowski*

## INTRODUCTION

Renal cell carcinoma is the most common neoplasm developing in the kidney and is diagnosed in approximately 31,000 individuals annually.[1] At time of diagnosis, 30% of patients have metastatic disease, and 40% of patients initially treated with surgery will develop metastases.[2] This tumor arises in the proximal renal tubular epithelium and histologically may contain clear cells, granular cells, or spindle cells.[3] The disease typically occurs in adults during the sixth to seventh decades of life, but it has been reported in young infants. The etiology of the neoplasm has not been defined, and both sporadic and hereditary forms have been described. This tumor was classically described as one of the great mimics in medicine because a variety of symptoms can develop that are not directly related to the tumor, such as anemia, erythrocytosis, and hepatomegaly.

In the presence of disease localized to the kidney, surgical removal is the only curative therapy. In patients with locally advanced stages or metastatic disease, therapy remains inadequate. In selected instances, surgery for removal of limited disease is utilized; however, in the majority of patients this is not possible. Systemic therapy with hormones or chemotherapy is ineffective. The recognition that the immune response may have antitumor effects in patients with renal cell carcinoma has resulted in a wide variety of approaches employing biologic therapy. The cytokines interferon-alpha (IFN-α) and interleukin 2 (IL-2) are widely utilized either alone or in combination. Response rates are generally less than 20%, but a subset of individuals having good performance status (defined as minimal or no symptoms) may develop durable complete regressions. Novel approaches employing adoptive transfer of immune cells, genetic-based vaccines, and new agents in combination with cytokines are under study. Experimental approaches remain an important component of therapy for this tumor.

**Figure 8–1:** The most common histologic type of renal cell carcinoma is the clear cell type *(A).* Between 1% and 6% of tumors contain spindle cells or pleomorphic giant cells and comprise the sarcomatoid variant *(B).* This latter variety is generally associated with a poorer prognosis.[4, 5] Most renal cell adenocarcinomas contain combinations of clear, granular, and spindle cells.[3]

**Figure 8–2: Unusual metastatic sites.** Patients with renal cell carcinoma frequently develop metastatic lesions in unusual locations. *A,* This patient with metastatic clear cell renal cancer presented with pain and tenderness over the right fifth metacarpal joint. The x-ray demonstrates a lytic lesion in the head of the fifth metacarpal bone. *B,* This magnetic resonance image (MRI) is from a patient with a primary renal cell carcinoma who presented with a soft-tissue mass in the proximal right lower extremity. The MRI demonstrates a metastatic tumor involving the medial aspect of the thigh; on biopsy, the tumor was found to be a clear cell carcinoma.

**Table 8–1: Staging of renal cell carcinoma.** Therapy of advanced renal cancer is dependent on stage, tumor location, comorbid factors in the patient, and patient acceptance. The staging systems utilized are illustrated in Table 8–1. The most commonly used system is the Robson Modification of the Flocks/Kadesky system.[6] In this system, advanced stages include IIIB (hilar lymph node [LN] involvement) or IV (local organ invasion/metastatic disease). The TNM classification discussed in Chapter 6 more accurately depicts the extent of tumor involvement, differentiates the extent of LN involvement (N1, N2, or N3), and includes in stage IV those patients with N2 or N3 lymph node disease.[7]

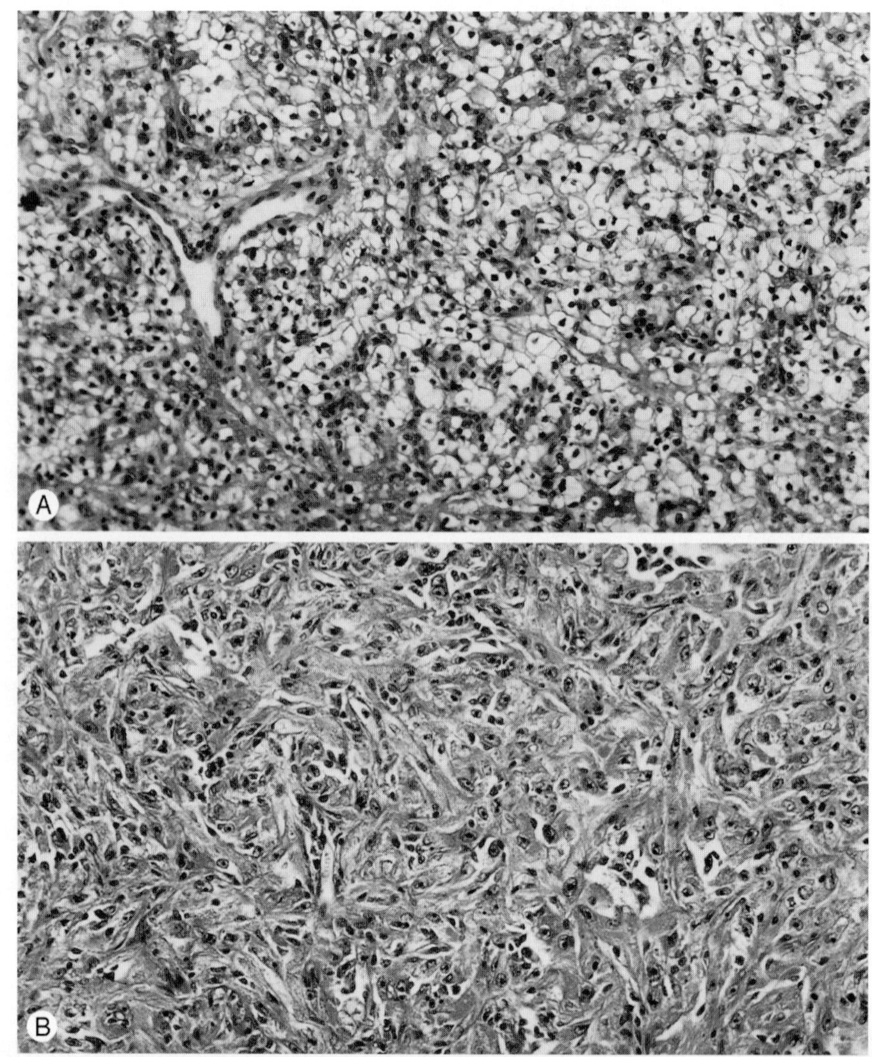

Figure 8–1

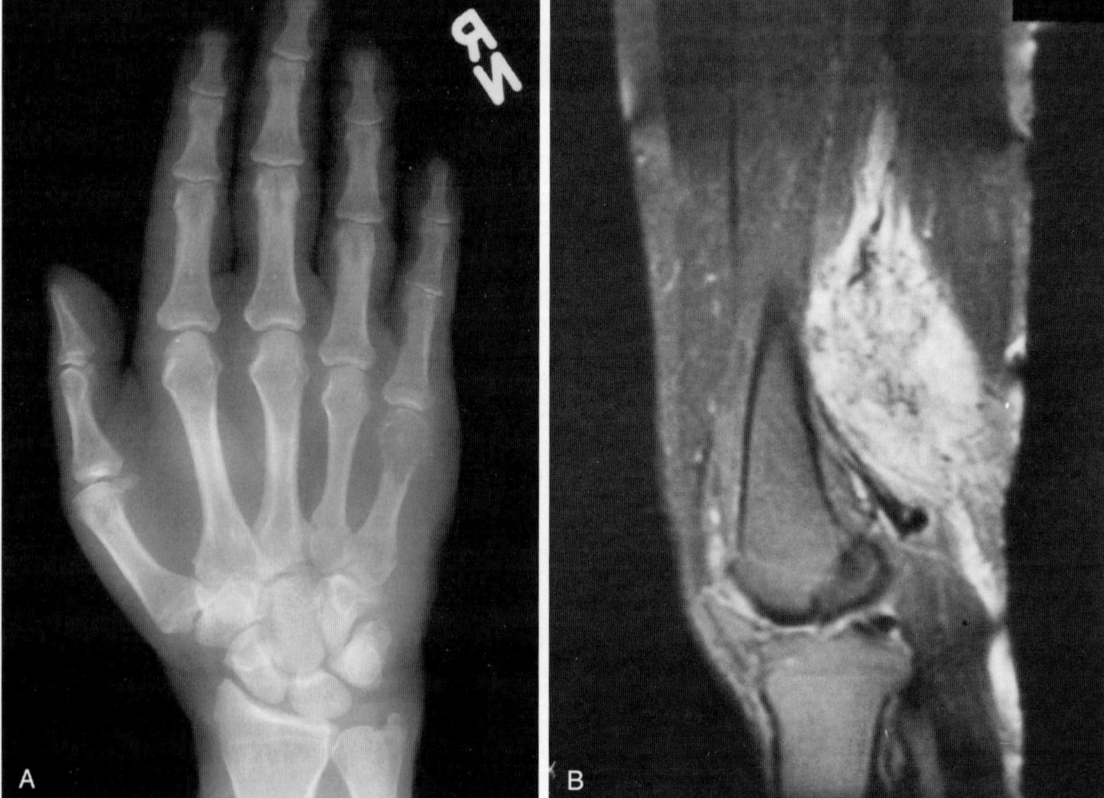

Figure 8–2

## TABLE 8–1

## RENAL CELL CARCINOMA STAGING SYSTEMS

| TNM CLASSIFICATION | | STAGE | TNM STAGES* | | | ROBSON MODIFICATION |
|---|---|---|---|---|---|---|
| T1 | ≤ 7.0 cm/limited to kidney | I | T1 | N0 | M0 | I |
| T2 | > 7.0 cm/limited to kidney | II | T2 | N0 | M0 | II |
| T3 | (a) Perinephric invasion | III | T1–2 | N1 | M0 | IIIB |
| | (b) Venous (major) invasion below diaphragm | | T3a-b | N0, 1 | M0 | IIIA or B |
| | (c) Venous invasion above diaphragm | | | | | |
| T4 | Invades Gerota's fascia | IV | T4 | N any | M0 | IV |
| N1 | Single ≤ 2 cm | | T any | N2, 3 | M0 | III or IV |
| N2 | Single > 2 cm ≤ 5 cm | | T any | N any | M1 | IV |
| N3 | Multiple ≤ 5 cm, single > 5 cm | | | | | |

*T = tumor, N = lymph nodes, M = metastases.
*Source*: Adapted from Guinan P, Sobin LH, Alggaba F, et al: TNM staging of renal cell carcinoma. Cancer 80:992, 1997.

**Table 8–2: Metastatic sites.** In patients who present with metastatic renal cell carcinoma, only 1% to 3% have solitary metastatic lesions.[9, 10] The majority have multiple sites. Lymphatic metastases to regional lymph nodes and sites of distant drainage such as the mediastinum and supraclavicular regions occur frequently. The major sites of hematogenous spread are the lung, bone, liver, and brain.[11] The frequencies of various metastatic sites for renal cell carcinoma are given in Table 8–2.

**Figure 8–3: Survival with metastatic renal cancer.** Survival statistics for patients with advanced renal cancer have not changed dramatically over the past 25 years. Patients with regional lymph node involvement (Robson stage IIIB) have limited 5- and 10-year survival rates. In patients with N2 and N3 disease 5-year survival rates are low, suggesting the systemic nature of this disease. In patients with metastatic disease (M1), 5-year survival rate is limited (<5%), with only occasional reports of individuals demonstrating long-term survival. Thus, patients with metastatic disease have a poor prognosis. Subgroups of patients with improved survival can be identified, however. Individuals developing metastases within 1 year of initial nephrectomy have 2-year survival rates approaching zero. In contrast, in those developing metastases 2 or more years after nephrectomy, a 20% 5-year survival rate is reported.[11, 12]

**Table 8–3: Prognostic factors.** Patients with metastatic renal cancer have a poor prognosis, and the overall 5-year survival rate is less than 5%.[13–17] Various factors can be identified, however, that predict im-

## TABLE 8–2

## METASTATIC SITE FREQUENCY IN PATIENTS WITH RENAL CELL CARCINOMA

| SITE | FREQUENCY |
|---|---|
| Pulmonary | 75% |
| Lymph nodes/soft tissue | 36% |
| Osseous | 20% |
| Liver | 10% |
| CNS | <10% |
| Skin | <10% |

*Source*: Data from Maldazys JD, DeKernion JB: Prognostic factors in metastatic renal carcinoma. J Urol 136:376–379, 1986.

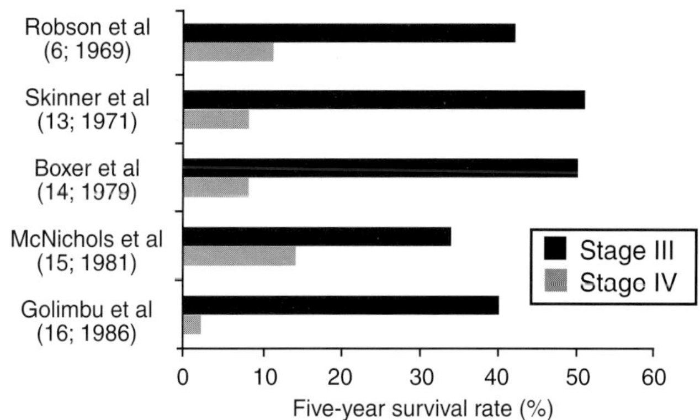


**Figure 8–3**

**TABLE 8–3**

## ANALYSES OF PROGNOSTIC VARIABLES IN PATIENTS WITH METASTATIC RENAL CELL CARCINOMA

| AUTHOR(S) | NO. OF PATIENTS | THERAPEUTIC REGIMEN(S) | FACTORS ASSOCIATED WITH IMPROVED SURVIVAL |
|---|---|---|---|
| Elson et al.[20] | 610 | Chemotherapy (multiple regimens) | PS, disease-free interval, number of metastatic sites, weight loss, prior chemotherapy |
| Maldazys et al.[11] | 181 | Multiple | Prior nephrectomy, disease-free interval, PS, lung metastases only |
| Palmer et al.[21] | 452 | IL-2 regimens | PS, time from Dx to Rx, number of metastatic sites |
| Minisian et al.[22] | 159 | IFN-α regimens | Prior nephrectomy, PS |
| Fossa et al.[23] | 295 | Chemotherapy, IFN-α | Sedimentation rate, weight loss |
| Landonio et al.[24] | 156 | Multiple | Prior nephrectomy, disease-free interval >24 mo, number of metastatic sites, PS |
| Fyfe et al.[25] | 255 | High-dose IL-2 trials | PS (predicts response) |
| Hänninen et al.[26] | 215 | IL-2, IL-2 and IFN-α | Sedimentation rate, LDH, hemoglobin, neutrophils, metastatic sites |

PS = performance status, Dx = diagnosis, Rx = treatment.

**TABLE 8–4**

## PROGNOSTIC FACTORS IN PATIENTS WITH METASTATIC RENAL CELL CARCINOMA

### CUMULATIVE RISK OF SURVIVAL AND PROGNOSTIC VARIABLES IN RENAL CANCER (HÄNNINEN ET AL.[26])

| Prognostic Variable | Risk Score | Risk Categories | Median Survival (months) |
|---|---|---|---|
| Sedimentation rate > 70 mm | 2 | Low (score 0) | 39.4 |
| LDH > 280 U/L | 2 | | |
| PMN > 6000/µl | 1 | Intermediate (score 1–3) | 15.0 |
| Hemoglobin < 100 g/L | 1 | | |
| Extrapulmonary metastases only | 1 | High (score ≥ 4) | 6.2 |
| Osseous metastases | 1 | | |

### PROGNOSTIC FACTORS FOR SURVIVAL IN RECURRENT OR METASTATIC RENAL CANCER (ELSON ET AL.[20])

| Risk Factor | No. of Risk Factors* | Risk Group | Median Survival (months) |
|---|---|---|---|
| ECOG PS (0, 1, etc.) | 0, 1 | 1 | 12.8 |
| Time from initial diagnosis (< 1 vs. ≥ 1 year) | 2 | 2 | 7.7 |
| Number metastatic sites (0, 1 vs. > 1) | 3 | 3 | 5.3 |
| Recent (≤ 6 mo) weight loss (no = 0, yes = 1) | 4 | 4 | 3.4 |
| Prior chemotherapy (no = 0, yes = 1) | ≥5 | 5 | 2.1 |

*Equals sum of ECOG performance status (PS) and other variables. If number of metastatic sites, weight loss, and prior chemotherapy all equal 1, the risk factor number is calculated by subtracting one.

proved survival. These characteristics include absence of symptoms (performance status), presence of pulmonary metastases only, and previous nephrectomy.[2, 3] Patients with hypercalcemia and stage IV disease also have a very poor prognosis, with median survival estimated as less than 50 days.[18] Finally, metastatic site is also a prognostic determinant, with liver[19] and multiple central nervous system sites predicting a poor outcome. Table 8–3 outlines a series of analyses that have been published identifying these poor prognostic determinants.

**Table 8–4: Models to predict survival.** Several authors have developed predictive models that can segregate patients with metastatic renal cell carcinoma into cohorts with different median survivals. Two of these systems were developed by Elson et al.[20] and Hänninen et al.[26] and are presented in Table 8–4. In the former, patients receiving various chemotherapeutic regimens were included, whereas in the latter, patients were treated with various cytokine regimens.

## TREATMENT

### Surgery for Metastatic Disease

**Figure 8–4:** The role of surgery in patients with metastatic disease is twofold. In the individual with an indolent growth pattern and a solitary metastatic site,[27] surgery to remove the metastasis may be associated with prolonged survival. Five-year survival rates over 30% have been reported and median survival times for this group of patients may exceed 3 years. In patients with multiple pulmonary metastases, surgical resection may also be employed. In a report by Cerfolio et al.,[28] patients in whom a solitary pulmonary metastasis was resected had a 5-year survival rate of 46%, and for those with two or more lesions resected the rate was 27%. This figure illustrates a patient who underwent nephrectomy and developed a solitary pulmonary metastasis 7 years later (A). Following resection, he remained disease-free for over 6 years (B). In patients with osseous metastases, radiation therapy plays a palliative role, but surgical resection should remain a potential option. In view of the vascular nature of some lesions, angioinfarction before resection is sometimes employed.

In patients presenting with multiple metastases who have their primary tumors in place, nephrectomy is considered a palliative measure. Symptoms such as pain, hematuria, and systemic complaints including fever and weight loss may be relieved.[29] Nephrectomy prior to therapy with cytokines is often employed. A recent randomized trial[30] has demonstrated that patients undergoing nephrectomy prior to treatment with IFN-α have a significant improvement in median survival compared with those receiving IFN-α alone (12.5 versus 8.1 months, $P = .033$).

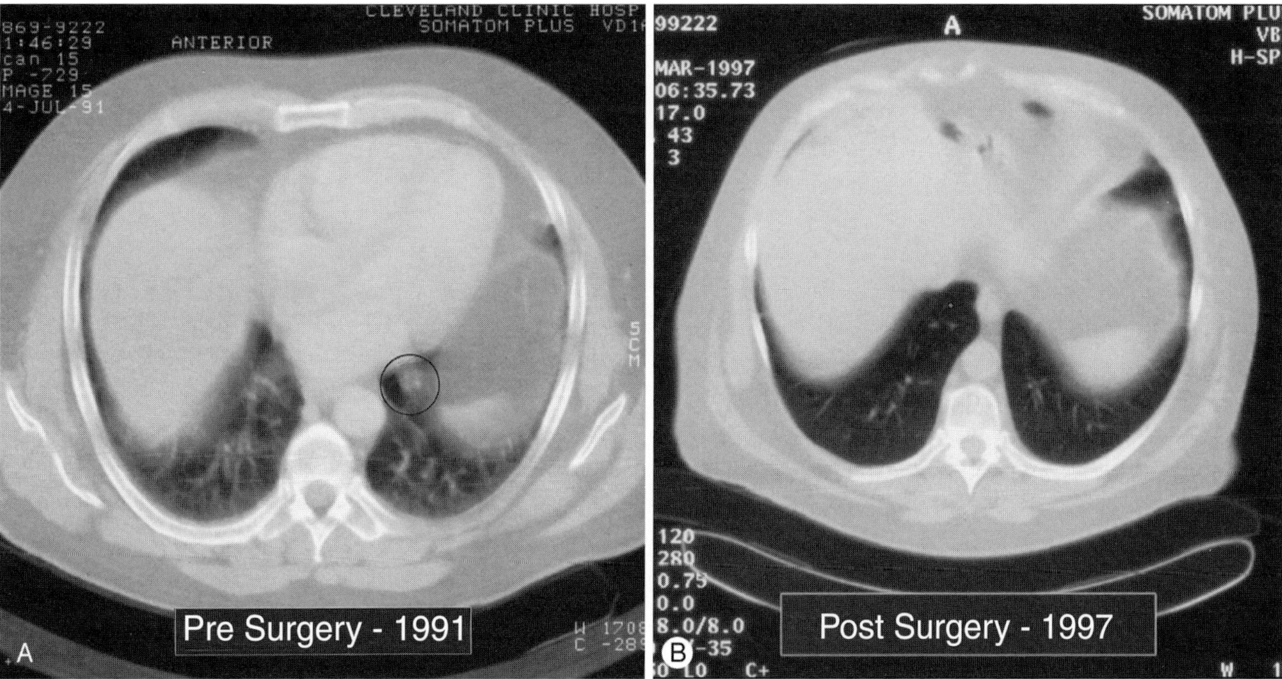


**Figure 8–4**

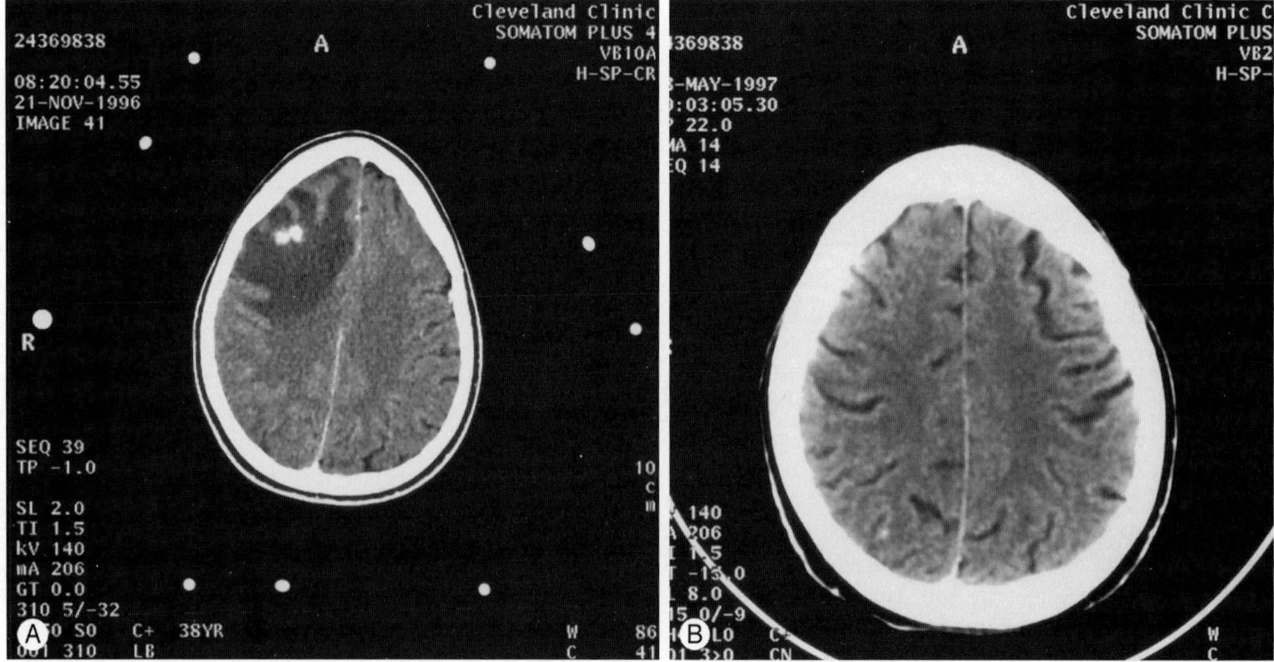

**Figure 8–5**

## Radiation

**Figure 8–5:** Radiation therapy in patients with symptomatic metastases is often employed for palliation. Objective or subjective responses are reported to occur in over 50% of patients treated with external beam therapy.[31] Doses utilized are commonly 3000 to 4000 cGy; however, 5000 cGy over a period of 5 to 6 weeks may be appropriate in selected situations, such as treatment of a solitary metastasis.[32, 33] Central nervous system metastases represent a significant problem in patients with advanced renal cancer. In the presence of a solitary lesion, a palliative resection should be utilized, if possible. Recently, stereotactic techniques and gamma knife radiotherapy have been employed. Whole brain radiotherapy has been used previously,[34, 35] but long-term sequelae, such as altered mentation, may be an undesirable consequence. This

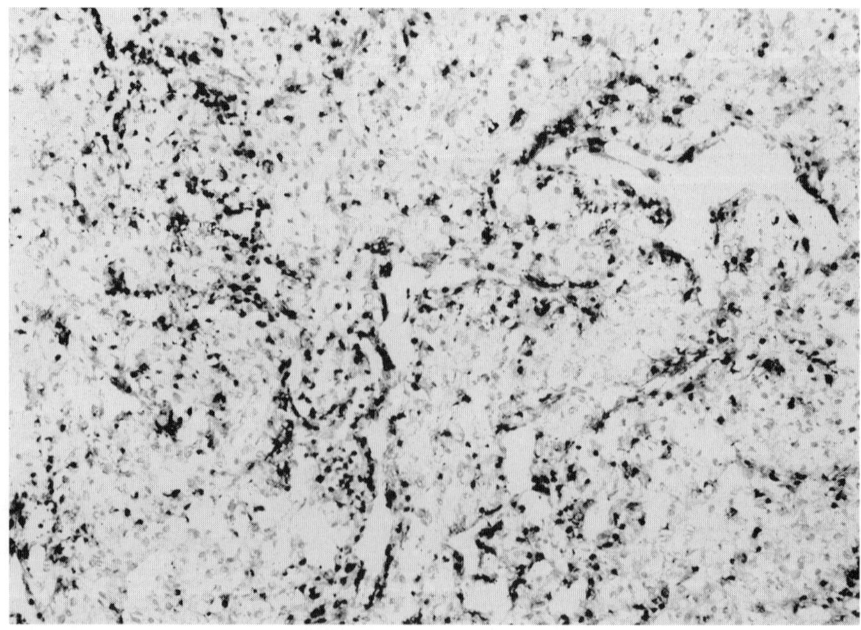

**Figure 8–6**

## HORMONES EMPLOYED IN RENAL CELL CARCINOMA PATIENTS

Estrogen antagonists: tamoxifen, nafoxidine
Progestational agents: Depo-Provera (methoxyprogesterone acetate), progesterone caproate
Androgens: fluoxymesterone, testosterone propionate

figure illustrates an individual with a central nervous system metastasis who received gamma knife radiotherapy and had an excellent response.

## Biologic Approaches

**Figure 8–6:** The observation that metastatic lesions may regress following nephrectomy provided a basis for the interest in therapy involving biologic approaches. The frequency of spontaneous regression is quite low,[36] but in a recent randomized trial comparing interferon-gamma with a placebo, a response rate of 6% was recorded in the placebo treatment arm.[37] The mechanisms responsible for these regressions are not clear, but enhancement of a pre-existing immune response has been suggested.[38] Additionally, the presence of CD3[+] tumor infiltrating T lymphocytes in renal neoplasms[38] as illustrated here suggests the existence of an active immune response. A clear cell tumor has been stained with monoclonal antibodies against the T-cell receptor (CD3ε chain), demonstrating an abundant infiltrate of T lymphocytes. Specific cytolytic T cells have also been found in this cell population.[39] Finally, the responses reported with various biologic therapeutic agents such as cytokines demonstrate the relevance of this approach.

## Therapy for Systemic Disease

### Hormones

**Table 8–5: Treatment of systemic disease: Hormone therapy.** Progestational agents and antiestrogen compounds have been utilized to treat patients with metastatic renal cell cancer based on a series of preclinical observations in a Syrian hamster model[40] indicating that an estrogen antagonist inhibited the growth of an estrogen-induced renal tumor. The collective experience with these agents has demonstrated they are of no value in the therapy of this disease. Agents such as megestrol acetate[41] and tamoxifen have overall response rates of less than 5%.[42] In a recent trial, patients received either chemoimmunotherapy (5-fluorouracil [5-FU], IL-2, IFN-α) or tamoxifen. No responses in the tamoxifen group were noted, and the median survival of this cohort was 14 months.[43] Agents such as megestrol acetate (Megace), however, may be of value for palliation of symptoms, such as weight loss.

### Chemotherapy

**Table 8–6: Treatment of systemic disease: Chemotherapy.** Metastatic renal cell carcinoma is a chemotherapy-resistant neoplasm. A review of over 3000 patients treated between 1983 and 1993 demonstrated an overall response rate of less than 5%.[44] Agents such as vinblastine are currently considered inactive, with objective response rates of less than 5% noted.[45] The antimetabolites 5-FU and floxuridine (FUDR) may have modest antitumor activity. The use of this latter agent as a circadian continuous infusion was associated with a response rate of 19.6% in early reports.[46] Subsequent phase II studies utilizing FUDR have not confirmed this finding[47, 48]; however, randomized trials are in progress. Currently, there is no standard accepted cytotoxic agent for the treatment of patients with metastatic renal cell carcinoma.



## VINBLASTINE AND FLOXURIDINE (FUDR): ACTIVITY IN METASTATIC RENAL CELL CARCINOMA

| AGENT | DOSE/SCHEDULE | NO. OF PATIENTS | RESPONSE RATE | REFERENCE |
|---|---|---|---|---|
| Vinblastine | 0.1 mg/kg IVB q 3 weeks | 81 | 2.5% | Pyrhönen et al.[41] |
| | 1.4–1.5 mg/kg CIV days 1–5 | 21 | 10% | Crivellari et al.[45] |
| | 0.1 mg/kg IVB q 3 weeks | 250 | 6.4% | Yagoda et al.[40] |
| FUDR | 0.15 mg/kg/day CIV days 1–14 | 56 | 19.6% | Von Roemeling et al.[42] |
| | 0.15 mg/kg/day CIV days 1–14 | 40 | 10% | Dexeus et al.[43] |
| | 0.15 mg/kg/day CIV days 1–14 | 28 | 8% | Sampaio et al.[44] |

IVB = intravenous bolus, CIV = continuous intravenous infusion.

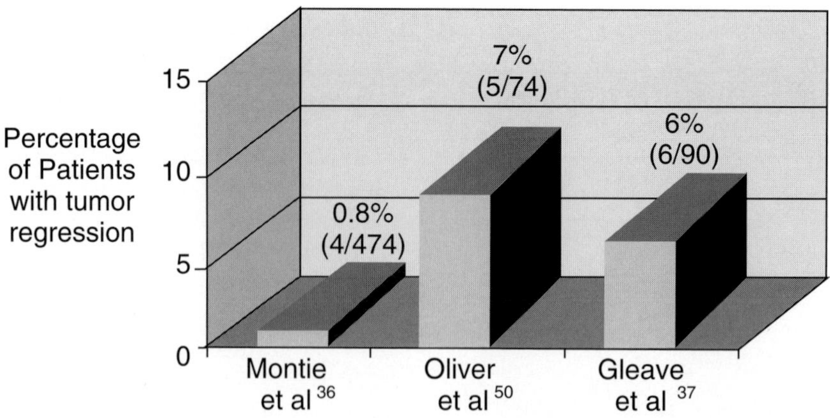



**Figure 8–7**

## Biologic Therapy

### Spontaneous Regression

**Figure 8–7:** Spontaneous regression of metastatic lesions in patients with renal cell carcinoma has been noted in two circumstances. In patients with a primary tumor in place and metastatic disease, regression of metastases following nephrectomy has been reported. In a review of 474 patients from nine series, only 4 patients (0.8%) could be characterized as having a spontaneous tumor response.[49] Alternatively, patients with metastatic disease receiving no active antitumor therapy have been reported to demonstrate regression of pulmonary metastases. In reports by two groups, the frequency of this finding is noted to be between 6% and 7%.[37, 50] The duration of these responses is generally short, but these observations are of interest and support the investigation of biologic therapy for this neoplasm.

### Interleukin 2

**Figure 8–8:** Interleukin 2 (IL-2) is a cytokine that supports the proliferation of antigen-specific cytolytic T cells.[51] The cDNA encoding human IL-2 was isolated,[52] and the molecular characteristics of this cytokine have been elucidated. It is a 15-kDa protein with a variable degree of glycosylation. The majority of IL-2 is produced by mature CD4$^+$ cells following antigenic stimulation.[53] Like most cytokines, rIL-2 has a short half-life,[54] and its pharmacokinetics vary with the route of administration. Schedules and routes of administration explored include intravenous bolus, subcutaneous, and continuous intravenous infusion. This agent was approved by the FDA in 1992 for the therapy of metastatic renal cell carcinoma. This figure presents a graphic representation of the IL-2 molecule. (From Bukowski RM, McLain D, Finke J: Clinical pharmaco-

kinetics of interleukin-1, interleukin-2, interleukin-4, tumor necrosis-factor and macrophage colony stimulating factor. In Chalner BA, Longo DL [eds]: Cancer Chemotherapy and Biotherapy—Principles and Practice. Philadelphia, Lippincott-Raven, 1996, pp 609–638.)

### rIL-2

**Table 8–7: High-dose therapy of rIL-2.** Approval of rIL-2 for therapy of metastatic renal cell carcinoma was based on the results of a series of phase II clinical trials in 255 patients utilizing single-agent therapy in a high-dose intravenous bolus schedule.[25] The schedule em-

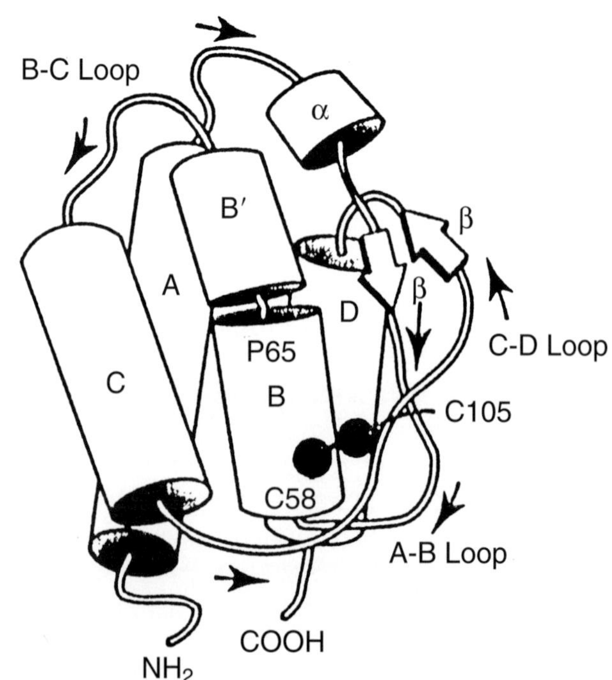



**Figure 8–8**

**TABLE 8–7**

**EFFICACY OF HIGH-DOSE rIL-2 THERAPY**

| TYPE OF RESPONSE | RESPONSE RATE | | RESPONSE DURATION (Months) | |
|---|---|---|---|---|
| | No. | Percentage | Median | Range* |
| Complete | 12/255 | 5 | NR | 5+ to 62+ |
| Partial | 24/255 | 9 | 19 | 3.0 to 57+ |
| Overall | 36/255 | 14 | 20.3 | 3.0 to 62+ |

*Plus signs mean ongoing.
NR = not reached.
*Source*: Data from Fyfe G, Fisher RI, Rosenberg SA, et al: Results of treatment of 255 patients with metastatic renal cell carcinoma: Risks and benefits in 215 consecutive single institution patients. J Urol 155:19, 1996.

ployed involved rIL-2 at a dose of 600,000 or 720,000 IU/kg as a 15-minute IV infusion every 8 hours over 5 days. A second cycle was administered following 5 to 9 days of rest, with therapy repeated after 6 to 12 weeks in patients who were responding or stable. The reported results are illustrated in Table 8–7. The durable 5% complete regression rate is notable. The toxicity of high-dose rIL-2 is substantial. A 4% drug-related mortality rate was reported, and over 50% of patients required administration of vasopressors to control hypotension. The patients treated in this manner represented a highly selected group of individuals, but the results are nevertheless of interest.

**Table 8–8: Randomized trials of rIL-2.** In view of the toxicity of high-dose rIL-2 and the highly selected nature of the patients treated, a randomized study has been conducted.[55] In this trial, 227 patients were randomized to receive high-dose rIL-2 or low-dose rIL-2.

Results demonstrate modest differences in response rates ($P$ = .059), with substantially less toxicity associated with the lower doses of rIL-2. No differences in response duration or median survival between the two treatment arms were found. The optimal rIL-2 regimen is therefore not clear. The substantial toxicity associated with high-dose rIL-2 in the absence of survival improvement suggests that lower dosage regimens should be explored. Currently, a study comparing these two rIL-2 regimens with one involving subcutaneous rIL-2 is in progress.

**TABLE 8–8**

**COMPARISON OF HIGH- AND LOW-DOSE rIL-2: INTERIM RESULTS**

| REGIMEN | TYPE OF RESPONSE | RESPONSE RATE | | RESPONSE DURATION* (Months) |
|---|---|---|---|---|
| | | No. | Percentage | |
| High Dose† (n = 115) | Complete | 9/115 | 8% | 19.0 to 61+ |
| | Partial | 13/115 | 17% | 4.0 to 21.0 |
| | Overall | 22/115 | 19% | — |
| Low Dose‡ (n = 112) | Complete | 5/112 | 5% | 3.0 to 61+ |
| | Partial | 6/112 | 5% | 4.0 to 23.0 |
| | Overall | 11/112 | 10% | — |

*Plus signs mean ongoing.
†rIL-2: 720,000 IU/kg IV bolus q 8 h × 5 days, repeat in 5 to 9 days if tolerated.
‡rIL-2: 72,000 IU/kg IV bolus q 8 h × 5 days, repeat in 5 to 9 days if tolerated.
*Source*: Data from Yang JC, Rosenberg SA: An ongoing prospective randomized comparison of interleukin-2 regimens for the treatment of metastatic renal cell carcinoma. Cancer J Sci Am 3:579, 1997.

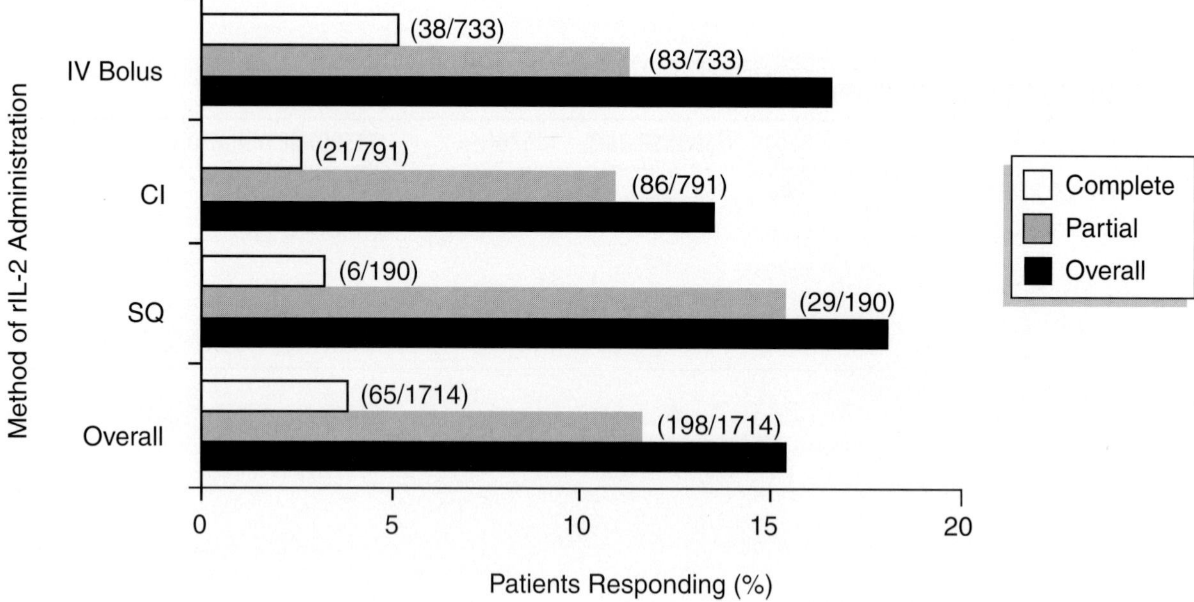



**Figure 8–9**

**Figure 8–9:** Because of the short half-life of intravenous bolus rIL-2, different routes including continuous intravenous infusion and subcutaneous administration have been studied. A recent review of 1714 patients treated with rIL-2 has been summarized[56] in which the overall response rate to rIL-2 was 15.4%, with a complete response rate of 3.8%. Major differences between the various schedules are not apparent. Randomized trials are required to determine if the schedule employed can influence complete response rates, response duration, time to progression, and survival. Numbers in parentheses refer to responses/total patients. SQ = subcutaneous, CI = continuous infusion. (From Bukowski RM: Natural history and therapy of metastatic renal cell carcinoma: Role of interleukin 2. Cancer 80[7]:1198–1220, 1997.)

## *Interferon-alpha*

**Table 8–9: Interferon-α.** The first cytokine to be utilized in patients with metastatic renal cell carcinoma was IFN-α.[57, 58] This family of molecules are inducible cellular glycoproteins with antiproliferative, antiviral, and immunomodulatory effects.[59] Studies with rIFN-α have involved a variety of doses varying between 1.0 MU and 50 MU/m$^2$ and schedules including both intermittent IV and subcutaneous administration. An overview of the results with various IFN-α preparations is illustrated in Table 8–9. Nineteen studies involving over 700 patients who received rIFN-α preparations are reviewed. Overall response rates in these trials varied from zero to 29%.[56] Response may not occur for 3 months, and its duration seldom exceeds 2

## TABLE 8–9

### SINGLE-AGENT IFN-α IN TREATMENT OF METASTATIC RENAL CELL CARCINOMA

| PREPARATION | NO. OF PATIENTS | COMPLETE RESPONSES (%) | PARTIAL RESPONSES (%) | OVERALL RESPONSE |
|---|---|---|---|---|
| Partially purified human leukocyte IFN-α[56] | 141 | 6 (4.3) | 20 (14.2) | 18.5% |
| Human lymphoblastoid IFN-α[56] | 398 | 4 (1.0) | 57 (14.3) | 15.3% |
| Recombinant IFN-α[56] | 767 | 14 (1.8) | 78 (10.2) | 12.0% |

**TABLE 8–10**

## RANDOMIZED TRIALS OF IFN-α THERAPY

| AUTHOR(S) | TREATMENT ARMS | NO. OF PATIENTS | RESPONSE RATE | TWO-YEAR SURVIVAL | MEDIAN SURVIVAL (Months) |
|---|---|---|---|---|---|
| Ritchie et al.[62] | IFN-α 10 MU SC TIW × 12 weeks | 167 | NS | 22% | 8.5* |
| | MPA 300 mg/day p.o. × 12 weeks | 168 | NS | 12% | 6.0* |
| Kriegmair et al.[63] | IFN-α 8 MU SC TIW and VBL 0.1 mg/kg IVB q 3 weeks | 41 | 20.5% | 20% | 16.0† |
| | MPA 500 mg/day p.o. | 35 | 0% | 20% | 10.0† |

*$P = .011$.
†$P = .19$.
MPA = medroxyprogesterone, NS = not stated, SC = subcutaneous, MU = million units, VBL = vinblastine, IVB = intravenous bolus, p.o. = orally, TIW = three times a week.

years.[60] Complete responses are seen, and are generally limited to patients with minimal pulmonary metastases. A recent review of published data suggests a dose of 5 to 10 MU/m$^2$ administered subcutaneously three to five times weekly produces optimal results,[56] and that chronic dosing is superior to intermittent high-dose IV administration. Subsets of patients with good performance status, lung predominant disease, and previous nephrectomy appear to respond most favorably to this agent.[22, 61]

**Table 8–10: Randomized trials.** Studies investigating the therapeutic efficacy of IFN-α compared with various cytokine- and non–cytokine-containing regimens have been conducted. The reports by Pyrhönen et al.,[45] Ritchie et al.,[62] and Kriegmair et al.[63] are of interest. In the latter two trials, patients with metastatic renal cell carcinoma were randomized to receive IFN-α with or without vinblastine or medroxyprogesterone.

The results of these two studies are summarized in Table 8–10. The findings by Pyrhönen[45] and Ritchie[63] suggest that IFN-α therapy may produce a modest enhancement of survival when compared to an inactive agent.

**Table 8–11: Interferon-α and 13-*cis*-retinoic acid.** The antitumor activity demonstrated by the combination of 13-*cis*-retinoic acid (CRA) and IFN-α in squamous cell carcinomas of the skin and cervix[64] resulted in phase II trials of this combination in metastatic renal cell cancer. A report by Motzer et al.[65] noted a response rate of 30% (findings in Table 8–11). Preliminary reports of additional phase II trials have appeared, and a phase III trial comparing IFN-α with and without CRA has been completed. This study demonstrated that the response rate and survival did not improve significantly with the addition of CRA.[66]

**TABLE 8–11**

## IFN-α AND 13-*CIS*-RETINOIC ACID (CRA) IN TREATMENT OF METASTATIC RENAL CELL CANCER

| NO. OF PATIENTS | COMPLETE RESPONSES (%) | PARTIAL RESPONSES (%) | OVERALL RESPONSE RATE | MEDIAN SURVIVAL |
|---|---|---|---|---|
| 44 | 3 (7%) | 10 (23%) | 30% (95% CI 16–44) | 15.5 months |

| AGENT | SCHEDULE |
|---|---|
| IFN-α | 3 MU SC daily |
| CRA | 1.0 mg/kg/day (divided doses) |

*Source:* Data from Motzer RJ, Schwartz L, Law TM, et al: Interferon alfa-2a and 13-*cis*-retinoic acid in renal cell carcinoma: Antitumor activity in a phase II trial and interactions in vitro. J Clin Oncol 13:1950, 1995.

TABLE 8–12

## COMBINATION rIL-2 AND IFN-α THERAPY IN METASTATIC RENAL CELL CARCINOMA

| METHOD OF rIL-2 ADMINISTRATION | NO. OF PATIENTS | CR (%) | PR (%) | OVERALL RESPONSE RATE |
|---|---|---|---|---|
| Subcutaneous | 675 | 34 (5.0) | 109 (16.2) | 21.2% |
| Continuous intravenous | 556 | 19 (3.4) | 92 (16.6) | 20.0% |
| Intravenous bolus | 180 | 9 (5.0) | 28 (15.5) | 20.5% |
| Totals | 1411 | 62 (4.4) | 229 (16.2) | 20.6% |

*Source:* Adapted from Bukowski RM: Natural history and therapy of metastatic renal cell carcinoma: Role of interleukin 2. Cancer 80(7):1198, 1997.

**Table 8–12: Interferon-α and rIL-2 combinations.** In preclinical murine tumor models, the synergistic antitumor effects of IFN-α and rIL-2 have been repeatedly demonstrated,[67] and have provided the rationale for clinical testing of this combination. Phase I studies demonstrated that this combination was tolerated. A series of phase II trials were then performed to investigate its efficacy in patients with metastatic renal cancer. rIL-2 was administered in a variety of schedules, and a summary of results in over 1400 patients is given in Table 8–12.[56] An overall response rate of 20.6%, with a complete response (CR) rate of 4.4%, was noted. The superiority of cytokine combinations compared with single-agent therapy has not been conclusively demonstrated in randomized studies, but available data suggest response rates may be slightly improved.

**Table 8–13: Outpatient rIL-2 and IFN-α regimens.** Outpatient regimens utilizing subcutaneous rIL-2 and IFN-α appear to produce responses in over 20% of patients. The schedule utilized by Atzpodien et al.[68] is illustrated in Table 8–13. A total of 152 patients were reported, with 9 complete (6%) and 29 partial (19%) responses. The toxicity of this regimen was characterized as moderate. The median duration of complete responses was 16+ months.

**Table 8–14: Biologic therapy.** Randomized trials of IFN-α, rIL-2, and combination continuous intravenous (CIV) therapy are shown in Table 8–14. Results from a French multicenter trial (CRECY) suggest that the combination of CIV rIL-2 and subcutaneous (SC) IFN-α may be superior to either cytokine alone.[69] In this study, 425 patients were randomized to therapy with rIL-2 (18 MIU/m²/day CIV on days 1 through 5, 12 through 15), IFN-α (18 MU SC three times per week), or the combination in which the IFN-α dose was decreased to 6 MU SC three times weekly from days 1 to

TABLE 8–13

## OUTPATIENT REGIMENS OF rIL-2 AND IFN-α IN TREATMENT OF RENAL CELL CARCINOMA*

| | WEEKS 1 AND 4 | | | | | WEEKS 2, 3, 5, 6 | | | | |
|---|---|---|---|---|---|---|---|---|---|---|
| | Day | | | | | Day | | | | |
| | 1 | 2 | 3 | 4 | 5 | 1 | 2 | 3 | 4 | 5 |
| **rIL-2** | | | | | | | | | | |
| 20 MIU/m² SC | — | — | ■ | ■ | ■ | — | — | — | — | — |
| 5 MIU/m² SC | — | — | — | — | — | ■ | — | ■ | — | ■ |
| **rIFN-α2** | | | | | | | | | | |
| 6 MU/m² | ■ | — | — | — | — | ■ | — | ■ | — | ■ |

*Cycles repeated every 8 weeks as tolerated.
■ = day of treatment, — = no therapy.
*Source:* Atzpodien J, Lopez-Hänninen E, Kirchner H, et al: Multiinstitutional home-therapy trial of recombinant human interleukin-2 and interferon alfa-2 in progressive metastatic RCC. J Clin Oncol 13:497, 1995.

**TABLE 8–14**

## RANDOMIZED TRIALS INVOLVING COMBINATION CYTOKINE THERAPY WITH rIL-2 AND IFN-α

| | | | | SURVIVAL | | |
| | | NO. OF | RESPONSE | Event-Free | | |
| AUTHOR(S) | TREATMENT | PATIENTS | RATE (%) | 1-Year | Two-Year | Median (Months) |
|---|---|---|---|---|---|---|
| Negrier et al.[69] | rIL-2 | 138 | 9 (6.5%)* | 15%† | 32% | NS |
| | IFN-α | 147 | 11 (7.5%)* | 12%† | 30% | NS |
| Henriksson et al.[70] | rIL-2 + IFN-α | 140 | 26 (18.6%)* | 20.9%† | 34% | NS |
| | rIL-2 + IFN-α + TMX | 65 | NS | NS | NS | 11.8 |
| | TMX | 63 | NS | NS | NS | 13.3 |

*$P < .01$.
†$P = .01$.
TMX = tamoxifen, NS = not stated.

17. The results suggest that the combination is superior to either agent alone both in terms of overall response rate and in event-free survival at 1 year. No differences in 2-year survival rates were noted.

A second trial by Henriksson et al.[70] compared the combination of subcutaneous rIL-2, IFN-α, and tamoxifen with tamoxifen alone. This study included 128 patients, and demonstrated no survival advantage for the cytokine-containing arm. Response evaluation was not a primary endpoint, but five complete responses were seen in the patients receiving rIL-2, IFN-α, and tamoxifen, compared with two patients given tamoxifen alone. A review of the available phase II trials and these randomized trials indicates that rIL-2 and IFN-α may improve response rates in patients with metastatic renal cell carcinoma. Effects on response duration and overall survival are unclear.

### Cytokines

**Table 8–15: Toxicity of cytokine regimens.** The toxicity associated with cytokine administration is dependent on the dose, route, and schedule of the cytokine. Although the effects may be dramatic, they resolve rapidly following discontinuation. The etiology of the various side effects seen with rIL-2 or IFN-α is unclear, but is thought to represent the effects of the cytokine cascades induced by administration of

**TABLE 8–15**

## COMPARATIVE TOXICITY OF VARIOUS CYTOKINE REGIMENS

| | TOXICITY REPORTED (%) | | |
| TOXIC REACTION | High-Dose rIL-2[55] (≥ Grade 3) | Subcutaneous rIL-2[71] | Subcutaneous rIL-2 and IFN-α[68] |
|---|---|---|---|
| Nausea/vomiting | 32% | 34% | 75% (4% ≥ Gr 3) |
| Diarrhea | 17% | — | 25% (≤ Gr 2) |
| Creatinine | 2% (≥ 8 mg/dl) | "Mild" | — |
| Oliguria (< 80 ml/8 hr) | 21% | — | — |
| Hypotension | 54% | 52% (11% BP < 90 mm Hg) | 28% (≤ Gr 2) |
| CNS toxicity | 12% | — | 9% (Gr 1) |
| Hyperbilirubinemia | 6% | 4% (Gr 1) | — |
| Arrhythmia | 4% | — | 2% (Gr 1) |
| Thrombopenia | 9% | — | — |
| Anemia | NS | NS | 34% (≤ Gr 2) |
| Pulmonary | 4% | — | 47% (7% ≥ Gr 3) |

NS = not stated, BP = blood pressure.

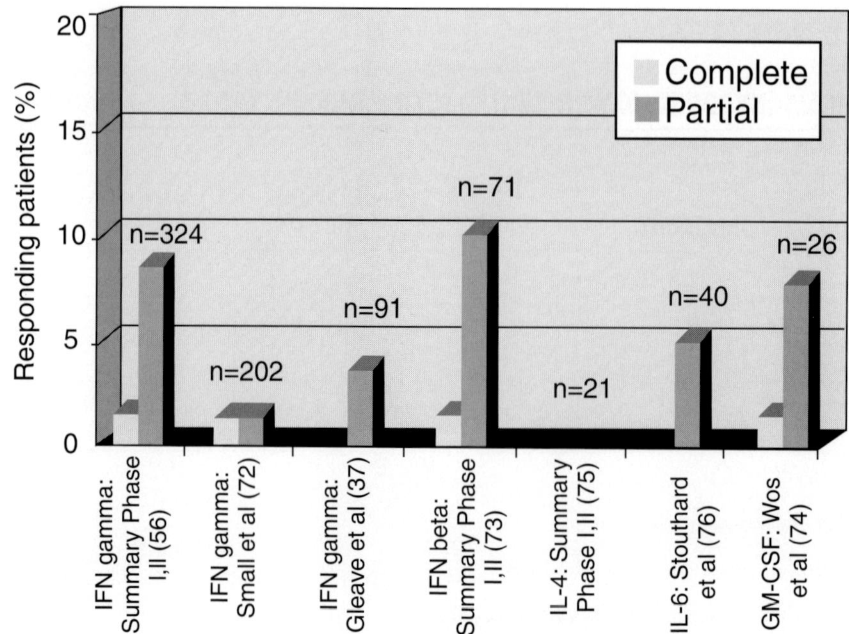


**Figure 8–10**

these proteins. Table 8–15 illustrates the spectrum of side effects seen with three different regimens including higher dose rIL-2,[55] low-dose subcutaneous rIL-2,[71] and an outpatient regimen of rIL-2 and IFN-α.[68] With all these regimens, fever, chills, malaise, and anorexia occur in the majority of patients. The use of higher dose rIL-2 is associated with a significant incidence of grade 3 or greater toxicity, requiring inpatient management. A variety of measures including antiemetics, fluids, pressor agents, and antidiarrheal agents can be utilized to control these effects. Familiarity with these side effects, and selection of patients with adequate pulmonary, cardiac, renal, and hematologic status, will minimize the morbidity of this type of therapy.

**Figure 8–10:** In view of the experience with rIL-2 and IFN-α, investigations of other cytokines have been conducted in patients with metastatic renal cell carcinoma. Reports utilizing IFN-β, IFN-γ, IL-4, IL-6, and GM-CSF are illustrated here. These studies include phase I, II, and III trials, and variable numbers of patients have been treated. Clinical responses to these biologic agents have been reported, but the antitumor effects appear limited and their overall role in therapy of renal cancer is not clear. Recently, the database with IFN-γ has been enlarged considerably by the preliminary reports of two studies utilizing low (60 μg/m²) but biologically active doses of this cytokine.[37, 72] The results of these studies indicate IFN-γ is not active in the therapy of metastatic renal cell carcinoma.

## TABLE 8–16

### RANDOMIZED CLINICAL TRIALS OF IFN-α AND VINBLASTINE IN RENAL CELL CARCINOMA THERAPY

| AUTHOR(S) | VINBLASTINE | IFN-α | VINBLASTINE (VBL) AND IFN-α |
|---|---|---|---|
| Fossa et al.[78] | | | |
| Dose/schedule | — | 18 MU TIW SC | VBL 0.1 mg/kg IV q 3 weeks<br>IFN-α 18 MU TIW SC |
| No. patients | — | 53* | 66* |
| % Responses | — | 11% | 24% |
| Median survival (months) | — | 12.0 | 12.0 |
| Pyrhönen et al.[41] | | | |
| Dose/schedule | 0.1 mg/kg IV<br>q 3 weeks | — | VBL 0.1 mg/kg IV q 3 weeks<br>IFN-α 18 MU TIW SC |
| No. patients | 81 | — | 79 |
| % Responses | 2.5% | — | 16% |
| Median survival (months) | 8.8 | — | 15.8 |

*178 patients entered, 119 evaluable.
IV = intravenous, TIW = three times weekly, SC = subcutaneous.

## TABLE 8–17

### CHEMOIMMUNOTHERAPY FOR TREATMENT OF METASTATIC RENAL CELL CANCER

| AUTHOR(S) | NO. OF PATIENTS | CR (%) | PR (%) | OVERALL RESPONSE RATE |
|---|---|---|---|---|
| Hänninen et al.[26] | 120 | 13 (10.8) | 34 (28.3) | 39.0% (31–47)* |
| Hoffmockel et al.[81] | 25 | 3 (9) | 10 (29) | 38.0% (22–56) |
| Dutcher et al.[83] | 36 | — | 7 (19) | 19.0% (9–33) |
| Sella et al.[82] | 19 | 3 (16) | 6 (32) | 48% (24–71) |
| Olencki et al.[84] | 39 | — | 3 (8) | 8% (NS) |

*95% CI.
NS = not stated.

## Chemotherapy and Cytokines

**Table 8–16: Chemoimmunotherapy with IFN-α and vinblastine.** In view of previous reports[40] indicating that vinblastine had antitumor activity in patients with metastatic renal cell carcinoma, it was combined with IFN-α. Preliminary data from phase II studies suggested that the combination might be useful, with response rates in excess of 30% reported by various groups.[77] Several randomized trials of this combination have been conducted and are summarized in Table 8–16. The report by Fossa et al.[78] demonstrated a higher response rate with IFN-α and vinblastine compared with IFN-α alone, but no effects on survival. A preliminary report by Pyrhönen et al.[45] indicates that vinblastine alone is inactive, and that the combination is superior. These findings suggest that IFN-α may potentially affect median survival in patients with metastatic renal cell carcinoma, and it appears that vinblastine alone or in combination with IFN-α is not a useful therapy.

**Table 8–17: Chemoimmunotherapy with rIL-2, IFN-α, and 5-FU.** Preclinical investigations have suggested that IFN-α may modulate the antiproliferative effects of antimetabolites such as 5-FU.[79] Studies in patients with various gastrointestinal neoplasms indicated therapeutic synergism[80]; therefore, interest in combining 5-FU with rIL-2 and IFN-α developed. A summary of results from phase II studies utilizing this combination is presented in Table 8–17. Response rates over 30% have been noted[26, 81, 82]; however, reports by other groups[83, 84] utilizing slightly different schedules of cytokine and 5-FU administration have been associated with lower response rates.

**Table 8–18: Chemoimmunotherapy.** The regimen reported by Hänninen et al.[26] is illustrated in Table 8–18. In this regimen rIL-2 and IFN-α are administered intermittently via the subcutaneous route, and 5-FU is administered during the last 4 weeks of each cycle. This approach represents an outpatient regimen with moderate toxicity.

## TABLE 8–18

### CHEMOIMMUNOTHERAPY REGIMEN FOR TREATMENT OF METASTATIC RENAL CELL CANCER

| AGENT | WEEKS 1 AND 4 | | | | | WEEKS 2 AND 3 | | | | | WEEKS 5 TO 8 | | | | |
|---|---|---|---|---|---|---|---|---|---|---|---|---|---|---|---|
| | Day 1 | Day 2 | Day 3 | Day 4 | Day 5 | Day 1 | Day 2 | Day 3 | Day 4 | Day 5 | Day 1 | Day 2 | Day 3 | Day 4 | Day 5 |
| IL-2 | | | | | | | | | | | | | | | |
| 10 MIU/m² SC BID | — | — | ■ | ■ | ■ | — | — | — | — | — | — | — | — | — | — |
| 5 MIU/m² SC | — | — | — | — | — | ■ | — | ■ | — | ■ | — | — | — | — | — |
| IFN-α | | | | | | | | | | | | | | | |
| 6 MU/m² SC | ■ | — | — | — | — | ■ | — | ■ | — | ■ | — | — | — | — | — |
| 9 MU/m² SC | — | — | — | — | — | — | — | — | — | — | ■ | — | ■ | — | ■ |
| 5-FU | | | | | | | | | | | | | | | |
| 750 mg/m² IV | — | — | — | — | — | — | — | — | — | — | ■ | — | — | — | — |

BID = twice daily, SC = subcutaneous, IV = intravenous bolus, ■ = day of treatment, — = no treatment.
*Source*: Adapted from Hänninen EL, Kirchner H, Atzpodien J: Interleukin-2 based home therapy of metastatic renal cell carcinoma: Risks and benefits in 215 consecutive single institution patients. J Urol 155:19, 1996.

**Table 8–19:** Table 8–19 shows the preliminary results from two trials[43, 85] in which patients were randomized to 5-FU/IL-2/IFN-α or a second treatment consisting of either tamoxifen or IL-2/IFN-α. The results vary and suggest that the schedule of drug administration or patient selection may be important. In the absence of randomized trials confirming the superiority of this approach, the value of chemoimmunotherapy remains unclear.

## Combined Modalities

**Figure 8–11:** The regressions produced by cytokine therapy in patients with metastatic renal cell carcinoma are generally partial. In patients with stable partial responses, the value of surgical removal of residual disease is being explored.[86–88] Alternatively, the value of cytoreductive surgery such as nephrectomy in patients with metastatic disease has also been studied.[89] At

### TABLE 8–19

#### RANDOMIZED TRIALS OF CHEMOIMMUNOTHERAPY FOR TREATMENT OF RENAL CELL CARCINOMA

| AUTHOR(S) | NO. OF PATIENTS | CR (%) | PR (%) | MEDIAN SURVIVAL (Months) |
|---|---|---|---|---|
| Atzpodien et al.[43] | | | | |
|   5-FU/IL-2/IFN-α | 41 | 7 (17) | 9 (22) | > 42* |
|   Tamoxifen | 38 | — | — | 14 |
| Negrier et al.[85] | | | | |
|   5-FU/IL-2/IFN-α† | 61 | — | 5 (8) | NS |
|   IL-2/IFN-α‡ | 70 | — | 1 (1.4) | NS |

*Median not reached after 42 months.

†rIL-2: 9 MIU SC days 1–6 weeks 1, 3, 5, 7; IFN-α: 6 MU SC days 1, 3, 5 weeks 1, 3, 5, 7; 5-FU: 600 mg/m² IV days 1–5, weeks 1 and 5.

‡rIL-2 and IFN-α only with doses and schedule as in other arm.

CR = complete response, PR = partial response, NS = not stated.

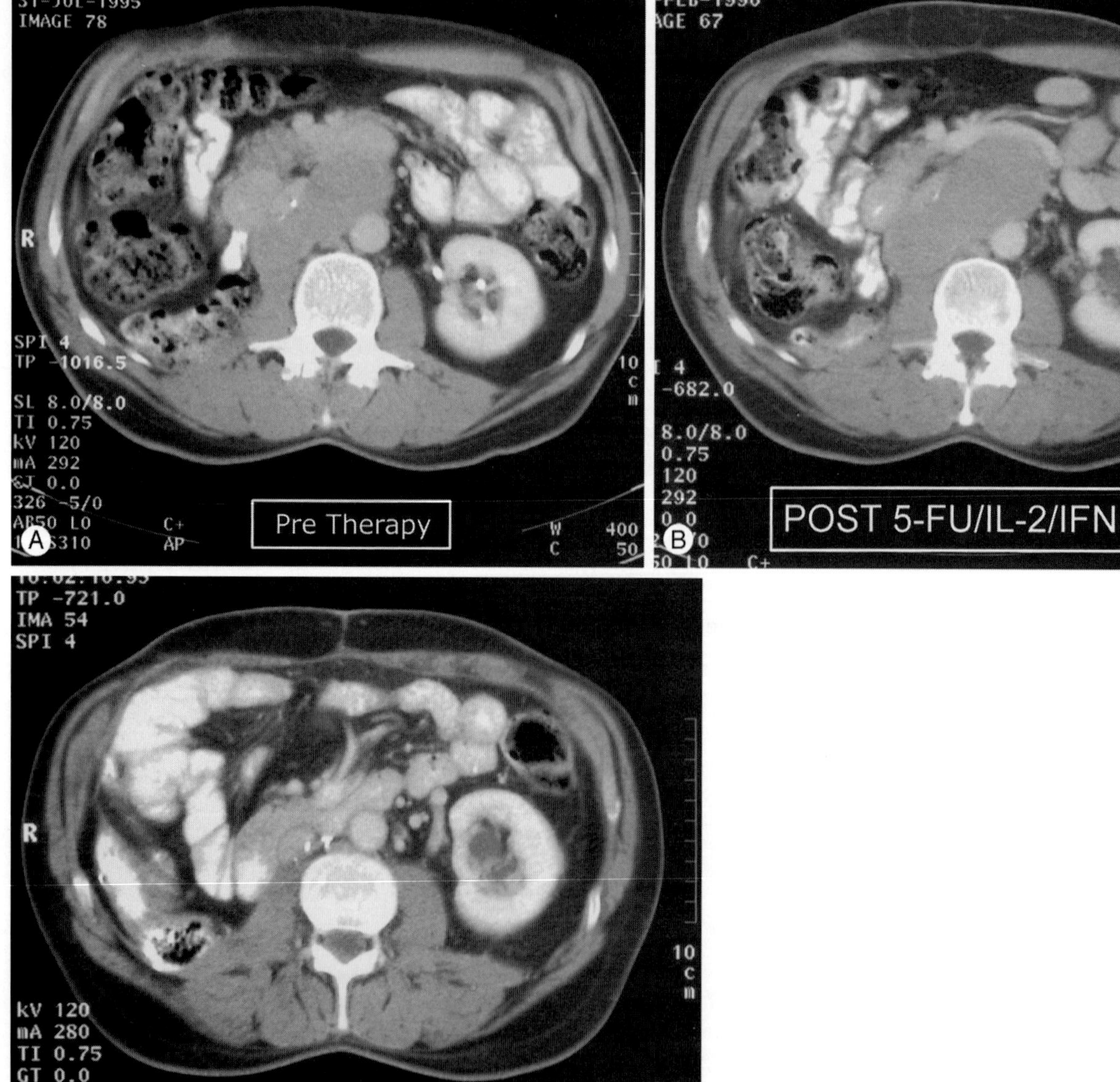


**Figure 8–11**

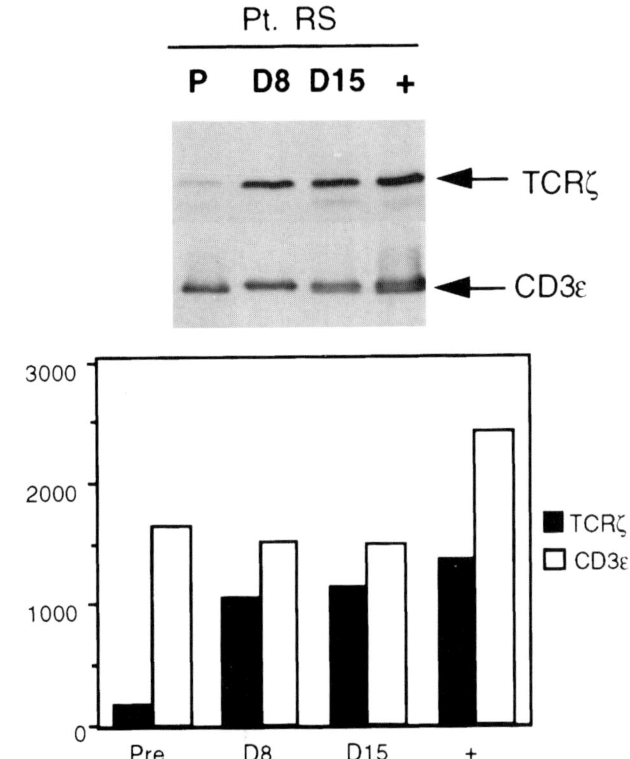


**Figure 8–12**

present, the value of either approach in enhancing outcomes such as disease-free survival or overall survival is unclear. All studies have been prospective, but the absence of a no surgery control does not permit critical evaluation of the combined modality approach because patient selection may play a crucial role in this type of treatment. A patient receiving 5-FU, rIL-2, and IFN-α is illustrated *(A)*, who had a minor regression of retroperitoneal lymph nodes *(B)*. The mass was ultimately resected *(C)*, and the patient remained disease-free for over 6 months.

### *Acquired Immune Dysregulation*

**Figure 8–12:** Impaired immune function in patients with advanced malignancies has been recognized for over 30 years.[90] In patients with renal cell carcinoma and metastatic or advanced disease, various abnormalities in T lymphocytes have now been described.[91, 92] Alterations of the T-cell antigen receptor (TCR) with decreases in TCRζ and various kinases involved in signal transduction have been reported.[93] This figure illustrates Western blots demonstrating differences in levels of TCRζ and CD3ε proteins (components of the T-cell receptor). In the lower panel densitometry was used to illustrate these differences. The patient received rIL-2, IFN-α, and 5-FU, and levels of TCRζ on days 8 and 15 are increased. Additionally, impaired nuclear translocation of transcription factors such as nuclear factor κB (NFκB) have been found.[94] It is possible that these acquired defects may impair responses to biologic therapy. The causes of these abnormalities may be multifactorial and may include secretion by the

tumor of various suppressive molecules,[94] enhanced T-cell apoptosis,[95] and local production of immunosuppressive cytokines such as IL-10.[96]

## Adoptive Immunotherapy

### *Tumor-Infiltrating Lymphocytes*

**Figure 8–13:** The significant infiltrate of T lymphocytes (TIL) present in renal tumors has also been a source of cells for adoptive immunotherapy (AIT). Tumors are digested *(A)*, and TIL are expanded in vitro with rIL-2 over a 3- to 4-week period.[97] The appearance of resulting cultures is illustrated *(B)*. Results of TIL infusions with rIL-2 or cytokine combinations have been variable.[98–100] This technique does not routinely produce a population of specific cytolytic T lymphocytes (CTLs).[98] The difficulties encountered in reproducibly culturing populations of T lymphocytes and the lack of reproducible clinical results make this approach of uncertain value. Another AIT approach involves culturing regional lymph nodes from patients immunized with autologous tumor cells and an adjuvant.[101] These results are preliminary. Finally, autolymphocyte therapy (ALT) is a technique employing peripheral blood T lymphocytes that have been activated ex vivo with a mixture of supernatant from lymphocytes activated for 72 hours with anti-CD3 monoclonal antibody.[102] Initial reports suggested a survival advantage for patients receiving ALT; this result was confined to males.[103] A confirmatory study comparing ALT to IFN-α has been completed, and results are pending.

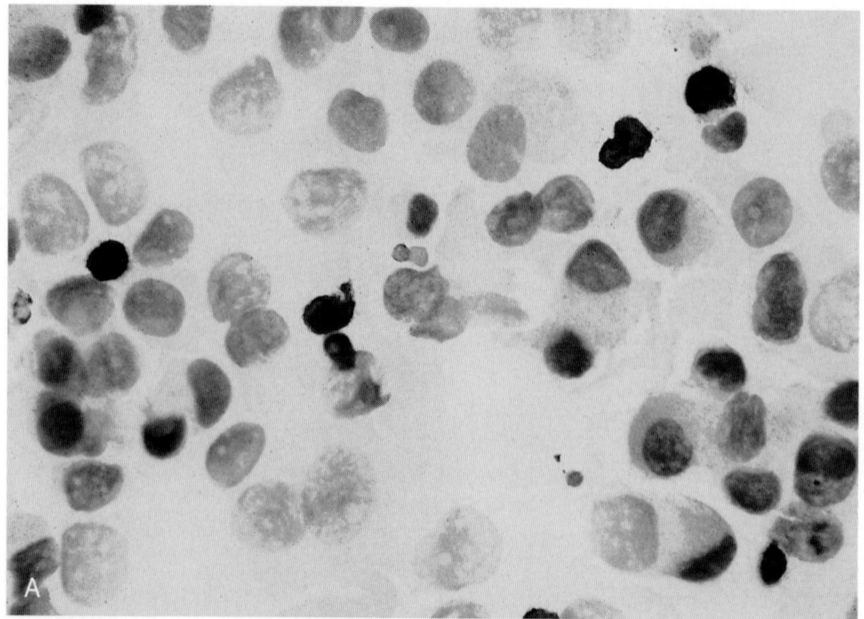

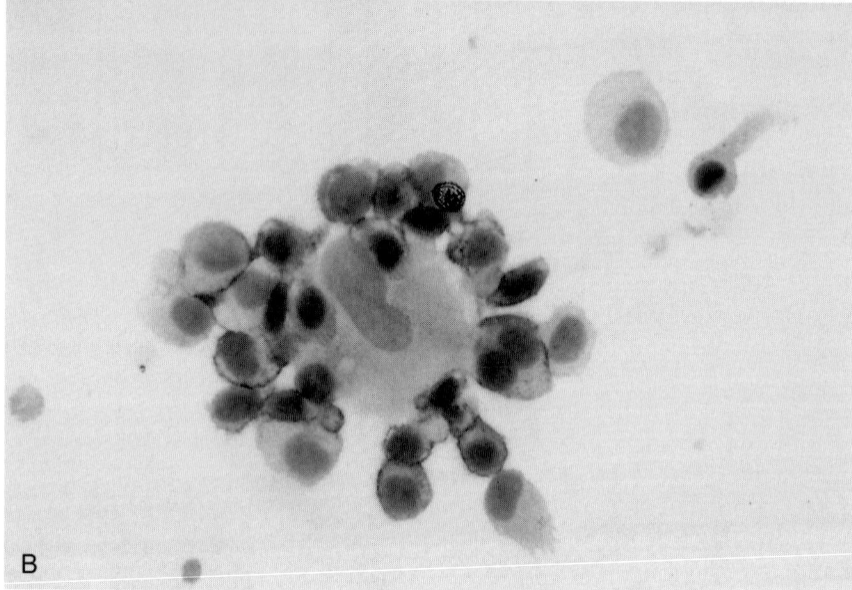

Figure 8–13

AIT remains an interesting approach to renal cell carcinoma, but the technical difficulties, lack of reproducible lymphocyte populations, and variable results make this approach investigational.

**Table 8–20:** The active transfer of immune lymphocytes to enhance cellular immunity has been investigated in renal cell carcinoma. Lymphokine-activated killer (LAK) cells represent the cell population that has been used most widely. LAK cells are derived by incubating peripheral blood mononuclear cells with rIL-2 (1000 IU/ml) for 72 to 96 hours.[103] Typically these cells have been administered with high doses of IL-2. Reported results are summarized in Table 8–20. This approach has been compared with rIL-2 alone, and a randomized trial from the National Cancer Institute did not demonstrate an increase in response rate or survival.[104] Clinical results reported with LAK cells and various methods of rIL-2 administration are also illustrated in this table.



## TABLE 8–20

### CLINICAL RESULTS WITH LAK CELLS AND rIL-2 IN TREATMENT OF METASTATIC RENAL CELL CARCINOMA

| METHOD OF rIL-2 ADMINISTRATION | NO. OF PATIENTS | CR (%) | PR (%) | OVERALL RESPONSE RATE |
|---|---|---|---|---|
| Continuous intravenous | 227 | 9 (4%) | 28 (12.3%) | 16.3% |
| Intravenous bolus | 216 | 20 (9.3%) | 39 (18.0%) | 27.3% |
| Totals | 461 | 29 (6.3%) | 68 (14.8%) | 21.0% |

*Source*: Adapted from Bukowski RM: Natural history and therapy of metastatic renal cell carcinoma: Role of interleukin 2. Cancer 80(7):1198, 1997.

## Vaccines

**Table 8–21:** Immunization with autologous cells to enhance the generation of specific immunity has been an immunotherapeutic approach utilized in the treatment of various tumors, including renal cell carcinoma. Irradiated autologous tumor cells with various adjuvants have been utilized, but results have not been remarkable.[105] The transfer of the cytokine gene GM-CSF into autologous tumor cells to enhance specific immune responses to these cells has been studied.[106, 107] The clinical results are illustrated in Table 8–21. The study by Simons et al.[100] demonstrated the feasibility of this approach and its lack of toxicity. One response was reported, resembling the reported results with systemic GM-CSF.[74] Vaccine approaches remain of interest, and isolation of tumor-associated antigens from renal cell carcinoma tumor would greatly facilitate this approach.

## Treating Metastatic Disease

**Figure 8–14:** Treatment with patients with metastatic renal cell carcinoma remains a challenge. The ap-

### TABLE 8–21

**PHASE I TRIAL OF AUTOLOGOUS RENAL CELL CANCER VACCINE GENERATED BY EX VIVO TRANSFER OF THE GM-CSF GENE**

| THERAPY | NO. OF PATIENTS | DOSE-LIMITING TOXICITY | CLINICAL RESPONSES |
|---|---|---|---|
| Irradiated autologous RCC* | 9 | None | 0 |
| Gene-modified irradiated autologous RCC* † | 7 | None | 1/7‡ |

*Vaccinations given intradermally or subcutaneously, and cell doses escalated in seclusive cohorts.

†MFG replication defective retroveral vector utilized.

‡Regression multiple pulmonary metastases.

*Source:* Data from Simons JW, Jaffee EM, Weber CE, et al: Bioactivity of autologous irradiated renal cell carcinoma vaccines generated by ex vivo granulocyte-macrophage colony-stimulating factor gene transfer. Cancer Res 57:1537, 1997.

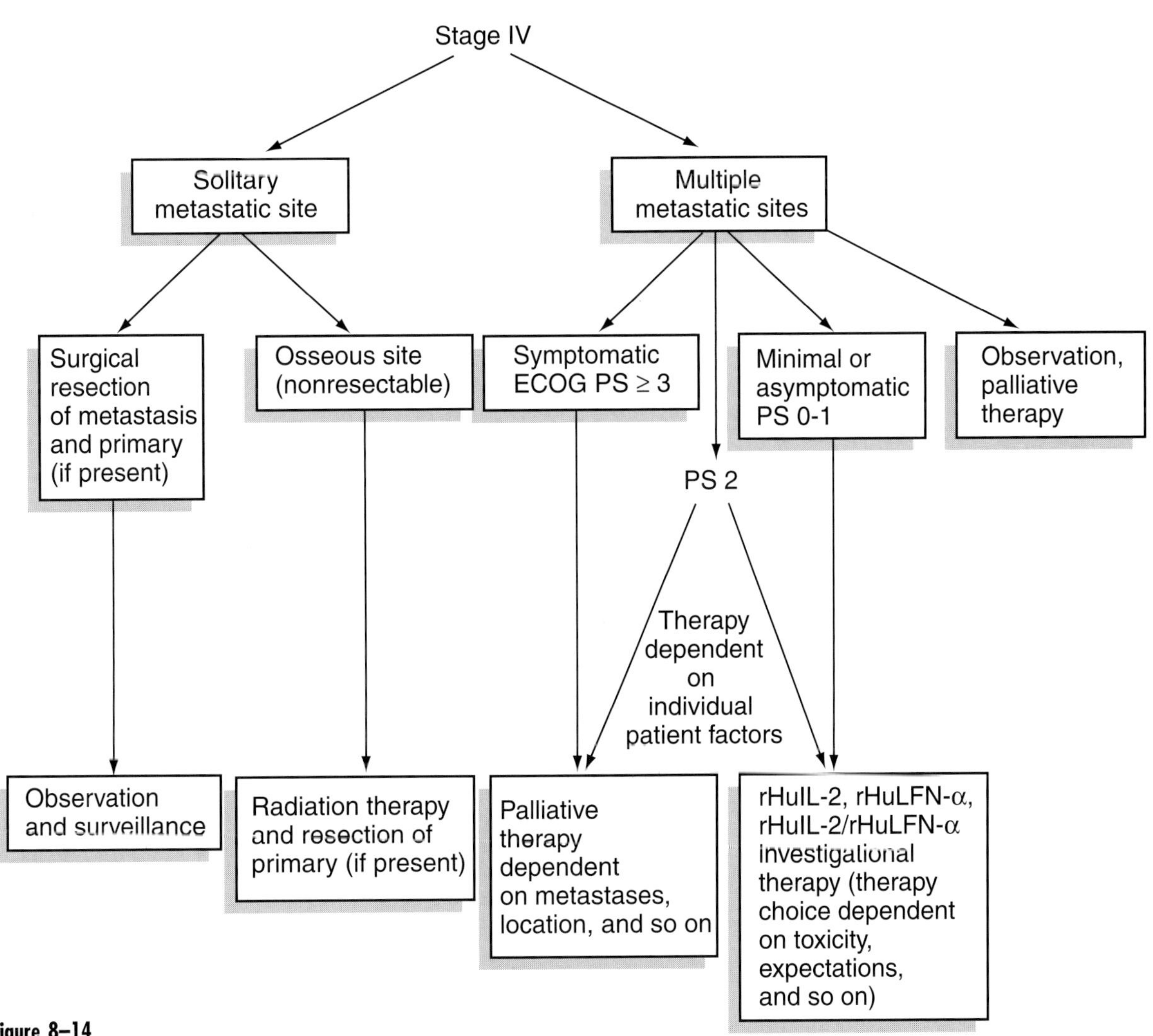


**Figure 8–14**

proaches available are associated with low response rates, and no universally accepted regimen exists. The cytokines rIL-2, IFN-$\alpha$, or the combination may produce meaningful antitumor responses in a subset of patients, but in general overall response rates are less than 20%. This figure outlines an approach to therapy of metastatic disease. Disease extent, comorbid disease, and patient expectations will modify the planned approach. (Data from Bukowski.[73])

# REFERENCES


1. Greenlee RT, Hill-Harmon M, Murray T, Thun M: Cancer statistics. CA Cancer J Clin 51(1):15–36, 2001.
2. Linehan WM, Shipley W, Parkinson D: Cancer of the kidney and ureter. In DiVita VT, Hellman S, Rosenberg SA (eds): Cancer: Principles and Practice of Oncology. Philadelphia, JB Lippincott, 1993, pp 1023–1051.
3. Robbins SL, Cotran RS: Pathologic Basis of Disease, 2nd ed. Philadelphia, WB Saunders, 1979.
4. Bertoni F, Ferri C, Benati A, et al: Sarcomatoid carcinoma of the kidney. J Urol 137:25–28, 1987.
5. Ro JY, Ayala AG, Sella A, et al: Sarcomatoid RCC: A clinicopathologic study of 42 cases. Cancer 59:516–526, 1987.
6. Robson CJ, Churchill BM, Anderson W: The results of radical nephrectomy for RCC. J Urol 101:297–301, 1969.
7. International Union Against Cancer (UICC): TNM Classification of Malignant Tumors, 4th ed. New York, Springer Verlag, 1987, pp 83–88.
8. Guinan P, Sobin LH, Alggaba F, et al: TNM staging of renal cell carcinoma. Cancer 80:992–993, 1997.
9. Middleton RG: Surgery for metastatic renal cell carcinoma. J Urol 97:973, 1967.
10. Tolia BM, Whitmore WF: Solitary metastasis from renal cell carcinoma. J Urol 114:836, 1975.
11. Maldazys JD, DeKernion JB: Prognostic factors in metastatic renal carcinoma. J Urol 136:376–379, 1986.
12. Stenzl A, DeKernion JB: Pathology, biology, and clinical staging of renal cell carcinoma. Semin Oncol 16 (suppl 1):3–11, 1989.
13. Skinner DG, Calvin RB, Vermillion CD, et al: Diagnosis and management of renal cell carcinoma. Cancer 28:1165–1177, 1971.
14. Boxer RJ, Waisman J, Leiber MM, et al: Renal carcinoma: Computer analysis of 96 patients treated by nephrectomy. J Urol 122:598–601, 1979.
15. McNichols DW, Segrura JW, DeWeerd JH: Renal cell carcinoma: Long-term survival and late recurrence. J Urol 126:17–23, 1981.
16. Golimbu M, Joshi P, Sperber A, et al: Renal cell carcinoma: survival and prognostic factors. Urology 27:291–301, 1986.
17. Cherri RJ, Goldman GG, Linder A, et al: Prognostic implications of vena caval extension of renal cell carcinoma. J Urol 128:910–912, 1982.
18. Fahn HJ, Lee YH, Chen MT, et al: The incidence and prognostic significance of humoral hypercalcemia in renal cell carcinoma. J Urol 145:248, 1991.
19. Droz JP, Rey A, Mahjoubi M, et al: Prognostic factors in metastatic renal cell carcinoma. In Klein EA, Bukowski RM, Finke JH (eds): Renal Cell Carcinoma: Immunotherapy and Cellular Biology. New York, Marcel Dekker, 1993, pp 11–24.
20. Elson PJ, Witte RS, Trump DL: Prognostic factors for survival in patients with recurrent or metastatic renal cell carcinoma. Cancer Res 48:7310–7313, 1988.
21. Palmer PA, Vinke J, Philip T, et al: Prognostic factors for survival in patients with advanced renal cell carcinoma treated with recombinant interleukin-2. Ann Oncol 3:475–480, 1992.
22. Minisian LM, Motzer RJ, Gluck L, et al: Interferon alpha 2-a in advanced renal cell carcinoma: Treatment results and survival in 159 patients with long-term follow-up. J Clin Oncol 11:1368–1375, 1993.
23. Fossa SD, Kramar A, Droz JP: Prognostic factors and survival in patients with metastatic renal cell carcinoma treated with chemotherapy or interferon-alpha. Eur J Cancer 30A:1310–1314, 1994.
24. Landonio G, Baiocchi C, Cattaneo D, et al: Retrospective analysis of 156 cases of metastatic renal cell carcinoma: Evaluation of prognostic factors and response to different treatments. Tumori 80:468–472, 1994.
25. Fyfe G, Fisher RI, Rosenberg SA, et al: Results of treatment of 255 patients with metastatic renal cell carcinoma who receive high dose recombinant interleukin-2 therapy. J Clin Oncol 13:688–696, 1995.
26. Hänninen EL, Kirchner H, Atzpodien J: Interleukin-2 based home therapy of metastatic renal cell carcinoma: Risks and benefits in 215 consecutive single institution patients. J Urol 155:19–25, 1996.
27. Kierney PC, van Heerdeen JA, Segura JW, et al: Surgeon's role in the management of solitary renal cell carcinoma metastases occurring subsequent to initial curative nephrectomy: An institutional review. Ann Surg Oncol 1:345–352, 1994.
28. Cerfolio RJ, Allen MS, Deschamps C, et al: Pulmonary resection of metastatic renal cell carcinoma. Ann Thorac Surg 57:339–344, 1994.
29. deKernion JB: Treatment of advanced renal cell carcinoma—Traditional methods and innovative approaches. J Urol 130:2, 1983.
30. Flanigan RC, Blumenstein BA, Salmon S, Crawford E: Cytoreduction nephrectomy in metastatic renal cancer: The results of Southwest Oncology Group Trial 8949 (abstract). Proc Am Soc Clin Oncol 19:2a, 2000.
31. Sundaresan N, Galicich JH, Baines MS: Vertebral body resection in the treatment of cancer involving the spine. Cancer 53:1393, 1984.
32. Onufrey V, Mohiuddin M: Radiation therapy in the treatment of metastatic renal cell carcinoma. Int J Radiat Oncol Biol Phys 11:2007–2009, 1985.
33. Fossa SD, Kjolseth I, Lund G: Radiotherapy of metastasis from renal cancer. Eur Urol 8:340, 1982.
34. Halperin EC, Harisiadis L: The role of radiation therapy in the management of metastatic renal cell carcinoma. Cancer 51:614, 1983.
35. Bukowski RM: The problem of metastases. In Montie JE, Pontes JE, Bukowski RM (eds): Clinical Management of Renal Cell Cancer. Chicago, Year Book Medical Publishers, 1990, pp 163–178.
36. Montie JE, Steward BH, Straffon RA, et al: The role of adjunctive nephrectomy in patients with metastatic renal cell carcinoma. J Urol 117:272, 1977.
37. Gleave M, Elhilali M, Frodet Y, et al: A multicenter randomized, double blind trial of autoimmune interferon gamma-1b (IFN$\gamma$) injection versus placebo for the treatment of metastatic renal cell carcinoma (mRCC) (abstract). Proc ASCO 16:317a, 1997.
38. Finke JH, Tubbs R, Connelly B, et al: Tumor-infiltrating lymphocytes in patients with RCC. Ann NY Acad Sci 532:387–394, 1988.
39. Finke JH, Rayman P, Hart L, et al: Characterization of TIL subsets from human renal cell carcinoma: Specific reactivity defined by cytotoxicity, IFN$\gamma$ secretion, and proliferation. J Immunother 15:91–104, 1994.
40. Harris DT: Hormonal therapy and chemotherapy of RCC. Semin Oncol 10:422–430, 1983.
41. Kjaer M: The role of medroxyprogesterone acetate (MPA) in the treatment of renal adenocarcinoma. Cancer Treat Rev 15:195–209, 1988.
42. Weiselberg L, Budman D, Vinciguerra V, et al: Tamoxifen in unresectable hypernephroma: A Phase II trial and review of the literature. Cancer Clin Trials 4:195–198, 1981.
43. Atzpodien J, Kirchner H, Franzke A, et al: Results of a randomized clinical trial comparing SC interleukin-2, SC alpha-2a-interferon, and IV bolus 5-fluorouracil against oral tamoxifen in progressive metastatic renal cell carcinoma patients (abstract). Proc ASCO 16:326a, 1997.
44. Yagoda A, Abi-Rached B, Petrylak D: Chemotherapy for advanced renal-cell carcinoma: 1983–1993. Semin Oncol 22:42–60, 1995.
45. Pyrhönen S, Salminen E, Lehtonem T, et al: Recombinant interferon alpha-2a with vinblastine vs. vinblastine alone in advanced renal cell carcinoma. A phase III study (abstract). Proc ASCO 15:244, 1996.

46. Von Roemeling RW, Hrushesky WJM: Circadian patterning of continuous floxuridine infusion reduces toxicity and allows higher dose intensity in patients with widespread cancer. J Clin Oncol 7:1710–1719, 1989.

47. Dexeus FH, Logothetis CJ, Sella A, et al: Circadian infusion of floxuridine in patients with metastatic renal cell carcinoma. J Urol 146:709–713, 1991.

48. Sampaio C, Olencki T, Murthy G, et al: Phase II trial of circadian infusion of the antimetabolite floxuridine in patients with metastatic RCC. J Inf Chemother 4:100–103, 1994.

49. Crivellari D, Tumolo S, Fustaci S, et al: Phase II study of five-day continuous infusion of vinblastine in patients with metastatic renal-cell carcinoma. Am J Clin Oncol 10:231–233, 1987.

50. Oliver RTD, Mehta A, Barnett MJ: A phase 2 study of surveillance in patients with metastatic renal cell carcinoma and assessment of response of such patients to therapy on progression. Mol Biother 1:14–20, 1988.

51. Gillis S, Union NA, Baker PF, et al: The in vitro generation and sustained culture of nude mouse cytolytic T-lymphocytes. J Exp Med 149:1460–1476, 1979.

52. Taniguchi T, Matsui H, Fujita T, et al: Structure and expression of a cloned cDNA for human interleukin-2. Nature 302:305–310, 1983.

53. Kroemer G, Andreu JL, Gonzalo JA, et al: Interleukin-2, autotolerance and autoimmunity. Adv Immunol 50:147–235, 1991.

54. Bukowski RM, McLain D, Finke J: Clinical pharmacokinetics of interleukin-1, interleukin-2, interleukin-4, tumor necrosis-factor and macrophage colony stimulating factor. In Chalner BA, Longo DL (eds): Cancer Chemotherapy and Biotherapy—Principles & Practice. Philadelphia, Lippincott-Raven, 1996, pp 609–638.

55. Yang JC, Rosenberg SA: An ongoing prospective randomized comparison of interleukin-2 regimens for the treatment of metastatic renal cell carcinoma. Cancer J Sci Am 3:579–584, 1997.

56. Bukowski RM: Natural history and therapy of metastatic renal cell carcinoma: Role of interleukin 2. Cancer 80(7):1198–1220, 1997.

57. Quesada JR, Swanson DA, Trindale A, et al: Renal cell carcinoma: Antitumor effects of leukocyte interferon. Cancer Res 43:940–947, 1983.

58. DeKernion JB, Sarna JB, Figlin R, et al: The treatment of renal cell carcinoma with human leukocyte alpha-interferon. J Urol 130:1063–1066, 1983.

59. Dorr RT: Interferon-alpha in malignant and viral diseases: a review. Drugs 45:177–211, 1993.

60. Gilewski T, Vogelzang NJ: Cost effectiveness and reimbursement issues in renal cell carcinoma. Semin Oncol 16 (suppl 1):20–26, 1989.

61. Figlin RA, Abi-Aad AS, Belldegrun A, et al: The role of interferon and interleukin-2 in the immunotherapeutic approach to renal cell carcinoma. Semin Oncol 18 (suppl 7):102–107, 1991.

62. Ritchie AWS, Griffiths G, Cook P, et al: Alpha interferon improves survival in patients with metastatic renal carcinoma—preliminary results of an MRC randomized controlled trial. Proc Am Soc Clin Oncol 17:310a, 1998.

63. Kriegmair M, Obemeder R, Hofstetter A: Interferon alpha and vinblastine versus medroxy-progesterone acetate in the treatment of metastatic renal cell carcinoma. Urology 45:758–762, 1995.

64. Lippman SM, Kavanaugh JJ, Paredes-Espinoza M, et al: 13-cis-retinoic acid plus interferon alpha-2a: Highly active systemic therapy for squamous cell carcinoma of the cervix. J Natl Cancer Inst 84:241–245, 1992.

65. Motzer RJ, Schwartz L, Law TM, et al: Interferon alfa-2a and 13-cis-retinoic acid in renal cell carcinoma: Antitumor activity in a phase II trial and interactions in vitro. J Clin Oncol 13.1950–1957, 1995.

66. Motzer RJ, Murphy BA, Bacik J, et al: Phase III trial of interferon alfa-2a with or without 13-cis-retinoic acid for patients with advanced renal cell carcinoma. J Clin Oncol 18:2972–2980, 2000.

67. Chikkala NF, Lewis I, Ulchaker J, et al: Interactive effects of α-interferon A/D and interleukin-2 on murine lymphokine-activated killer activity: Analysis at the effector and precursor level. Cancer Res 50:1176–1182, 1990.

68. Atzpodien J, Lopez-Hänninen E, Kirchner H, et al: Multiinstitutional home-therapy trial of recombinant human interleukin-2 and interferon alfa-2 in progressive metastatic RCC. J Clin Oncol 13:497–501, 1995.

69. Negrier S, Escudier B, Lasset C, et al: Recombinant human interleukin-2, recombinant interferon alfa-2a or both in metastatic renal cell carcinoma. N Engl J Med 338:1272–1278, 1996.

70. Henriksson R, Nilsson S, Colleen S, et al: Survival in renal cell carcinoma—a randomized evaluation of tamoxifen vs. interleukin 2, α-interferon (leucocyte) and tamoxifen. Br J Cancer 77:1311–1317, 1998.

71. Sleijfer DTH, Janssen RJ, deVries EGE, et al: Phase II study of subcutaneous interleukin-2 in unselected patients with advanced renal cell cancer on an outpatient basis. J Clin Oncol 10:1119–1123, 1992.

72. Small EJ, Weiss G, Dutcher J, et al: A multicenter open-label trial of autoimmune interferon-gamma-1b injection (IFNg) for the treatment of metastatic renal cell carcinoma (mRCC) (abstract). Proc Am Soc Clin Oncol 16:343a, 1997.

73. Bukowski RM, Novick AC: Clinical practice guidelines: renal cell carcinoma. Cleveland Clin J Med 64 (1):1–44, 1997.

74. Wos E, Olencki T, Tuason L, et al: Phase II trial of subcutaneously administered granulocyte-macrophage colony-stimulating factor in patients with metastatic renal cell carcinoma. Cancer 73:1149–1153, 1996.

75. Stadler WM, Rybak ME, Vogelzang NJ: A phase II study of subcutaneous recombinant human interleukin-4 in metastatic renal cell carcinoma. Cancer 76:1629–1633, 1995.

76. Stouthard JML, deVries EGE, deMulder PH, et al: Recombinant human interleukin 6 in metastatic renal cell cancer: A phase II trial. Br J Cancer 73:789–793, 1996.

77. Bollack C, Jacqmin D, Bergerat JP, et al: Recombinant interferon alpha plus vinblastine in metastatic renal cell cancer: updated results. In Debruyne FMJ, Bukowski RM, Pontes JE, deMulder PHM (eds): Immunotherapy of Renal Cell Carcinoma. Berlin, Springer Verlag, 1991, pp 75–81.

78. Fossa SD, Martinelli G, Otto U, et al: Recombinant interferon alfa-2a with or without vinblastine in metastatic renal cell carcinoma: Results of a European multi-center phase III study. Ann Oncol 3:301–305, 1992.

79. Houghton JA, Morton CL, Adkins DA, et al: Locus of the interaction among 5-fluorouracil, leucovorin, and interferon-α2a in colon carcinoma cells. Cancer Res 53:4243–4250, 1993.

80. Wadler SW, Schwartz EL, Goldman M: Fluorouracil and recombinant interferon-α-2A: An active regimen against advanced colorectal carcinoma. J Clin Oncol 7:1769–1775, 1989.

81. Hoffmockel G, Langer W, Theiss M, et al: Immunochemotherapy for metastatic renal cell carcinoma using a regimen of interleukin-2, interferon-α and 5-fluorouracil. J Urol 156:18–21, 1996.

82. Sella A, Zukiwski A, Robinson E, et al: Interleukin-2 (IL-2) with interferon-α (IFN-α) and 5-fluorouracil (5-FU) in patients (PTS) with metastatic renal cell cancer (RCC) (abstract). Proc Am Soc Clin Oncol 13:237, 1994.

83. Dutcher J, Logan T, Gordon M, et al: 5FU + subcutaneous (sc) interleukin-2 (IL2) plus sc Intron (IFN) in metastatic renal cell cancer (RCC) patients (PTS). A CWG study (abstract). Proc Am Soc Clin Oncol 15:272, 1996.

84. Olencki T, Bukowski RM, Budd GT, et al: Phase I/II trial of simultaneously administered rIL-2/rHuIFNα2a and 5-FU in patients (PTS) with metastatic renal cell carcinoma (RCC) (abstract). Proc Am Soc Clin Oncol 15:263, 1996.

85. Negrier S, Escudier B, Dovillard JY, et al: Randomized study of interleukin-2 (IL2) and interferon (IFN) with or without 5-FU (FUCY study) in metastatic renal cell carcinoma (MRCC) (abstract). Proc Am Soc Clin Oncol 16:326a, 1997.

86. Sella A, Swanson DA, Ro JY, et al: Surgery following response to interferon-alpha-based therapy for residual renal cell carcinoma. J Urol 149:19–22, 1991.

87. Sella A, Swanson D, Amato R, et al: Evidence for a favorable effect of surgical resection of residual metastatic renal cell carcinoma (RCC) following biological therapy (BT) (abstract). Proc Am Soc Clin Oncol 12:246, 1993.

88. Rackley R, Novick A, Klein E, et al: The impact of adjuvant nephrectomy on multi-modality treatment of metastatic renal cell carcinoma. J Urol 152:1399–1403, 1994.

89. Walther MM, Alexander RB, Weiss GH, et al: Cytoreductive

surgery prior to interleukin-2-based therapy in patients with metastatic renal cell carcinoma. Urology 42:250–258, 1993.

90. Broder S, Waldmann TA: The suppressor-cell network in cancer. N Engl J Med 299:1281–1284, 1978.

91. Miescher S, Whitesides TL, Carrel C, et al: Functional properties of tumor-infiltrating and blood lymphocytes in patients with solid tumors: Effects of tumor cells and their supernatants on proliferative responses of lymphocytes. J Immunol 136:1899–1907, 1986.

92. Finke JH, Zea A, Stanley J, et al: Loss of T-cell receptor zeta chain and p56[lck] in T-cells infiltrating human RCC. Cancer Res 53:5613–5616, 1993.

93. Li X, Liu J, Park JK, et al: T cells from renal cell carcinoma patients exhibit an abnormal pattern of kappa B-specific DNA-binding activity: A preliminary report. Cancer Res 54:5424–5429, 1994.

94. Kolenko V, Wang Q, Riedy MC, et al: Tumor induced suppression of T-lymphocyte proliferation coincides with inhibition of JAK3 expression and IL-2R signaling: Role of soluble products from human renal cell carcinomas. J Immunol 159:3057–3067, 1997.

95. O'Mahony AM, O'Sullivan GC, O'Connell J, et al: An immune suppressive factor derived from esophageal squamous cell carcinoma induces apoptosis in normal and transformed cells of lymphoid lineage. J Immunol 151:4847–4856, 1993.

96. Wang Q, Redovan C, Tubbs R, et al: Selective cytokine gene expression in RCC tumor cells and tumor infiltrating lymphocytes. Int J Cancer 61:1–6, 1995.

97. Rosenberg SA, Speiss P, Lafreniere R: A new approach to the adoptive immunotherapy of cancer with tumor-infiltrating lymphocytes. Science 233:1318–1321, 1986.

98. Bukowski RM, Sharfman W, Murthy S, et al: Clinical results and characterization of tumor-infiltrating lymphocytes with or without recombinant interleukin-2 in human metastatic renal cell carcinoma. Cancer Res 51:4199–4205, 1991.

99. Rayman P, Finke JH, Olencki T, et al: Adoptive immunotherapy utilizing IL-2 and IL-4 for expansion of tumor-infiltrating lymphocytes in renal cell carcinoma. In Chang AE, Shu S (eds): Immunotherapy of Cancer with Sensitized T Lymphocytes. Boca Raton, RG Landes, 1994, pp 123–129.

100. Figlin RA, Thompson JA, Bukowski RM, et al: Multi-center, randomized, phase III trial of CD8 (+) tumor-infiltrating lymphocytes in combination with recombinant interleukin-2 in metastatic renal cell carcinoma. J Clin Oncol 17:2521–2527, 1999.

101. Chang AE, Aruga A, Cameron MJ, et al: Adoptive immunotherapy with vaccine-primed lymph node cells secondarily activated with anti-CD3 and IL-2. J Clin Oncol 15:796–807, 1996.

102. Osband ME, Lavin PT, Babayan RK, et al: Effect of autolymphocyte therapy on survival and quality of life in patients with metastatic renal-cell carcinoma. Lancet 335:994–998, 1990.

103. Rosenberg SA, Lotze MT, Yang JC, et al: Experience with the use of high dose interleukin-2 in the treatment of 652 cancer patients. Ann Surg 210:474–485, 1989.

104. Rosenberg SA, Lotze MT, Yang JC, et al: Prospective randomized trial of high-dose interleukin-2 alone or in conjunction with lymphokine-activated killer cells for the treatment of patients with advanced cancer. J Natl Cancer Inst 85:622–632, 1993.

105. Galligioni E, Francini M, Quaia M, et al: Randomized study of adjuvant immunotherapy with autologous tumor cells and BCG in renal cancer. In Bystryn J, Ferrone S, Livingston P (eds): Specific Immunotherapy of Cancer with Vaccines. New York, NY Academy of Sciences, 1993, pp 367–369.

106. Jaffee EM, Pardoll DM: Gene therapy: Its potential applications in the treatment of renal-cell carcinoma. Semin Oncol 22:81–91, 1995.

107. Simons JW, Jaffee EM, Weber CE, et al: Bioactivity of autologous irradiated renal cell carcinoma vaccines generated by ex vivo granulocyte-macrophage colony-stimulating factor gene transfer. Cancer Res 57:1537–1546, 1997.

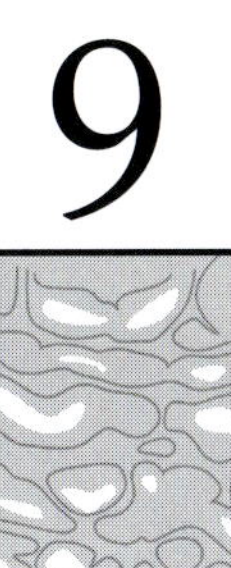

# Nonseminomatous Germ Cell Tumors: Surgical Management


*Elliot Fagelman*

*Ihor S. Sawczuk*

*Mitchell C. Benson*


Retroperitoneal lymph node dissection serves to provide pathologic staging of nonseminomatous germ cell tumors (NSGCT) as well as a known therapeutic benefit. Retroperitoneal lymph node dissection (RPLND) is considered in patients who have clinical stage I disease and are at high risk for relapse under surveillance and those with an embryonal cell tumor or vascular invasion.[1] The therapeutic benefit varies, depending on the stage of the disease. RPLND can be curative in up to 70% of patients with stage IIA NSGCT. The cure rate declines as the volume of retroperitoneal involvement increases.[2] Another role of RPLND is surgical removal of residual nodal or extranodal masses after initial chemotherapy or as an alternative to chemotherapy in patients with low volume retroperitoneal disease.

Retrograde ejaculation is a potential problem that may result from RPLND. Prior to modified RPLND and nerve-sparing RPLND, approximately 90% of those patients undergoing complete bilateral RPLND either developed retrograde ejaculation or became anejaculators. The preservation of the lumbar sympathetic nerve fibers is important in maintaining antegrade ejaculation and involves understanding the anatomy of the nerves and the pattern of lymph node metastasis. On the right side, the postganglionic nerve fibers travel posterior to the inferior vena cava (IVC) to join the hypogastric plexus of nerves anterior to the abdominal aorta. On the left side, the sympathetic fibers run dorsal and left of the aorta to join the preaortic decusation of nerve trunks. The nerves then travel anterior to the iliac vessels to enter the pelvis.[3, 4] Using the modified and nerve-sparing RPLND, antegrade ejaculation can be preserved in approximately 90% of patients.[3]

## Preoperative Evaluation

Preoperative evaluation includes a complete history and physical examination. Laboratory work-up includes a complete blood cell count, serum electrolytes, renal function tests, liver function tests, coagulation profile, and tumor markers (alpha-fetoprotein, human chorionic gonadotropin, and lactic acid dehydrogenase). Imaging studies must include a computed tomographic (CT) scan of the abdomen and pelvis as well as a chest x-ray. Routine CT scans of the chest are not mandatory in patients with low volume disease. However, in patients with positive lymphadenopathy seen on abdominal imaging, a CT scan of the chest can be beneficial.[5] In addition, patients should have a preoperative mechanical bowel preparation with antibiotics.

This chapter reviews the surgical techniques underlying the modified and nerve-sparing RPLND in low volume retroperitoneal disease for NSGCT, as well as its complications and results.

**Figure 9–1:** Primary sites of lymphatic drainage from the left testis, as defined by early lymph node metastases from left-sided testis tumors.[6] The distribution of nodal metastases in NSGCTs has been described by Donohue.[7] The preaortic and left para-aortic areas are the most common sites of left testicular tumor

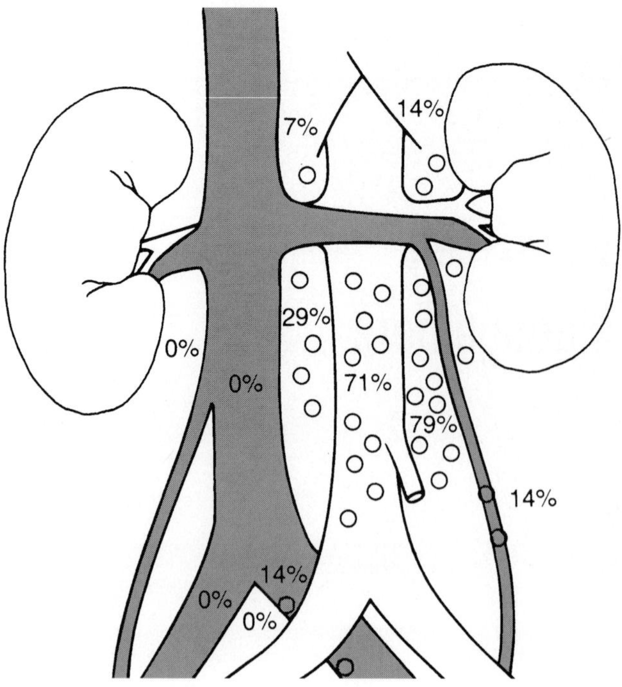


**Figure 9–1**

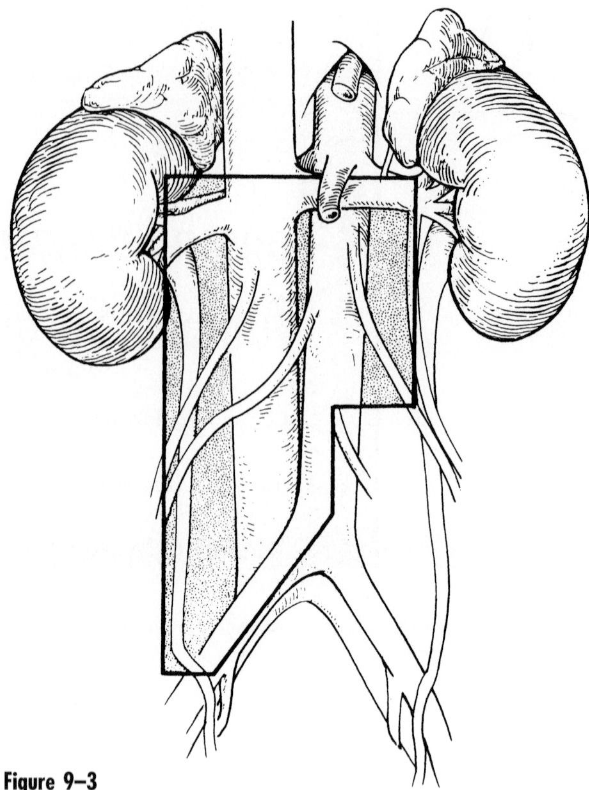

**Figure 9–3**

spread. (From Donohue JP: Metastatic pathways of nonseminomatous germ cell tumors. Semin Urol 2:217, 1984.)

**Figure 9–2:** Primary sites of lymphatic drainage from the right testis, as defined by early lymph node metastases from right-sided testis tumors. (From Donohue JP: Metastatic pathways of nonseminomatous germ cell tumors. Semin Urol 2:217, 1984.)

**Figure 9–3:** Template for modified right-sided retroperitoneal lymph node dissection (RPLND). The dissection is complete above the level of the inferior mesenteric artery but limited to the ipsilateral side below the level of the inferior mesenteric artery.[3] The rationale

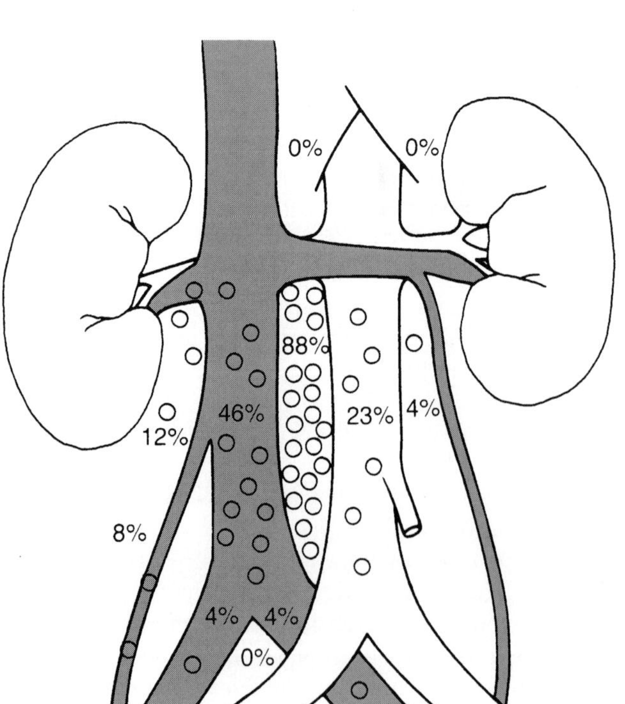


**Figure 9–2**

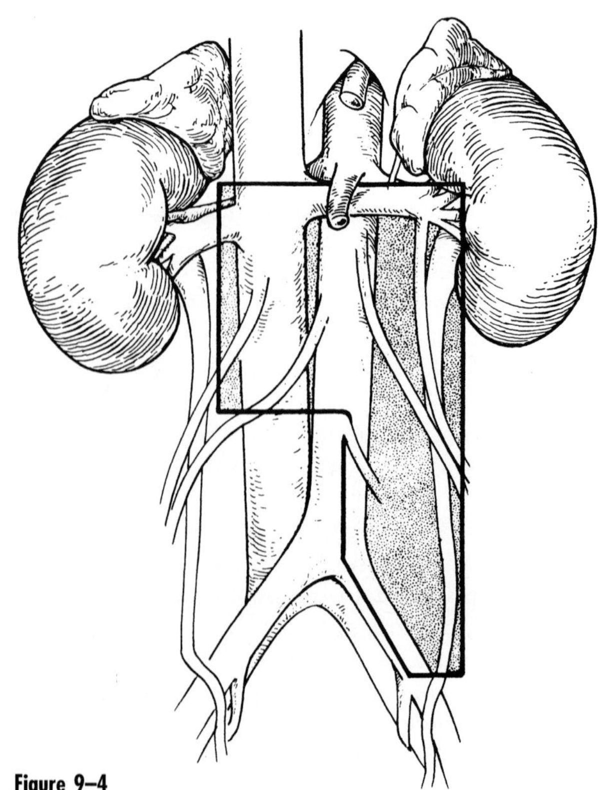

**Figure 9–4**

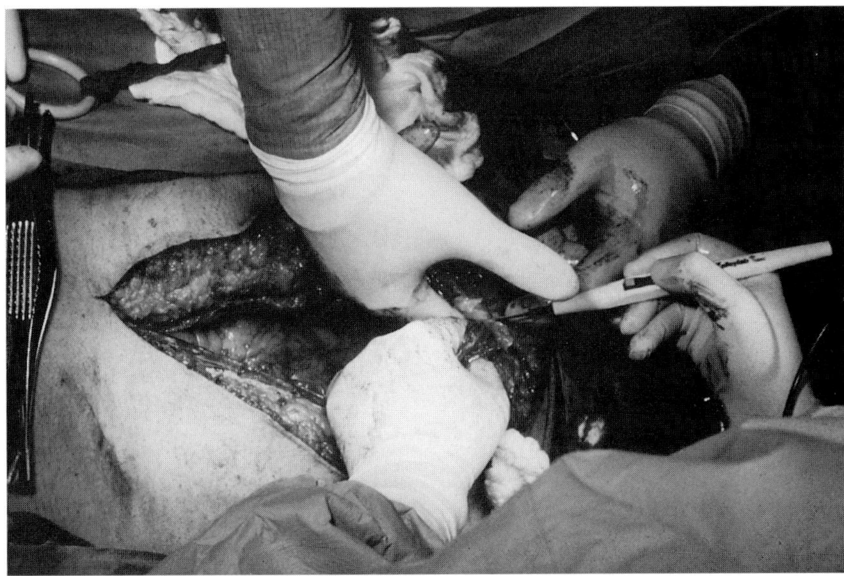

Figure 9–5

for a modified RPLND comes from significant separation of the hypogastric plexus, anterior to the aortic bifurcation, and the predictable landing sites for lymph node metastases. The template RPLND limits the dissection below the inferior mesenteric artery to the side ipsilateral to the tumor to preserve neural pathways involved with antegrade ejaculation. Richie in 1990 reported the preservation of antegrade ejaculation in 75 of 88 patients (88%).[8] (From Richie JP· Neoplasms of the testis. In Walsh PC, Retik AB, Vaughan ED, Wein AJ (eds): Campbell's Urology, 7th ed. Philadelphia, WB Saunders, 1998, p 2431.)

**Figure 9–4:** Template for modified left-sided retroperitoneal lymph node dissection.[3] (From Richie JP: Neoplasms of the testis. In Walsh PC, Retik AB, Vaughan ED, Wein AJ (eds): Campbell's Urology, 7th ed. Philadelphia, WB Saunders, 1998, p 2431.)

**Figure 9–5:** The patient is positioned supine, and a Foley catheter is inserted to monitor urine output. A transabdominal approach is used. A generous midline incision from the xiphoid process to the pubic symphysis is demonstrated in this figure.

**Figure 9–6:** The incision is deepened using cautery or sharp dissection and the fascia is incised in the midline. The peritoneum is entered carefully so as to avoid injury to the underlying bowel. After the peritoneum is entered, a self-retaining retractor is placed. We prefer an Omni retractor, as shown in this figure.

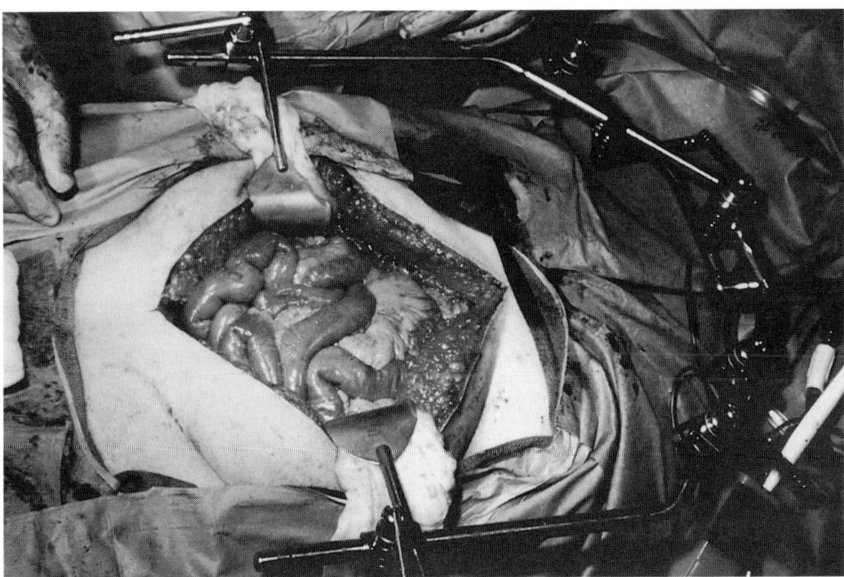

Figure 9–6

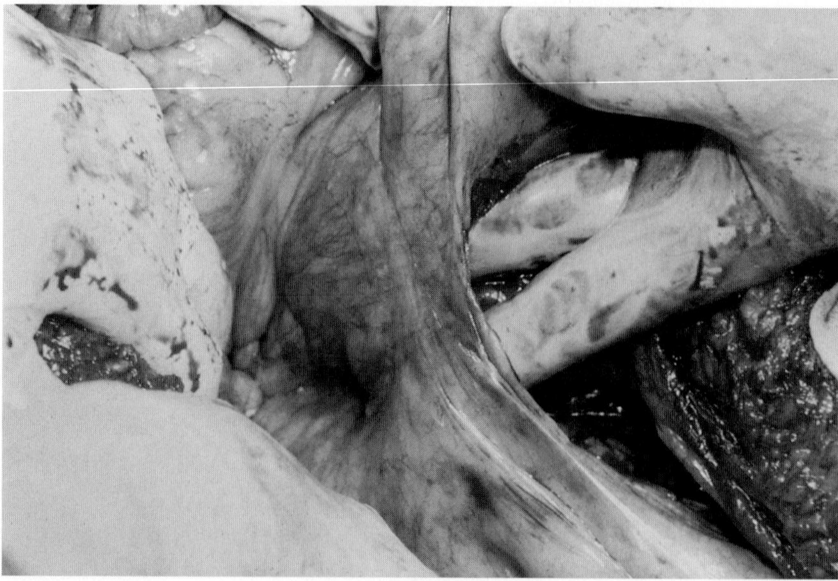

**Figure 9–7**

**Figure 9–7:** The abdomen is inspected and the retroperitoneum palpated to evaluate for extensive lymphadenopathy. The posterior peritoneum is incised along the white line of Toldt. The root of the mesentery is incised to the ligament of Treitz. In order to gain full mobilization of the bowel and adequate exposure of the retroperitoneum, it may be necessary to divide the inferior mesenteric vein (IMV).

**Figure 9–8:** After mobilization of the small and large bowel, the intestinal contents are placed into a bowel bag.

**Figure 9–9:** After the small and large bowel are placed in a bowel bag, exposure of the retroperitoneum is achieved, with the inferior vena cava and aorta being visualized.

**Figure 9–10:** The "split and roll" technique is used to remove the lymphatic tissue. The technique is shown schematically in this figure. (From Donohue JP: Radical orchiectomy and retroperitoneal lymph node dissection. In Richie JP: Urologic Oncology. Philadelphia, WB Saunders, 1997, p. 526.)

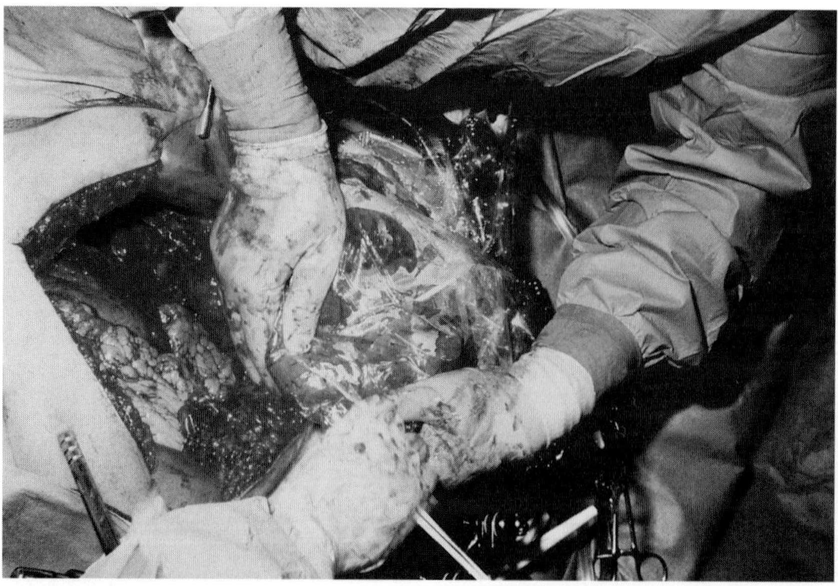

**Figure 9–8**

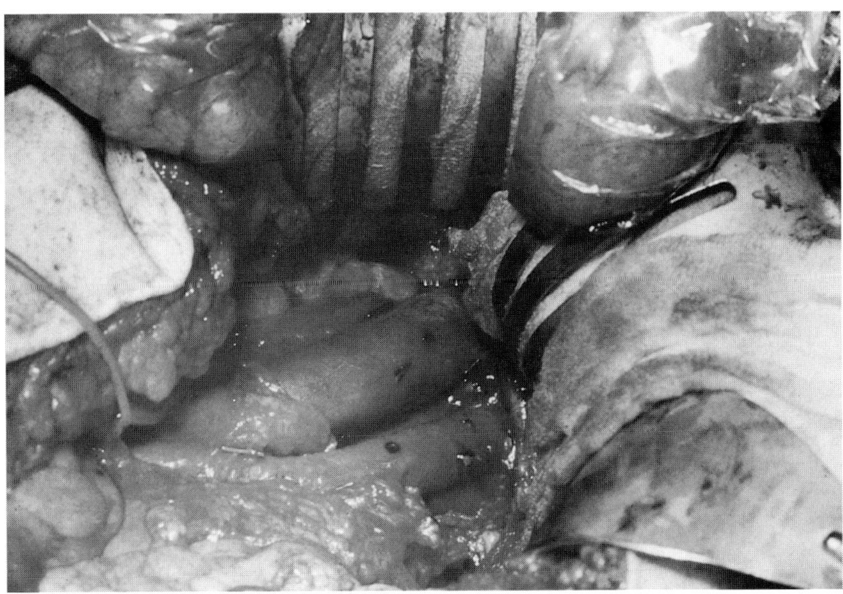

Figure 9–9

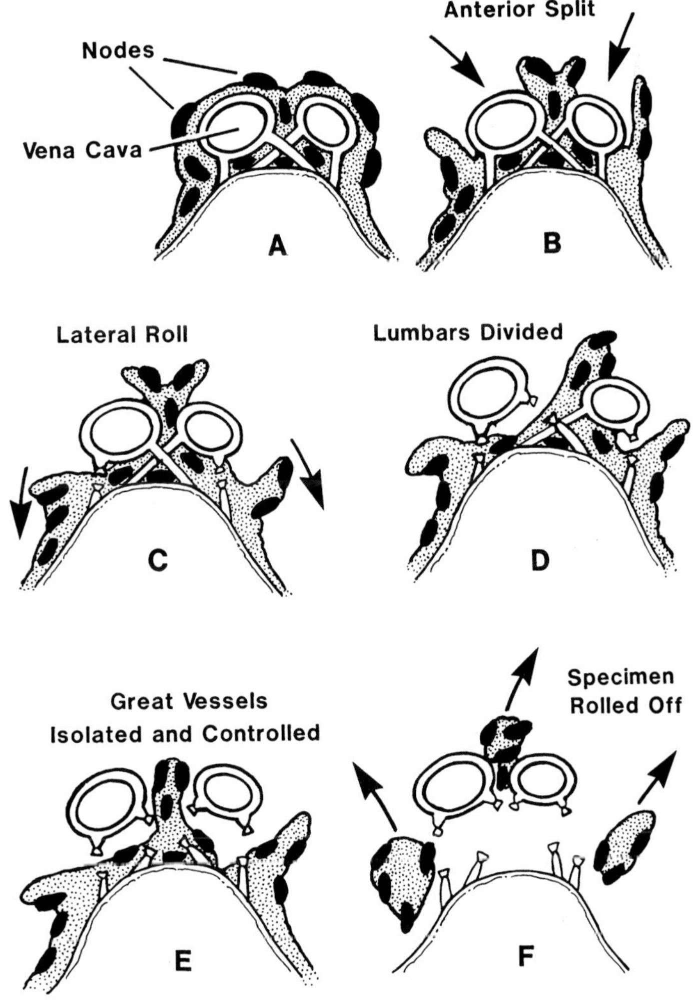


Figure 9–10

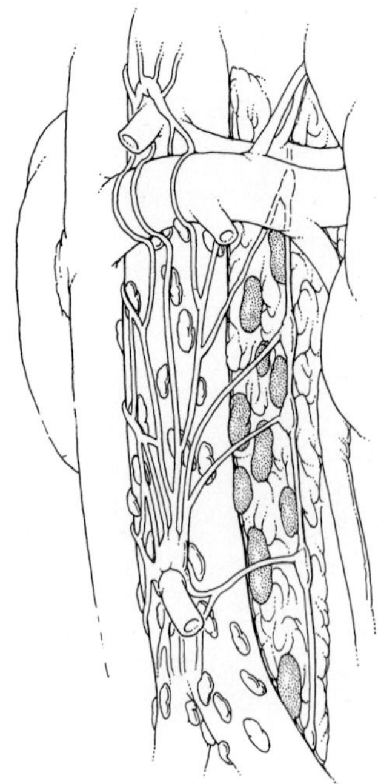

**Figure 9–11**

**Figure 9–11:** Another approach is a nerve-sparing RPLND, in which the lumbar postganglionic sympathetic nerve fibers are identified and preserved during the operation. This technique is more time consuming than is the template RPLND. With this technique, antegrade ejaculation has been preserved in 100% of patients.[4] The initial step in a nerve-sparing RPLND is exposure of the lumbar sympathetic chain by dissecting posterolateral to the aorta. The L1–L3 nerve roots course medial and inferior and join the contralateral sympathetic branches and splanchnic sympathetic fibers, which course anterior to the aorta. These relationships are demonstrated in this figure, in which the left sympathetic fibers from the L1–L4 ganglia of the sympathetic chain dorsal and left of the aorta join the preaortic decussation of nerve trunks.[7] (From Donohue JP, Foster RS: Retroperitoneal lymphadenectomy in staging and treatment. The development of nerve-sparing techniques. Urol Clin North Am 25:465, 1998.)

**Figure 9–12:** As described by Donohue and Foster, after the sympathetic chain and nerve roots are identified, the anterior retroperitoneal lymph nodes are dissected from the nerve roots.[7] The posterior nerve roots are dissected to allow removal of the nodal package lying in the sulcus bounded by the aorta medially, the spinous ligaments posteriorly, and the nerve roots, which lie ventral to the nodes. This figure shows the left-sided nerve-sparing technique after clearance of the posterior set of lymph nodes.[7] (From Donohue JP, Foster RS: Retroperitoneal lymphadenectomy in staging and treatment. The development of nerve-sparing techniques. Urol Clin North Am 25:465, 1998.)

**Figure 9–13:** Nodal tissue anterior to the great vessels is dissected free and clipped using surgical clips.

**Figure 9–14:** After the nodal tissue anterior to the great vessels is dissected, the nodal package is rolled laterally. This provides exposure of the lumbar vessels. In this figure, a lumbar artery is isolated and ligated.

**Figure 9–15:** Following ligation of the lumbar veins, the inferior vena cava (IVC) is fully mobilized as shown in the figure. Nodal tissue can then be removed posterior to the IVC.

**Figure 9–16:** The lateral and medial extent of a template-sparing RPLND is demonstrated. The renal vessels represent the superior extent of the dissection. The medial limit of the dissection is the midline of the IVC. The left ureter in the vessel loop represents the lateral extent of dissection. The inferior mesenteric artery (IMA) is also demonstrated and represents the most inferior aspect of the dissection on the right side.

## Complications

**Table 9–1:** Complications of primary RPLND were reported for 478 patients who underwent RPLND.[9] There were a total of 53 complications. The complications of RPLND included wound infection, bowel injury or obstruction, ureteral injury, vascular injury, inci-

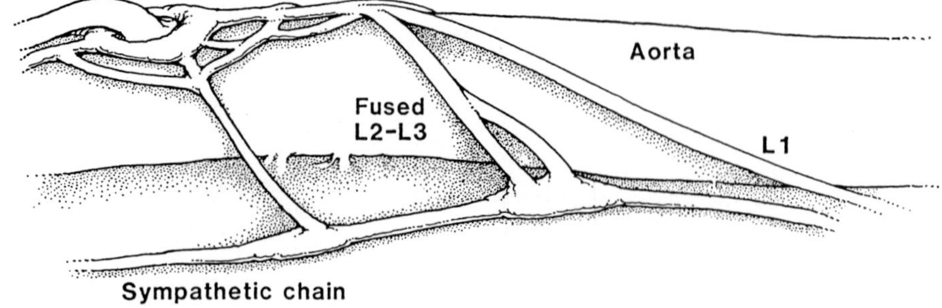


**Figure 9–12**

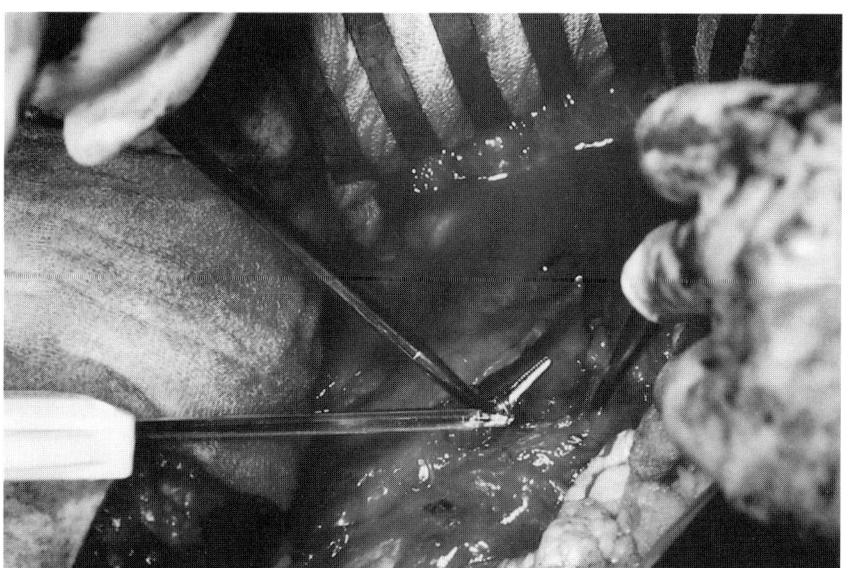

**Figure 9–13**

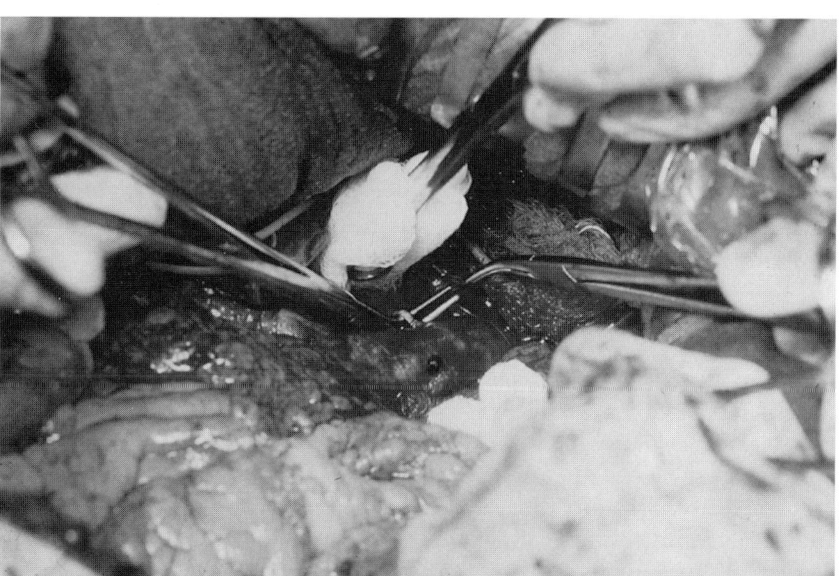

**Figure 9–14**

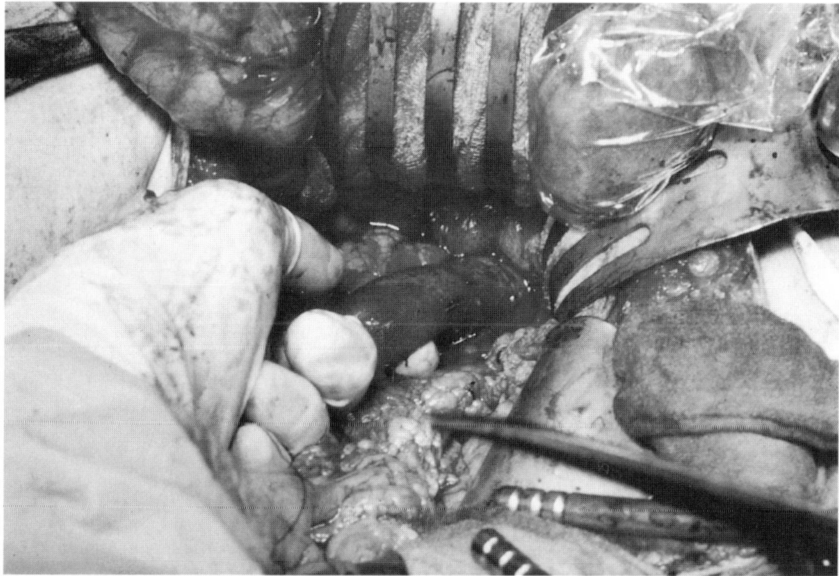

**Figure 9–15**

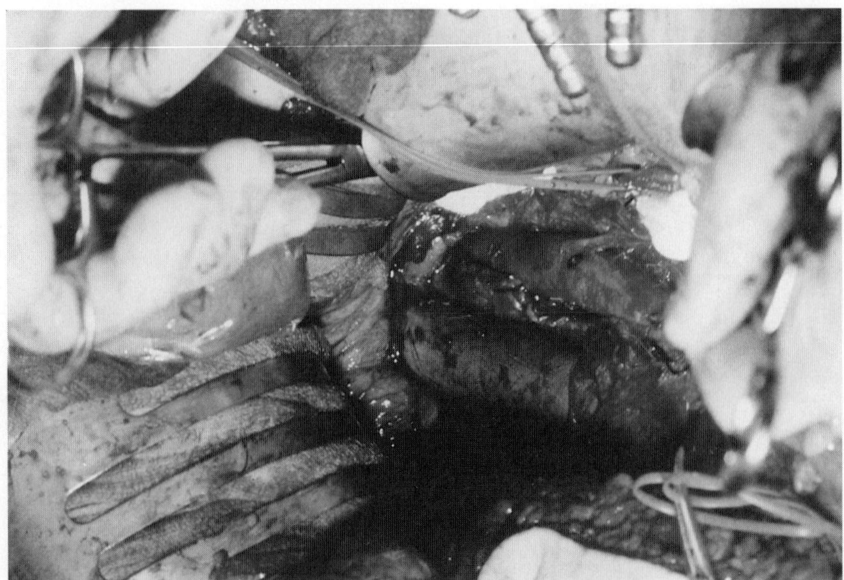

**Figure 9–16**

sional hernia, hematoma, infection, atelectasis, pneumonia, ileus, lymphocele, and pancreatitis.

**Table 9–2:** Complications of RPLND after chemotherapy were reported for in 603 patients.[10] There were a total of 144 complications. Following chemotherapy for testicular cancer, RPLND can be complicated by fibrosis around the great vessels and renal hilum. RPLND after chemotherapy is associated with an increased number of complications, especially pulmonary ones. The adult respiratory distress syndrome may occur and is associated with the pulmonary toxicity of bleomycin. The risk of this complication increases with increasing inspired oxygen concentration and fluid overload. Patients who undergo RPLND after receiving bleomycin should have preoperative pulmonary function tests.

## Other Techniques

**Figure 9–17:** Exposure of the retroperitoneum for advanced disease following chemotherapy. Via a thoracoabdominal approach, the posterior peritoneum is in-

## TABLE 9–1

### COMPLICATIONS OF RETROPERITONEAL LYMPH NODE DISSECTION

| COMPLICATION | NUMBER (%) |
|---|---|
| 1. Wound infection | 23 (4.8%) |
| 2. Small bowel obstruction | 11 (2.3%) |
| 3. Urinary tract infection | 10 (2.1%) |
| 4. Ascites (chylous) | 3 |
| 5. Lymphocele | 1 |
| 6. Pancreatitis | 1 |
| 7. Rectus sheath hematoma | 1 |
| 8. Scrotal hematoma | 1 |
| 9. Ureteral injury | 1 |
| 10. Ventral hernia | 1 |

## TABLE 9–2

### COMPLICATIONS OF RETROPERITONEAL LYMPH NODE DISSECTION AFTER CHEMOTHERAPY

| COMPLICATION | NUMBER |
|---|---|
| 1. Pulmonary | 46 |
| 2. Wound infection | 29 |
| 3. Small bowel obstruction | 14 |
| 4. Chylous ascites | 12 |
| 5. Lymphocele | 10 |
| 6. Neural injury | 7 |
| 7. Pancreatitis | 6 |
| 8. Ureteral injury | 6 |
| 9. Urinary tract infection | 5 |
| 10. Renal infarction | 3 |
| 11. Gastrointestinal bleeding | 3 |
| 12. Retroperitoneal bleeding | 2 |
| 13. Colon necrosis | 1 |

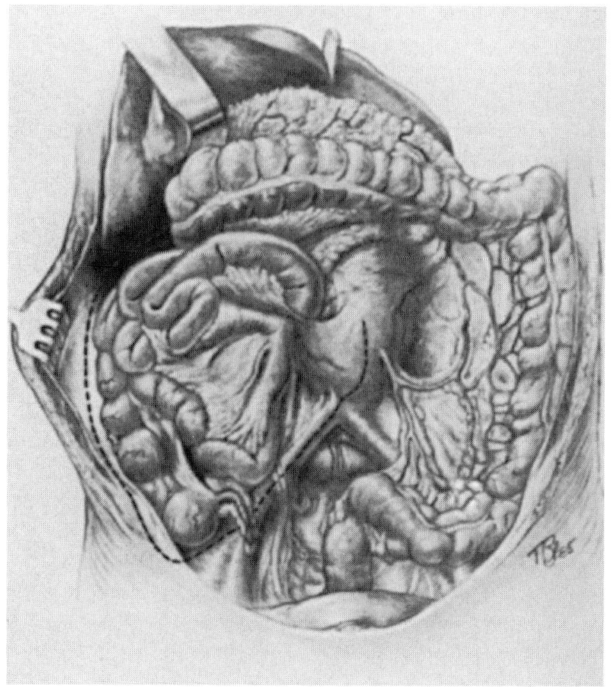

**Figure 9–17**

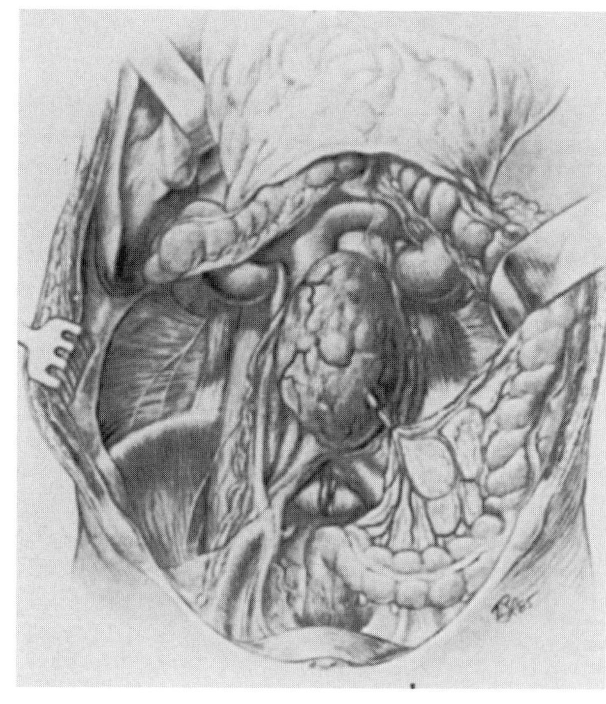

**Figure 9–18**

cised from the ligament of Treitz down along the root of the mesentery, around the cecum, and up the right gutter. This maneuver allows all of the small bowel and ascending colon to be placed into a plastic bag on the chest.[11] (From Skinner EC, Skinner DG: Surgery of testicular neoplasms. In Walsh PC, Retik AB, Vaughan ED, Wein AJ (eds): Campbell's Urology, 7th ed. Philadelphia, WB Saunders, 1998, p 3428.)

**Figure 9–18:** The inferior mesenteric artery, which often is encased in the mass, is divided. The left colon is mobilized off Gerota's fascia. The sigmoid mesentery may be adherent to the mass and can be resected, provided that the marginal artery remains intact.[11] (From Skinner EC, Skinner DG: Surgery of testicular neoplasms. In Walsh PC, Retik AB, Vaughan ED, Wein AJ (eds): Campbell's Urology, 7th ed. Philadelphia, WB Saunders, 1998, p 3429.)

**Figure 9–19:** Laparoscopic RPLND has been utilized. The potential benefits include smaller incisions, decreased postoperative pain, and faster recovery.[12] The location of port sites (for an RPLND) is shown. At this time, we believe that a traditional open approach is the standard of care. (From Winfield HN: Laparoscopic retroperitoneal lymphadenectomy for cancer of the testis. Urol Clin North Am 25:41, 1998, Fig. 1.)

**Table 9–3:** Observation following RPLND for stage II NSGCT indicated that the results of RPLND depend on the volume of disease present in the retroperitoneum. In pathologic stage I disease, a 90% relapse-free survival can be achieved after orchiectomy and RPLND. As shown in Table 9–3, when there is a large volume of disease, the relapse rate is very high.[13]

**Table 9–4:** Adjuvant chemotherapy following RPLND for stage II NSGCT patients. Adjuvant chemotherapy after RPLND for stage II disease has dramatically improved disease-free survival. The results of two series are shown in Table 9–4.[13]

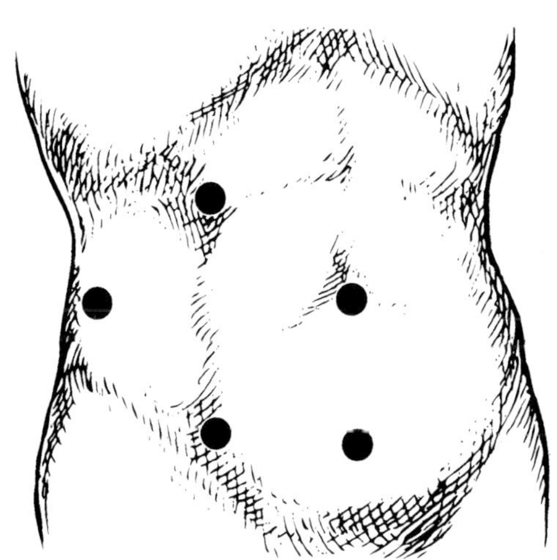

**Figure 9–19**

**TABLE 9–3**

**OBSERVATION FOLLOWING RETROPERITONEAL LYMPH NODE DISSECTION FOR STAGE II NONSEMINOMATOUS GERM CELL TUMORS**

| AUTHOR | EXTENT OF NODAL DISEASE | NO. OF PTS | RELAPSE (%) |
| --- | --- | --- | --- |
| Richie, 1991[14] | Nodes ≤ 2 cm, < 6 nodes, no extranodal extension | 39 | 3 (8) |
| Williams et al., 1987[15] | Microscopically positive nodes | 30 | 12 (40) |
| | Nodes < 2 cm, no extranodal extension | 17 | 9 (53) |
| | Nodes > 2 cm, no extranodal extension | 43 | 26 (60) |
| | Extranodal extension | 5 | 1 (20) |
| Fraley et al., 1985[16] | Stage IIA (not defined by authors) | 12 | 5 (42) |
| | Stage IIB, "small retroperitoneal metastases" | 14 | 13 (93) |
| | Stage IIC, "large but resectable metastases" | 3 | 3 (100) |

*Source:* Adapted from Frohlich MW, Small EJ: Stage II nonseminomatous testis cancer: The roles of primary and adjuvant chemotherapy. Urol Clin North Am 25:453; 1998.

**TABLE 9–4**

**ADJUVANT CHEMOTHERAPY FOLLOWING RETROPERITONEAL LYMPH NODE DISSECTION FOR STAGE II NONSEMINOMATOUS GERM CELL TUMOR PATIENTS**

| AUTHOR | REGIMEN AND # OF CYCLES | PATIENTS | DFS (%) | MEDIAN F/U (mos) |
| --- | --- | --- | --- | --- |
| Motzer et al., 1995[17] | EP X 2 | 50 | 100 | 42 |
| Behnia et al., 1996[18] | BEP X 2 | 86 | 99 | 47 |

EP = etoposide and cisplatin; BEP = bleomycin, etoposide, and cisplatin.
*Source:* Adapted from Frohlich MW, Small EJ: Stage II nonseminomatous testis cancer: The roles of primary and adjuvant chemotherapy. Urol Clin North Am 25:454, 1998.

# REFERENCES


1. Albers P, Miller GA, Orazi A: Immunohistochemical assessment of tumor proliferation and volume of embryonal carcinoma identify patients with clinical stage A nonseminomatous testicular germ cell tumor at low risk for occult metastasis. Cancer 75:844, 1995.
2. Jewett MAS, Incze P: Retroperitoneal lymphadenectomy: The traditional treatment option. Semin Urol Oncol 14:24–29, 1996.
3. Richie JP: Neoplasms of the testis. In Walsh PC, Retik AB, Vaughan ED, Wein AJ (eds): Campbell's Urology, 7th ed. Philadelphia, WB Saunders, 1998, pp 2411–2452.
4. Donohue JP, Foster RS, Rowland RG, et al: Nerve-sparing retroperitoneal lymphadenectomy with preservation of ejaculation. J Urol 144:287–292, 1990.
5. Gatti JM, Stephenson RA: Staging of testis cancer. Combining serum markers, histologic parameters, and radiographic imaging. Urol Clin North Am 25:397–403, 1998.
6. Kaplan JN: Surgical anatomy of the retroperitoneum, kidneys, and ureters. In Walsh PC, Retik AB, Vaughan ED, Wein AJ (eds): Campbell's Urology, 7th ed. Philadelphia, WB Saunders, 1998, pp 49–88.
7. Donohue JP, Foster RS: Retroperitoneal lymphadenectomy in staging and treatment. The development of nerve-sparing techniques. Urol Clin North Gem 25:461–468, 1998.
8. Richie JP: Clinical stage 1 testicular cancer: The role of modified retroperitoneal lymphadenectomy. J Urol 144:1160–1163, 1990.
9. Baniel J, Foster RS, Rowland RG, et al: Complications of primary retroperitoneal lymph node dissection. J Urol 152:424–427, 1994.
10. Baniel J, Foster RS, Rowland RG, et al: Complications of post chemotherapy retroperitoneal lymph node dissection. J Urol 153:976–980, 1995.
11. Skinner EC, Skinner DG: Surgery of testicular neoplasms. In Walsh PC, Retik AB, Vaughan ED, Wein AJ (eds): Campbell's Urology, 7th ed. Philadelphia, WB Saunders, 1998, pp 3410–3432.
12. Winfield HN: Laparoscopic retroperitoneal lymphadenectomy for cancer of the testis. Urol Clin North Am 25:469–478, 1998.
13. Frolich MW, Small EJ: Stage II nonseminomatous testis cancer: The roles of primary and adjuvant chemotherapy. Urol Clin North Am 25:451–459, 1998.
14. Richie JP, Kantoff PW: Is adjuvant chemotherapy for patients with stage B1 testicular cancer? J Clin Oncol 9:1393, 1991.
15. Williams SD, Stablein DM, Einhorn LH, et al: Immediate adjuvant chemotherapy versus observation with treatment at relapse in pathological stage II testicular cancer. N Engl J Med 317:1433, 1987.
16. Fraley EE, Narayan P, Vogelzang NJ, et al: Surgical treatment of patients with stage I and II nonseminomatous testicular cancer. J Urol 134:70, 1985.
17. Motzer RJ, Sheinfeld J, Mazumdar M, et al: Etoposide and cisplatin adjuvant therapy for patients with pathologic stage II germ cell tumors (see comments). J Clin Oncol 13:2700, 1995.
18. Behnia M, Foster R, Roth B, et al: Adjuvant bleomycin, etoposide and cisplatin in fully resected stage B nonseminomatous testicular cancer. Proc Am Soc Clin Oncol 15:249, 1996.

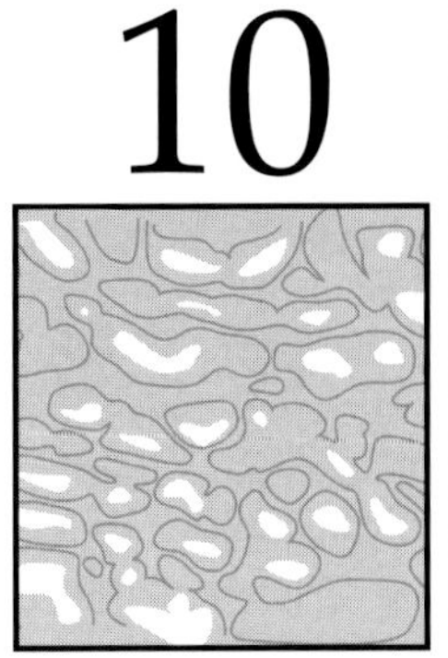

# Nonseminomatous Germ Cell Tumors: Systemic Issues

*Gary Hudes*

*Scott Saxman*

## INTRODUCTION

In general, the management of nonseminomatous germ cell tumors is more challenging than that of seminomas (reviewed in Chapter 11). Figure 10–1 shows the International Germ Cell Collaborative Group prognostic classification system. Whereas 90% of patients with seminoma fall under the "good prognosis" group, only half of the patients with nonseminomatous tumors fall into this category.

Eighty percent of germ cell tumors that grow in culture possess excess genetic material from the short arm of chromosome 12, which serves as a cytogenetic marker for a germ cell malignancy (Fig. 10–2). The mainstay of therapy in patients with metastatic testicular nonseminomatous germ cell tumor remains chemotherapy, typically with cisplatin, etoposide, and other agents, depending on the extent of metastatic disease (Figs. 10–3 to 10–5). This chapter presents several images of illustrative clinical vignettes related to the systemic management of nonseminomatous germ cell tumors.

## PROGNOSTIC CLASSIFICATION

**Figure 10–1:** International germ cell collaborative group prognostic classification system developed from survival data on more than 5800 patients with metastatic germ cell tumors treated with chemotherapy. PFS = progression-free survival. Prognosis is determined by readily available clinical data including primary tumor site, location of metastases, and extent of tumor markers, such as α-fetoprotein (AFP), human chorionic gonadotropin (β-hCG), and lactate dehydrogenase (LDH) elevations.[1]

**Figure 10–2:** The presence of excess genetic material from the short arm of chromosome 12 is a nonrandom, cytogenetic marker of germ cell malignancy. An isochromosome of the short arm of chromosome 12

| GOOD PROGNOSIS | |
| --- | --- |
| NONSEMINOMA | SEMINOMA |
| Testis/retroperitoneal primary<br>***and***<br>No nonpulmonary visceral metastases<br>***and***<br>*Good markers - all of:*<br>*AFP < 1000 ng/ml and*<br>*hCG < 5000 iu/l (1000 ng/ml) and*<br>*LDH < 1.5 x upper limit of normal* | Any primary site<br>***and***<br>No nonpulmonary visceral metastases<br>***and***<br>Normal AFP, any hCG, any LDH |
| **56% of nonseminomas**<br>**5 year PFS 89%**<br>**5 year survival 92%** | **90% of seminomas**<br>**5 year PFS 82%**<br>**5 year survival 86%** |
| INTERMEDIATE PROGNOSIS | |
| NONSEMINOMA | SEMINOMA |
| Testis/retroperitoneal primary<br>***and***<br>No nonpulmonary visceral metastases<br>***and***<br>*Intermediate markers - any of:*<br>*AFP ≥ 1000 and ≤ 10,000 ng/ml or*<br>*hCG ≥ 5000 iu/l and ≤ 50,000 iu/l or*<br>*LDH ≥ 1.5 x N and ≤ 10 x N* | Any primary site<br>***and***<br>Nonpulmonary visceral metastases<br>***and***<br>Normal AFP, any hCG, any LDH |
| **28% of nonseminomas**<br>**5 year PFS 75%**<br>**5 year survival 80%** | **10% of seminomas**<br>**5 year PFS 67%**<br>**5 year survival 72%** |
| POOR PROGNOSIS | |
| NONSEMINOMA | SEMINOMA |
| Mediastinal primary<br>***or***<br>Nonpulmonary visceral metastases<br>***or***<br>Poor markers - any of:<br>*AFP > 10,000 ng/ml or*<br>*hCG > 10,000 iu/l (10,000 ng/ml) or*<br>*LDH > 10 x upper limit of normal* | **No patients classified as poor prognosis** |
| **16% of nonseminomas**<br>**5 year PFS 41%**<br>**5 year survival 48%** | |

**Figure 10–1**

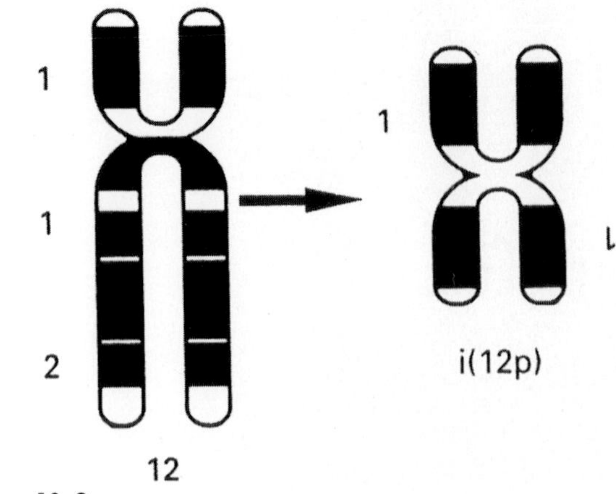



**Figure 10–2**

[i(12p)], composed of two short arms in tandem, is found in approximately 80% of germ cell tumors (GCTs) that grow in culture.[2] Germ cell tumors that lack i(12)p usually have abnormally banded marker chromosomes containing multiple copies of 12p.[2, 3]

**Figure 10–3:** *A* and *B*, Abdominal CT images demonstrating a large left-sided retroperitoneal mass and multiple hepatic metastases in a 22-year-old male with mixed testicular nonseminomatous GCT containing elements of embryonal carcinoma, choriocarcinoma, seminoma, and mature teratoma. The patient also had multiple pulmonary metastases. This patient was in the poor prognosis category based on liver metastases and extreme tumor marker elevation.

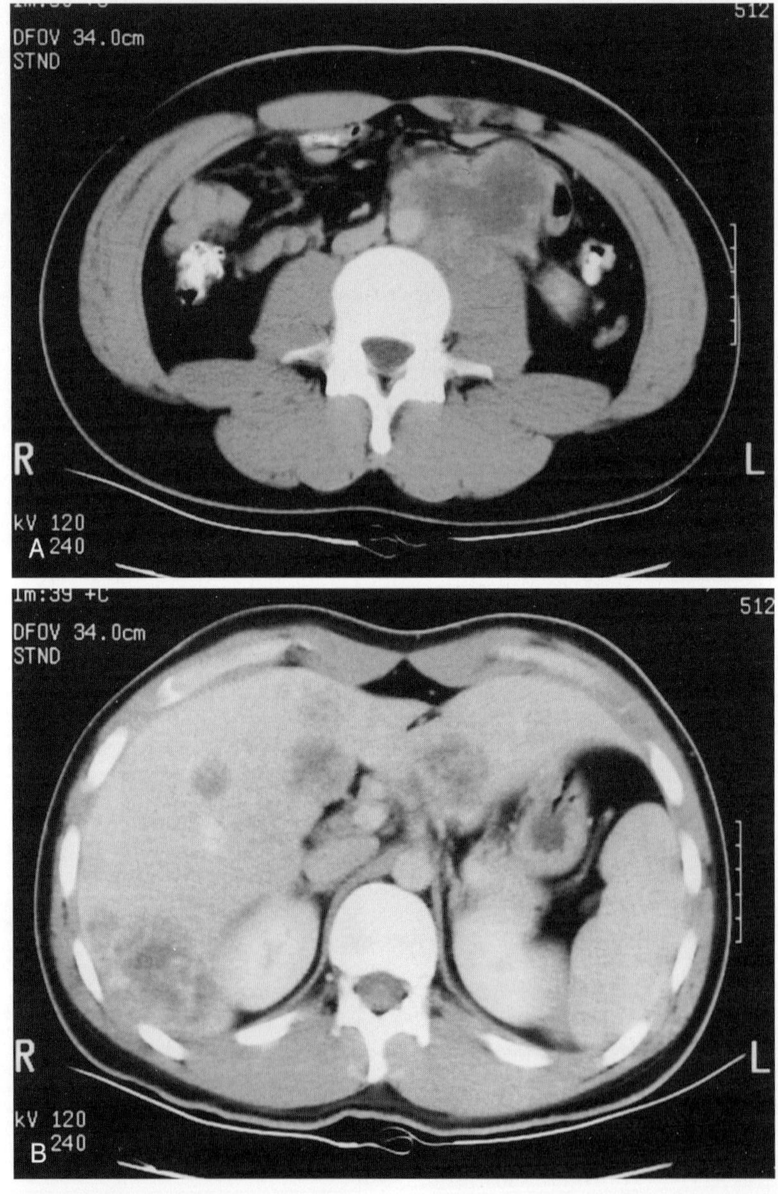



**Figure 10–3**

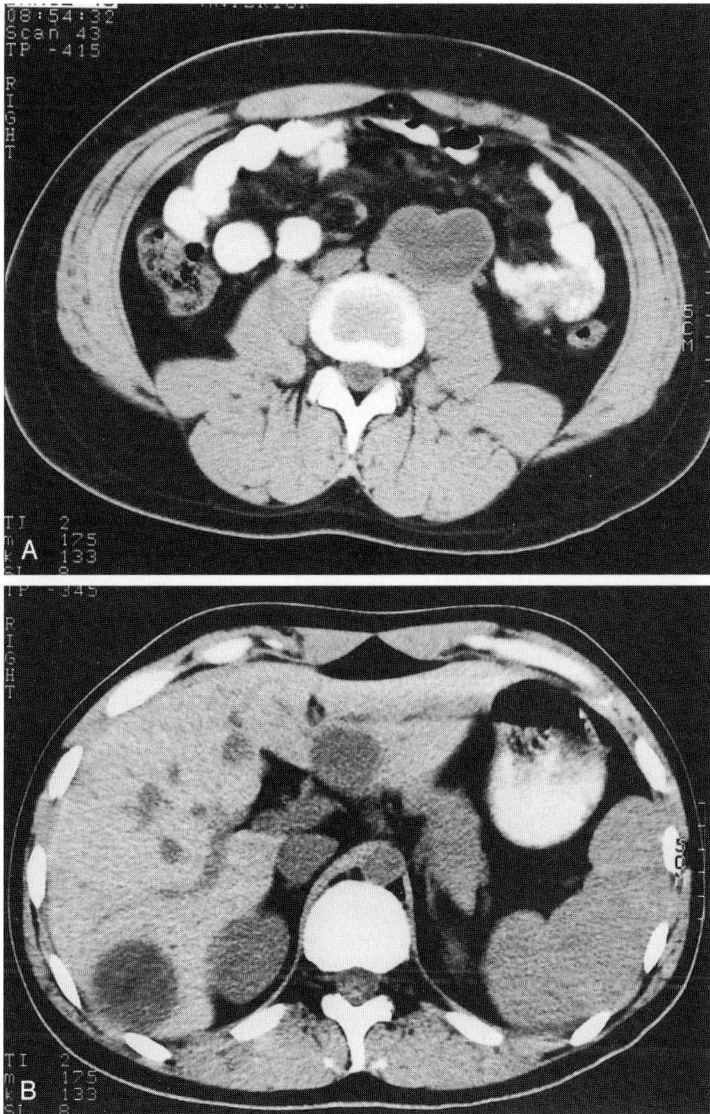

**Figure 10–4**

## RESIDUAL MASSES FOLLOWING CHEMOTHERAPY

**Figure 10–4:** CT images in the same patient described in Figure 10–3 following four cycles of chemotherapy with bleomycin, etoposide, and cisplatin. The retroperitoneal mass is smaller and more cystic in appearance *(A)*, and the liver metastases have decreased in size and have a low-density, cystic appearance *(B)*. Resection of the residual liver lesions yielded necrotic material without viable carcinoma. The retroperitoneal mass contained mature teratoma, but no carcinoma. Residual masses in patients with nonseminomatous GCTs consist of necrosis (45%), teratoma (45%), or residual carcinoma (10%). Because teratoma can enlarge over time and undergo malignant transformation, abnormalities shown radiologically that persist after chemotherapy should be surgically removed.

**Figure 10–5:** Tumor marker response to chemotherapy in the same patient in Figures 10–3 and 10–4. The patient's serum β-hCG level declined approximately 10-fold with each cycle of chemotherapy but remained elevated at the completion of the fourth cycle of therapy. With further follow-up, the β-hCG level continued to decline to low normal values, at which time the patient underwent resection of residual masses (Fig. 10–4), 4 months after completing chemotherapy. The patient remains continuously free of tumor recurrence at 5 years following surgical resection of residual masses, with undetectable levels of tumor markers. Normalization of β-hCG by the end of the fourth cycle of chemotherapy occurs in only 10% of patients who present with very high (>50,000 mIU/ml) levels of this tumor marker. Such patients should be monitored monthly, with initiation of salvage therapy if there is evidence of tumor progression.[4]

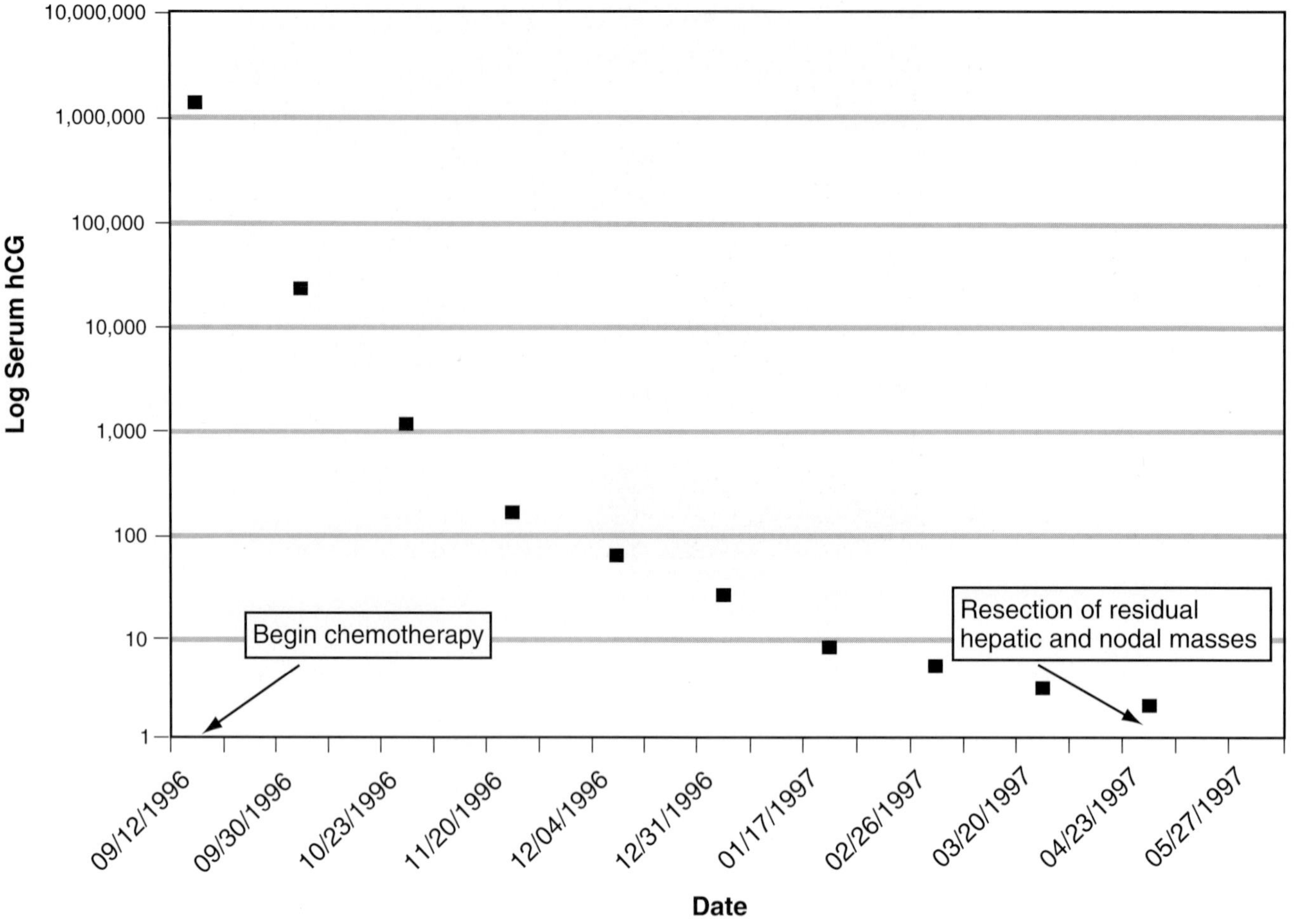

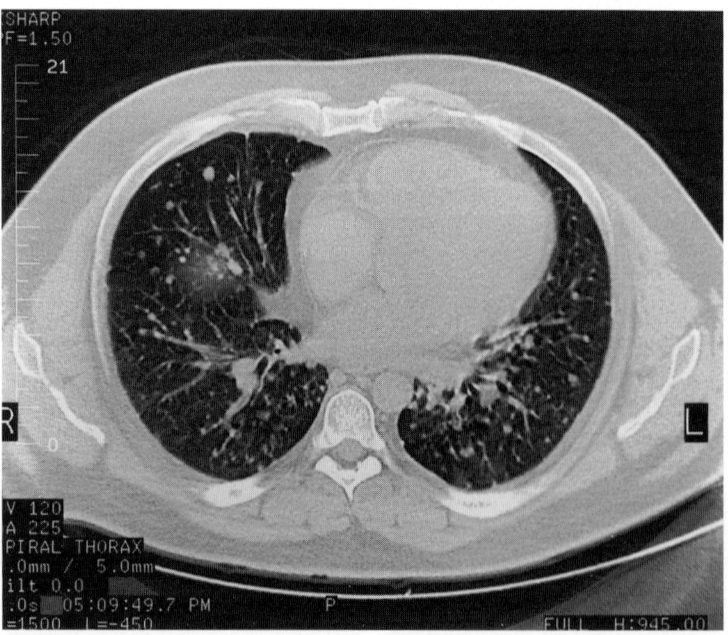



Figure 10–5



Figure 10–6

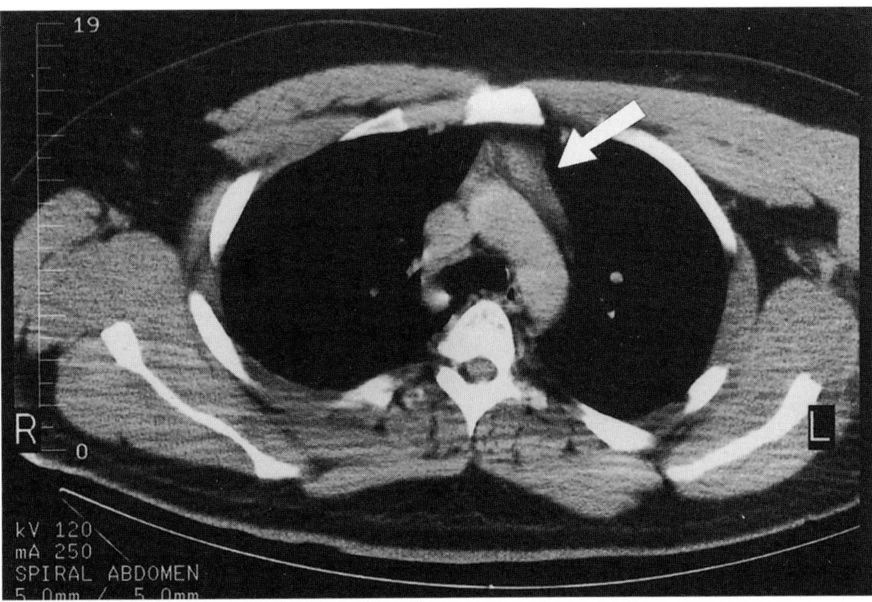

**Figure 10–7**

## PULMONARY SARCOIDOSIS MIMICKING METASTATIC GERM CELL TUMOR

**Figure 10–6:** Pulmonary sarcoidosis mimicking metastatic GCT. This patient presented with testicular seminoma, primary tumor invading vascular spaces, and rete testis. Thoracic CT scan revealed several pulmonary nodules that had not appeared on a prior scan obtained approximately 1 year preceding cancer diagnosis. Abdominal CT scan was negative. Nodules regressed following three cycles of bleomycin, etoposide, and cisplatin chemotherapy, but increased in number and size in the second year of follow-up. Serum levels of angiotensin-converting enzyme (ACE) were markedly elevated, and multiple lung biopsies revealed noncaseating granulomas typical of sarcoidosis. Nodules and pulmonary function remain stable 4 years later. Paratracheal adenopathy or pulmonary nodules that occur in the absence of retroperitoneal disease or marker elevation, particularly in patients with seminoma, should be biopsied before malignancy is assumed.[5]

## THYMIC EFFECT OF CHEMOTHERAPY

**Figure 10–7:** Thymic rebound following chemotherapy for GCT. CT images of the chest revealed complete regression of multiple pulmonary nodules, together with the appearance of a new anterior mediastinal "mass" (*arrow*) 1 month following completion of chemotherapy for a stage IIIB testicular nonseminomatous GCT in a 20-year-old male. The location was typical of thymic enlargement, which may occur in young patients following cytotoxic therapy. Correlation with tumor markers and initial sites of disease, overall tumor response, and close follow-up will distinguish this phenomenon from tumor recurrence or progression.

## EXTRAGONADAL GERM CELL TUMOR

**Figure 10–8:** Chest x-ray demonstrating mediastinal widening in a patient with a mediastinal germ cell tumor. Extragonadal GCTs can occur in multiple locations; however, most commonly arise in the retroperitoneum or anterior mediastinum. Mediastinal nonseminomatous GCTs are associated with the Klinefelter syndrome and with hematologic malignancies, particu-

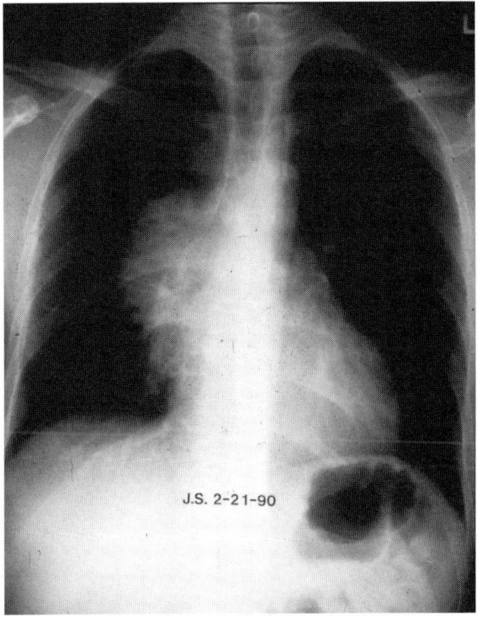

**Figure 10–8**

larly acute megakaryocytic leukemia. The surgical and chemotherapeutic management of extragonadal GCTs is identical to that for advanced testicular cancer, but the overall curability of these tumors is lower, and second-line chemotherapy is less effective than in patients with a testicular primary GCT.[6]

## REFERENCES


1. International Germ Cell Cancer Collaborative Group: International germ cell consensus classification: A prognostic factor-based staging system for metastatic germ cell cancers. J Clin Oncol 15:594–603, 1997.
2. Bosl GJ, Ilson DH, Rodriguez E, et al: Clinical relevance of the i(12p) marker chromosome in germ cell tumors. J Natl Cancer Inst 86:349–355, 1994.
3. Rodriguez E, Houldsworth J, Reuter VE, et al: Molecular cytogenetic analysis of i(12p)-negative human male germ cell tumors. Genes Chromosomes Cancer 8:230–236, 1993.
4. Zon RT, Nichols C, Einhorn L: Management strategies and outcomes of germ cell tumor patients with very high human chorionic gonadotropin levels. J Clin Oncol 16:1294–1297, 1998.
5. Toner GC, Bosl GJ: Sarcoidosis, "sarcoid-like lymphadenopathy," and testicular germ cell tumors. Am J Med 89:651, 1990.
6. Nichols CR, Roth BJ, Heerema N, et al: Hematologic neoplasia associated with primary mediastinal germ-cell tumors. N Engl J Med 322:1425, 1990.

## 11

# Radiotherapy in the Management of Seminoma

*Matthew T. Ballo*

*Kathleen M. Shadle*

*Alan Pollack*


According to the National Cancer Institute Surveillance, Epidemiology and End Results (SEER) Program data from 1995 the incidence of testicular cancer is rising and affects 4.5 of every 100,000 men.[1] Testicular cancer is the most common solid tumor found in men between the ages of 20 and 35. Greater than 95% of testicular tumors originate from germ cells within the testicle. These germ cells fall into one of two clinicopathologic groups: seminomatous and nonseminomatous germ cell tumors. Forty percent of men with testicular cancer will have seminoma, and of these men, approximately 75% will have disease confined to the testicle.

Seminoma is exquisitely sensitive to both chemotherapy and radiotherapy and is highly curable with modern treatment. In the year 2001, there are estimated to be 7200 cases of testicular cancer in the United States, with only 400 deaths.[2] The standard treatment for early stage disease has been radical inguinal orchiectomy followed by radiotherapy to the potentially involved lymph nodes. Some patients with seminoma may be cured with surgery alone. Patients with advanced stage disease are usually treated successfully with platinum-based chemotherapy regimens.

This chapter reviews the epidemiology, anatomy, staging, pathology, and treatment of testicular seminoma. Radiographic imaging studies are included to illustrate clinical findings commonly seen. Conventional management of seminomas is reviewed, as well as emerging treatment strategies.

## EPIDEMIOLOGY

**Figure 11–1:** SEER data on the incidence and mortality rates for testicular cancer in the United States from 1973 to 1995.[1] Incidence rates are per 100,000 population and are age-adjusted to the 1970 U.S. standard

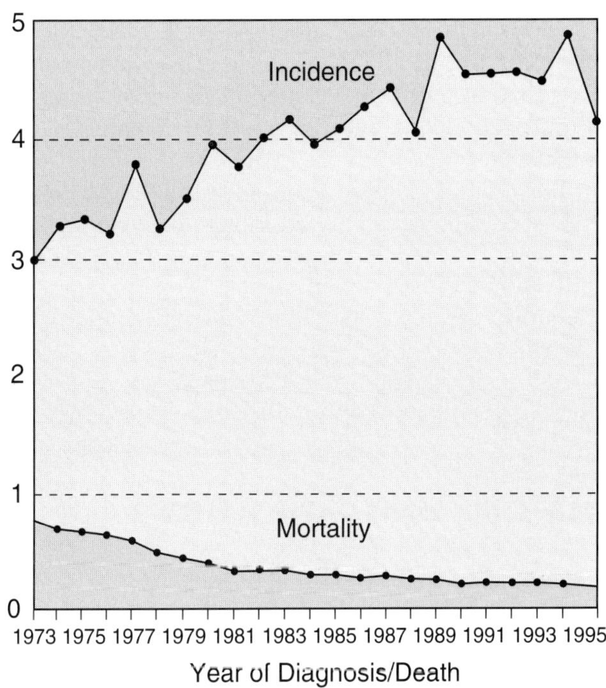


**Figure 11–1**

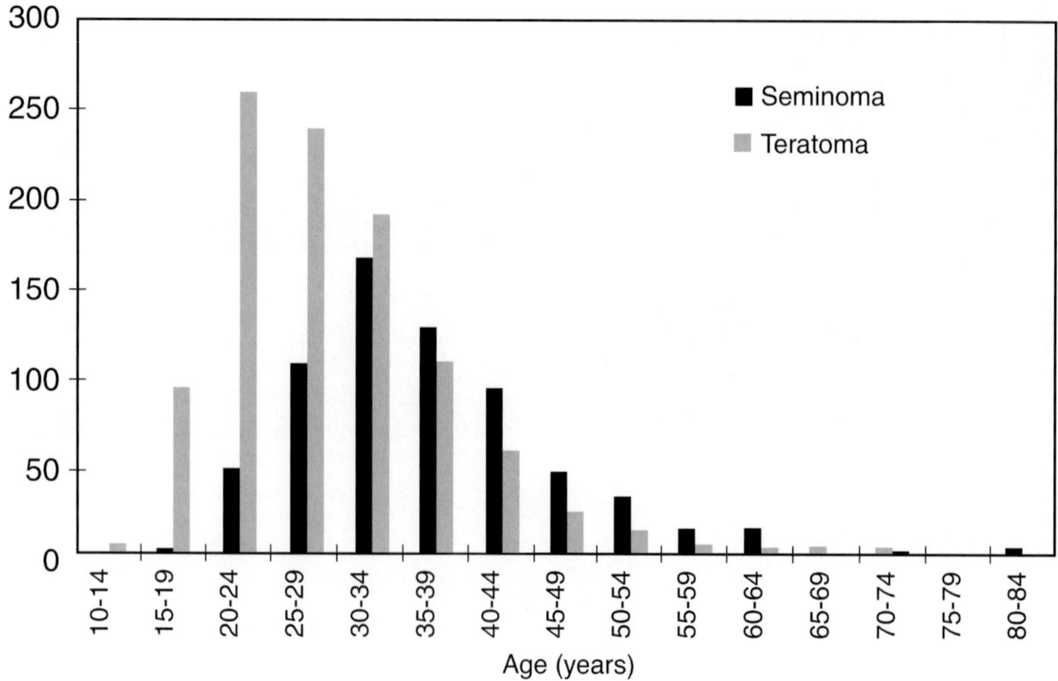



**Figure 11–2**

population. The lifetime risk of developing testicular cancer for men is 0.34%, and the risk for death from testicular cancer is only 0.02%. The incidence of testicular cancer has increased by about 45% from 1973 to 1995. The factors that are responsible for this increase are not fully understood. Despite the increase in the incidence of testicular cancer, the 5-year survival rate has improved from 78.7% in 1973 to 95.3% by the late 1980s. The improvement in survival is a result of the development of effective chemotherapeutic regimens.

**Figure 11–2:** The age distribution of patients with testicular germ cell tumors treated at the Royal Marsden Hospital in London from 1980 to 1994.[3] The incidence of seminoma is greatest in men between the ages of 20 and 45 years. The median age of diagnosis is 37 years. Seminomas are seen in men over the age of 50 to a much greater extent than are nonseminomatous germ cell tumors. (Redrawn from Harwich A: Testicular Cancer: Investigation and Management. Baltimore, Williams & Wilkins, 1991.)

## ANATOMY AND PATHOLOGY

**Figure 11–3:** The primordial germ cells in the developing embryo descend from the posterior abdominal wall into the scrotal sac. During the development of the pelvis and growth of the trunk, little elongation of the gubernaculum testis occurs. The testes then undergo descent relative to the body wall and come to lie in close proximity to the inguinal region. The testes remain in the abdominal region of the inguinal canal

until the seventh month of fetal life, after which they descend into the scrotal sac. The lymphatic drainage descends with the developing testicle. During the descent of the testicle there is the potential for ectopic testicular rests along its path.

Cryptorchidism and ectopic testicular tissue are clearly etiologic factors that contribute to the development of seminoma. With cryptorchidism, the testicle is arrested along the path of normal descent. With ectopy, the testicle has deviated from the normal path of descent. Examples of locations of ectopic and cryptorchid testes are illustrated here. The prepubic testicle is the most common site for a cryptorchid testicle, and the superficial inguinal region is the most common site for an ectopic testicle. (From Kogan S: Cryptorchidism. In Kelalis PP, King LR, Belman AB [eds]: Clinical Pediatric

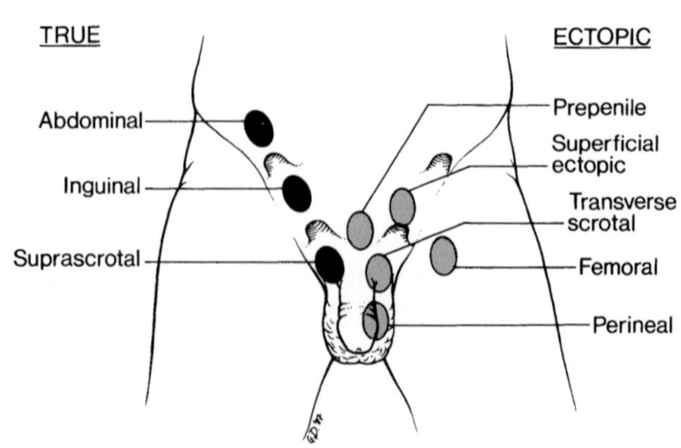



**Figure 11–3**

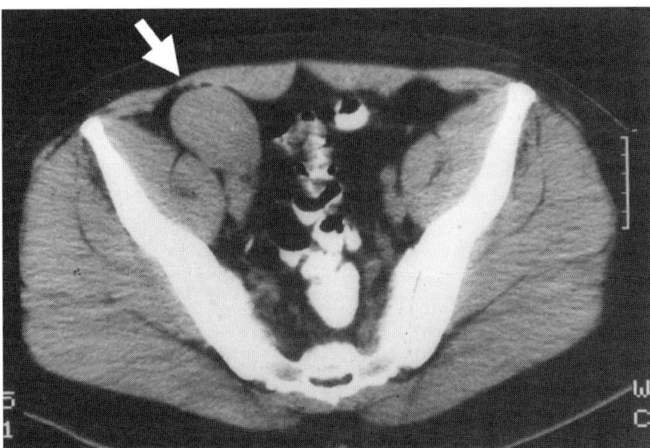

**Figure 11–4**

Urology, 3rd ed. Philadelphia, WB Saunders, p. 1050, 1992, Fig. 23–5.)

**Figure 11–4:** Cryptorchidism is seen in 10% of patients who develop seminoma and is the most consistently associated risk factor for the development of a seminoma. The impact of age at the time of surgical correction of the cryptorchid testicle was reviewed by the United Kingdom Testicular Study Group[4] in a case-controlled study. The results suggest that surgical correction of the cryptorchid testicle in early childhood reduced the risk of development of seminoma. Shown

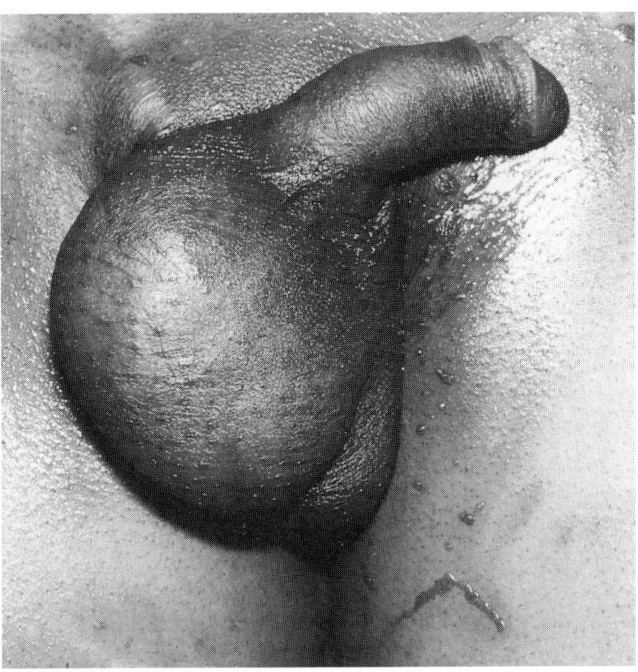

**Figure 11–6**

here is a right pelvic testicle *(arrow)* that did not have surgical correction and in which a seminomatous germ cell tumor subsequently developed.

**Figure 11–5:** A lateral view of the testis with the tunica vaginalis reflected. (From Moore KL: Clinically Oriented Anatomy, 3rd ed. Baltimore, Williams & Wilkins, 1992, Fig. 2–19A.)

**Figure 11–6:** A scrotal mass in a patient prior to an inguinal orchiectomy.

**Figure 11–7:** Intraoperative site of an inguinal orchiectomy. An inguinal incision with high ligation of the spermatic cord and vascular supply at the internal inguinal ring should be performed. This method prevents potential lymphatic and vascular dissemination of tumor cells. Trans-scrotal biopsies of testicular masses should be avoided, as they may result in spillage of tumor cells and aberrant lymphatic spread.

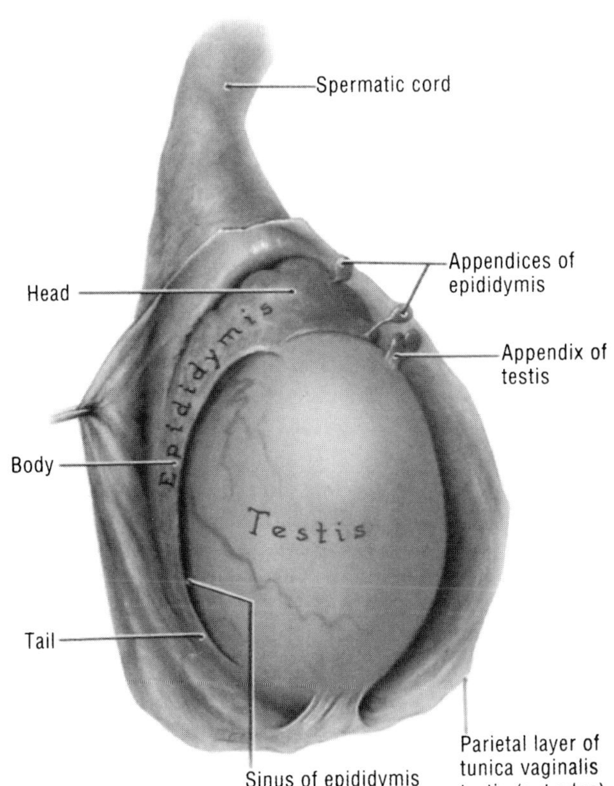


**Figure 11–5**

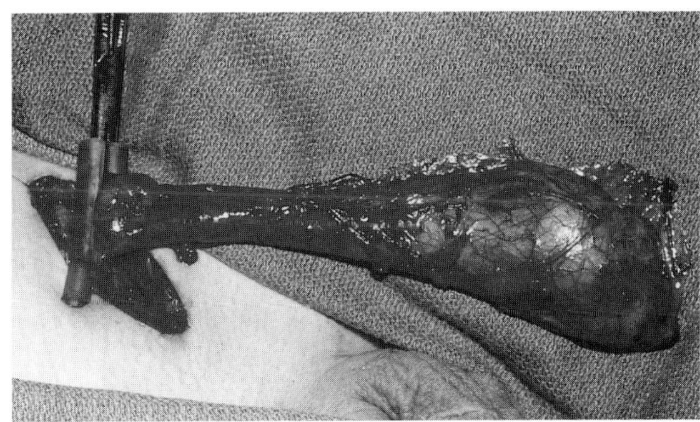

**Figure 11–7**

## COMPARISON OF CLINICAL STAGING SYSTEMS IN SEMINOMA

| DISEASE EXTENT | MD ANDERSON[6] | WALTER REED[7] | ROYAL MARSDEN[8] |
|---|---|---|---|
| Testicle | I | IA<br>IB (+RPLND) | I |
| Retroperitoneal lymph nodes | IIA (<10 cm)<br>IIB (≥10 cm) | II | IIA (<2 cm)<br>IIB (2–5 cm)<br>IIC (5–10 cm)<br>IID (>10 cm) |
| Supradiaphragmatic lymph nodes | III | III | III |
| Visceral metastases | IV | III | IV |

RPLND = retroperitoneal lymph node dissection.

*Source:* Adapted from Ritchie JP: Neoplasms of the testis. In Walsh PC, Retik AB, Stamey TA, Vaughn ED (eds): Campbell's Urology, 6th ed. Philadelphia, WB Saunders, 1992.)

## CLASSIFICATION

**Table 11–1:** There are many different staging systems that are used to classify testicular seminoma. For the 1997 American Joint Committee on Cancer (AJCC) staging system, refer to Chapter 6. MD Anderson Hospital, Walter Reed Hospital, and the Royal Marsden Hospital have all developed staging systems. These clinical staging systems have been developed at institutions that have treated large numbers of patients with seminoma. In general, a stage I tumor is limited to the testicle, stage II seminoma includes infradiaphragmatic lymph nodes, and stage III tumor is nodal disease found to extend above the diaphragm. It is particularly important to note the differences in the staging systems for stage II disease when comparing results from different institutions.

The staging evaluation in the patient with seminoma should include pathologic review of the orchiectomy specimen, computed tomographic (CT) scan of the abdomen, and a chest x-ray. CT scan of the chest is indicated in patients with evidence of nodal involvement on CT scan of the abdomen. Serum β-hCG (human chorionic gonadotropin) and AFP (alpha-fetoprotein) should be obtained preoperatively and postoperatively. Elevation of β-hCG postoperatively in a patient with stage I disease (allowing for the 24-hour half-life) suggests microscopic nodal involvement and a prognosis similar to that for stage II disease.

**Figure 11–8:** Cross section of this testicle reveals the tumor present in the lower pole of the testicle.

**Figure 11–9:** The majority of patients are diagnosed with early stage seminoma limited to a single testicle. The stage distribution of 398 patients with seminoma treated at MD Anderson Cancer Center from 1960 to 1991 is shown.

**Figure 11–8**

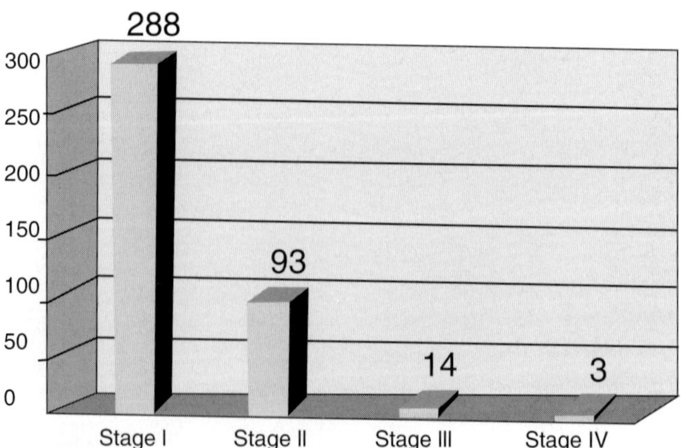


**Figure 11–9**

## LYMPH NODE SPREAD

**Figure 11–10:** The primary route of spread of testicular seminoma is to the para-aortic lymph nodes. A right testicular lymphangiogram shows the lymphatic vessels following the path of the spermatic cord and testicular artery. After passing through the inguinal ring, the lymphatics continue on an upward course, terminating in the para-aortic lymph nodes between the level of the renal vessels superiorly and the aortic bifurcation inferiorly. The lymphatics terminate in the interaortocaval, precaval, and preaortic nodes. The lymphatics from the right testicle can cross the midline, and contralateral lymph node involvement can be seen. Left-sided lymphatic drainage, on the other hand, does not cross the midline. Lymphangiography is no longer necessary in the management of testicular tumors. Microscopic lymph node metastases not seen on CT scan are adequately treated with radiotherapy doses of 20 to 25 Gy.

**Figure 11–11:** Schematic illustration of the lymphatic drainage.[5] Note the lymphatics of the scrotum and scrotal skin drain to the superficial inguinal lymph nodes and potentially can be involved if the scrotum has been violated either by previous scrotal surgery or by trans-scrotal biopsy. (From Moore KL: Clinically Oriented Anatomy, 3rd ed. Baltimore, Williams & Wilkins, 1992, Fig. 2–22.)

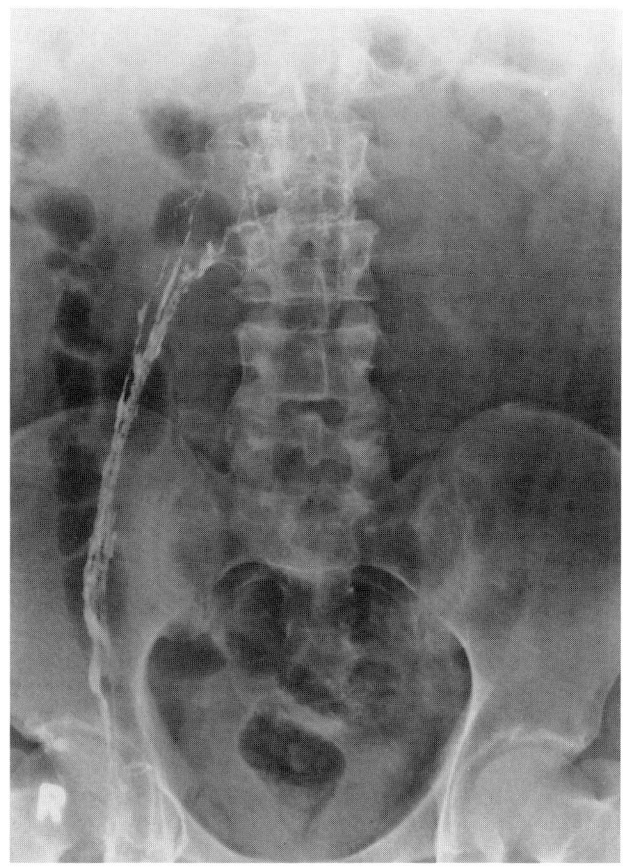

**Figure 11–10**

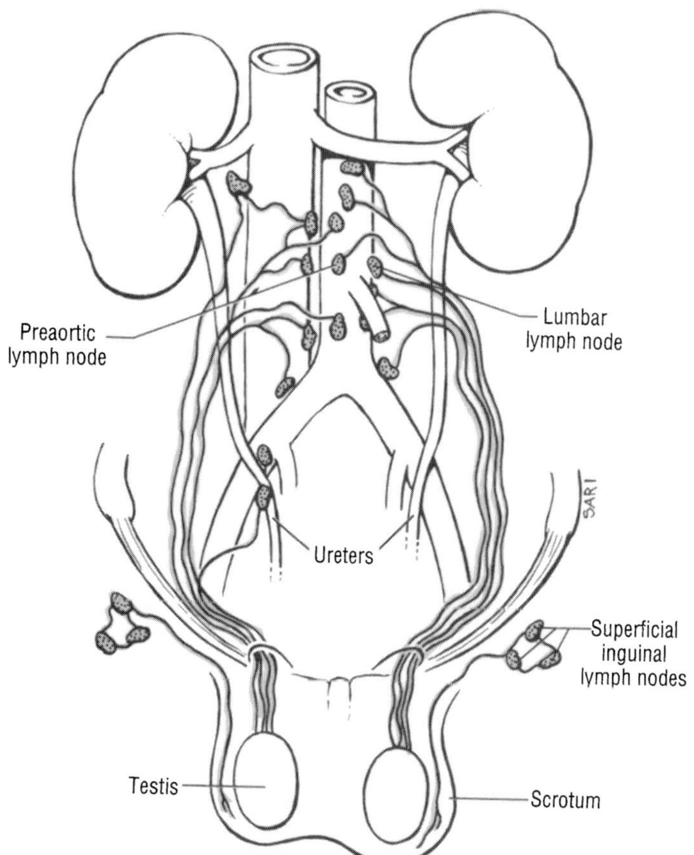


**Figure 11–11**

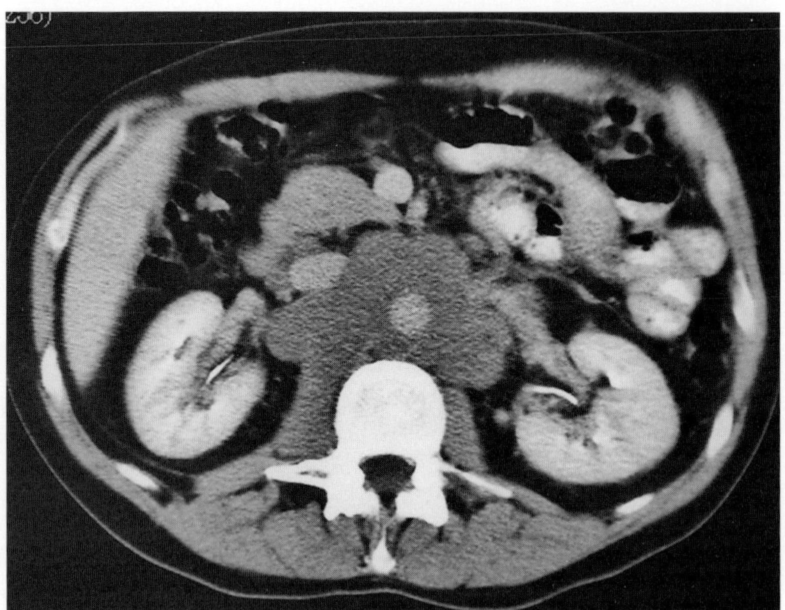

**Figure 11–12**

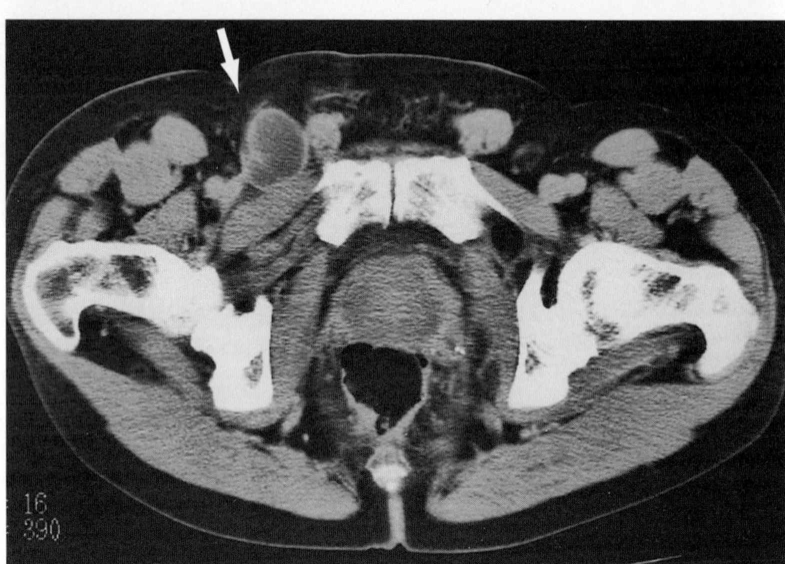

**Figure 11–13**

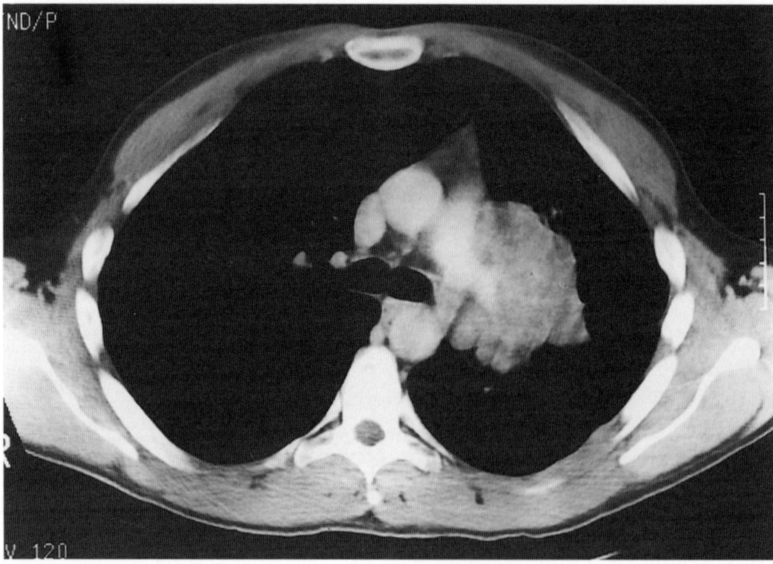

**Figure 11–14**

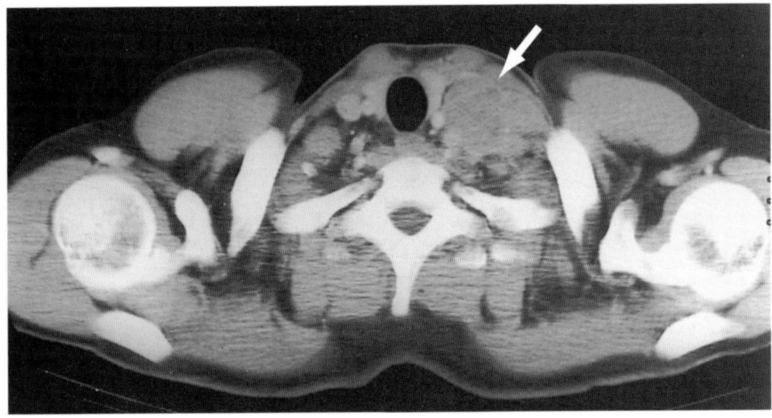

**Figure 11–15**

**Figure 11–12:** CT scan of the abdomen demonstrating enlarged para-aortic lymph nodes at the level of the renal hilum.

**Figure 11–13:** CT scan of the pelvis with an enlarged right inguinal lymph node *(arrow)*. Subsequent biopsy confirmed seminoma. Altered pelvic lymphatic drainage from prior scrotal surgery predisposes patients to inguinal or pelvic lymph node metastasis.

**Figure 11–14:** Mediastinal lymph node metastases can be seen in patients with advanced disease.

**Figure 11–15:** Virchow's node in the left supraclavicular fossa *(arrow)* can be a site of metastatic disease, on presentation or at relapse, due to lymphatic drainage of the para-aortic nodes into the thoracic duct.

## TREATMENT

**Table 11–2:** The standard postorchiectomy treatment for stages I and II seminoma has been irradiation of the para-aortic and ipsilateral pelvic lymph nodes. The majority of patients with stage I seminoma in whom surveillance fails develop para-aortic lymph node recurrences. Because these lymph nodes are at the greatest risk of harboring residual disease, there is increasing evidence that limited para-aortic irradiation is sufficient to provide excellent long-term results (Table 11–2).

**Figure 11–16:** Fossa and Horwich randomized 478 men with stage I seminoma to traditional pelvic and para-aortic irradiation ("dog-leg") versus para-aortic irradiation alone. The relapse-free survival rates were 97% and 96%, respectively, although there were more pelvic failures in the para-aortic irradiation-only group.[13] (Redrawn from Fossa SD, Horwich A, Russell JM, et al: Optimal planning target volume for stage 1 testicular seminoma. A Medical Research Council randomized trial. J Clin Oncol 17:1146–1154, 1999.)

**Figure 11–17:** *A,* The classic para-aortic treatment field extends from the top of T10 to the bottom of L5 and is treated with an anterior and posterior parallel-opposed technique using high-energy photons generated by a megavoltage linear accelerator. The patient is treated daily, Monday through Friday, to a dose of 25 to 30 Gy in 15 fractions. There is a trend to treat smaller fields (T11 or T12 to L5, as shown) using lower doses (20 Gy in 10 fractions). *B,* The ipsilateral hemipelvis is included for prior orchiopexy or disruption of the nor-

## TABLE 11–2

### STAGE I SEMINOMA: EXPERIENCE OMITTING HEMIPELVIC TREATMENT

| AUTHOR | NO. OF PATIENTS | FOLLOW-UP PERIOD | FIELD | DOSE | 5-YEAR DISEASE-FREE RATE |
|---|---|---|---|---|---|
| Read[10] | 94 | 34 mo | T12–L4 | 20 Gy | 1 relapse |
| Kiricuta[11] | 86 | 63 mo | L1–L5 | 30 Gy | 95.3% |
| Sultanem[12] | 35 | 40 mo | T11–L5 | 25 Gy | 0 relapse |
| Fossa[13] | 236 | 54 mo | T11–L5 | 30 Gy | 96.0%* |
|  | 242 | 54 mo | Dog-leg | 30 Gy | 96.6% |

*Four pelvic failures and one death.

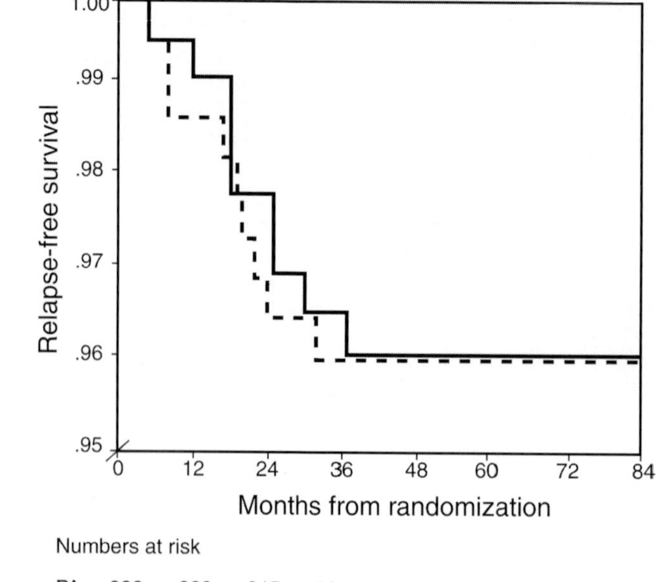



**Figure 11–16**

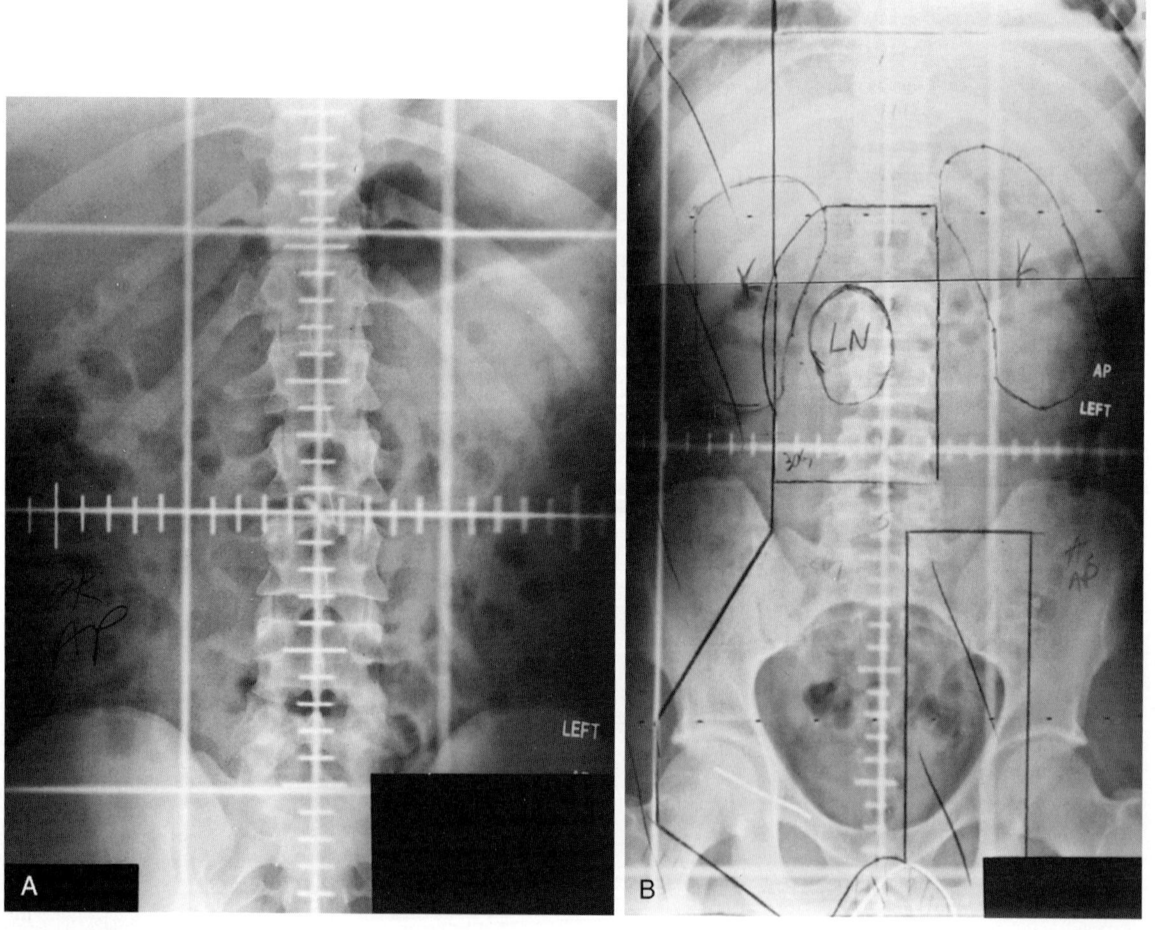



**Figure 11–17**

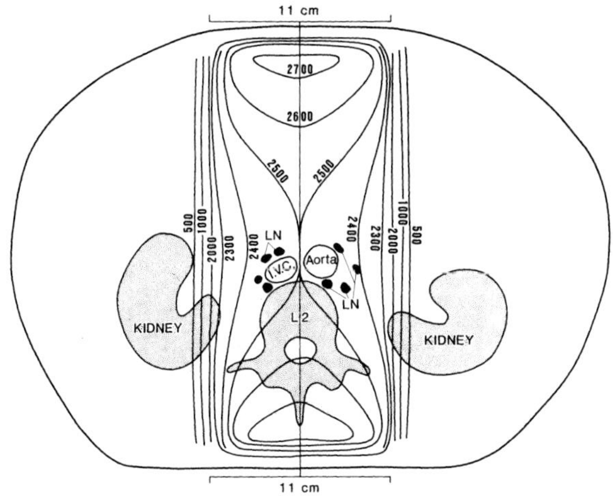


**Figure 11–18**

mal lymphatic drainage (prior trans-scrotal surgery or herniorrhaphy). A 5-Gy boost may be given to areas of gross disease.

**Figure 11–18:** A cross section of a treatment plan from the para-aortic field with the isodose curves indicating the dose to the lymph nodes, with sparing of the kidneys.

**Tables 11–3 and 11–4:** The results using postorchiectomy irradiation for stages I and II seminoma have been excellent, with a long-term disease-free survival rate of 97%.

**Table 11–5:** Despite excellent results with radiotherapy, there is increasing interest in postorchiectomy surveillance. The side effects associated with radiotherapy include a 20% incidence of nausea, vomiting, and diarrhea during treatment. Oligospermia can develop, but

## TABLE 11–3
### STAGE I DISEASE CONTROL

| NO. OF PATIENTS | NO. RELAPSED | NO. SALVAGED | SEMINOMA DEATHS | SERIES |
|---|---|---|---|---|
| 42 | 1 | 1 | 0 | Epstein, 1990[14] |
| 132 | 6 | 5 | 1 | Bayens, 1992[15] |
| 184 | 4 | 0 | 4 | Giacchetti, 1993[16] |
| 282 | 8 | 5 | 3 | Dosmann, 1993[6] |
| 95 | 2 | 2 | 0 | Lai, 1993[17] |
| 102 | 2 | 1 | 1 | Amichetti, 1994[18] |
| 79 | 4 | 3 | 1 | Oliver, 1994[19] |
| 101 | 3 | 2 | 1 | Niewald, 1995[20] |
| 86 | 4 | 4 | 0 | Kiricuta, 1996[11] |
| 188 | 1 | 1 | 0 | Hültenschmidt, 1996[21] |
| 81 | 5 | 3 | 2 | Stein, 1993[22] |
| 27 | 1 | 0 | 1 | Miki, 1998[23] |
| 169 | 5 | 4 | 0 | Bauman, 1998[24] |
| 1568 | 46 (2.9%) | 31 (67%) | 14 (0.9%) | Total |

## TABLE 11–4
### STAGE II DISEASE CONTROL

| NO. OF PATIENTS | LYMPH NODE SIZE | NO. RELAPSED | NO. SALVAGED | SEMINOMA DEATHS | SERIES |
|---|---|---|---|---|---|
| 16 | <5 cm | 0 | 0 | 0 | Epstein, 1990[14] |
| 35 | <5 cm | 8 | 5 | 2 | Bayens, 1992[15] |
| 55 | <10 cm | 7 | 4 | 3 | Dosmann, 1993[6] |
| 33 | <5 cm | 2 | 1 | 1 | Lai, 1993[17] |
| 15 | <10 cm | 1 | 1 | 0 | Speer, 1995[25] |
| 37 | <5 cm | 4 | 4 | 0 | Hültenschmidt, 1996[21] |
| 31 | <5 cm | 2 | 2 | 0 | Whipple, 1997[26] |
| 39 | <5 cm | 3 | 2 | 0 | Bauman, 1998[24] |
| 261 | | 27 (10%) | 19 (70%) | 6 (2%) | Totals |

## TABLE 11–5

### SURVEILLANCE FOR STAGE I DISEASE

| STUDY | NO. OF PATIENTS | FOLLOW-UP (Months) | TIME TO RELAPSE* | RELAPSE RATE |
|---|---|---|---|---|
| DATECA[27] | 261 | 48 | 14 mos | 20% |
| PMH[28] | 172 | 50 | 16 mos | 18% |
| Royal Marsden[29] | 103 | 62 | NA | 18% |

NA = not available.
*Median.

most patients will recover normal sperm counts within 18 months of treatment. The most serious long-term complication is the development of radiation-induced malignancy. This occurs in less than 1% of patients undergoing irradiation.

Patients who undergo observation must be followed with imaging studies and physical examination at regular intervals. Approximately 20% of patients with stage I disease will develop evidence of metastatic relapse. The majority of these metastases will occur in para-aortic lymph nodes. Results of salvage using either radiotherapy or platinum-based chemotherapy is excellent, with 99% long-term survival.

**Figure 11–19:** When the cost of elective irradiation was compared with that of surveillance, including long-term follow-up studies and salvage therapy, surveillance generated 39% more medical costs with no difference in outcome.[30] (From Sharda NN, Kinsella TJ, Ritter MA: Adjuvant radiation versus observation: A cost analysis of alternate management schemes in early-stage testicular seminoma. J Clin Oncol 14:2936, 1996, Fig. 2.)

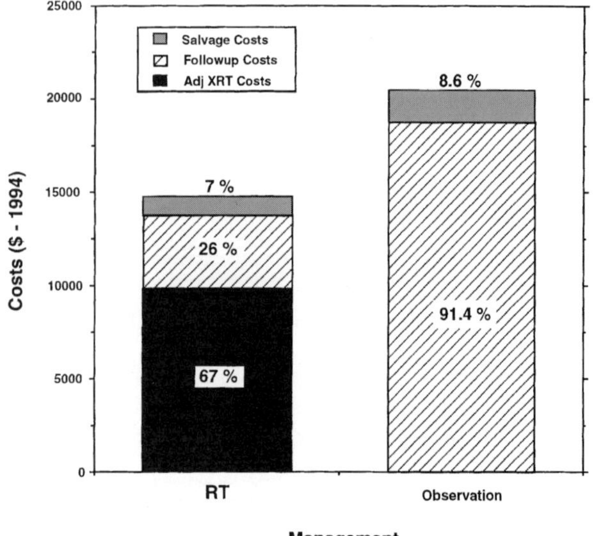


**Figure 11–19**

## TABLE 11–6

### ADJUVANT CARBOPLATIN FOR TREATMENT OF STAGE I SEMINOMA

| SERIES | NO. OF PATIENTS | CYCLES | FOLLOW-UP (Months) | RELAPSES |
|---|---|---|---|---|
| Kratzik, 1993[31] | 56 | 2 | 31 | 1 |
| Oliver, 1994[19] | 54 | 2 | 62 | 2 |
| | 65 | 1 | 29 | 0 |
| Dieckmann, 1996[32] | 22 | 2 | 24 | 0 |
| | 60 | 1 | — | 1 |
| Krege, 1997[33] | 43 | 2 | 28 | 0 |

*Source:* Adapted from Fiveash J, Sandler HM: Controversies in the management of stage I seminoma. Oncology 12:1203–1212, 1998.

**Table 11–6:** There has also been interest in treating postorchiectomy stage I patients with adjuvant chemotherapy alone. Seminomas are highly sensitive to platinum-based chemotherapeutic agents, and excellent disease-free survival rates have been achieved with one or two cycles of carboplatin (Table 11–6). In one nonrandomized study, radiotherapy, surveillance, and one or two courses of adjuvant carboplatin were retrospectively reviewed.[19] The outcome for all patients regardless of treatment was excellent, with a long-term disease-free survival rate of 96% or greater.

**Table 11–7:** Despite the fact that the disease in some patients with stage IIC is adequately controlled with primary radiotherapy, most patients are now treated with chemotherapy. The failure rate following radiotherapy in patients with nodal metastases between 5 cm and 10 cm (Royal Marsden Stage IIC) is higher than for those with nodes measuring 5 cm or less (Table 11–7). This difference was statistically significant in the series at the Princess Margaret Hospital.[34] Platinum-containing chemotherapy regimens with bleomycin and VP-16 (BEP) or vinblastine and bleomycin (PVB) are frequently employed. The PVB regimen is being replaced with BEP due to its decreased toxicity, yet equal efficacy.

## TABLE 11–7

### FAILURE OF PRIMARY RADIATION THERAPY FOR STAGE II SEMINOMA BY BULK OF ABDOMINAL DISEASE

| SERIES | STAGE IIA-B (<5 cm) | STAGE IIC (5–10 cm) | *p* VALUE |
|---|---|---|---|
| Dosmann, 1993[6] | 2/13 | 2/3 | NS |
| Warde, 1998[34] | 7/64 | 9/16 | <0.0001 |

NS = not significant.

**TABLE 11–8**

**POSTCHEMOTHERAPY RESIDUAL MASS AND HISTOLOGIC CORRELATION**

| CT SCAN FINDING | NO. OF PTS. | RESECTION | BIOPSY | HISTOLOGICALLY POSITIVE |
|---|---|---|---|---|
| Mass >3 cm | 27 | 21 | 6 | 8 (30%) |
| Mass <3 cm | 28 | 11 | 17 | 0 |

*Source:* Adapted from Herr HW, Sheinfeld J, Puc HS, et al: Surgery for postchemotherapy residual mass in seminoma. Urology 157:860–862, 1997.

**Table 11–8:** The management of residual masses after chemotherapy for advanced seminoma is controversial. Several authors have reported that failures after chemotherapy are seen in areas of initial bulk disease. A review of patients treated at the Memorial Sloan-Kettering Cancer Center who had surgery for postchemotherapy residual para-aortic masses was recently reported.[35, 36] Thirty percent of patients with residual masses greater than 3 cm had viable tumor on pathologic review compared with 0% viable tumor if the residual mass was less than 3 cm. Royal Marsden Hospital, however, reported only 1 failure out of 11 patients with residual masses at 3 cm or more who were observed; this compared favorably with the 1 failure in 7 patients who received adjuvant irradiation.[37] If treatment of a postchemotherapy residual mass is pursued, as is done at M.D. Anderson Cancer Center, 20 to 25 Gy is a reasonable treatment approach that has limited morbidity.

# REFERENCES


1. Surveillance, Epidemiology and End Results (SEER) Cancer Statistics Review, Section 24, 1996.
2. Greenlee RT, Hill-Harmon M, Murray T, Thun M: Cancer statistics. CA Cancer J Clin 51(1):15–36, 2001.
3. Horwich A: Testicular Cancer: Investigation and Management. Baltimore, Williams & Wilkins, 1991.
4. Forman D, Chilvers C, Oliver R, et al: The aetiology of testicular cancer: Association with congenital abnormalities, age at puberty, infertility and exercise. Br Med J 308:1393–1399, 1994.
5. Moore KL: Clinically Oriented Anatomy, 3rd ed. Baltimore, Williams & Wilkins, 1992.
6. Dosmann MA, Zagars GK: Postorchiectomy radiotherapy for stages I and II testicular seminoma. Int J Radiat Oncol Biol Phys 26:381–390, 1993.
7. Maier JG, Sulak MH: Radiation therapy in malignant testis tumors, Part 1: Seminoma. Cancer 32:1212–1216, 1973.
8. Thomas G, Jones W, Van Oosterom A, et al: Consensus statement on the investigation and management of testicular seminoma 1989. Progr Clin Biol Res 357:285–294, 1990.
9. AJCC Cancer Staging Manual, 5th ed. Philadelphia, Lippincott-Raven, 1998.
10. Read G, Johnston RJ: Short duration radiotherapy in stage I seminoma of the testis: Preliminary results of a prospective study. Clin Oncol 5:364–366, 1993.
11. Kiricuta IC, Sauer J, Bohndorf W: Omission of the pelvic irradiation in stage I testicular seminoma: A study of postorchiectomy para-aortic radiotherapy. Int J Radiat Oncol Biol Phys 35:293–298, 1996.
12. Sultanem K, Souhami L, Benk V, et al: Para-aortic irradiation only appears to be adequate treatment for patients with stage I seminoma of the testis. Int J Radiat Oncol Biol Phys 40:455–459, 1998.
13. Fossa SD, Horwich A, Russell JM, et al: Optimal planning target volume for stage I testicular seminoma: A Medical Research Council randomized trial. J Clin Oncol 17:1146–1154, 1999.
14. Epstein BE, Order SE, Zinreich ES: Staging, treatment, and results in testicular seminoma: A 12-year report. Cancer 65:405–411, 1990.
15. Bayens YC, Helle PA, Van Putten WLJ, et al: Orchidectomy followed by radiotherapy in 176 stage I and II testicular seminoma patients: Benefits of a 10-year follow-up study. Radiother Oncol 25:97–102, 1992.
16. Giacchetti S, Raoul Y, Wibault P, et al: Treatment of stage I testis seminoma by radiotherapy: Long-term results—A 30-year experience. Int J Radiat Oncol Biol Phys 27:3–9, 1993.
17. Lai PP, Bernstein MJ, Kim H, et al: Radiation therapy for stage I and II testicular seminoma. Int J Radiat Oncol Biol Phys 28:373–379, 1993.
18. Amichetti M, Fellin G, Bolner A, et al: Stage I seminoma of the testis: Long-term results and toxicity with adjuvant radiotherapy. Tumori 80:141–145, 1994.
19. Oliver RTD, Edmonds PM, Ong JYH, et al: Pilot study of 1 and 1 course carboplatin as adjuvant for stage I seminoma. Should it be tested in a randomized trial against radiotherapy? Int J Radiat Oncol Biol Phys 29:3–8, 1994.
20. Niewald M, Waziri A, Walter K, et al: Low-dose radiotherapy for stage I seminoma: Early results. Radiother Oncol 37:164–166, 1995.
21. Hültenschmidt B, Budach V, Genters K, et al: Results of radiotherapy for 230 patients with stage I-II seminomas. Strahlenther Onkol 172:186–192, 1996.
22. Stein ME, Kessel I, Luberant N, et al: Testicular seminoma stage I: Treatment results and long-term follow-up (1969–1988). J Surg Oncol 53:175–179, 1993.
23. Miki T, Nonomura N, Saiki S, et al: Long-term results of adjuvant irradiation or surveillance in stage I testicular seminoma. Int J Urol 5:357–360, 1998.
24. Bauman GS, Venkatesan VM, Ago CT, et al: Postoperative radiotherapy for stage I/II seminoma: Results for 212 patients. Int J Radiat Oncol Biol Phys 42:313–317, 1998.
25. Speer TW, Sombeck MD, Parsons JT, et al: Testicular seminoma: A failure analysis and literature review. Int J Radiat Oncol Biol Phys 33:89–97, 1995.
26. Whipple GL, Sagerman RH, van Rooy EM: Long-term evaluation of postorchiectomy radiotherapy for stage II seminoma. Am J Clin Oncol 20:196–201, 1997.
27. Von der Maase H, Specht L, Jacobsen GK, et al: Surveillance following orchidectomy for stage I seminoma of the testis. Eur J Cancer 29A:1931–1934, 1993.
28. Warde P, Gospodarowicz MK, Panzarella T, et al: Stage I testicular seminoma: Results of adjuvant irradiation and surveillance. J Clin Oncol 13:2255–2262, 1995.
29. Horwich A, Alsanjari N, A'Hern R, et al: Surveillance following orchidectomy for stage I testicular seminoma. Br J Cancer 65:775–778, 1992.
30. Sharda NN, Kinsella TJ, Ritter MA: Adjuvant radiation versus

observation: A cost analysis of alternate management schemes in early-stage testicular seminoma. J Clin Oncol 14:2933–2939, 1996.

31. Kratzik C, Kuhrer I, Wiltsche C, et al: Carboplatin-monotherapie bei seminomen im stadium I. Acta Chir Aust 25:27–28, 1993.

32. Dieckmann KP, Krain J, Kuster J, et al: Adjuvant carboplatin treatment for seminoma clinical stage I. J Cancer Res Clin Oncol 122:63–66, 1996.

33. Krege S, Kalund G, Otto T, et al: Phase II study: Adjuvant single-agent carboplatin therapy for clinical stage I seminoma. Eur Urol 31:405–407, 1997.

34. Warde P, Gaspodarowicz M, Panzarella T, et al: Management of stage II seminoma. J Clin Oncol 16:290–294, 1998.

35. Herr HW, Sheinfeld J, Puc HS, et al: Surgery for a post-chemotherapy residual mass in seminoma. J Urol 157:860–862, 1997.

36. Puc HS, Heelan R, Mazumdar M, et al: Management of residual mass in advanced seminoma: Results and recommendations from the Memorial Sloan-Kettering Cancer Center. J Clin Oncol 14:454–460, 1996.

37. Horwich A, Paluchowska B, Norman A, et al: Residual mass following chemotherapy of seminoma. Ann Oncol 8:37–40, 1997.

<h1>Index</h1>

Note: Page numbers followed by the letter f refer to figures, and those followed by t refer to tables.


## A

ABCD staging system, 117
Acrolein, 77
ACTH (adrenocorticotropic hormone), 5f
Adenocarcinoma
bladder, 128
prostate, 2f, 122
renal, 132
Adenoid cystic carcinoma, 2f, 122
Adenoma
adrenal, 153t
renal, 129, 131
villous, 125
Adenosquamous carcinoma, 2f
Adrenal glands
anatomy of, 144–146, 146f
androgen from, 5f
removal of, 151–152, 152f
Adrenal tumors, 144–154, 145f–153f. *See also*
*specific types, e.g.,* Pheochromocytoma.
diagnosis of, 147f
treatment of, 153t
Adrenocorticocarcinoma, 144
CT of, 152–153, 153f
diagnosis of, 147
histology of, 154
treatment of, 153t
Adrenocorticotropic hormone (ACTH), 5f
Adriamycin. *See* Doxorubicin.
AFP (alpha-fetoprotein), 134–137, 199f, 208
African Americans
bladder cancer and, 75, 76f
prostate cancer and, 3f, 19, 20t
AGNORs (argyrophilic nucleolar organizing
regions), 122
Aldosterone, 144, 145f
Aldosteronoma, 144
Alpha-fetoprotein (AFP), 134–137, 199f, 208
American Indians, bladder cancer and, 76f
Amphiregulin, 11f
Anaplasia, 133
Anastomosis, bladder, 32f, 36f

Androgen(s)
ablation of, 1, 6f
blockade of, 6, 121–122
epidermal growth factor and, 5–6, 6f, 11f
receptor for, 7f
mutations of, 8, 9f
synthesis of, 4–5, 5f
Androgen-dependent transcriptional
activation, 5–6, 6f
Angiogenesis, in prostate cancer, 13f
Angiomyolipoma (AML), 134
Antiandrogens, 6, 123
nonsteroidal, 6f
Apoptosis
*bcl-2* oncogene and, 10–11, 11f, 16f
p53 tumor suppressor gene and, 10, 11f,
16f
Argyrophilic nucleolar organizing regions
(AGNORs), 122
Asians, bladder cancer and, 76f

## B

Bacillus Calmette-Guérin (BCG)
for bladder cancer, 75
for kidney cancer, 164–165
Basal cell carcinoma, prostate, 122
*bcl-2* oncogene, 10–11, 11f, 16f
Benign prostatic hypertrophy (BPH)
PSA levels and, 22
surgery for, 17
Benzidine, 76
Bicalutamide, 6
Biologic therapy, for renal cell carcinoma,
172f–176f, 173–180, 175t–179t, 180f
Bladder
anastomosis of, 32f, 36f
outlet obstruction of, 53t
nonepithelial tumors of, 128
nonpapillary noninfiltrating flat lesions of,
127–128
papillary noninfiltrating epithelial tumors
of, 125–127

Bladder *(Continued)*
replacement of, 86f–90f
Bladder cancer, 75–90, 123–128
characterization of, 124
chemotherapy for, 75–76, 84, 103–113,
104f–112f, 104t–109t
neoadjuvant, 107t, 107–109, 108f, 109t
radiotherapy with, 100–101, 101f, 102f,
102t, 103t
clinical features of, 124–125
cystoscopy for, 84, 85f
diagnosis of, 80f–85f, 81–84
epidemiology of, 75–76, 76f
histopathology of, 78f–81f
imaging for, 82–84, 83f–85f, 91f, 92f
in situ, 78f, 127
invasive, 80f, 81
metastatic, 98t, 102t, 103t, 126–127
molecular biology of, 77t
prognosis for, 98t, 124
radiotherapy for, 95–103, 96f–102f, 101t–
103t
chemotherapy with, 100–101, 101f, 102f,
102t, 103t
risks for, 76–77, 106f
sonography for, 82, 83f
squamous cell, 76, 128
staging of, 77f–81f, 96, 97f, 98t, 123–124,
123f
superficial, 79f
survival after, 75–76, 86–87, 97f, 98t, 101t,
106f
treatment of, 84–90, 85f–90f, 95–96, 96f
undifferentiated, 128
upper urinary tract disease with, 91f, 91–
92, 92f
Bleomycin
for germ cell tumors, 198t, 201, 203
for seminoma, 214
Bone metastases
biology of, 15f, 15–16
from prostate cancer, 15f, 22
from RCC, 169t
Bosniak classification, 156–159, 157f, 158f

BPH (benign prostatic hypertrophy), 17, 22
Brachytherapy
　for bladder cancer, 96
　for prostate cancer, 45, 46f, 67
Breast cancer, 147

## C

Cadherins, 12–13, 13f, 16f
CAG trinucleotide repeats, 7–8, 8t
Cancer. *See at anatomic site, e.g.,* Bladder
　cancer.
Carboplatin
　for bladder cancer, 105t
　for seminoma, 214t
Carcinoma in situ (CIS)
　bladder, 78f, 127
　testicular, 137
Carcinosarcoma. *See specific type, e.g.,* Renal
　cell carcinoma.
Catecholamine, 144, 145f
CD3⁺ tumor-infiltrating T lymphocytes,
　172f, 173
CDC (collecting duct carcinoma), 132
Chemoimmunotherapy, 181t, 181–183, 182t,
　183f
Chemotherapy. *See also specific drugs, e.g.,*
　Vinblastine.
　for bladder cancer, 103–113, 104f–112f,
　　104t–109t
　　radiotherapy with, 100–101, 101f, 102f,
　　　102t, 103t
　for germ cell tumors, 196t, 197, 198t, 201,
　　202f
　for renal cell carcinoma, 173t, 181t, 181–
　　183, 182t, 183f
　for seminoma, 214t, 215t
　retroperitoneal lymph node dissection
　　and, 196t, 197, 198t
　thymic effect of, 203f
Choriocarcinoma, 136
Chromophobe cells, 131
CIS (carcinoma in situ), 78f, 127, 137
Cisplatin
　for bladder cancer, 100–104, 101f, 102f,
　　102t–104t, 109t
　for germ cell tumors, 198t, 201, 203
Clear cell adenocarcinoma, of bladder, 128
Clear cell renal cancer, 131, 167, 168f
Clear cell sarcoma, 133
Collecting duct carcinoma (CDC), 132
Colorectal cancer, 19f, 19t
Computed tomography (CT)
　of adrenals, 146f
　of adrenocorticocarcinoma, 152–153, 153f
　of bladder cancer, 82–83, 84f, 91f, 109, 110f
　of bladder cancer radiotherapy, 99–100,
　　100f
　of germ cell tumors, 200f, 201f
　of prostate cancer, 48f–50f, 48–51
　of renal cell carcinoma, 156f, 156–157,
　　158f, 159
　of seminoma metastases, 210f, 211f
　of transitional cell cancer, 163, 164f
Condyloma acuminatum, 125
Conformal radiation therapy, 48f–52f
Cortisol, 144, 145f
Cowden disease, 10
Cryotherapy, for prostate cancer, 39–42,
　40f–42f, 41t, 67
Cryptorchidism, 138
　seminoma and, 206f, 206–207, 207f
CT. *See* Computed tomography (CT).
Cushing's disease, 147

Cushing's syndrome, 153
　adrenal tumor with, 144
Cyclin-dependent kinases (CDKs), 111f
Cyclophosphamide, 77, 104t, 105t
Cyst(s)
　dermoid, 136
　multilocular, 133
　renai, 156–159, 157f, 158f
Cystectomy, 75–76, 84–87, 85f, 86f
　chemotherapy with, 101f, 102f, 109t
　metastases and, 98t
　partial, 109
　reconstruction after, 86f–90f
　transurethral resection and, 95
Cystic nephroma, 133
Cystic tumor, 132
Cystoscopy, 84, 85f
Cystourethritis, 53t

## D

Dehydroepiandrosterone (DHEA), 5f
Denonvilliers' fascia, 24–25, 26f
Dentato-rubro-pallido-luysian atrophy, 7–8,
　8t
Dermatitis, after radiotherapy, 53t
Dermoid cyst, 136
Diethylstilbestrol (DES), 6f
Digital rectal examination (DRE), 20–21
Dihydrotestosterone (DHT), 5–6, 6f
　5α-reductase and, 8f
Docetaxel, for bladder cancer, 105t, 106t
Dopamine, 145f
Doxorubicin, 75, 103–104, 104t, 105t, 109t

## E

E-cadherin, 12–13, 13f, 16f
Embryonal carcinoma, 135–136, 200f
Endodermal sinus tumor, 135–136
Endometrioid carcinoma, 121–122
Endothelin-1, 11f, 12f
Enteritis, after radiotherapy, 53t
Epidermal growth factor (EGF)
　androgens and, 5–6, 6f, 11f
　receptor for, 111–112, 112f
Epinephrine, 144, 145f
Epithelial tumors
　classification of, 124
　papillary noninfiltrating, 125–127
Estradiol, 145f
Estrogen receptor, 7f
　mutations of, 8, 9f
Estrogen therapy, 123
Etoposide, 198t, 201, 203
External beam radiation, candidates for,
　46–47, 47f

## F

Fibroblast growth factor 7 (FGF-7), 11f
Flocks/Kadesky classification, 167, 169t
5-Fluorouracil (5-FU)
　for bladder cancer, 100–103, 102f, 102t,
　　104t
　for renal cell carcinoma, 181t, 181–182,
　　182t
Flutamide, 6, 8, 9f

## G

Gallium nitrate, 105t, 106t

Gemcitabine, 105t, 106t
Germ cell tumors, 137–139
　age distribution for, 206f
　chromosome 12 and, 199–200, 200f
　extragonadal, 203f, 203–204
　extratesticular, 137
　intratubular, 137
　location of, 206f
　nonseminomatous
　　chemotherapy for, 196t, 197, 198t, 201,
　　　202f
　　surgery for, 189–197, 190f–197f, 196t,
　　　198t
　　systemic issues with, 199f–203f, 199–204
　prognosis for, 137
　pulmonary sarcoidosis vs., 202f, 203
　testicular, 134–137
Gleason score, 2, 3f, 121
　prostatectomy and, 22–23, 23f
　radiotherapy and, 46
Glucocorticoid receptor, 7f
Gonadoblastoma, 139
Goserelin, 65–66
Granulocyte-macrophage colony-stimulating
　factor (GM-CSF) gene, 185t
Granulosa cell tumors, 138
Growth factors, 15
　androgens and, 5–6, 6f, 11f
　bladder cancer and, 111–112, 112f
Gynecomastia, 138, 153

## H

Halsted, William H., 17
Hamartoma, 10
hCG. *See* Human chorionic gonadotropin
　(hCG).
Hereditary prostate cancer 1 (HPC1) locus,
　4f, 16f
Hispanics
　bladder cancer and, 76f
　prostate cancer and, 20t
Hormone therapy
　for prostate cancer, 47f, 63–66, 64f–66f, 68f
　for renal cell cancer, 173t
Human chorionic gonadotropin (hCG), 199f
　testicular tumors and, 136–137, 208
　urothelial carcinoma and, 126–127
Human papillomavirus (HPV), 125
Huntington's disease, 7–8, 8t
Hyperaldosteronism, 153
Hyperparathyroidism, 147t
Hypothalamic-pituitary-gonadal axis, 4–5, 5f
Hypoxia-induced factor 1 (HIF-1), 15

## I

IFN-α. *See* Interferon-alpha (IFN-α).
Ifosfamide, 105t, 106t
IGF (insulin-like growth factor), 11f
IL-2. *See* Interleukin 2 (IL-2).
Ileal conduit urinary diversion, 87f
Immune dysregulation, with malignancies,
　183f
Immunotherapy, for RCC, 144, 161, 163f,
　183–184, 184f, 184t
Implants, transperineal, 60f, 60–61, 61t
Impotence
　after cystectomy, 87
　after prostatectomy, 17, 18, 36–37, 37t
　after radiotherapy, 54–55, 55t
Infiltrating tumors, 125
Insulin-like growth factor (IGF), 11f

Interferon-alpha (IFN-α)
  for RCC, 167, 176t–182t, 176–182, 180f
    nephrectomy with, 171
      prognosis with, 170t
    5-FU with, 181t, 181–182, 182t
    IL-2 with, 178t, 178–179, 179t–182t
    medroxyprogesterone with, 177t
    preparations of, 176f
    13-*cis*-retinoic acid with, 177t
    toxicity of, 179t, 179–180
    vinblastine with, 177t, 180t
Interferon-gamma, 180f
Interleukin 2 (IL-2)
  5-fluorouracil with, 181t, 181–182, 182t
  for RCC, 144, 161, 163f, 167, 174f
    prognosis with, 170t
    recombinant, 174–176, 175t
      administration of, 176f
      IFN-α and, 178t, 178–179, 179t–182t
      lymphokine-activated killer cells and,
        184t
      toxicity of, 179t, 179–180
Interleukin 4 (IL-4), 180f
Interleukin 6 (IL-6), 180f
Intratubular malignant germ cells (ITMGC),
  136. *See also* Germ cell tumors.
Intravenous pyelogram (IVP), 82, 83f, 91f

### K

Kennedy syndrome, 7–8, 8t
Kidney tumors, 143–144. *See also* Renal cell
  carcinoma (RCC); Renal medullary
  carcinoma.
  diagnosis of, 154f
  metastatic, 147
  staging of, 129, 130f
  TILs in, 172f, 173, 183–184, 184f
  types of, 130–134
Klinefelter syndrome, 138

### L

Lactate dehydrogenase (LDH), 199f
LAK (lymphokine-activated killer) cells, 163,
  184t
Latinos
  bladder cancer and, 76f
  prostate cancer and, 20t
Leiomyosarcoma, bladder, 128
Leydig cells, 4–5, 137–139
Lipid cell carcinoma, 127
Lung cancer, 19f, 19t, 169t, 171f
Luteinizing hormone–releasing hormone
  (LHRH), 6
Lymphadenectomy, 22, 27f. *See also*
  Retroperitoneal lymph node dissection
  (RPLND).
Lymphoepithelioma-like carcinoma, 126
Lymphokine-activated killer (LAK) cells,
  163, 184t
Lymphoma
  *bcl-2* oncogene and, 10–11, 11f
  prostate, 2f
  testicular, 139

### M

Machado-Joseph disease, 7–8, 8t
Macropapillary urothelial carcinoma, 127
Magnetic resonance imaging (MRI)
  of bladder cancer, 83, 84f, 92f
  of pheochromocytoma, 149–150, 150f

Magnetic resonance imaging (MRI)
    *(Continued)*
  of vena caval thrombus, 160f
Mainz pouch, 90f
Medroxyprogesterone, 177t
Melanoma, 124, 147
MEN (multiple endocrine neoplasia), 147t
Mesoblastic nephroma, 133
Metaiodobenzylguanidine (MIBG) scan,
  148–149, 149f
Metanephric adenoma, 131
Methotrexate, 103–104, 104t, 105t, 109t
Microcystic urothelial carcinoma, 127
Mitomycin C, 75, 104t
MRI. *See* Magnetic resonance imaging
  (MRI).
Mucinous adenocarcinoma, 122. *See also*
  Adenocarcinoma.
Multilocular cyst, 133
Multiple endocrine neoplasia (MEN), 147t

### N

2-Naphthylamine, 76
Nelson, Joel, 12
Nephrectomy
  for renal cell carcinoma, 160–162, 161f,
    161t, 171
  for transitional cell carcinoma, 164–165
Nephroblastic lesions, 132–134
Nephroblastoma, 131, 132–133
  metastatic, 137
Nephroma, 133. *See also* Kidney tumors.
Nephroureterectomy, 91–92, 92f
Nested urothelial carcinoma, 127
Neuroendocrine carcinoma, small cell, 122
Neurofibromatosis, 147t
Neurotensin, 11f
Nilutamide, 6
Nonepithelial tumors, 12
Nonpapillary noninfiltrating flat lesions,
  127–128
Nonseminomatous germ cell tumors
  (NSGCT). *See also* Germ cell tumors.
  chemotherapy for, 196t, 197, 198t, 201,
    202f
  prognosis for, 199f, 199–200, 200f
  surgery for, 189–197, 190f–197f, 198t
  systemic, 199f–203f, 199–204
Nontransitional cell carcinoma, 127–128. *See
  also* Transitional cell carcinoma (TCC).
Norepinephrine, 144, 145f
NSGCT. *See* Nonseminomatous germ cell
  tumors (NSGCT).
Nuclear transcription factors, 7f

### O

Oat cell carcinoma, 122
Oncocytoma, 129, 131
Oncogene, *bcl-2*, 10–11, 11f, 16f
Orchiectomy, 207f
  radiotherapy after, 211t, 211–215, 212f–
    214f, 213t–215t
Orthotopic reservoirs, 88f–89f

### P

Paclitaxel, 105t, 106t
PAP (prostatic acid phosphatase), 2, 122, 123
Papillary adenoma, 129
Papillary epithelial tumors, 125–127

Papilloma
  renal cell carcinoma and, 132
  squamous, 125, 128
  urothelial, 125
Para-aortic radiotherapy, 211–213, 212f
Paraganglioma, 124
PDGF. *See* Platelet-derived growth factor
  (PDGF).
Pelvic lymphadenectomy, 22, 27f
p53 gene
  bladder cancer and, 95, 109–113, 110f–112f
  prostate cancer and, 10, 11f, 16f
Phenacetin
  bladder cancer and, 77
  TCC and, 144
Phenoxybenzamine, 150
Phenylalanine, 145f
Pheochromocytoma, 144
  diagnosis of, 147–150, 148f–150f
  hereditary syndromes with, 147t
  histology of, 148, 149f
  hypertension with, 144, 150–151
  metaiodobenzylguanidine scan for, 148–
    149, 149f
  surgery for, 150–152, 151f, 152f, 153t
  symptoms of, 147–148, 148f
PIN (prostatic intraepithelial neoplasia), 2f,
  120
Planning target volume (PTV), 51
Plasmacytoid urothelial carcinoma, 127
Platelet-derived growth factor (PDGF)
  bladder cancer and, 111–112, 112f
  prostate cancer and, 5–6, 6f
Polyembryoma, 136
Polymorphic chain reaction (PCR), 82f
Prazosin, 150
Proctitis, after radiotherapy, 53t, 54f, 55f
Progesterone receptor, 7f
  mutations of, 8, 9f
Propranolol, 150–151
Prostate
  anatomy of, 1f, 24f
    surgical, 24f–26f
  blood supply to, 25f
  cell types of, 119
  nerve supply to, 26f
Prostate cancer
  5α-reductase in, 8f, 16f
  androgen receptor mutations in, 8, 9f
  angiogenesis in, 13f
  *bcl-2* oncogene and, 10–11, 11f, 16f
  biology of, 7f–16f
  brachytherapy for, 45, 46f
  cryotherapy for, 39–42, 40f–42f, 41t, 67
    complications after, 42f
  diagnosis of, 119–120
  endocrinology of, 4–6, 5f, 6f
  epidemiology of, 2–3, 3f
  familial, 4f
  Gleason score for, 2, 3f, 22–23, 23f, 121
  grading of, 2, 3f, 22–23, 23f, 121
  growth factors and, 5–6, 6f, 11f
  histology of, 119
  hormone therapy for, 47f, 63–66, 64f–66f,
    68f, 123
  hypermethylation in, 8–9, 9f, 16f
  hypoxia in, 14f, 15
  immunopathology of, 122–123
  incidence of, 1, 3f, 18–19, 19f, 19t
  indolent, 20, 21f
  location of, 24f
  metastatic, 12, 13f, 20, 21f
    bone scan for, 15f, 22
    palliation of, 70
    patterns of, 24
    radiotherapy for, 47

Prostate cancer *(Continued)*
    survival rates for, 66–67, 67t
    tests for, 22–23, 23f
mortality from, 1–3, 3f, 19f, 20, 21f
multicentricity of, 121
paracrine-endocrine cells and, 122
pathology of, 2f
p53 tumor suppressor gene and, 10, 11f,
    16f
precursor lesions of, 120
prostatic intraepithelial neoplasia and, 2f,
    120
race and, 3f, 19, 20t
radiotherapy for, 45–70, 46f–70f. *See also*
    Radiotherapy, for prostate cancer.
ras mutations in, 12f, 16f
retinoblastoma gene and, 9f, 9–10
risks for, 4f, 19, 20t
squamous cell, 2f, 122
staging of, 2, 3f, 22–23, 23f, 117–120, 118f
surgery for, 17–42, 18f–42f
trinucleotide repeats in, 7–8, 8t
tumor suppressor genes in, 8, 9f
tumor volume and, 121
types of, 2f, 121–122
WHO classification for, 121
Prostatectomy, 17–42, 18f–42f
anatomy for, 24–26, 25f, 26f
bladder anastomosis in, 32f, 36f
complications from, 17–20, 35f, 35–37, 36f,
    36t, 37t, 39t
history of, 17–18, 18f
impotence after, 17, 18, 36–37, 37t
incontinence after, 17, 18, 36t, 39t
indications for, 18, 20–24, 23f
nerve-sparing, 30f
perineal, 17, 18f, 33, 34f
prostate-specific antigen assays after, 37t,
    37–38, 38f
radiotherapy after, 47, 68–70, 69t
radiotherapy vs., 45, 47f, 59t, 60
results with, 37–38
retropubic, 17, 18f, 26–33, 27f–33f
    management after, 32–33, 33f
    patient position for, 27f
    preparation for, 26–27
salvage, 38–39, 39t, 67, 68f
transfusions for, 26–27, 35
Prostate-specific antigen (PSA), 1, 18,
    122–123
adenocarcinoma and, 122
prostatectomy and, 37t, 37–38, 38f
radiotherapy and, 45–47, 56f, 59t, 62f
values for, 21–23, 23f
Prostatic acid phosphatase (PAP), 2, 122, 123
Prostatic intraepithelial neoplasia (PIN), 2f,
    120
PSA. *See* Prostate-specific antigen (PSA).
PTEN tumor suppression gene, 10f
PTV (planning target volume), 51


**R**

Radiotherapy
after orchiectomy, 211t, 211–215, 212f–214f,
    213t–215t
after prostatectomy, 47, 68–70, 69t
after TURB, 100–102, 101f, 101t
conformal, 48f–52f
for bladder cancer, 95–103, 96f–102f, 101t–
    103t
    chemotherapy with, 100–101, 101f, 102f,
    102t, 103t
for prostate cancer, 45–70, 46f–70f
    body cast and, 52f

Radiotherapy *(Continued)*
    chemotherapy with, 45–46, 68–70, 69t
    dose escalation and, 63
    early, 57–61, 58f, 58t–61t, 60f
    hormone therapy with, 47f, 63–66, 64f–
    66f, 68f, 123
    impotency after, 54–55, 55t
    incontinence after, 54f, 54t
    locally advanced, 61–67, 62f–66f, 62t, 67t
    management after, 53t
    metastatic, 66–67, 67t, 68f, 70f
    patient selection and, 46–48, 47f, 47t
    planning target volume for, 51
    prostatectomy after, 38–39, 39t
    prostatectomy vs., 45, 47f, 59t, 60
    PSA test and, 45–47, 56f, 59t, 62f
    residual carcinoma after, 123
    results from, 56–67
    side effects of, 52f–55f, 53t–55t, 60
    survival with, 58t
    younger patients with, 60f
for renal cell carcinoma, 172f, 172–173
for seminoma, 205f–214f, 205–215, 208t–
    215t
history of, 46f
para-aortic, 211–213, 212f
transperineal implant, 60f, 60–61, 61t
Ras mutations, 12f, 16f
Rb. *See* Retinoblastoma (Rb) gene.
RCC. *See* Renal cell carcinoma (RCC).
Receptor tyrosine kinases (RTKs), 111–112,
    112f
Reinke crystal, 137
Renal adenoma, 129, 131
Renal cell carcinoma (RCC), 131–132. *See
    also* Kidney tumors.
adrenal cancer vs., 153
diagnosis of, 154f–158f, 154–159, 155t
genetics of, 154, 155f
histology of, 155, 167, 168f
imaging for, 156f–158f, 156–159
immunotherapy for, 144, 161, 163f
incidence of, 143, 167
metastatic, 162f, 162–163, 163f, 167–186,
    168f–185f
    algorithm for, 185f, 185–186
    biologic therapy for, 172f–176f, 173–180,
    175t–179t, 180f
    chemotherapy for, 173t, 181t, 181–183,
    182t, 183f
    hormone therapy for, 173t
    immunotherapy for, 144, 161, 163f, 183–
    184, 184f, 184t
    prognosis for, 169–171, 172t
    radiotherapy for, 172f, 172–173
    sites for, 167, 168f, 169t
    spontaneous regression with, 174f
    surgery for, 171f
    survival with, 169f
    vaccines for, 185t
presentation of, 143–144
staging of, 167, 169t
survival with, 161
symptoms of, 155t
systemic therapy for, 167–186, 168f–185f
treatment of, 144, 160f–163f, 160–163, 161t
vena caval thrombus with, 159f, 159–160,
    160f
Renal cysts, 156–159, 157f, 158f
Renal medullary carcinoma, 132
Reservoirs, orthotopic, 88f–89f
Retinoblastoma (Rb) gene
bladder cancer and, 95, 109–111, 110f, 111f
prostate cancer and, 9f, 9–10
13-*cis*-Retinoic acid, 177t
Retinoic acid receptor, 7f

Retroperitoneal lymph node dissection
    (RPLND), 189–197, 190f–197f, 196t, 198t
chemotherapy after, 196t, 197, 198t
complications with, 189, 194–196, 196t
nerve-sparing, 194f, 195f
staging and, 208f
Rhabdoid tumor, 134
Rhabdomyosarcoma
bladder, 128
metastatic, 137
Robson classification, 167, 169t
RPLND. *See* Retroperitoneal lymph node
    dissection (RPLND).
RTKs (receptor tyrosine kinases), 111–112,
    112f


**S**

Sarcoidosis, 202f, 203
Sarcoma
    clear cell, 133
    prostate, 2f
    undifferentiated, 137
Schiller-Duval bodies, 136
*Schistosoma haematobium,* 76
Scrotal mass, 207t
SEER Program, 205
Seminoma, 134–136. *See also* Testicular
    tumors.
age distribution for, 206f
chemotherapy for, 214t
cryptorchidism and, 206f, 206–207, 207f
diagnosis of, 208f
epidemiology of, 205f, 205–206
metastatic, 209f–211f
mortality with, 211t–214t
prognosis for, 199f, 199–200, 200f, 211t–
    214t
radiotherapy for, 205f–214f, 205–215, 208t–
    215t
spermatocytic, 135
staging of, 208t
Sertoli cell tumors, 138–139
Sickle cell disorder, 132
Small cell carcinoma, 2f
Smoking
    bladder cancer and, 76
    TCC and, 144
Sonography. *See* Ultrasonography.
Spermatocytic seminoma, 134–136
Spindle cell carcinoma, 128
    renal, 131–132
    urothelial, 127
Spinocerebellar ataxia, 7–8, 8t
Squamous cell carcinoma
    bladder, 76, 128
    prostate, 2f, 122
Squamous papilloma, 125, 128
Stauffer's syndrome, 155
Steroids, 144, 145f
    adrenocorticocarcinoma and, 153
    receptors for, 7f
Stoma, after cystectomy, 86f–90f
Surveillance, Epidemiology and End Results
    (SEER) Program, 205
Syncytiotrophoblasts, 136–137


**T**

Tamoxifen, for RCC, 179t, 182t
TCC. *See* Transitional cell carcinoma (TCC).
T-cell antigen receptors (TCR), 183f. *See also*
    Tumor-infiltrating lymphocytes (TILs).

Teratoma, 136
    age distribution for, 206f
    classification of, 136
    metastatic, 137
Testicular tumors. *See also specific types, e.g.,*
        Germ cell tumors.
    anatomy for, 207f
    classification of, 208f
    epidemiology of, 205f, 205–206
    prognosis for, 137
    retroperitoneal lymph node dissection for,
        189–197, 190f–197f, 196t, 198t
    staging of, 134, 135f, 208t
    types of, 134–139
Testosterone, 145f
    5α-reductase and, 8f
    metabolism of, 5f
    synthesis of, 4–5, 5f
TGF-β (transforming growth factor β),
        11f
Theca cell tumors, 138
Thiotepa, 75
Thrombus, vena caval, 159f, 159–160, 160f
Thymic effect, of chemotherapy, 203f
Thyroid cancer, 147t
Thyroid hormone receptor, 7f
TILs (tumor-infiltrating lymphocytes), 144,
        161, 163f, 184–185, 185f
TNM. *See* Tumor-node-metastasis (TNM)
        system.
Transforming growth factor β (TGF-β), 11f
Transitional cell carcinoma (TCC)
    benign, 125
    bladder, 75, 77f
        malignant, 126–127
        other cell types with, 128
        urothelial, 126–127
        variants of, 127
    diagnosis of, 163, 164f
    histology of, 164
    prostate, 2f, 122
    renal, 143–144
    risks for, 144
    staging of, 77f–81f
    treatment of, 164–165, 165f
    upper urinary tract, 91f
    ureterorenoscopy for, 91
Transitional cell papilloma, 125
Transperineal implants, 60f, 60–61, 61t
Transrectal ultrasound (TRUS), 22
    cryosurgery with, 40f, 42f

Transrectal ultrasound (TRUS) *(Continued)*
    radiotherapy and, 47–48
Transurethral resection of bladder (TURB),
        75–76, 84–86, 85f
    adjuvant therapies with, 95–96, 96f, 107t
    chemotherapy with, 101f, 101–103, 102f,
        102t, 103t
    radiotherapy with, 96–97, 97f, 100–102,
        101f, 101t
Transurethral resection of prostate (TURP),
        26
Transurethral sonography, 82. *See also*
        Ultrasonography.
Trimetrexate, 106t
Trinucleotide repeats, 7–8, 8t
TRUS. *See* Transrectal ultrasound (TRUS).
Tubulopapillary adenoma, 129
Tumor suppressor gene(s)
    inactivation of, 8, 9f
    p53
        bladder cancer and, 95, 109–113, 110f–
            112f
        prostate cancer and, 10, 11f, 16f
    PTEN, 10f
Tumor-infiltrating lymphocytes (TILs), 144,
        161, 163f, 184–185, 185f
Tumor-node-metastasis (TNM) system
    for bladder cancer, 122–123, 123f
    for prostate cancer, 117–119, 118f
    for renal carcinoma, 128–130, 129f
    for renal cell carcinoma, 167
    for testicular cancer, 134, 135f
TURB. *See* Transurethral resection of bladder
        (TURB).
TURP (transurethral resection of prostate),
        26
Tyrosine, 145f

**U**

Ultrasonography
    of bladder cancer, 82, 83f
    of renal cell carcinoma, 156f, 158f, 159
    of transperineal implants, 60f, 60–61, 61t
    transrectal, 22
    transurethral, 82
Urachal adenocarcinoma, 128
Ureter, TCC of, 91f, 91–92, 92f
Ureterorenoscopy, 91

Urethral sphincter, 26f
Urinary diversion, 86–90f
Urinary tract
    calculi in, 81
    reconstruction of, 86f–90f
    transitional cell carcinoma of, 144
    upper, 91f, 91–92, 92f
Urothelial carcinoma, 126–127
Urothelial papilloma, 125
Urothelial cells, 81f, 81–82

**V**

Vascular endothelial growth factor (VEGF),
        15
Vena caval thrombus, 159f, 159–160, 160f
Villous adenoma, 125
Vinblastine
    for bladder cancer, 103–104, 104t, 105t,
        109t
    for RCC, 177t, 180t, 181
    for seminoma, 214
Vincristine, 104t
von Hippel–Lindau disease, 143
    genetics of, 154, 155f
    nephrectomy and, 161
    pheochromocytoma with, 147t

**W**

Wilms' tumor, 131, 132–133
    metastatic, 137
World Health Organization (WHO)
        classification system
    for prostate cancer, 121
    for teratoma, 136

**Y**

Yolk sac tumor, 135–136. *See also* Testicular
        tumors.
Young, Hugh Hampton, 17

**Z**

Zoladex, 65–66

ISBN 0-7216-8738-5